c Mental Health
s, systems, and practice

Forensic Mental Health
Concepts, systems, and practice

Edited by

Annie Bartlett

Gill McGauley

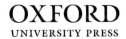

OXFORD
UNIVERSITY PRESS

OXFORD

UNIVERSITY PRESS

Great Clarendon Street, Oxford ox2 6DP

Oxford University Press is a department of the University of Oxford.
It furthers the University's objective of excellence in research, scholarship,
and education by publishing worldwide in

Oxford New York

Auckland Cape Town Dar es Salaam Hong Kong Karachi
Kuala Lumpur Madrid Melbourne Mexico City Nairobi
New Delhi Shanghai Taipei Toronto

With offices in

Argentina Austria Brazil Chile Czech Republic France Greece
Guatemala Hungary Italy Japan Poland Portugal Singapore
South Korea Switzerland Thailand Turkey Ukraine Vietnam

Oxford is a registered trade mark of Oxford University Press
in the UK and in certain other countries

Published in the United States
by Oxford University Press Inc., New York

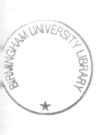

25302337

British Library Cataloguing in Publication Data
Data available

Library of Congress Cataloging in Publication Data
Data available

Typeset in Minion
by Cepha Imaging Private Ltd., Bangalore, India
Printed in UK
on acid-free paper by
CPI Antony Rowe, Chippenham, Wiltshire

ISBN 978-0-19-856685-4 (Pbk)

10 9 8 7 6 5 4 3 2 1

Oxford University Press makes no representation, express or implied, that the drug
dosages in this book are correct. Readers must therefore always check the product
information and clinical procedures with the most up-to-date published product
information and data sheets provided by the manufacturers and the most recent codes of
conduct and safety regulations. The authors and the publishers do not accept responsibility
or legal liability for any errors in the text or for the misuse or misapplication of material in
this work. Except where otherwise stated, drug dosages and recommendations are for the
non-pregnant adult who is not breast-feeding.

To Sandra and Freddie
To Tim, Sarah and Jessica

With thanks to Estela Welldon for her encouragement and enthusiasm in our early meetings at The Groucho Club

Foreword

I have long worked at the interface between law and psychiatry. Although a large part of my practice involves political cases, the other significant part of my work has involved domestic killing - mothers of their children, spouses of their partners, victims of their abusers. As a criminal lawyer, it seemed clear to me that, when people offended against society's norms, explanation would often be found in the mental processes at play. The law recognizes this need to consider the workings of the human mind because to establish guilt of a crime it is necessary to prove not only the actus reus or the thing done but also the mens rea or mental element. However, in the bad old days judges insisted that jurors were perfectly capable of working out these issues themselves using their common sense and made clear their determination that no expert was going to usurp the jury's function by bringing their 'hocus pocus' into the court.

When I started practising at the criminal Bar over thirty years ago, forensic psychiatry still played a limited role. Indeed it was only in the previous decade – 1960 to be precise – that the statutory defence of diminished responsibility had been created, which reduced murder to manslaughter on the grounds of mental abnormality.

In the last twenty years forensic psychiatry has become much more central to the criminal justice system, largely because of the changes which have taken place within society. Our communities have become increasingly interested in the contribution that the psychological sciences can make to human understanding and people are more honest about mental illnesses such as schizophrenia, bi-polar disorder, and depression.

Some of the taboos in our society have also been shattered, particularly around illegitimacy, sexual abuse, familial violence, and homosexuality and it has been recognized that silence on these issues has often led to mental ill health and even tragic events which bring people before the courts. This has expanded the role of the psychiatrist, psychologist, and other mental health professional in the family courts and within the criminal trial, particularly at sentencing. One of my own areas of work where the forensic psychiatrist has played a crucial role has been in extending the defence of provocation to situations of domestic violence and sexual abuse, explaining the long term mental health consequences for many victims of violation and trauma. Indeed, the editors of this book are well known to me professionally as they have both helped me develop my own understanding of psychiatry and been instrumental in edging the law towards more human outcomes, especially for women.

The great change in forensic mental health has been that, with far greater frequency, specialists are now called upon to share their expertise in order to help the jury evaluate motivation, diminished responsibility, provocation, or to assist the judge in making an appropriate disposal in the sentencing process. The judicial resistance to the expert has largely melted, so long as it is clear that the final decision in criminal cases still rests with the judge or the jury.

However, other factors have played their part in the growing role of forensic mental health within the legal system. While risk-taking is an important element in human progress, citizens in developed societies are increasingly risk averse. They feel entitled to live in safety and believe that all reasonable steps should be taken to reduce risk.

There was a time when risk was an accepted part of life. Misfortune, God's will and providence were all invoked to explain the calamities that befell us. Living was a risky business and the ravaging losses which families and communities suffered were deemed to be outside the ordinary person's control. In our stumbling advances towards a just society, we reached for legal concepts of liability to compensate for the losses and personal injuries people suffered. Workers were compensated for the risks they took for masters; consumers acquired the right not to be harmed by poisonous foodstuffs or faulty goods; property owners became liable for the safe passage of their visitors. There slowly evolved the right not to be exposed to unfair risk.

This social empowerment of citizens went hand in hand with the advance of rationalism and the belief that effects usually have causes and inexplicable "acts of God" are rare. This has meant that explanations are now sought for everything that goes wrong. As the mysteries of life have been unravelled so the human spirit of inquiry reaches for an understanding about whatever we experience. We want to know why something occurred and whether it was preventable. Are there people to be held responsible and possibly punished or made to pay?

Reducing risk is a sane objective in a sophisticated society but liberty is also an important value. Failing to take steps to protect others or to behave in a way that is mindful of another's safety should have consequences. However, the question we must face is where lines should be drawn – what is an acceptable level of risk?

Heightened anxiety about the future and growing insecurity has contributed to a culture of fear in our society. As a result we have seen increased panic about safety and an enthusiasm to blame whoever comes into the frame. We have seen a ratcheting up of sentences and the doubling of the prison population in less than twenty years, with many who are mentally ill ending up in jail. Another consequence is that the professionalism of doctors, nurses, teachers, social workers, and a whole slew of public servants is being undermined because of fear of litigation. When people seek security at all costs, opportunities for progress are often forfeited and trust between people can be destroyed.

In recent times mental health professionals have come under increased pressure because of a heightened level of anxiety about mental patients presenting a threat to public safety. In reality, few do. However, the government's response to this public concern, which is often fuelled by the tabloid press, has included attempts to introduce wider powers of preventive detention and to require clinicians to complete lengthy risk assessment forms on each contact with a patient. These initiatives have stimulated a vital debate about how professionals can best care for their patients while at the same time fulfilling their duty to protect the public.

This is an important book. All the issues I have mentioned and many more are discussed within its chapters. Anyone who works with mentally disordered offenders will find it an invaluable resource, packed with insight and information. However, the reader will also discover a thought-provoking and discursive critique of what is happening to our society. Mental health professionals play a crucial role within our system of justice; the specialists who work with offenders are at a particularly challenging coal face. This book will undoubtedly become the text to which they all turn for guidance and sustenance and I warmly welcome its publication.

Baroness Helena Kennedy QC
Honorary Fellow of the Royal College of Psychiatrists

Contents

Section 3 **Law**

Section 4 **Ethical aspects**

Section 5 **Social policy**

Introduction and acknowledgements

Annie Bartlett and Gill McGauley

A quarter of a century ago we did not imagine that our careers would focus so frequently on decisions about people's personal freedom and the possible deprivation of their liberty. Yet decisions of this kind are being taken on a daily basis by us and by other professionals working in different parts of the forensic world. Many professionals working with mentally disordered offenders (MDOs) might neither see this as their central task nor necessarily is it so. The primary role of a community psychiatric nurse is to care for and treat patients on a day-to-day basis; yet they may find themselves involved in decisions about someone being compulsorily recalled to hospital. Defence lawyers may see their role as maintaining their clients' liberty, but they participate in proceedings which may lead to their clients' imprisonment. Other professionals, judges or consultant forensic psychiatrists, more obviously have the final say about a person's liberty. The fact that you are reading this book probably means that you are involved to some degree in a system that exists to decide who is allowed to remain in society and who is not. These decisions have not only criminological, legal and psychiatric rationales, but also humanitarian and moral dimensions.

It is important for any society to decide who and why someone gets locked up, what happens to them when they are locked up and for how long they should be locked up. Our own answers to these questions may be important measures of our humanity. Certainly those of us brought up in the shadow of Soviet gulags or the Nazi concentration camps would be inclined to think so. We find ourselves, in England and Wales, living and working in a society that has the highest rate of imprisonment per head of population in the old European Union;[1] England and Wales have their highest prison population ever.[2] Many of that prison population have treatable mental health problems.[3] England and Wales have also detained more people than ever before in secure hospitals on Ministry of Justice Restriction Orders.[4] It is timely, in particular, to consider the legitimacy of the forensic enterprise and the dialectic of care and custody. We must examine, as responsible professionals, why we are doing what we are doing.

The origins of this book lie in our wish to explore this question from a range of academic and clinical perspectives. This process does not necessarily answer any questions but has generated thought-provoking contributions from professionals working across the forensic world, in health, criminal justice, social care, legal and voluntary sector arenas. We hope this book is neither a manual for forensic work nor just another academic text. We hope it will be thought-provoking. We do not want it to determine a particular train of thought or dictate a particular

---

[1] Walmsley, R. 2003 World Prison Population List (fourth edition) Findings 188 www.rds.homeoffice.gov.uk/rds/pdfs2/r188.pdf

[2] Home Office 2007 Population in Custody 2006 www.homeoffice.gov.uk/rds/omcs.html

[3] Singleton, N., Meltzer, H. and Gatward, R. 1998 Psychiatric Morbidity among Prisoners in England and Wales. London: ONS.

[4] Ly, L. and Foster, S. 2005 Statistics of Mentally Disordered Offenders 2004. Home Office Statistical Bulletin. www.homeoffice.gov.uk/rds

course of action. The ethos of the book is to challenge and test professional concepts and explore their value. It is agnostic in intent.

We are very grateful that we have had the opportunity to incorporate the diverse views of our contributors, each of whom is an expert in their field. We have been fortunate that many of the ideas in the book have been scrutinized by those whom we and other contributors of this book have taught in the Diploma and MSc in Forensic Mental Health at St George's, University of London. Students in these courses come from all over the forensic world and over the last decade have brought their own knowledge to the teaching process. This book is the distillation of that process, one that has given us the confidence that we might know what our readers want and need to know. We thank not only our authors but also the several hundred students who have helped us refine our thinking.

One of the central difficulties of the forensic world is that it is rarely thought of as a single entity, and it is harder still to make it function as one. More than 15 years ago, the Reed Committee[5] observed that it was difficult to co-ordinate all the agencies involved, or potentially involved, in an offender's care. Government departments, health and social care and voluntary sector organizations, as well as frontline criminal justice and penal institutions, are all engaged in the definition, management and processing of the MDO, the person with the unfortunate combination of offending behaviour and mental health problems.

MDOs are caught in a spider's web of a system. They are often in contact with many parts of the system at once, with little idea of their options or their likely future. Sadly, many of them will continue to need the combination of care and custody these agencies provide for much of their lives. The effective and efficient operation of the forensic system is complicated by the legitimately different perspectives of the agencies involved. Their capacity to provide care and exert control is varied and follows from fundamentally distinct frameworks and traditions.

These issues of difference underpin this book. We do not lay out a single argument. We do encourage debate by laying out the different positions of the professions who have a part to play in the life of an MDO. The authors' contributions and styles of writing are distinctive and appropriate to their topics. Although there is a degree of uniformity, we have allowed authors flexibility in how they introduce key ideas.

As each of the six sections has an introduction to orientate the reader, we provide here only a brief description of how the text is organized. The opening section, on Violence, Dangerousness covers a range of ideas from the disciplines of criminology, sociology, psychiatry and psychology that contribute to an understanding of these concepts. The second section, on Forensic Psychotherapeutic Approaches to MDOs, details the contributions of both cognitive and psychodynamic psychotherapies to understanding and managing the psychopathology, risk and interpersonal interactions of MDOs. In addition to describing some of the types of psychotherapy available for MDOs, in both the health care and prison systems, the section addresses the psychological impact on staff and services of treating and containing these individuals. Legislation, both statutory and case law, has changed substantially in relation to MDOs over the last decade, and the third section, on Law, discusses these changes, as well as the fierce debate that has surrounded them. This debate has informed both statute law and the way in which health professionals should address legal issues. The fourth section, on Ethics, develops some of these ideas on capacity, autonomy, vulnerability and responsibility. It describes common ethical dilemmas for professionals in

---

5 Department of Health and Home Office. 1992 Review of Health and Social Services for Mentally Disordered Offenders and Others Requiring Similar Services. (The Reed Committee) Final Summary Report. HMSO, London, 1992. Command Number 2088.

forensic settings as it lays out the different duties involved in the different professional roles intrinsic to multi-agency working. The fifth section, on Social Policy, discusses the development of the concept of the MDO and the way that penal, health and social care institutions are designed to meet their needs. It illustrates how much has changed, especially in the last 15 years, and how much of that change has been driven by the risk agenda. The book concludes with an International section. We explore the ways in which other countries think about antisocial and violent behaviours and how their circumstances and dilemmas have led to approaches to MDOs both similar to and different from those of England and Wales. We have had to be selective in the range of material for this section but believe that such comparisons are valuable and assist us in a measured analysis of our local situation.

We would like to thank all our section editors for their additional work and introductory contributions and Tim Hucker for his editorial input. We are especially grateful to Carol Maxwell and Martin Baum at Oxford University Press for supporting this endeavour and for their quiet and steady encouragement and guidance. We are indebted to Greg Hughes for his expert and patient proof reading and to Evelyn Bowman for all her help in the final stages of the project. We would also like to thank Jose Vazquez Cereijo for his kind permission to use Un Dia de mi Diario (A Day in my Diary) for our front cover. In conclusion, we hope that this book will make a serious contribution to forensic mental health thought and will be valuable to practitioners working in the field.

Annie Bartlett
Gill McGauley
July 2009

Biographies

Annie Bartlett is a Reader in Forensic Psychiatry at St George's University of London (SGUL) and Honorary Consultant Forensic Psychiatrist in Central North West London Foundation Trust. She is Clinical Lead for Offender Care (Mental Health) in the Trust and works clinically in HMP Holloway. She was previously Clinical Director of the South West London and St George's Forensic Service. She is an experienced university teacher and has been Course Director of the MSc and Diploma in Forensic Mental Health since setting them up at SGUL in 1996. She has an MA in English from Cambridge University where she also graduated in Medicine MB BChir. Her research training was funded by a Wellcome Trust Health Services Fellowship and she has a PhD (Cantab) in Social Anthropology. She has published widely on mental health and social exclusion (with particular reference to women and to gay and lesbian issues). She also continues to research culture and practise in secure institutions. She has been Chair of the Royal College of Psychiatrists Gay and Lesbian Special Interest Group. She is now Clinical Adviser (women and personality disorder) to the London Specialist Commissioning Group (Offender Care) for the London Primary Care Trusts.

Gill McGauley (BSc, MBBS, FRCPsych, PGCert HE) is a Reader and Consultant in Forensic Psychotherapy. She has developed the discipline of forensic psychotherapy both clinically and through postgraduate teaching, scholarship and research. She works clinically in Broadmoor Hospital, West London Mental Health NHS Trust, where she established the first forensic psychotherapy service in a high secure hospital. As a Reader in the Division of Mental Health at St George's University of London (SGUL), she is heavily involved in postgraduate and undergraduate teaching. She has had a significant role in developing the Diploma and MSc in Forensic Mental Health at SGUL, working with Annie Bartlett, and has been lead for undergraduate teaching in psychiatry. Her research interests include the application of psychological therapies for personality disordered forensic patients and the contribution of psychological therapies to assessing personality and risk in forensic patients. She has developed national and international training and educational initiatives in forensic psychotherapy as Chair of the National Reference Group for Training and Education in Forensic Psychotherapy; through membership of postgraduate training committees of The Royal College of Psychiatrists and through her work for the International Association for Forensic Psychotherapy as Secretary and as past President. In 2009 she was awarded a National Teaching Fellowship Individual Award by the Higher Education Academy in recognition of individual excellence in teaching in higher education in England and Northern Ireland.

Gwen Adshead (MBBS, MA, FRCPsych) is a forensic psychiatrist and psychotherapist. She has worked as a consultant psychotherapist at Broadmoor High Secure Hospital for the last 10 years and also holds an honorary lecturer's post at St George's University of London. She has a masters degree in medical law and ethics and has published widely in the field of ethics in mental health. Her book, Ethical Issues in Forensic Mental Health Research, was co-edited with Dr Christine Brown and published by Jessica Kingsley Publishers. Her most recent book, co-edited with Dr Caroline Jacob, is also published by Jessica Kingsley and is entitled Personality Disorder: The Definitive Reader.

Gill Aston is a lecturer in the Department of Midwifery, Women and Child Health at the Florence Nightingale School of Nursing and Midwifery and a member of the Division of Health and Social Care Research, King's College London UK. Gillian is a midwife and undertook her original midwifery education and training at King's College Hospital, London. Included in her academic discipline and areas of expertise are social sciences and the arts. Her doctoral studies were undertaken at the University of Manchester, UK under the supervision of Professor Rebecca Emerson Dobash and she was awarded a PhD for a thesis entitled 'From the margins into the centre: women's experiences of domestic violence during pregnancy'. Her research includes an evaluation of a multi-agency domestic violence service based in maternity and sexual health services.

Loraine Bacchus completed a PhD in Psychiatry at St George's Hospital Medical School, now St George's University of London, in 2002. Her thesis was the first UK study to explore routine screening for domestic violence by midwives, as part of the Economic and Social Research Council's UK Violence Research Programme. Following this she worked on a survey of the prevalence of domestic violence in pregnancy and associated mental health and obstetric outcomes. In 2003 she joined Kings College London where she was the Principal Investigator on a theory-based evaluation of a multi-agency domestic violence intervention based in maternity and sexual health settings. In her non-academic role Loraine has worked as a domestic violence advocate in general practice and health visiting and developed clinical guidelines for addressing domestic violence in a range of healthcare settings. She was the coordinator of the UK national forum Health Ending Violence and Abuse Now (HEVAN) for four years and currently serves on the Board of the Nursing Network on Violence Against Women International (NNVAWI). In 2008 she joined the Gender Violence and Health Centre at the London School of Hygiene & Tropical Medicine where she is a Research Fellow.

Stephen Blumenthal is a consultant adult psychotherapist and clinical psychologist at the Portman Clinic, Tavistock and Portman NHS Foundation Trust, London, UK. The Portman Clinic specializes in the psychoanalytic treatment of people with problems of violence, sexual perversion, criminality and delinquency. He is a psychoanalytic psychotherapist and is also involved in research on violence and perversion. He is involved in teaching and training and runs a course on psychodynamic approaches to assessing and managing risk.

Tina Burke (LLB (Hons), BSc (Hons), MSc, PG Cert HEd, RMN) is a Senior Lecturer and Programme Director of the MSc in Forensic Mental Health Care run by the Faculty of Health and Social Care, London South Bank University. Ms Burke worked as a nurse practitioner in forensic services and was Clinical Lead at South West London and St George's Mental Health NHS Trust before her academic appointment. She works with a number of organizations helping to shape and improve services for people with mental health needs in forensic settings.

John Crichton (BMedSci, BM BS (Nottm), PhD (Cantab), MRCPsych, FHEA) is consultant forensic psychiatrist at the Orchard Clinic, Royal Edinburgh Hospital, Scotland's first medium secure unit. After studying psychology and medicine at Nottingham University he completed initial training in Psychiatry at Cambridge. In 1993 he was appointed Nightingale Research Scholar at Trinity Hall, Cambridge University, and at the Institute of Criminology he completed a PhD investigating the management of violence and other challenging behaviour involving psychiatric inpatients. He has published over 40 peer review papers and book chapters, editing *Psychiatric Patient Violence: Risk and Response* in 1995. He has provided expert evidence in a number of important legal cases, including *Bournewood*. In 2000 Dr Crichton was awarded the Lettsom prize by the Royal Society of Medicine and the Medical Society of London for the paper *The physical, mental and moral health of prisoners.* He has held academic posts in Cambridge and Edinburgh and recently has been Medical Director of the Forensic Network and State Hospitals' Board for Scotland. In 2008 Dr Crichton was appointed the foundation national Training Programme Director in forensic psychiatry. He is a Honorary Fellow in law at Edinburgh University.

Bridget Dolan Before she was called to the Bar in 1997 Bridget Dolan (PhD, C.Psychol, Barrister-at-law) was a forensic psychologist and lecturer at St George's Hospital Medical School, now St George's University of London, where she specialized in severe personality disorders. As a barrister she specializes in all aspects of mental health law, medical law and inquests. She has acted as counsel in several high-profile inquiries involving homicides by psychiatric patients and deaths in secure psychiatric care. She also sits as a part-time Tribunal Judge in the First Tier Tribunal (Mental Health).

Nigel Eastman is a Professor of Law and Psychiatry at the University of London and Head of Forensic Psychiatry at St George's University of London. He is both a doctor and a lawyer, being a member of Gray's Inn. He is also an Honorary Consultant Forensic Psychiatrist in the National Health Service with extensive experience of clinical forensic psychiatry, assessing and treating patients with severe mental disorders who have committed serious offences and/or who are facing serious criminal charges. He previously established a regional forensic mental health service and was, for 10 years, its clinical director. He has carried out empirical and scholarly research and published widely, on the relationship between law and psychiatry, as well as concerning services and policy for mentally disordered offenders. He has been an advisor to the Law Commission and has other substantial experience of conducting work on public policy in relation to law and psychiatry; for example, he has been a Member of the Mental Health and Disability Committee of the Law Society since 1989 and has given evidence to Parliamentary Select Committees on law and psychiatry. He has extensive experience of acting as an expert witness in both criminal and civil proceedings, in this jurisdiction and in the jurisdictions of other countries. He is an expert member of the Foreign Secretary's International Death Penalty Panel.

Ceri Evans is Clinical Director of the Canterbury Regional Forensic Psychiatric Service and a Clinical Senior Lecturer with the Christchurch School of Medicine and Health Sciences in New Zealand. He holds academic qualifications including Bachelor of Medicine and Bachelor of Surgery with distinction from the University of Otago, Master of Arts in Experimental Psychology from Oxford University via a Rhodes Scholarship, Master of Science with Merit in Psychiatric Research and Methods from the University of London and a PhD in Forensic Psychiatry from the University of London. He trained in psychiatry at the Maudsley Hospital in London. He became a Member of the Royal College of Psychiatrists in 1998 and completed specialist training as a forensic psychiatrist on the South Thames training scheme. He returned to New Zealand in 2003 to work as a Senior Lecturer in Forensic Psychiatry at the University of Auckland, also working part time as a consultant forensic psychiatrist at the Mason Clinic. In 2005 he took up his current post with the Canterbury District Health Board. He has led national initiatives on behalf of the Ministry of Health and Department of Corrections on violence risk assessment and prison screening for mental illness. His academic interests include perpetrators' memories of violent offending, violence risk assessment, abnormal homicide, and prison psychiatry. He is Course Convener for the University of Otago postgraduate course in forensic psychiatry based in Christchurch, New Zealand.

Rob Ferris is a Fellow of the Royal Australian and New Zealand College of Psychiatrists. He trained in medicine and both general adult and forensic psychiatry in Adelaide, South Australia, and also worked for a period in Darwin in Australia's Northern Territory. He then worked as a Consultant Forensic Psychiatrist at Broadmoor High Secure Hospital for four years before taking up a Consultant post in 1993 in what is now the Thames Valley Forensic Mental Health Service. Based initially at the Wallingford Clinic in South Oxfordshire he was the lead clinician involved in the planning and development of the Oxford Clinic, moving there when it opened in 1999. He was Clinical Director of the Service between 2000 and 2004.

He is a former member of the board of the International Academy of Law and Mental Health and a member of the advisory board of the Centre for Capital Punishment Studies at the University of Westminster. His interests include psychiatric ethics, particularly relating to Capital Punishment, forensic psychotherapy, prison mental health care and teaching. He currently holds a Consultant Forensic Psychiatrist post based at the Oxford Clinic Medium Secure Unit in Oxford and is a member of the Forensic Mental Health Inreach team at HMP Bullingdon

Nerida Harford-Bell read English Literature at East Anglia (BA Hons,) then completed an MA in Literature at Sussex. She then read Law and was called to the Bar in 1984. She practises exclusively in criminal defence. She has been instructed in cases involving murder, manslaughter, rape and other sexual offences and also serious drug crime. Her practice includes judicial review, inquests and civil actions against police. Mental health issues arise frequently in her cases, particularly those with female defendants.

Val Hawes is a Consultant Forensic Psychiatrist at the Fens Unit, HMP Whitemoor. After spending the first part of her medical career in primary care work in East Malaysia (1970–79), then Nepal (1983–91), Val trained in psychiatry in East London before starting higher specialist training in the psychiatry of learning disability at St George's Hospital Medical School. She was in the first group to complete the Diploma in Forensic Mental Health in 1997, then in the first group to complete the MSc in 1999. Meanwhile, Val moved into forensic psychiatry, completing her higher training in early 2001. She started work at the Dangerous and Severe Personality Disorder (now the Fens) Unit at HMP Whitemoor soon after it opened in September 2000. In addition to providing psychiatric assessment and care for prisoners on the Unit she is fully involved in the psychological treatment programme of the Unit.

Julia Houston (BSc, MSc, C.Psychol) is a Consultant Clinical and Forensic Psychologist at the Forensic Mental Health Services, Shaftesbury Clinic in London, UK, where she is lead for Psychology and Psychotherapies and team leader of the multi-disciplinary Sex Offender Service. She has over 20 years, experience in working with mentally disordered offenders and with sex offenders. Previous publications include *Making Sense with Offenders: Personal Constructs, Therapy and Change* (Wiley, 1998) and *Sexual Offending and Mental Health: Multi-disciplinary Management in the Community* (Edited with Sarah Galloway. Jessica Kingsley, 2008).

Darrick Jolliffe is a Senior Lecturer in Criminology at the University of Leicester. He has a BSc in Psychology from McMaster University and an MPhil and PhD in Criminology from the University of Cambridge and is a Chartered Scientist with the British Psychological Society. His main research interests are the relationship between empathy and offending, the development of offending through the life course and evaluations research.

Sue Kesteven is a Tribunal Member of the First Tier Tribunal (Mental Health) and an independent member of the Parole Board of England and Wales. She graduated with a BA (Hons) from

Exeter University in 1978 after which she worked in the field of professional regulation in relation to doctors and dentists. She obtained a Certificate (1996) and Diploma (1997) in Criminology from Birkbeck College before switching to a career in mental health and criminal justice, working for Nacro's Mental Health Unit. She has a Diploma in Forensic Mental Health from St George's Hospital Medical School and is author of *Women who challenge: women offenders and mental health issues* (2002) and joint author of *Information sharing: challenges and opportunities* (2004).

Sarah Lerner is a solicitor and partner in the firm Hereward & Foster, a legal aid practice based in London's East End. She specialises in Mental Health, Child Care and Community Care Law. She is accredited to the Solicitors' Regulation Authority Mental Health Review Tribunal Scheme and Children Panel. She has extensive experience of acting for children and parents in care proceedings and has represented many patients before the Mental Health Review Tribunal. She has taught regularly for Mind, the leading mental health charity in England and Wales, and is a former committee member of the Mental Health Lawyers Association. She has had conduct of a number of reported cases and has rights of audience in the higher courts.

Madleina Manetsch (MD) is a Consultant Psychiatrist working in a Child and Adolescent Forensic Psychiatry service attached to the Department of Child and Adolescent Psychiatry at the University of Zurich, Switzerland. She studied Medicine at the University of Basel, Switzerland, and completed her specialisation in Psychiatry and Psychotherapy at the Psychiatric Clinics, University of Basel, and the Forensic Mental Health Service at South West London and St George's Mental Health NHS Trust in London, UK. Her main clinical and research interests lie in developing psychotherapeutic interventions for emotionally and behaviourally disturbed adolescent offenders.

Gill Mezey (MBBS, FRCPsych) is a Reader and Consultant in Forensic Psychiatry at St George's University of London. Her research interests include psychological trauma and psychiatric aspects of domestic violence and sexual assault. She was the Principal Investigator on two Research Council-funded studies exploring the prevalence and health impact of domestic violence during pregnancy. She chaired the Royal College of Psychiatrists' working groups on Domestic Violence and on Rape and was an advisor to the Department of Health's Victims of Violence and Abuse Prevention Programme. Her publications include books on Male Rape, Psychological Trauma and Violence Against Women and over 60 papers in peer-reviewed journals.

Derek Perkins is a Consultant Clinical and Forensic Psychologist and the Head of Psychological Services for the forensic services of West London Mental Health NHS Trust, including Broadmoor Hospital. He has worked in prison, community and forensic mental health services for about 40 years and was involved in the early development of the national 'Dangerous and Severe Personality Disorder' services. He has been involved in the development of sex offender treatment programmes in forensic mental health, prison and community settings and has published a number of papers and book chapters on this subject. He was a member of the Howard League Working Party on sexual offence legislation reform in the 1980s, during which time he also worked with the police on research into sex offender profiling. He has provided advice and consultancy to the now Ministry of Justice on sexual homicide cases and was recently part of an international forum on sexual homicide and paraphilias, which is published as a book of the same name by the Correctional Service Canada. His clinical work is with sex offenders at Broadmoor High Secure Hospital, including psychophysiological assessment of sexual interests through penile plethysmography (PPG) assessment. He and a prison service colleague Christopher Dean have published on PPG assessment and research (Prison Service Journal) and also contributed to national guidelines on PPG work through the British Psychological Society. His research interests include psychophysiological assessment of sexual arousal and the assessment and treatment of sadistic sexual offending and sexual homicide.

Sharon Prince (BSc Psychology, MSc Clinical Psychology) is a Consultant Clinical and Forensic Psychologist and the Clinical Lead of the Leeds Personality Disorder Clinical Network; a multi-disciplinary and multi-agency service working with individuals with significant personality difficulties or disorder. The service was originally funded as one of the Department of Health pilot sites in community specific personality-disordered services. Previously she worked for 10 years in a forensic mental health service in south London, which also included developing and co-facilitating a group for Black Male inpatients (a brief and interesting experience). Sharon has been a lecturer on the Diploma in Forensic Mental Health, St George's University of London and has taught on both the Surrey and Leeds Doctoral Clinical Psychology training courses.

Daniel Riordan (MA, MBBS, MRCPsych, FRANZCP) is a consultant forensic psychiatrist and psychotherapist working at Long Bay Hospital and Silverwater Women's Correctional Centre in Sydney. Daniel trained at the London Hospital Medical College in East London and worked in general medicine before training in psychiatry at St George's Hospital in South London. Inspired by the therapeutic endeavours of staff at Henderson Hospital with difficult-to-treat patients he trained in psychotherapy, undergoing his own individual and then group analysis. He trained in forensic psychiatry and has worked in secure hospitals and English prisons before taking up a post in Sydney where he works in a high secure hospital and various correctional centres in New South Wales. Daniel has a special interest in group analysis, medical law and ethics as well as in teaching at both undergraduate and postgraduate levels.

Crystal Romilly After graduating in Economics from LSE, Crystal studied Medicine at Guy's Hospital and subsequently trained in psychiatry and forensic psychiatry. She has been a Consultant Forensic psychiatrist at South West London and St George's Mental Health NHS Trust for six years, first as Inreach Consultant at Wandsworth prison and now at the Shaftesbury Clinic Regional Secure Unit. Crystal has written on male genital self-mutilation, restriction orders, sexual behaviour in high security and prison mental health.

Trudie Rossouw is a consultant child psychiatrist working in North East London Foundation Trust where she is also the associate medical director for specialist services. She is also a qualified psycho analyst registered with the British Psychoanalytical Society. Previously she worked in South Africa and her chapter refers to her work as a police doctor in 1988 in Cape Town, South Africa.

Jaydip Sarkar is a consultant forensic psychiatrist working in Arnold Lodge Medium Secure Unit, East Midlands Centre for Forensic Mental Health in Leicester. He works with both male and female personality disordered patients across four care-streams. He is part of two national pilots: Women's Enhanced Medium Secure Services and step-down services for male patients with Dangerous and Severe Personality Disorder. His areas of clinical interest are helping clients develop an understanding of their impulses and emotions through affect regulation therapies, the nature of personality disorder and its classification and management, and holistic approaches to mental health care. He is piloting new ways of managing behaviours involving harm to self and others. He is keen on integrating different ways of managing affects and behaviour and is a proponent of 'Integrative Eclecticism' as an approach to treatment and interventions in the NHS. His research interests are trauma and its processing, bio- and neurofeedback to manage impulsivity and arousal and neurobiological underpinnings of psychopathy. He peer-reviews for mainstream mental health, criminological and forensic journals and is co-editing a book on the nature, theory and therapeutic interventions in personality disorders. He is keen to pilot approaches derived from findings from work on neuroscience of psychotherapy.

Lib Skinner is a solicitor and team leader of the Family and Child Care team at Hereward and Foster solicitors in East London. She is a member of the Children Panel and Family Law Panel and has rights of audience in the higher courts. She qualified in 1993 and before that worked in local government as a welfare rights officer for 12 years. Prior to that she worked with ex-prisoners, homeless and young unemployed people. She has represented many clients with mental health difficulties in family proceedings.

Emma van Hoecke After qualifying as a doctor Emma obtained a BA in Women's Studies from the University of Leuven, Belgium, and subsequently completed the Diploma and Masters in Forensic Mental Health at St George's University of London. Emma developed her interest in transcultural psychiatry through working as a psychiatrist in India and The Netherlands and as a forensic psychiatrist working in both The Netherlands and the UK at Broadmoor High Secure Hospital.

Cleo Van Velsen qualified as a doctor in London and pursued her postgraduate education as a psychiatrist at St George's Hospital. Prior to becoming a senior registrar at the Maudsley Hospital in psychotherapy she spent one year working at the Medical Foundation for the Care of Victims of Torture where she completed research on posttraumatic stress disorder and trauma. In 1994 Dr Van Velsen became a Consultant Psychiatrist in Psychotherapy at the Maudsley Hospital, with sessions within Forensic Psychiatry. She further developed her interest in forensic psychotherapy and, in 1999, took up a full-time post as Consultant Psychiatrist in Forensic Psychotherapy at the John Howard Centre, a medium secure service in East London. Dr Van Velsen was involved in the outpatient assessment, treatment and management of complex patients, both within the hospital setting and in community sectors.

In May 2008, Dr Van Velsen became the Responsible Clinician for a 10-bed ward, based within the Millfields Unit, a pilot project for the national Dangerous and Severe Personality Disorder Programme. Dr Van Velsen has written several chapters, co-edited a book on forensic psychotherapy with Dr Estela Welldon, and was also section editor on the Edinburgh Encyclopaedia of Psychoanalysis. She has an interest in understanding violence through film. Although working in a service unlike that of clinical psychoanalysis she has always felt underpinned and maintained by her training as a psychoanalyst at the British Institute of Psychoanalysis.

Martin Wrench (MA, MSW) is Principal Social Worker and Lead for Training and Consultation at the Henderson Hospital Therapeutic Community, UK. He was a senior forensic social worker in South West London for 10 years until taking up his current post in 1999. He was course tutor responsible for the law module on the Diploma in Forensic Mental Health at St George's University of London from 1998 to 2005. Martin has considerable experience as a trainer, supervisor and consultant on forensic mental health and personality disorder and as an organisational consultant to a wide range of health service providers. In addition, Martin is a Cognitive Analytic Therapist.

Martin has particular expertise with regard to personality disorder and in working with this client group in both forensic and non-forensic settings. He has recently been course leader on the Post Graduate Certificate in Working with Personality Disorder, a course run in conjunction with the Cassel Hospital, The University of East London and Experts by Experience.

Section 1

Violence and dangerousness

Chapter 1

Introduction to violence and dangerousness

Annie Bartlett

Only sometimes are violence and dangerousness the business of psychiatry; this section teases out when and why. It explains and explores the various theoretical approaches to different kinds of violence. Its purpose is to help the reader decide when a particular approach might be analytically persuasive, empirically robust and/or useful.

The section begins with two key chapters. Both are probably essential reading if the rest of the section is to make sense. The first, 'Medical Models of Mental Disorder', explains how medicine, and therefore psychiatry, thinks about abnormality. This is important because clinical psychiatry continues to be governed by medical model thinking; it is the most powerful single paradigm in mental health work. The second chapter, 'Violence in a Criminological Context', outlines the criminological approach to the categorization and measurement of crime, and violence in particular, as well as how social science might understand its occurrence. These chapters provide the foundations on which the rest of the section is built.

Chapter 4, 'Psychiatric Disorder: Understanding Violence', drills down into the common mental disorders, disorders that form much of the work of mental health services; it considers the nature and frequency of the relationship of these individual disorders to acts of violence. This level of detail about psychiatric disorders is what many people might see as 'core business'.

The chapters 'Race and Culture; the relationship of Complex Social Variables to the Understanding of Violence' and 'Gender, Crime and Violence' address a crucial issue in forensic mental health, that is, how to explain and understand, in societal terms, the apparently different rates of violence in different social groups. These are issues where those involved in forensic mental health often have strong views; these chapters attempt to weigh up the evidence on inequality in these sensitive areas.

The section also considers what might be thought of as 'test cases' for the value of different explanatory models. Domestic violence, sexual offending and responses to trauma (Chapters 7, 8 and 9) are areas in which many academic disciplines have something to say. These three chapters evaluate, in each case, the relevance of psychological, psychiatric, sociological, criminological and anthropological thinking to these topics.

Chapter 2

Medical models of mental disorder

Annie Bartlett

Aim

This chapter introduces the reader to the medical model, which is the dominant conceptual model in forensic mental health practice.

Learning objectives

- To understand the elements of a medical model of illness
- To be able to describe the strengths and weaknesses of the medical model as applied to mental health problems
- To evaluate the medical model as applied to two common disorders in forensic mental health practice, that is, schizophrenia and psychopathy
- To outline the historical development of the medical model in evolving mental health services
- To consider the historical and contemporary critiques of the medical model and its application both in general and forensic mental health practice

---

Introduction

This chapter will describe the medical model and go on to consider its strengths as a model for mental disorders. Mental disorders are very varied, and our understandings of the disorders have changed dramatically in the last century. It is reasonable to ask whether the medical model is equally helpful with regard to all psychiatric disorders or whether there are some psychiatric disorders where it is more useful. This leads on to a more detailed consideration of the value of the model in relation to the common mental disorders affecting the forensic population, namely schizophrenia and psychopathy.

This chapter then critiques the medical model from several perspectives. The model developed in the context of evolving psychiatric services that invariably involved compulsory admission. Dissatisfaction with institutionally based psychiatric services left the model open to a sociologically informed critique. Since the advent of deinstitionalization, a number of other critiques have developed, that is, cultural, gender-based and service user, and all are relevant to forensic practice. The key question, running through the chapter, is the extent to which the medical model is adequate for forensic practice.

Medical model thinking

There is no complete agreement as to what constitutes a medical model of illness but the following components are often mentioned:

- Aetiology (causes)
- Symptoms and signs
- Investigations
- Diagnosis
- Treatment plans
- Prognosis (outcome)

These are commonly discussed in relation to notions of *illness* or *disease*.[1] Not everybody referring to a medical model will have in mind exactly the same list of processes. However, the common use of more or less similar terms reflects the fact that medical practitioners need to communicate effectively about the patients they see and ensure that this structure works well. It is also based on scientific evidence about disease process, and this provides legitimacy for the interventions of medicine. The actions of medicine would otherwise break the taboos associated with both the touching and invasion of the body, and practitioners working without such legitimacy would be open to criticism as well as legal process.

Illnesses or diseases affect individuals or numbers of individuals. *Aetiological factors* identified by the medical model are predominantly biological, for example, infectious agents causing tuberculosis or the genetic basis of bipolar disorder. Widening of aetiological factors to include aspects of the individual's environment, be they psychological or social factors, is commonly done within psychiatry. Equally, there is an argument that a proper understanding of non-psychiatric disorders can be enhanced by including an awareness of associated social factors, for example, the link between tuberculosis and poverty or gastrointestinal disorders and the water supply. *Symptoms and signs* are elicited in physical disorders and there are parallels within certain psychiatric disorders—for example, subjective feelings of elation and irritability in hypomania accompanied by signs of over activity. *Investigations* in physical illness are usually technological, for example, blood tests, X-rays. Investigations within psychiatry are occasionally technological—for example, ECGs and MRI scans—but will usually include social investigation, for example, family structure and functioning and psychological investigation such as aspects of personality or intellectual functioning. *Diagnoses* within psychiatry are generally made by medical members of a multidisciplinary team. The value of diagnosis is debated among members of the multidisciplinary team and can be seen as a substitute for more detailed thinking. It exemplifies a reductionist approach to the totality of the individual concerned. It has the advantage, within a strict medical model, of providing a basis on which to organize the treatment plan. *Treatment* plans in psychiatry usually include physical, psychological and social aspects of treatment. Aspects of the individual, his or her presenting complaint and response to treatment will allow a judgement to be made about *prognosis* which relates to existing research evidence both within physical and mental disorders.

Psychiatry's attachment to medical model thinking is evident in its use of both the ICD-10 (WHO 1992) and DSM-IV (APA 1994) classificatory systems. Both systems incorporate, at least in relation to some disorders, many elements of the medical model described above. They are the most comprehensive approaches to diagnosis within psychiatry to date and come under regular

---

[1] There is an interesting sociological debate on distinctions between illness and disease, but this will not be touched on further in this chapter.

review in the context of both a changing evidence base and evolving professional opinion. Both ICD-10 and DSM-IV have expanded the number of disorders they describe. The emergence of classificatory systems of this kind is a response to concerns about the reliability of psychiatric diagnosis (Spitzer and Fleiss 1974). Within DSM-IV there are currently five Axes, though in clinical practice few people would routinely use anything other than an Axis I or Axis II diagnosis, that is, the axes focused on mental illness and personality pathology. Currently there are more than 300 diagnostic categories within DSM-IV, despite the relative poverty of the therapeutic armoury when compared to the range of interventions in other branches of medicine.

Problems with the medical model within psychiatry

These include the following, described in detail in Text Box 2.1.

The subjective experience of the patient or the client plays second fiddle to the views of the medical experts. Symptoms and signs equate with particular illness categories, that is, different symptoms and signs indicate the presence or absence of different illness syndromes. The patient's own experience, which will not necessarily be expressed within the language of symptoms and signs, can be ignored in search of a diagnosis. Thomas et al (1996) argued that the subjective experience of symptoms and signs is relegated to second place behind the perceived usefulness of separating out different mental illnesses.

The meaning of symptoms can be lost by strict adherence to a medical model. The preference among psychiatrists for detailed phenomenological descriptions of aspects of people's mental state—for example, of hallucinations or delusions – means that the particular meaning of the symptom to the individual person can be lost. This includes how symptoms can be contextualized in important aspects of someone's life. For example, if a woman patient complains of voices outside her head—in the voice of a man who says that she is 'bad'—then this may simply be construed, phenomenologically, as evidence of second person auditory hallucinations. The real significance of this kind of phenomenology could be the woman's experience of sexual abuse by a man. There are historic examples where attending only to the *kinds* of phenomena elicited from patients has led to problems. Rosenhan (1973) reported the hospitalization of individual researchers who reported voices saying 'thud' and 'thump'. These researchers continued to be detained in hospital after some period of time, despite showing no other evidence of mental abnormality. Their life histories were then cited as further evidence of psychiatric problems even though they did not suffer from any.

Box 2.1 Problems with the medical model in psychiatry

- Neglect of the patient's subjective understanding of their state of mind
- Adherence to a phenomenological approach to symptoms can lead to indifference to content
- Research bias towards biological explanation with less interest in social causes of psychiatric morbidity
- The absence of physiological correlates for many mental disorders
- Political abuse has followed from the interpretation of political protest and other social attitudes as signs of mental disorder
- Treatments introduced as efficacious have been seen to be lacking efficacy and often to generate problems in their own right

There is considerable research into the biological basis of psychiatric disorder, which is to be welcomed. Financial support from the pharmaceutical industry, which has an interest in developing biological interventions, often underpins such research. Biology is often the end-point for more complex causation. For example, seratonin and noradrenalin reuptake inhibitors increase the availability of both of the key neurotransmitters involved in depression. This is not to say that the sole cause of depression is abnormal neurotransmitters. Brown et al's (1977) work on the social origins of depression emphasized, inter alia, the importance of early life experiences in working class women. The medical model is concerned predominantly with biology in much of medicine. There is a risk, when it is applied to psychiatry, of confusing biology as a substrate for affective experience with biology as the primary cause of mood disorders. It is easy to forget that the neurochemistry of the brain responds, at least in part, to the environment in which a person finds himself or herself. Spitzer and Wilson (1975) have discussed whether psychiatric disorders meet the criteria for physiological dysfunction. They have argued that for the most part they do not, giving the following reasons.

First, for most psychiatric disorders there is no real understanding of specific aetiology. They are most often considered to be multifactorial, their main determinants being hard to identify. There are, of course, honourable exceptions to this, for instance, Huntington's Chorea, a genetic disorder. Second, the features of psychiatric disorders are not always qualitatively different from some aspects of normal functioning. What they mean by this is that 'coughs' and 'heart pain' are not part of the ordinary experience of being well. It is of course much less clear that feeling anxious, for example, before an examination or feeling mildly depressed, for example, before starting the working week are not just part of the ordinary range of human emotion. Clearly, phenomena such as delusions or hallucinations are much more obviously qualitatively different. Third, they suggested that to demonstrate physiological disorder there should be a demonstrable physical change in the person. In cases of lung cancer you would expect to see a tumour on a chest X-ray. There are areas of psychiatry where this is the case. Abnormal MRI scans of the brain are common in people with dementia. In other areas of psychiatry there is more debate, both about the presence of specific biological variation and its significance. The role of predisposing genetic factors in personality disorder is a good example of this (Tobena 2000). Fourth, Spitzer and Wilson argued that internal processes of physiological dysfunction should, once initiated, proceed independent of environmental conditions. There seems to be no very clear evidence that this could be demonstrated in mental disorder, in contrast for instance to the routine physiological resolution of chest infections. In the course of their debate, Spitzer and Wilson also pointed out that not all physical illnesses would meet this criterion and argued that the value of the medical model for mental disorder may be independent of logic. They have also argued that the medical model may be the least bad option, and it would not be clear what would replace were it to be abandoned.

Societal response to mental illness has at times been brutal. There are historical and contemporary examples that suggest that even if mental distress does not fit easily into a disease model, a broadly medically based approach may have the advantage of being more humanitarian than alternatives. Thus, for instance, previous responses to mental disorder within British society have included the persecution of witches, the incarceration of individuals within prisons and workhouses and the construction of the mad person as evil, thus requiring religious approaches (Porter 1987:8–38; Porter 1990:33–109). Against this argument is the idea that if the diagnostic terms are insufficiently rigorous, there is considerable scope for political abuse. Two clear examples of this were the incarceration of individuals within Soviet asylums as a result of the widespread use of the term 'schizophrenia'. The World Psychiatric Association concluded this was politically motivated and Soviet All-Union Group of Psychiatrists resigned from the World Psychiatric Association in 1983 and were readmitted only in 1989 (Gordon and Meux 2000). Similarly, the inclusion of the 'homosexualities' within diagnostic manuals until the mid-1970s indicated both a prevailing societal view about same-sex relationships and also provided justification for what purported to be the appropriate treatment of "sexual deviance"(King and Bartlett 1999; King et al 2004; Rosenhan 1975; Smith et al 2004).

It is a reasonable prerequisite of a medical model that the treatments entailed be beneficial. Anything else undermines the legitimacy of an intervention. Historically, this has not been clear in relation to psychiatric interventions. Notable examples of discredited treatment interventions include insulin coma therapy and leucotomy, as well as the kinds of purging and drenching in cold water characteristic of early nineteenth century psychiatry (Porter 1990:169–228). These did not work and were either dangerous or unpleasant. More recently, drug treatments have been subject to scrutiny. Benzodiazepines, used to manage anxiety, have come to be seen as addictive and unsuitable for prolonged prescription and ineffective over a long period. Neuroleptic medication has been recognized in recent years as associated with a small number of sudden deaths (Appleby et al 2000). The side-effects of medication are a major source of concern to patients and off-putting in terms of long-term prophylactic treatment. Even new anti-psychotic drugs have important side-effects. Clozapine can affect white blood cells and routine blood tests are required to monitor this. Electroconvulsive therapy (ECT) is recommended for a smaller number of psychiatric disorders than in the past and was the focal point of a passionate debate between the profession of psychiatry and the users' movement (MIND 2003). Disputes about efficacy are important, as in many cases drug treatment and physical treatment is given coercively, that is, through the use of the compulsory powers of the 1983 Mental Health Act to detain and treat. In these instances, the discrepancy between the subjective experience of the patient and the action indicated by the medical model can be considerable and unbridgeable. A further major criticism of drug treatments in psychiatry is that they may control symptomatology but they do not cure underlying disease. This is the weakest of the criticisms as this is also true of many chronic physical diseases, for example, rheumatoid arthritis.

Schizophrenia and psychopathy are important concepts in forensic practice. Text boxes 2.2 and 2.3 rehearse some of the key issues in the application of medical model thinking to these concepts; it is up to the reader to weigh up in their own mind how well the model fits. There is no final verdict.

The institution of psychiatry

The emergence of the medical model did not happen in isolation from changes in the care of the mad (Miller 1986; Treacher and Baruch 1981). The nineteenth century and early twentieth century saw the gradual development of specific medical expertise in madness; these practitioners contributed to and used medical understandings of madness as asylums were created in large numbers. It may well have seemed the least bad option.

A wave of political investigation into conditions in private madhouses and the small number of public asylums in England at the start of the nineteenth century was accompanied by a rethink as to the nature of 'insanity' and appropriate responses to it, both at an individual and a societal level. Jones (1993) carefully documented the progress of the parliamentary inquiries into allegations of brutality, notably at the Bethlem Hospital. There was evidence that some patients were chained to the wall and kept in insanitary circumstances.

> Once witchcraft, sorcery and conjuration had died out and most people lost faith in exorcism, the methods traditionally used by medical practitioners were the only ones left with any credibility until the development of moral treatment at the Retreat.
>
> (Jones 1993: 39)

Box 2.2 The case of schizophrenia

Definition: Exact meaning has changed over time but now defined in DSM-IV and ICD-10

Aetiology: Known to have significant genetic loading but assorted environmental factors also identified

Symptoms: Acute illness commonly involves disorders of perception and belief

Signs: Clinicians often rely on behavioural observation of soft signs such as apathy, social withdrawal, lack of conversation or thought disorder

Investigations: Physical investigations only to exclude organic disorder that may mimic some of the presentation. Social investigation to establish course of illness and family background

Treatment: Contemporary practice often confined to medication and contact with mental health workers for social and psychological support. Evidence base of family intervention or cognitive behavioural approaches to symptoms seldom used

Prognosis: Well researched

Problems with the model:

1. Concern about the value of the diagnosis across cultures both internationally and in United Kingdom in multi-cultural contexts

2. Stigma and overemphasis in public discourse of risk

3. Previous use of diagnostic term politically abusive

4. Previously an unreliable diagnosis

5. Many patients frame their problems differently and there is a gulf between the understanding of the patient and the professionals

6. Historical treatments brought the profession of psychiatry into disrepute

Jones is referring to the use of bromides and other basic drugs with no specific psychological effect that were utilized by medical practitioners who had responsibility for the insane. The case of George III who went mad when on the throne of England is enlightening. The indignities of these ineffective treatments are well illustrated in the film *The Madness of King George* (Porter 1987: 39–59). Ironically, he suffered from porphyria, a physical disorder, then unidentified, which can give rise to episodic mental symptoms. It is evident that at the start of the nineteenth century there was no established psychiatric profession and no interventions that affected the natural history of mental disorders.

Following a wave of enquiries into existing madhouse conditions, the government both legislated and financed the expansion of the public asylum system in England and Wales. The total number of patients and the number of county and city asylums as well as their average number of occupants increased dramatically over the course of more than 100 years (Jones 1993:116) with the average number of individuals held in an asylum as well as the number of asylums rising by a factor of 10. Certainly the rise in asylum detentions exceeded that expected by the increase in overall population (Jones 1993:115). This occurred at a time of huge social change in England with the creation of an industrial workforce and displacement of populations from the countryside to the town and an increase in the population overall.

The expansion noted above was explained in several ways. First, insanity was becoming more common. This can be seen as comprehensible in view of a rapidly changing society.

Box 2.3 The case of psychopathy

Definition: There are a wealth of terms, that is, psychopathy (historical), Antisocial Personality Disorder (DSM-IV), Dissocial Personality Disorder (ICD-10), Psychopathic Disorder (Mental Health Act category), Dangerous and Severe Personality Disorder (new government inspired category of DSPD)

Aetiology: Some genetic evidence that criminality and antisocial personality disorder run in families. Violence, a key aspect of the clinical syndrome, is linked with male gender. Environmental factors have been postulated to relate to the development of adult antisocial behaviour, for example, physical abuse in childhood

Symptoms: Few individuals with pronounced personality traits of this kind seek help spontaneously

Signs: Diagnostic frameworks emphasize unwanted behaviours

Investigations: Personality inventories and tools such as the Psychopathy Checklist have enhanced the likelihood of a standardized approach

Treatment: Evidence that the therapeutic community model can achieve reductions in service usage and subjective improvement

One-third of high secure patients are held under a diagnosis of Psychopathic Disorder, despite concerns about treatment potential. New DSPD units have been set up at considerable cost and are under evaluation

Prognosis: Re-offending can be construed as prognosis and there is an increasing body of evidence about the prediction of risk in relation to extreme antisocial histories

Problems with the model:

1. Repeated doubts have been expressed about the place of any of these categories in mental health

2. Many professionals are confused as to the existence of a core concept; this inhibits effective communication

3. The clinical syndromes were not reliably or rigorously diagnosed in the past and the value of diagnosis doubted, with doctors using it as synonymous with untreatable

4. Prisons contain many individuals with diagnosable disorders who are not offered treatment

Second, institutionalizing individuals was appropriate in view of the success of 'moral treatment'. Moral treatment was a more humane approach to patients, giving them adequate food and exercise rather than either locking them up in small crates or attaching manacles over long periods. It was initially propounded by the Quakers at the York Retreat. It was then taken up within the public asylum system by John Connolly. The advent of moral treatment was also linked with the advent of non-restraint. Scull (1979) argued that an expansion in the size of the asylum population in the United Kingdom, which was interestingly matched by a similar increase in other countries (notably in the United States), could not be justified on the basis of an increase in the numbers of the insane. Scull saw it rather as a convenient mechanism to distil out from mainstream society a large number of social deviants identified as such based on class, race and gender. Jones (1978) has drawn attention to the way in which asylum doctors coped administratively with these increasing numbers, while being viewed negatively by other doctors.

Twentieth century developments and medical psychiatry

During the time that the asylum population continued to expand, there was increasing enthusiasm for medical models of mental illness based on the belief that physical and mental illnesses had more in common than previously thought.

The Mental Treatment Act of 1930 instituted a number of important changes in society's responses to mental disorders. In particular, the term 'asylum' was replaced with that of 'mental hospital'; the term 'lunatic' was replaced with the term 'person of unsound mind'. Psychiatric outpatient departments were established and voluntary treatment, rather than compulsory detention in hospital, became possible for the first time (see Jones 1993:135). By 1945 psychiatry was established as a branch of medicine but inpatient numbers were still rising because of the continuing inadequacy of any therapeutic methods to decrease the asylum population. The structure of services to people with mental disorder might mimic that for physical disorder but the interventions did not; the salaries of psychiatrists rose.

In 1954, a Private Member's Bill (Parliamentary Debates 1954) brought before Parliament highlighted issues of overcrowding, staff shortages and stagnation within large-scale mental hospitals, noting in particular the presence of many, many long-term patients. This was the start of the move towards deinstitutionalization. Raftery (1992) noted that, at its peak in 1954, the asylum population was 4 in 1,000 of the UK population. The creation of effective anti-psychotic medication certainly provided an impetus (Jones 1982). So too did changes in legislation exemplified by the 1959 Mental Health Act and alterations in service structure; the will of the politicians also led to the implementation of the revolutionary policy of deinstitutionalization. Services began to be located in the communities in which people lived, as opposed to being asylum-based.

Accompanying and perhaps, in part, propelling these changes in outlook was the emergence of an intellectual critique from both inside and outside psychiatry. This addressed how psychiatry was conceptualizing mental disorder and how it was conducting itself, particularly the way in which it had created stagnant asylum populations. Goffman (1961), Szasz (1961), Foucault (1967) and Scheff (1966, 1981) wrote independently, but their ideas resonate with each other's views. Taken together they still represent a formidable assault on established practice. They are considered in greater detail in the following section.

The development of the anti-psychiatry movement

Goffman (1961), in a highly influential monograph, generated a highly determinist but satisfyingly complete model of the 'total institution'. This was based on a period of social research in a large US mental hospital in which the author emphasizes shared aspects of institutional life. He draws attention to similarities between mental hospitals, army barracks, concentration camps and prisons. He describes the social processes within institutions that predispose an individual to lose any sense of their own identity. He compares medical interventions to assault, focusing on the treatment interventions of the day, ECT and psychosurgery. The concept of the 'total institution' relates to institutions that are cut off from mainstream society. Goffman sees asylums as abnormal social environments that are inherently anti-therapeutic.

Like Goffman, Szasz has written frequently on the subject of mental illness. He (Szasz 1961) equates mental illness to 'problems in living', undermining the organic basis to mental disorders that at the time was less well established than now. His theoretical position is that mental illness serves psychiatrists much as witchcraft served theologians, that is, as a set of beliefs that created a need for experts. He considers that people suffering from mental illness abdicate a degree of personal responsibility. Patients impersonate the sick role, and psychiatrists play the role of medical therapists. Szasz has been taken to task by numerous other authors, including Anthony Clare (1980), who argued that there is no empirical evidence for his assertions. Clare pointed out that to deny the reality of the suffering of those with mental illness is unfair. Szasz is also criticized by Jones (1993:175–178) for supporting capitalist values, being opposed to state psychiatry and advocating private psychotherapy.

The essence of Scheff's (1966, 1981) critique of the theory of psychiatry is that diagnostic formulations neglect the accompanying social processes. Thus, psychiatric symptoms are considered to be contrary to ordinary social norms and established, long-term illness not to be a consequence of an intrinsic disorder but an adaptive social role determined by the response of society to the flouting of the rules of ordinary life.

The focus is not so much 'one-off' episodes of illness but chronic illness. Scheff argued that mental illness is best seen as a metaphor and that it is more useful to examine the idea of 'deviant behaviour' violating accepted social norms. He further argued that deviance is rendered permanent if the following conditions are satisfied: first, that one is defined as mentally ill; second, if one acquires deviant status; and third, if one involuntarily or otherwise adopts the social role of the mentally ill. This theory is now quite old, and like Szasz's, is undermined by recent advances in our understanding of the organic changes that accompany some major mental health problems, but it is linked with the modern debate on stigma. Scheff continued that the negative public discourse on madness provides readily accessible labels which can be attached to the mentally ill. He also stated that there are a certain number of rewards for accepting the role of the deviant person. In particular, individuals are in a position to develop 'insight', something valued by psychiatrists. Fighting the role of the deviant is fairly futile. The deviant role jeopardises access to work, accommodation and education. Accepting the role of the deviant may also be one resolution of the emotional turmoil involved in wanting to 'know' the nature of the problem. It may be simpler and less traumatic to accept the proffered role. The role of the deviant resolves that which is otherwise incomprehensible but in a different way from the medical model.

Foucault (1967), writing as a historian, charted madness from the late sixteenth century to the eighteenth century. In contrast to Goffman, Scheff and Szasz, who are writing about their own periods and about the United States, Foucault wrote a social history of France. The argument he put forward has come to be seen to be more important than the historical facts. It centres on a notion of the 'great confinement' which, he argued, predates that of the development of asylums in nineteenth century England and North America. The great confinement was a rounding up of everybody who did not fit into society. They would then be located either in prisons or hospitals. His argument was that this confinement was not based on notions of illness but rather on protestant influences, the 'work ethic' in particular. Thus the confinement of the mad was not about 'curing the sick', rather it was about the 'condemnation of idleness' in which those in power in society control the movement and location of the powerless. In his work on madness and in other volumes (Foucault 1989) Foucault went on to argue that hospitals themselves create disease. He argued (Foucault 1979) that institutions such as factories, schools, mental hospitals and prisons were designed primarily as mechanisms of social control. Both hospitals and prisons have a major deterrent value; they are unpleasant enough for people to want to avoid incarceration.

All these writers display considerable cynicism about the motives of staff involved in institutional care and the frameworks the helping professions use to understand and care for those with mental health problems. The mass institutionalization of largely poor individuals at a time of therapeutic impotence did no favours to the evolving mental health professions. These authors are right to point out that mental hospitals became less humane than Tuke ever intended and that public images of the mad have an effect on their lives.

Although Goffman, Szasz, Scheff and Foucault are the grand old men of the anti-psychiatry movement, their ideas are still relevant, and the contemporary debate on stigma (Crisp 2003) and the incorporation of ideas on stigma and labelling into the concept of social exclusion (Leff and Warner 2006:19–40) show the enduring power of the sociological concepts and also of medical model thinking.

Contemporary critiques of psychiatry

More contemporary critiques from multiple authors are also of value to current practice in psychiatry. These are listed below as follows:

- Cultural critique
- Gender critique
- User critique

What all three of these critiques have in common is that they dispute the value of the medical model and in different ways highlight value systems implicit in medical judgement. In all of these critiques we hear echoes of earlier writers.

Cultural critique

The clinical classificatory systems, ICD-10 (WHO 1992) and DSM-IV (APA 1994) have been developed in Europe and North America with relatively little input from practitioners elsewhere. The discipline of anthropology, in particular, had led a critique that attacks the model's assumption of universality. Anthropologists have argued that Western diagnostic categories may not apply outside of the West for the following reasons:

- Different cultures have different concepts of person, thus different ideas about appropriate social relations, for example, independence, separation and individuation
- Behaviours viewed as mad by the West may not be so construed indigenously
- Notions of a mind/body dichotomy may not be shared by other societies

This critique is exemplified by the writing of Kleinman (1977, 1980, 1987) and countered by Leff (1988, 1990). Kleinman argued that the Western gaze neglects local understandings of illness, and its categories do not fit with indigenous models of distress. Leff argued that the core concepts of major diagnostic categories such as schizophrenia, like physical illness, can be found throughout the world. The consequence is a polarized debate between social anthropology and psychiatry as to the value of extending Western designed and developed diagnostic systems throughout the rest of the world. This has implications for the design and acceptability of certain services.

This debate has acquired local meaning in the United Kingdom as society has become ethnically and culturally more complex. In the United Kingdom the focus of this debate has been on the involvement of ethnic minorities in psychiatric care, where there are examples both of the over-representation and under-representation of ethnic minorities in patient populations (Davies et al 1996). Multiple explanations for this phenomenon have been brought forward, predominantly to explain the overrepresentation of young black men in inpatient facilities (Littlewood and Lipsedge 1988). The kinds of explanations that have been offered are as follows:

- Practitioners of psychiatry are racist

- Individuals from ethnic minorities are alienated from mainstream, predominantly white-run services
- The stress of migration as it applies to particular historical groups gives rise to an increase in the prevalence of certain psychiatric disorders
- The stress of living in a predominantly racist society as a member of an ethnic minority group is more likely to generate mental disorder
- There is misdiagnosis because of lack of cultural congruity between patient and doctor or other mental health worker
- There are biological differences within particular ethnic minority groups that give rise to different prevalence of mental disorder

The importance of these critiques lies in the fact that they are a challenge to the apparently scientific basis of the medical model, both psychiatric theory and practice, and also because these explanations do not generate a consensus, rather an acrimonious debate about psychiatry's approach to ethnic minority groupings (McKenzie and Bhui 2007; Murray and Fearon 2007; Patel and Heginbotham 2007; Singh 2007). This relates most particularly to the issue of compulsory detention and the overrepresentation most particularly of individuals of Afro-Carribean and African origin within secure hospital services (Coid et al 2000; see also Prince this volume pp 67–78).

Gender critique

Historically, it has been true that there are far more female than male patients in psychiatry. In the nineteenth century, by 1850, there were more women detained than men; in the twentieth century, women outnumbered men in private hospitals, public hospitals, outpatient departments and psychotherapy services (Ussher 1991). Formal admissions—that is, compulsory admissions to hospital—are now different: for both Parts II and III of the 1983 Mental Health Act, male admissions outnumber female admissions (NHS Information Centre for Health and Social Care 2008.

Showalter (1987) has provided the most coherent and intellectually stimulating approach to issues of gender in historical and contemporary psychiatry. She has argued that, historically, women have been construed as irrational, closer to nature and symbolically linked with the body. This echoes much anthropological writing about more contemporary concepts of women cross culturally (Ortner 1974; MacCormack and Strathern 1980). Men are associated with reason, culture and intellectual discourse. The essence of her argument is that madness is the "historical label applied to female protest and revolution", because women have been excluded from domains of reason and thus their avenues of protest are distorted into ill health. She points out that the most authoritative critics of psychiatry such as Foucault and Goffman never looked at gender, and argues that changing diagnostic fashions within psychiatry, based on a medical model, have disguised a very basic problem, which is that women are still more frequently the ones deemed ill. In the nineteenth century they suffered from hysteria; in the twentieth from depression (Nolen-Hoeksema 1987). Psychiatry has substantially accepted the role of gender specific social factors in generating certain psychiatric disorders (Harris et al 1991). Showalter (1987) notes that women are much more frequently prescribed psychotropic drugs as well as being more likely to be the recipients of care. She relates the diagnostic bias to a feminist analysis of society, and observes that the writers of psychiatric text books, the professors of psychiatry, are usually men and that the dynamics of patient/mental health worker relationships often mimic those of women to men. Thus she relates power balances within psychiatry to those in wider society as well as to those within the woman's micro environment. The difficulty, however, is that distress, however conceptualized, is not going away. Showalter poses dilemmas for mental health workers confronted with distressed patients for whom there may be an obvious social solution but one that is impossible to achieve.

Many of the ideas expounded by Showalter are evident within the forensic arena and have become well accepted. Women in prison have high rates of early abuse, usually by men, and the dynamics of prison environments run the risk of replicating the hierarchical relationships of gendered violence (Bartlett 2007). Forensic services have conspicuously moved towards holistic care for women in secure hospitals with an emphasis on integrating female roles into care (DH 2002, 2003) (see Bartlett, this volume pp. 53–66).

User critique

The user critique is heterogeneous in nature. This term signifies the range of ideas that constitute a commentary on mental health services and their theoretical justification. Part of this critique is based on empirical research on levels of satisfaction with services (e.g. Golding 1997; Raleigh et al 2007). Much of it emerges through the third sector, for example, Mind, Survivors Speak Out and some through eloquent individual users of services, for example, Millett (1990).

A key theme in this area is inequality between patients and experts, an inequality bolstered by the nature of mental health legislation that gives experts power over patients. Chamberlain (1988) commented on the difference between the individual users' subjective experience versus the medical account of their condition. She noted that coercion is particularly important in areas of disagreement around diagnosis and treatment plans. She observed psychiatric services as non-individualized and abusive in the absence of patient controlled alternatives.

Just as some elements of other critiques look dated, so too do some elements of the user critique. There are now some patient-led services, for example, the Sun Project in South-West London. Patient involvement in the systems of the NHS is now a routine; there are examples of this even in high secure care where patients are involved in Patients' Councils. Abuse of patients receives little attention by comparison with earlier periods (Martin 1984). Dangerousness is now flavour of the month and the Mental Health Act (2007) united in opposition to it both user organizations and professional bodies, dismayed at the illiberal tone of draft Bills and the final Act.

Taken in historical perspective the most surprising thing about the user critique is that it exists; in the last 200 years much has changed in terms of conditions of care, advocacy and self-advocacy.

Conclusion

The early and late critiques of medical model thinking and its practical consequences are cogent and have much to recommend them. They have had an impact. Mental health practice has not been, and is not, impervious either to criticism or constructive comment. There have been huge changes in the scope of mental health theory and practice in 200 years. The medical model is resilient. There is no sign of it dissolving away when confronted with important challenges and arguably it has grown stronger with time, with new support offered for biopsychosocial approaches (Shah and Mountain 2007). This may reflect both an increasing evidence base and the fact that it is embedded within a powerful profession. It may also reflect the fact that the model is intrinsically robust and can adapt to changes in thinking but still provide a framework of understanding for what is now multidisciplinary practice. It has the robustness and flexibility of good models which are not supposed to limit thought but to facilitate it, in this case in order to help patients. The medical model in its current form is not a strait-jacket. Nor is it perfect – it is only a model.

Key points

- ♦ The power of the medical model in mainstream medicine and mental health is that it legitimizes therapeutic intervention
- ♦ The value of the medical model in mental health is compromised by, among other factors, inadequate biological understanding of the origin of common mental health problems and its difficulty incorporating the patient's experience of their difficulties
- ♦ There is a parallel between the historical development of the medical model, concepts of mental health practitioners, legal understandings of madness and provision of care
- ♦ Detailed examination of common forensic mental health problems, that is, schizophrenia and psychopathy, illustrates the varying degree of robustness of the medical model within mental health practice

References

APA 1994 American Psychiatric Association Diagnostic and Statistical Manual 4th Edition. Washington DC: American Psychiatric Association.

Appleby, L., Thomas, S., Ferrier, N., Lewis, G., Shaw, J. and Amos, T. 2000 Sudden Unexplained Death in Psychiatric In-patients. British Journal of Psychiatry 176: 405–406.

Bartlett, A. 2007 Women in Prison: Concepts, Clinical Issues and Care Delivery. Psychiatry 6, 11: 444–448.

Brown, G., Harris, T. and Copeland, J.R. 1977 Depression and Loss. British journal of Psychiatry 130: 1–18.

Chamberlain, J. 1988 On Our Own London: MIND.

Clare, A. 1980 Psychiatry in Dissent. London: Tavistock.

Coid, J.W., Kahtan, N., Gault, S. and Jarman, B. 2000 Ethnic Differences in Admissions to Secure Psychiatric Services 177: 55–61.

Crisp, A. 2003 Every Family in the Land: Understanding Prejudice and Discrimination Against People with Mental Illness. London: RSM Press.

Davies,S., Thornicroft, G., Leese, M., Higgingbotham, A. and Phelan, M. 1996 Ethnic Differences in Risk of Compulsory Psychiatric Admission among Representative Cases of Psychosis in London. British Medical Journal 312: 533–537.

Department of Health. 2002 Women's Mental Health: Into the Mainstream. London: Department of Health.

Department of Health. 2003 Mainstreaming Gender and Women's Mental Health: Implementation Guidance. London: Department of Health.

Foucault, M. 1967 Madness and Civilisation: A History of Insanity in the Age of Reason. (Trans. Howard, R.) Harmondsworth: Penguin.

Foucault, M. 1979 Discipline and Punish: The Birth of a Prison (Trans. Sheridan, A.M.) Harmondsworth: Penguin.

Foucault, M. 1989 The Birth of the Clinic. London Routledge. First published 1963 Presses Universitaires de France.

Goffman, E. 1961 Asylums: Essays on the Social Situations of Mental Patients and Other Inmates. New York: Anchor Books (reprinted Harmondsworth: Pelican 1968).

Golding, J. 1997 Without Prejudice: Mind – Lesbian, Gay and Bisexual Mental Health Awareness Research. London: MIND.

Gordon, H. and Meux, C. 2000 Forensic Psychiatry in Russia: Past, Present and Future. Psychiatric Bulletin 24: 121–123.

Harris, T., Surtees, P. and Bancroft, J. 1991 Is Sex Necessarily a Risk Factor to Depression. British Journal of Psychiatry 158: 708–712.

Hansard, Vol 523, column 2293–2371 19th February 1954.

Jones, K. 1978 Society Looks at the Psychiatrist. British Journal of Psychiatry 132: 321–332.

Jones, K. 1982 Scull's Dilemma. British Journal of Psychiatry 141: 221–226.

Jones, K. 1993 Asylums and After: A Revised History of Mental Health Services from the Early Eighteenth Century to the 1990s. London: Athlone.

King, M. and Bartlett, A. 1999 British Psychiatry and Homosexuality. British Journal of Psychiatry 175: 106–113.

King, M, Smith, G. and Bartlett, A. 2004 Treatments of Homosexuality in Britain since the 1950s– an Oral History: The Experience 0f Professionals. British Medical Journal 328: 429–432.

Kleinman, A. 1977 Culture, Depression and the 'New' Cross Cultural Psychiatry. Social Science and Medicine 11: 3–11.

Kleinman, A. 1980 Core Clinical Functions and Explanatory Models 71–118 in Patients and Healers in the Context of Culture. Berkeley: University of California Press.

Kleinman, A. 1987 Anthropology and Psychiatry: the Role of Culture in Cross Cultural Research on Illness. British Journal of Psychiatry 151: 447–454.

Leff, J. 1988 Psychiatry Around the Globe: A Transcultural View. London: Gaskell.

Leff, J. 1990 The 'New Cross-cultural Psychiatry': A Case of the Baby and the Bathwater. British Journal of Psychiatry 156: 305–307.

Leff, J. and Warner, R. 2006 Social Inclusion of People with Mental Illness. Cambridge: Cambridge University Press.

Littlewood, R. and Lipsedge, M. 1988 Culture Bound Syndromes 105–142 in Recent Advances in Clinical Psychiatry 5 (Granville-Grossman, K. Editor) Edinburgh: Churchill Livingstone.

MacCormack, C. and Strathern, M. (Editors) 1980 Nature, Culture and Gender. Cambridge: Cambridge University Press.

Martin, L. 1984 Hospitals in Trouble. Oxford: Blackwell.

McKenzie, K. and Bhui, K. 2007 Institutional Racism in Mental Health Care. British Medical Journal 334: 649–650.

Miller, P. 1986 Critiques of Psychiatry and Critical Sociologies of Madness 12–42 in The Power of Psychiatry (Miller, P. and Rose, N. Editors) Cambridge: Polity.

Millett, K. 1990 The Loony Bin Trip. New York: Simon and Schuster.

MIND 2003 Making Sense of ECT. London: MIND.

Murray, R.M. and Fearon, P. 2007 Searching for Racists under the Psychiatric Bed: Commentary on . . . Institutional Racism in Psychiatry. Psychiatric Bulletin 31: 365–366.

NHS Information Centre for Health and Social Care 2008. Inpatients formally detained in hospital under the Mental Health Act 1983 and other legislation, England 1997–98 to 2007–08. www.ic.nhs.uk.

Nolen-Hoeksema, S. 1987 Sex Differences in Unipolar Depression: Evidence and Theory. Psychological Bulletin 101: 259–282.

Ortner, S.B. 1974 Is Female to Male as Nature Is to Culture? 67–88 in Woman, Culture and Society (Rosaldo, M.Z. and Lamphere, L. Editors) Stanford: Stanford University Press.

Patel K. and Heginbotham, C. 2007 Institutional Racism in Mental Health Services Does not Imply Racism in Individual Psychiatrists: Commentary on . . . Institutional Racism in Psychiatry. Psychiatric Bulletin 31: 367–368.

Porter, R. 1987 A Social History of Madness. London: Weidenfeld and Nicolson.

Porter, R. 1990 Mind Forged Manacles: A History of Madness in England from the Restoration to the Regency. London: Penguin (first published by Athlone).

Raftery, J. Mental Health Services in Transition: The United States and United Kingdom. British Journal of Psychiatry 1621: 589–593.

Raleigh, V.S., Irons, R., Hawe, E. et al 2007 Ethnic Variations in the Experiences of Mental Health Service Users in England: Results of a National Patient Survey Programme. British Journal of Psychiatry 191: 304–312.

Rosenhan, D.L. 1973 On Being Sane in Insane Places. Science 179: 250–258.

Rosenhan, D.L. 1975 The Contextual Nature of Psychiatric Diagnosis. Journal of Abnormal Psychology 84: 462–474.

Scheff, T.J. 1966 Being Mentally Ill: A Sociological Theory. Chicago: Aldine.

Scheff, T.J. 1981 The Role of the Mentally Ill and the Dynamics of Mental Disorder: A Research Framework 54–62 in the Sociology of Mental Illness (Grusky, O. and Pollner, M. (Editors) New York: Holt, Rinehart and Winston.

Scull, A. 1979 Museums of Madness: The Social Organisation of Insanity in Nineteenth Century England. London: Allen Lane.

Shah, P. and Mountain, D. 2007 The Medical Model Is Dead – Long Live the Medical Model. British Journal of Psychiatry 191: 375–377.

Showalter, E. 1987 The Female Malady: Women, Madness and English Culture 1839–1980. London: Virago.

Singh, S.P. 2007 Institutional Racism in Psychiatry: Lessons from Inquiries. Psychiatric Bulletin 31: 363–365.

Smith, G., Bartlett, A. and King, M. 2004 Treatments of Homosexuality in Britain since the 1950s – an Oral History: The Experience of Patients. British Medical Journal 328: 427–429.

Spitzer, R.L. and Wilson 1975 cited (p. 37) in Kiesler, D.J. 1999 Beyond the Disease Model of Mental Disorder. Westport: Praeger/Greenwood.

Szasz, T.S. 1961 The Myth of Mental Illness: Foundations of a Theory of Personal Conduct. New York: Dell.

Thomas, P., Romme, M.A.J. and Hemmelinjk, J. 1996 Psychiatry and the Politics of the Underclass. British Journal of Psychiatry 169: 401–404.

Tobena, A. 2000 Aetiopathogenesis of Personality Disorder (from Genes to Biodevelopmental Process) 964–968 in Oxford Textbook of Psychiatry Vol 1 (Gelder, M., Lopez Ibor, J.J. and Andreasen, N.C. Editors). Oxford: Oxford University Press.

Treacher, A. and Baruch, G. 1981 Towards a Critical History of the Psychiatric Profession 120–149 in Critical Psychiatry: The Politics of Mental Health (Ingleby, D. Editor) Harmondsworth: Penguin.

Ussher, J. 1991 Women's Madness: Misogyny or Mental Illness. London: Harvester Wheatsheaf.

WHO (World Health Organisation) 1992 International Classification of Diseases. 10th Edition. Classification of Behavioural and Mental Disorders: Clinical Descriptions and Diagnostic Guidelines. Geneva: WHO.

Chapter 3

Violence in a criminological context

Darrick Jolliffe

Aim

To introduce a criminological approach to the measurement and understanding of violence

---

Learning objectives

- To explain how violence is measured
- To describe estimates of the frequency and nature of violence in England and Wales
- To outline social factors that have been found to increase the likelihood of violence taking place

---

Introduction

Criminology is the study of crime. This definition, however, is somewhat simplistic, as criminology is a complex and multi-faceted area of enquiry. That is, crime can be considered from a number of perspectives, including legal, political, sociological, psychological or even philosophical. For example, criminology can encompass the study of what crime is, including how the definitions of crime are developed and how they change with time, as well as how they might be applied to specific groups or segments of the population as opposed to others (Lauritsen and Sampson 1998). Criminology also includes scope to investigate features of the criminal process, including the characteristics of the actors involved (both the 'criminal' and the 'victim'), the setting in which the act took place and the social response to this act (e.g. Hollin 1989). This chapter is particularly concerned with examining the concept of violence within this broad criminological framework.

Although variations in the definition of violence do exist, it can be defined as a behaviour that is intended to cause and/or actually causes physical or psychological injury (Farrington 2001a). Within this definition, some researchers feel it is important to subdivide violence based on its intended goal. Expressive violence is used to describe violence that is not explicitly directed at achieving an external goal. An example of expressive violence would be a scenario in which an individual becomes involved in a dispute at a pub and hits out to hurt another person. Instrumental violence is used to describe violence used as a means to an end. An example of this would be threatening someone with the purpose of getting money (Blackburn 1995). Distinctions have also been drawn between proactive violence (when the opportunity for violence is actively sought out) and reactive violence (when one responds violently to an emotionally charged or antagonistic situation) (Crick and Dodge 1996). It is important to note these sub-definitions of violence. However, it can prove more difficult in practice to classify particular violent incidents reliably. This is because real-life violence often contains elements of each sub-type (Cornell et al 1996). Clearly, however, the most important violent offences defined by criminal law are homicide, assault, robbery and rape.

Measuring violence

There are three main tools that provide some insight into how much violence might be taking place. These are official records, victimization surveys and self-reports of offending behaviour. Each of these measures has benefits and limitations for measuring violence. These might be best illustrated by considering the movement in stages from the commission of a violent offence through conviction and incarceration for this offence by the criminal justice system.

A criminal justice system involves a successive funnelling process, shown here in a simplified form:

- Violence committed
- Reported to police
- Recorded by police
- Offender convicted
- Sentenced to custody

Of all violent acts committed, only some are reported to the police. Of all violent acts reported, only some are recorded by the police. Of all violent acts recorded, only some lead to the detection of an offender and to a conviction in court. Of all offenders found guilty in court, only some are sentenced to custody. Of course, there are many other possible stages that could have been shown, and many disposals other than incarceration, but these are some of the more important stages relevant to the current chapter.

The three main measures of violence are relevant to different levels of this funnelling process. Official records refer to all offences recorded by the police as well as records of convictions and sentences to periods of incarceration. Official records of violence have been collected for many years in England and Wales, and currently most of these official records are collected, collated and published by the Home Office. The Home Office is responsible for matters of criminal law as well as the police, prison and probation services in England and Wales (Chapman and Nivem 2000). For example, according to Home Office figures, there were 1.5 robberies per 1,000 population recorded by the 43 police forces in England and Wales in 1999. Similarly, in 1999 there were 0.12 persons per 1,000 population convicted of robbery, and 0.09 persons per 1,000 sentenced to prison for robbery (Farrington and Jolliffe 2005).

Victimization surveys involve asking people to report on their experiences of being a victim of crime in a specified time period (usually the previous 12 months). Individuals are usually identified through public registers and requested to answer questions either over the phone or in an interview at their home. Victimization surveys provide information about the first two stages of the crime funnel described above: crime committed and crime reported to the police. The first national victimization survey in England and Wales (the British Crime Survey or BCS) was conducted in 1982, and measured crime committed in the calendar year 1981. Subsequent national victimization surveys were carried out at two-year or four-year intervals up to 1999. Beginning in 2001 (measuring crimes committed in 2000), the BCS has been conducted annually. Because it captures offences not necessarily reported to the police or recorded by the police, the BCS is usually regarded as a more accurate measure of certain types of violence. For example, in comparison to the official figures given for robbery in 1999 of 1.5 per 1,000 population, according to the BCS there were 8.24 robbery offences per 1000 population, and of these, 2.5 per 1,000 population were reported to the police (Farrington and Jolliffe 2005).

Self-reports have been widely used by criminologists and have the benefit of providing information about violence that may not be part of official sources (Farrington 2001b). These devices involve asking people to report if they have committed any of the specified offences; and if so, how many times, in a set time period. There have been three nationally representative self-reported offending surveys conducted by the Home Office. In the first of these studies, Graham and Bowling (1995) sampled 1,648 young people aged 14 to 25 and found that 9% of males and 4% of females reported having committed violence[1] in the past 12 months. The second national survey in England and Wales reported the prevalence of violence for those aged between 12 and 30 (in the past 12 months) to be 4% for males and less than 1% for females (Flood-Page et al 2000). The survey carried out in 2003 suggested that 7% of males and 4% of females aged 10 to 65 had committed assault in the past 12 months (Budd et al 2005). Based on population estimates for 2003, this would be the equivalent of approximately 25 violent female offenders per 1,000 female population and 50 violent male offenders per 1,000 male population.

From these brief descriptions of the three main tools for measuring violence, it is easy to see that official records provide a very diluted measure of violence. For various reasons (e.g. fear of revictimization, perception that the violence was not serious, low confidence in police) not all violence will be reported to the police; of those violent offences that are reported, some may not be recorded by the police (e.g. because police decide there is too little evidence to proceed), meaning these violent offences would not be reflected in the official records. However, the benefits of official records are that they have been collected regularly over a long period and thus allow for changes in violence over time to be assessed. Also, if we were interested in identifying violent people for the purposes of examining the causes of violence, official records of convictions and incarcerations for violence would be useful. These official measures provide confidence that an individual has acted violently (i.e. they have been proven guilty in a court) and that this offence was serious enough to warrant incarceration. Many studies of violent individuals use official records as their evidence for violence having taken place (Jolliffe and Farrington 2004).

Victimization surveys provide a much less biased picture of the amount of violence than official records, in most instances as they collect information from an earlier stage of the criminal justice process. In addition, victimization measures have similar definitions to official records of many violent offences, and have been available in England and Wales since 1981. Therefore, victimization measures can be used to provide a complementary picture of the how rates of violence have changed over time.

Limitations of victimization measures include how the sample of respondents was obtained, how the victimization survey was administered to the respondents and also issues of memory or concealment. For example, using public registers to identify respondents means that some individuals at risk of being violently victimized (e.g. the homeless) are missed. Also, it is easy to envisage how certain approaches to victimization measures (e.g. anonymous calls over the phone) might provide more accurate information about sensitive issues such as violent victimization than others (e.g. personal interview in the respondent's home). Related to this issue of the validity of reporting, this measure of violence is unsubstantiated by supplementary evidence and therefore solely dependent on the memory of the respondent. Some violent incidents may be forgotten (or concealed), whereas other incidents might be exaggerated.

Further difficulties with victimization measures are more specifically related to violence, and might be less of an issue when obtaining information about other types of offences such as burglary or car theft. There is evidence to suggest that there is differential reporting with respect to certain details of violent events. For example, individuals appear more likely to report being the victim of theft than violence (Farrington and Jolliffe 2004). However, even within the category of violence it appears that individuals are more likely to report being assaulted violently than being

---

[1] This involved offences that might have been classified as robbery, assault and wounding.

assaulted sexually (Walby and Allen 2004). In addition, individuals appear more likely to report violence if the perpetrator is a stranger as opposed to a family member (Ellis and Walsh 1999).

Similar to victimization measures, the main benefit of self-report measures is that they appear to provide more accurate information about violence than official records (Farrington 2001b). Unlike victimization measures, however, which only identify the number of violent offences, self-reports are especially important in identifying the number of violent individuals involved in certain types of violence, and the frequency of involvement of these individuals (Farrington et al 2003). Self-reports are also relatively inexpensive and easy to use, which has made them a popular method in most forms of criminological research (Farrington 2001b).

A major limitation of self-reports is that they tend to be limited by the representativeness of the sample who complete the self-report measure. That is, self-reports tend to be administered to samples of individuals convenient for research purposes; therefore a great deal of research has been carried out on university undergraduates and school students (e.g. Jolliffe and Farrington 2006), but in all likelihood this methodology misses the most violent individuals, as they tend to have low educational attainment and are likely to be truant from school (Farrington 1995).

The method of administering these measures might also influence the validity of self-reports. Although most self-report measures are administered in a way that allows the respondent to respond anonymously (e.g. filling in an anonymous questionnaire in a classroom where the researcher doesn't know the students), there is some evidence to suggest that if respondents feel their anonymity might be compromised they are less honest. It has been suggested that the very low prevalence of violence that was evident in the Youth Lifestyle Survey carried out by the Home Office in 1999 (4% of males and less than 1% of females reported acting violently in the past year) was a result of the method of administration (e.g. Wikstrom 2002). In this study, the researchers went to the individual's house and asked them about self-reported offending. In many cases, other individuals were in the house at the same time the questionnaire was being administered, and often in the same room. In most cases, that individual was the respondent's mother, which is certainly not a recipe for obtaining the most honest responses.

Obviously the issue of memory or concealment is an important factor with self-reports. Like victimization measures, self-reports tend to rely exclusively on what an individual says they have done. However, research has shown that those who have committed the most offences have a distinct tendency to underreport their involvement (Farrington 2001b). This might be because they have committed so many offences they cannot remember them all, or that these individuals fail to report accurately to 'play it safe'.

A further issue with self-reports is that they tend to do a good job of assessing less serious forms of offending (e.g. truanting, shoplifting, fighting) as opposed to more serious types of offending (e.g. robbery, sexual violence). This is likely because of a general unwillingness to report taking part in these more serious forms of violence and because of the relative infrequency of these more serious types of violence (Farrington 2001b). Generally, self-reports have been shown to be more valid when they use information from a number of sources. For example, research has suggested that when self-reports are 'triangulated', that is, they combine information from a respondent as well as the respondent's mother and teacher, they provide more valid information than reports from the respondent only (Farrington 1997).

Combining measures

The comparison between self-reports and official records gives some indication of the probability of a violent offender being caught and convicted. For example, in the Cambridge Study of 411 South London boys followed up from the age of 8 to 48, 45% of boys admitted starting a fight or using a weapon in a fight between ages 15 and 18, but only 3% were convicted of assault between these ages (Farrington 1989). Hence, only 7% of self-reported violent offenders between ages 15 and 18 were convicted. Self-reported violence also had predictive ability. That is, 10% of those who admitted assault up to age 18 were subsequently convicted of assault, compared to 5% of those who did not report committing assault (Farrington 1991).

Similarly, in a Seattle prospective longitudinal study, Farrington et al (2003) compared official records to self-reports for a number of different offences for more than 800 children from age 5 to 18. The results showed that 18% of those who reported assaulting someone were referred to court for assault, whereas only 13% of those who reported robbery were referred to court for robbery. Moreover, when the actual number of assault and robbery offences was considered, less than 4% of assault offences and 2.5% of robbery offences ended up with a corresponding referral to court.

Changes in violence over time

There are a number of limitations that need to be considered when examining changes in the rates of violence over time. For example, with official records the legal definitions of certain categories of violence may change over time, which might make different years of the study incomparable. In addition, specific political initiatives affecting the criminal justice system may mean that certain violent offences are more likely to make an appearance in official statistics one year rather than another (e.g. policing targeted at street robbery). For victimization measures, changes in the wording of questions or the method of administration (for example, changing from phone calls to personal interviews) might influence reporting rates. General social changes such as the greater acknowledgement of sexual victimization by acquaintances might also alter the public's rate of reporting this offence. All of these potentially biasing factors might result in changes to the violent crime rate, but make it difficult to determine if changes in the violent crime rate reflect a change in an offence coming to our attention (i.e. either official or victimization measures) or a real increase in that type of violent offence (Farrington and Jolliffe 2005).

Acknowledging these limitations, there is evidence from official records to suggest that rates of violent crime have been increasing in England and Wales. The most comprehensive work in the area was carried out by Farrington and Jolliffe (2004), who examined trends in crime in England and Wales from 1981 to 1999. The results show that homicide had increased from 559 cases in 1981 to 746 in 1999 (from 1.1 to 1.4 per 100,000 population). Robbery had increased substantially from 20,282 cases in 1981 to 78,884 in 1999 (from 0.4 to 1.5 per 1,000 population), whereas rape of a female had increased sevenfold from 1,068 to 7,707 (4 to 29 per 100,000 females). Assaults appeared to have increased from 98,021 to 218,433 (2.0 per 1,000 population to 4.1 per 1,000 population).

It is difficult to determine how the official violent crime rate has changed since 1999, because of some significant changes in the counting of offences and the collection of data by the Home Office. These changes include moving from recording offences on a calendar year basis to a financial year basis in 1998–1999, the introduction of new counting rules for certain offences in 1998 and the introduction of the National Crime Recording Standard in 2002 (Coleman et al 2005). The authors of the most recent volume of *Crime Statistics* published by the Home Office suggested that the impact of these changes is still being reflected in the current official figures (Nicholas et al 2005).

With these limitations in mind, the official records appear to suggest that violent crime has continued to increase slowly since 1999. In 2004–2005, the Home Office reported 859 homicides (1.6 per 100,000 population), 88,710 robberies (1.7 per 1,000 population) and 12,867 rapes of females (49 per 100,000 females).

Examination of the national victimization survey (BCS) also suggests that violence has increased in England and Wales. Robberies increased from 162,641 in 1981 to 345,994 in 1999 (4.2 to 8.2 per 1,000 population. Assault increased from 507, 286 in 1981 up to a peak of 810,994 in 1995, but declined to 585,949 in 1999 (from 13.1 to 19.7 and then to 14.0 per 1,000 population; Farrington and Jolliffe 2004). However, according to the BCS, in 2004–2005 the rates of violence have been decreasing. In 2004–2005, the number of violent incidents reported in the BCS fell by 11% based on comparisons with the 2003–2004 BCS (Nicholas et al 2005). There were 56.5 violent offences per 1,000 population and 8.1 muggings[2] per 1,000 population. The authors suggested that the difference between the official records (showing increases in violence) and victimization measures (showing substantial decreases in violence) is the result of both an increase in the public's willingness to report violence and an increase in police recording of these reports, but not an increase in the actual amount of violence (Nicholas et al 2005).

Violent offenders

Violent crime, like other crimes, arises out of a complex interaction between the offender and the victim in a specific situation. In some cases, violence probably arises within a relatively normal individual faced with a situation that is conducive to violence. However, there is evidence to suggest there are some factors that increase a person's probability of acting violently in any given situation (Farrington 2001a). The remainder of this chapter will discuss a selection of these factors. Within a single chapter it is impossible to review all that is known about violent offenders; for more extensive information see Loeber and Farrington (1998) and Flannery and Huff (1999).

Gender and violence

The single most important factor associated with violence is gender. Males are more likely than females to commit violence, and when they do it is more frequent and serious than the violence committed by females (Farrington 2001a). In 2004, 62,500 males were convicted or cautioned for violence against the person compared with 13,200 females, yielding a gender (male:female) ratio of 4.7 to 1 (Home Office 2005: 111). For robbery, the gender ratio was even higher, with 7,000 males being convicted compared with 900 females (7.8 to 1).

Interestingly, self-report surveys yield much lower gender ratios than official sources. The gender ratio of violence (in the last 12 months) in the major national self-report surveys conducted by the Home Office were 2.3 to 1 (Graham and Bowling 1995; ages 14 to 25), 1.8 to 1 (Flood-Page et al 2000; ages 12 to 30) and 1.8 to 1 (Budd et al 2005; ages 10 to 65). A number of explanations were put forward to explain the apparent discrepancy in the official and self-reported gender ratios. Most suggest that self-reported offences tend to be less serious and also imply the possibility that the police and courts might discriminate in favour of females (especially if they are pregnant or have small children (Daly and Bordt 1995).

Numerous explanations exist for gender differences in violence. Maccoby and Jacklin (1974) suggested that these differences may be in part innate. They pointed out that gender differences in aggression are seen early in life, before any differential reinforcement of aggression in boys and girls. Furthermore, they suggested males are more aggressive than females in all societies for which evidence was available, that similar gender differences in aggressiveness were found in sub-human primates as in humans, and that aggression is related to levels of testosterone, which is

---

[2] Mugging involves theft from a person and is similar to robbery.

much higher in males. It follows that because males are on average bigger and stronger than females, males are better equipped to commit offences that benefit from the use of, or appearance of, physical strength.

Another possible explanation for the difference in rates of violence by males and females is that the two genders are socialized differently by their parents. In general, girls are supervised more closely and tend to stay at home more often, meaning parents are well placed to notice and react to unwanted behaviours, including aggression. Adults are generally more tolerant of aggressive behaviour in boys than in girls, and they may tacitly encourage boys to be 'tough' and take risks. Based on the theory that the strength of the conscience depends on the reinforcement of appropriate behaviour and the punishment of socially disapproved acts (e.g. Eysenck 1996), it follows that girls will develop a stronger conscience and be less likely to commit violent acts than boys.

Age and violence

Age is also strongly associated with violence. Most evidence suggests that individuals are most likely to be violent in their mid- to late teenage years. Table 3.1 shows the convictions per 1,000 males and females for three violent offences in 2004. For violence against the person, the peak age for convictions for males was 18 to 20 (6.4 per 1,000 males) and for females it was 15 to 17 (0.8 per 1,000 females). Similarly, the peak age of convictions for robbery was 15 to 17 for both males and females (1.8 per 1,000 males and 0.3 per 1,000 females). The peak age of convictions for sexual offences was relatively similar across the mid- to late teens for males, whereas females were rarely convicted of sexual offences.

Similar results are obtained in self-report surveys. For example, in the Offending Crime and Justice Survey of Budd, Sharp and Mayhew (2005), the peak age of violence was 14 to 17 for males

Table 3.1 Convictions for violence (per 1,000 males/females) 2004

Age range	Per 1,000 males Violence against the person	Per 1,000 females Violence against the person
12–14	0.85	0.3
15–17	4.73	0.82
18–20	6.36	0.64
21+	1.23	0.12
	Robbery	Robbery
12–14	0.57	0.1
15–17	1.83	0.31
18–20	1.44	0.11
21+	0.14	0.01
	Sexual offences	Sexual offences
12–14	0.19	*
15–17	0.39	*
18–20	0.31	*
21+	0.2	0.005

* Numbers too small to make estimation.
Based on data provided in Home Office (2005) and population estimates from the Office of National Statistics (2006).

and females. For males, the percentage admitting violence decreased from 33% at age 14–15 to 18% at 18–19 and 9% at 20–25; for females, the figures were 18%, 11% and 6%, respectively.

Many theories have been proposed to explain why violence (especially by males) peaks in the teenage years. For example, violence has been linked with testosterone levels in males, which increase during adolescence and early adulthood and decrease thereafter (Archer 1991). Other explanations focus on changes with age in physical capabilities and opportunities to commit crime linked to changes in 'routine activities' (Cohen and Felson 1979), such as going to pubs in the evenings with other males. The most influential explanation emphasizes the importance of social influences (Farrington 1986). From birth, children are under the influence of their parents, who generally discourage offending. However, during their teenage years, juveniles gradually break away from the control of their parents and become influenced by their peers, who may encourage offending. After age 20, violent offending declines as peer influences give way to a new set of influences in the form of spouses and female partners.

Changeable factors associated with violence

Although both gender and age are clearly associated with violence, neither of these factors provides a useful point of intervention to reduce violence. We cannot selectively incarcerate all males, or all those between the ages of 15 and 20, no matter how appealing that might be to some. There are, however, some risk factors that have been identified that are changeable. To determine whether a changeable risk factor is a predictor or a possible cause of violence, the risk factor needs to be measured before the violence, which is why longitudinal studies are so important. Below is a selection of findings regarding some changeable social and family risk factors from some of the more famous longitudinal studies in criminology.

Social factors associated with violence

Having delinquent friends has consistently been associated with violence. For example, in the Rochester Youth Development Study (a longitudinal study of 1,000 adolescents through their early adult years), peer delinquency was found to be strongly related to self-reports of youth violence (Thornberry et al 1995). However, it is difficult to determine how far the link between delinquent friends and delinquency might be a consequence of co-offending, which is very common under the age of 21 (Reiss and Farrington 1991). There is some evidence to suggest that acting in a delinquent manner increases the likelihood of having delinquent friends and that having delinquent friends increases the likelihood of an individual acting delinquently (Elliott and Menard 1996). Farrington et al (2002) found that delinquent peers were more likely to be a consequence of offending rather than a cause of offending.

In general, coming from a low socio-economic status (SES) family is associated with an increased probability of violence. For example, in the US National Youth Survey, a nationally representative US sample of more than 1,700 adolescents aged 11 to 17, self-reported felony assault and robbery were about twice as common among lower class youths than middle class youths. The relationship between low SES and violence has also been found in studies in countries such as Sweden, Denmark, New Zealand and England (Farrington, 1998; Henry et al 1996; Hogh and Wolf 1983; Wikstrom 1985). Those living in high-crime neighbourhoods appear to be more violent than those living in low-crime neighbourhoods. In the Rochester Youth Development Study, living in a high-crime neighbourhood was significantly related to self-reported violence (Thornberry et al 1995). Similarly, in the Pittsburgh Youth Study, a study of more than 1,500 boys in the first, fourth and seventh grades in public schools in Pittsburgh, living in a 'bad neighbourhood' (either as rated by the mother or based on census measures of poverty, unemployment and female-headed households) was significantly related to both official and self-reports of violence (Farrington 1998).

Family factors

Numerous family factors predict violence. In her follow-up of 250 Boston boys in the Cambridge–Somerville longitudinal study, McCord (1979) found that the strongest predictor at age 10 of later convictions for violence (up to age 45) were poor parental supervision, parental aggression (including harsh, punitive discipline) and parental conflict. McCord (1977) also demonstrated that fathers convicted for violence tended to have sons convicted of violence. In the Cambridge (England) study, the strongest childhood predictor of adult convictions of violence was having a convicted parent (Farrington 2001c).

Similar results have been obtained in other studies. In the Chicago Youth Development Study, which is a longitudinal follow-up of nearly 400 inner-city boys initially studied from age 11 to 13, poor parental monitoring and low family cohesion predicted later self-reported violence (Gorman-Smith et al 1996). Poor parental monitoring and low attachment to parents predicted self-reported violence in the previously mentioned Rochester Youth Development Study (Thornberry et al 1995). Disrupted families between birth and age 10 predicted convictions of violence up to age 21 in the British National Survey, which was a follow-up study of more than 5,000 individuals born in one week in March 1946 (Wadsworth 1978). Disrupted families also predicted official violence in the Cambridge Study (Farrington 1998), but subsequent analysis suggested the cause of the disruption and the post-disruption trajectory were important factors. That is, delinquency rates were similar in disrupted families and in intact families with high levels of conflict, and family disruptions caused by marital disharmony were more damaging than disruptions caused by parental death (Juby and Farrington 2001).

Harsh physical punishment by parents and child physical abuse typically predict violent offending (Malinosky-Rummell and Hansen 1993). Harsh parental discipline also predicted official and self-reported violence in the Cambridge Study (Farrington 2001c). In the Columbia County Study, a study of more than 800 third-grade children in Columbia County, New York, Eron et al (1991) reported that parental punishment at age 8 predicted not only arrests for violence up to age 30 but also the severity of men's punishment of their own children at age 30 as well as their history of spousal assault.

In the Pittsburgh Youth Study, harsh physical punishment predicted violence for Caucasians but not for African Americans (Farrington et al 2003). It has been suggested that this is because physical discipline is associated with neglect and coldness in Caucasian families but with concern and warmth in African-American families (e.g. Kelley et al 1992).

In a longitudinal study of more than 900 abused children and nearly 700 controls in Indianapolis, Widom (1989) discovered that recorded child physical abuse and neglect predicted later arrests for violence, and this was true for both males and females and for those of different races. Child sexual abuse also predicted adult arrests for sex crimes (Widom and Ames 1994). In the Rochester Youth Study, Thornberry et al (1995) showed that recorded childhood maltreatment under the age of 12 predicted self-reported violence between the ages of 14 and 18 equally well for males and females, for those of different races and for those of both higher and lower SES.

Large family size (number of children) was found to predict youth violence in both the Cambridge Study and the Pittsburgh Youth Study (Farrington 1998). There are a number of possible reasons that a large number of siblings might increase the risk of a child's delinquency. In general, as the number of children increases, the amount of parental attention that can be given to each child decreases. Additionally, as the number of children increases, the household tends to become more overcrowded, possibly leading to increases in frustration and conflict. In the

Cambridge Study, large family size did not predict delinquency for boys living in the least crowded conditions (two or more rooms than there were children). This suggests that household over-crowding might be an important factor mediating the association between large family size and offending (West and Farrington 1973).

Conclusion

In criminology, violence is studied using official records, victimization measures and self-reports. Each of these measures has strengths and weaknesses when examining violence, and the most valid information comes from combining these measures. According to official records, violence has been increasing in England and Wales since 1981, and according to victimization measures, violence has increased from the levels in 1981 but has declined recently. It has been suggested that this discrepancy between official records of violence (continuing to rise) and victimization measures of violence (decreasing violence) is the result of the public's greater willingness to report violence and the greater willingness of the police to record violence, rather than an actual increase in the amount of violence committed.

A number of factors have been found to be associated with an increase in the likelihood of violence, and some of these have been reviewed in this chapter. Males are more likely to be involved in violence than females, and those in their mid- to late teenage years appear most likely to be involved in violence. A number of social and family factors have also been found to increase the likelihood of violence. These include having delinquent friends, coming from a family of low SES, living in a bad neighbourhood, the type and quality of parenting, parental convictions, disrupted families, physical punishment and abuse, and large family size. Interestingly, these social and family risk factors have been consistently reported in a number of different studies in different countries. This suggests that interventions designed to address these factors would significantly reduce violence (e.g. Welsh and Farrington 2000).

References

Archer, J. 1991 The Influence of Testosterone on Human Aggression. British Journal of Psychology 82: 1–28.

Blackburn, R. 1995 Violence 357–373 in Handbook of Psychology in Legal Contexts (Bull R. and Carson D. Editors) London: Wiley.

Budd, T., Sharp, C. and Mayhew, P. 2005 Offending in England and Wales: First Results from the 2003 Crime and Justice Survey. Home Office Research Study. London: Home Office.

Chapman, B. and Niven, S. 2000 A Guide to the Criminal Justice System in England and Wales. London: Home Office.

Cohen, L.E. and Felson, M. 1979 Social Change and Crime Rate Trends: A Routine Activity Approach. American Sociological Review 44: 588–608.

Coleman, K., Finney, A. and Kaiza, P. 2005 Violent Crime 71–89 in Crime in England and Wales 2004/2005, Home Office Statistical Bulletin (Nicholas, S., Povey, D., Walker, A. and Kershaw, C. Editors) London: Home Office.

Cornell, D.G., Warren, J., Hawk, G., Stafford, E., Oram, G. and Pine, D. 1996 Psychopathy in Instrumental and Reactive Violent Offenders. Journal of Consulting and Clinical Psychology 64: 783–790.

Crick, N.R. and Dodge, K.A. 1996 Social Information Processing Mechanism in Reactive and Proactive Aggression. Child Development 67: 993–1002.

Daly, K. and Bordt, R.R. 1995 Sex Effects and Sentencing: An Analysis of the Statistical Literature. Justice Quarterly 12: 141–176.

Elliott, D.S. and Menard, S. 1996 Delinquent Friends and Delinquent Behavior. Temporal and Developmental Patterns 28–67 in Delinquency and Crime: Current Theories (Hawkins, J.D. Editor) Cambridge: Cambridge University Press.

Ellis, L. and Walsh, A. 1999 Criminology: A Global Perspective. New York: Allyn and Bacon.

Eron, L.D., Huesmann, L.R. and Zelli, A. 1991 The Role of Parental Variables in the Learning of Aggression1 69–188 in The Development and Treatment of Childhood Aggression (Pepler D.J. and Rubin K.J. Editors) Hillsdale NJ: Lawrence Erlbaum.

Eysenck, H.J. 1996 Personality and Crime: Where Do We Stand? Psychology, Crime and Law 2: 143–152.

Farrington, D.P. 1986 Age and Crime 189–250 in Crime and Justice Vol 7 (Tonry, M. and Morris, N. Editors) Chicago: Chicago University Press.

Farrington, D.P. 1989 Self-reported and Official Offending from Adolescence to Adulthood 99–425 in Cross-National Research I Self-Reported Crime and Delinquency (Klein, M. Editor) Dordrecht: Kluwer.

Farrington, D.P. 1991 Childhood Aggression and Adult Violence: Early Precursors and Later Life Outcomes 5–29 in The Development and Treatment of Childhood Aggression (Pepler D.J. and Rubin K.H. Editors) Hillsdale NJ: Lawrence Erlbaum.

Farrington, D.P. 1995 The Development of Offending and Antisocial Behaviour from Childhood: Key Findings from the Cambridge Study of Delinquent Development. Journal of Child Psychology and Psychiatry 36: 929–964.

Farrington, D.P. 1997 Human Development and Criminal Careers 361–408 in The Oxford Handbook of Criminology 2nd Edition (Maguire, M., Morgan, R. and Reiner, R. Editors) Oxford: Clarendon Press.

Farrington, D.P. 1998 Predictors, Causes and Correlates of Male Youth Violence 421–475 in Youth Violence (Tonry M. and Moore M.H. Editors) Chicago: University of Chicago Press.

Farrington, D.P. 2001a The Causes and Prevention of Violence 57–95 in Violence in Health Care: Understanding, Preventing and Surviving Violence—A Practical Guide for Health Professionals (Shepherd, J. Editor) Oxford: Oxford University Press.

Farrington, D.P. 2001b What Has Been Learned from Self-reports about Criminal Careers and the Causes of Offending? London: Home Office Online Report www.Homeoffice.Gov.Uk/Rds/Pdfs/Farrington.Pdf

Farrington, D.P. 2001c Predicting Adult Official and Self-Reported Violence 66–88 in Clinical Assessment of Dangerousness: Empirical Contributions (Pinard, G-F. and Pagani, L. Editors) Cambridge: Cambridge University Press.

Farrington, D.P. and Jolliffe, D. 2004 England and Wales in Cross National Studies 1–38 in Crime and Justice (Farrington, D.P., Langan, P.A. and Tonry, M. Editors) Washington DC: Bureau of Justice Statistics.

Farrington, D.P. and Jolliffe, D. 2005 Crime and Justice in England and Wales, 1981–1999. Crime and Justice 33: 41–81.

Farrington, D.P., Jolliffe, D., Hawkins, J.D., Catalano, R.E., Hill, K.G. and Kosterman, R. 2003 Comparing Delinquency Careers in Court Records and Self-reports. Criminology 41: 933–958.

Farrington, D.P., Loeber, R. and Stouthamer-Loeber, M. 2003 How Can the Relationship between Race and Violence be Explained? 213–237 in Violent Crime: Assessing Race and Ethnic Differences (Hawkins, D.F. Editor) Cambridge: Cambridge University Press.

Farrington, D.P., Loeber, R., Yin, Y. and Anderson, S.J. 2002 Are Within-individual Causes of Delinquency the Same as between Individual Causes? Criminal Behaviour and Mental Health 12: 53–68.

Flannery, D.J. and Huff, C.R. (Editors) 1999 Youth Violence: Prevention, Intervention and Social Policy. Washington DC: American Psychiatric Press.

Flood-Page, C. Campbell, S. Harrington, V. and Miller, J. 2000 Youth Crime: Findings from the 1998/99 Youth Lifestyles Survey. Home Office Research Study 209 London: Home Office.

Gorman-Smith, D., Tolan, P.H., Zelli, A. and Huesmann, L.R. 1996 The Relation of Family Functioning to Violence among Inner-City Minority Youth. Journal of Family Psychology 10: 115–129.

Graham, J. and Bowling, B. 1995 Young People and Crime, Home Office Research Study 145 London: Home Office.

Henry, B., Caspi, A., Moffitt, T.E. and Silva, P.A. 1996 Temperamental and Familial Predictors of Violent and Non-violent Criminal Convictions: Age 3 to Age 18. Developmental Psychology 32: 614–623.

Hogh, E. and Wolf, P. 1983 Violent Crime in a Birth Cohort: Copenhagen 1953–1977 249–267 in Prospective Studies of Crime and Delinquency (Van Dusen, K.T. and Mednick, S.A. Editors) Boston: Kluwer.

Hollin, C.R. 1989 Psychology and Crime: An Introduction to Criminological Psychology. London: Routledge.

Home Office 2005 Criminal Statistics 2004 England and Wales. Home Office Statistical Bulletin. London: Home Office.

Jolliffe, D. and Farrington, D.P. 2004 Empathy and Offending: A Systematic Review and Meta-analysis. Aggression and Violent Behavior 9: 441–476.

Joliffe, D. and Farrington, D.P. 2006 The Development and Validation of the Basic Empathy Scale. Journal of Adolescence 29: 589–611.

Juby, H. and Farrington, D.P. 2001 Disentangling the Link between Disrupted Families and Delinquency. British Journal of Criminology 41: 22–40.

Kelley, M.L., Power, T.G. and Wimbush, D.D. 1992 Determinants of Disciplinary Practices in Low-income Black Mothers. Child Development 63: 573–582.

Lauritsen, J.L. and Sampson, R.J. 1998 Minorities, Crime and Criminal Justice 241–268 in The Handbook of Crime and Punishment (Tonry, M. Editor) New York: Oxford University Press.

Loeber, R. and Farrington, D.P. (Editors) 1998 Serious and Violent Juvenile Offenders: Risk Factors and Successful Interventions. Thousand Oaks CA: Sage.

Maccoby, E.E. and Jacklin, C.N. 1974 The Psychology of Sex Differences. Stanford: Stanford University Press.

Malinosky-Rummell, R. and Hansen, D.J. 1993 Long-term Consequences of Childhood Physical Abuse. Psychological Bulletin 114: 68–79.

Mccord, J. 1977 A Comparative Study of Two Generations of Native Americans 83–92 in Theory in Criminology: Contemporary Views (Meier, R.F. Editor) Beverly Hills CA: Sage.

Mccord, J. 1979 Some Child-rearing Antecedents of Criminal Behavior in Adult Men. Journal of Personality and Social Psychology 37: 1477–1486.

Mccord, J. 1996 Family as Crucible for Violence: Comment on Gorman-Smith et al. Journal of Family Psychology 10: 147–152.

Nicholas, S., Povey, D., Walker, A. and Kershaw, C. 2005 Introduction in 7–9 Crime in England and Wales 2004/2005 (Nicholas, S., Povey, D., Walker, A. and Kershaw, C. Editors) Home Office Statistical Bulletin. London: Home Office.

Office of National Statistics 2006 www.Statistics.Gov.Uk

Reiss, A.J. and Farrington, D.P. 1991 Advancing Knowledge of Co-offending: Results from a Prospective Longitudinal Survey of London Males. Journal of Criminal Law and Criminology 82: 360–395.

Thornberry, T.P., Huizinga, D. and Loebder, R. 1995 The Prevention of Serious Delinquency and Violence: Implications from the Program of Research on the Causes and Correlates of Delinquency 213–237 in Howell, J.C., Krisberg, B., Hawkins, J.D. and Wilson, J.J. Editors) Sourcebook on Serious, Violent and Chronic Juvenile Offenders, Thousand Oaks CA: Sage.

Wadsworth, M.E.J. 1978 Delinquency Prevention and Its Uses: The Experience of a 21-Year Follow-up Study. International Journal of Mental Health 7: 43–62.

Walby, S. and Allen, J. 2004 Domestic Violence, Sexual Assault and Stalking: Findings from the British Crime Survey. Home Office Research Study 276. London: Home Office.

Welsh, B.C. and Farrington, D.P. 2000 Monetary Costs and Benefits of Crime Prevention Programs 305–361 in Crime and Justice Vol 27 (Tonry, M. Editor) Chicago: University of Chicago Press.

West, D.J. and Farrington, D.P. 1973 Who Becomes Delinquent? London: Heinemann.

Widom, C.S. 1989 The Cycle of Violence. Science 244: 160–166.

Widom, C.S. and Ames, M.A. 1994 Criminal Consequences of Childhood Sexual Victimization. Child Abuse and Neglect 18: 303–318.

Wikstrom, P.O. 2002 Adolescent Crime in Context: A Study of Gender, Family Social Position, Individual Characteristics, Community Context, Life-Styles, Offending and Victimization. Home Office Research Study. London: Home Office.

Wikstrom, P-O., H. 1985 Everyday Violence in Contemporary Sweden. Stockholm: National Council For Crime Prevention.

Chapter 4

Psychiatric disorder: understanding violence

Tina Burke

Aim

To explain how psychiatric disorder contributes to an understanding of violence.

Learning objectives

- Outline and examine the various studies that link violence and mental disorder
- Consider evidence for and against the factors identified by research, to be associated with violence
- Explore processes for predicting and assessing risk

Introduction

In recent years, societal fears and the response of the government to the perceived dangerousness of individuals with mental illness have contributed to a change in the policy and practice of forensic mental health care. Risk assessment and management have been emphasized. Legislative guidelines and administrative documentation have been introduced, which imply that the priority of mental health services is to reduce risk (DOH 1999; SCMH 2001). The fulfilment of this responsibility in forensic services requires practitioners to predict and, moreover, prevent future violent behaviour, so that risk assessment is now widely assumed to be one of their core skills (Monahan 2001; NIMHE 2003).

This chapter examines the evidence that links violence and mental disorder. It also considers critically the processes for predicting and assessing risk.

The link between mental illness and violence – nature and extent of the evidence

Until comparatively recently there has been widespread rejection of the notion that a relationship exists between mental illness and violence, or indeed between crime in general and mental disorder (Gunn 1977). In a review of studies on patients discharged from psychiatric hospitals, Monahan and Steadman (1983: 211) found that there was no support for the premise that people with mental illness were more dangerous than the demographically matched general population. Similar findings have been reported elsewhere (Hafner and Boker 1992: 89).

However, more recent research, including prospective and longitudinal studies, supports the contention that there is a link between mental disorder and violence, albeit a modest one.

The nature of this research has been dominated by studies into the prevalence and connection between psychiatric disorders and violence, and it falls into four broad categories:

- Studies that have examined levels of violence prior to admission to psychiatric hospital, during hospitalization and post discharge
- Studies that examine the frequency of mental illness among those who have exhibited violent behaviour
- Community studies where the presence of mental illness and levels of violence are established separately and the relationship between the two analysed
- Birth cohort studies, where large random population samples are studied over time and the relationship between variables such as diagnosis and the likelihood of committing violence are analysed

The studies have yielded differing prevalence rates.

Violence before, during and after hospitalization

High rates of violent behaviour by people with mental illness have been reported prior to admission to hospital. These range from 12% 48 hours prior to admission (Rossi et al 1986), 19% in the month prior to admission (Johnston et al, 1986) and 26% in the 6 months previous to admission (Binder and McNiel 1988). A large number of studies into inpatient violence have been conducted, which have generally supported relatively high rates of violence among psychiatric inpatients. These range from 7% to 10% of patients involved in violent incidents in a 1- to 3-month observational period (Kay et al 1988), 10% to 40% from 3-month to 4-year observational periods, (Monahan 1992) and 59% over a 17-year observational period (Gudjonsson et al 1999).

Studies that have followed up individual hospitalized patients on discharge have also reported high rates of violence. For example, a review of the literature comparing the arrest rate of discharged patients with that of the general population (Link et al 1992) concluded that ex-psychiatric patients' arrest rates were 200% greater than the average for the general population. Similarly, Lindqvist and Allebeck (1990) reported that conviction rates for violent offences, over a 15-year period, by individuals who were discharged from hospital with a diagnosis of schizophrenia, were four times higher than the general population average. Similar findings have been reported in other studies (Belfrage 1998a).

However, a study by Steadman et al (1998) involving 1,136 patients in the United States, who were observed for a year post-discharge from hospital and followed up every 10 weeks, reported that prevalence rates (17.9%) of violence for people with a major mental disorder were indistinguishable from the matched neighbourhood sample. Similar findings from the McArthur Community Risk Study (Monahan et al 2001), have reported that the prevalence of violence among people discharged from psychiatric hospital, who do not have symptoms of substance abuse are similar to prevalence rates for violence among other people living in their community.

Mental illness and violence in prison

A number of studies have reported on prevalence of mental illness among prison detainees. For example, Singleton et al (1998) interviewed 3,142 male and female remanded and sentenced prisoners in 131 prisons in the United Kingdom. They identified high rates of functional psychosis among both categories of prisoner. In an earlier study, Taylor and Gunn (1984) reported that the incidence of schizophrenia in a random sample of 1,241 males remanded to Brixton prison was 6%, compared with the estimated rate in the South London population at that time of 0.5% (Wessely 1997). The prevalence of mental illness in populations of convicted violent offenders in prison has also been reported as 6%, more than three times that estimated in the general US population (Monahan 1992), and 11% of individuals convicted of violent crime in a British prison had schizophrenia (Taylor and Gunn 1984). Other studies have also reported a high incidence of mental disorder among individuals convicted of violent crime including homicide in Denmark (Gottlieb et al 1987) and Finland (Eronen et al 1996).

Community studies

The most convincing study of the existence of an association between mental disorder and violence is a community study conducted by Swanson et al (1990). This involved a retrospective analysis of data gathered from over 10,000 interviews, carried out, in three locations in the United States, as part of the Epidemiological Catchment Area Survey (ECAS). The Diagnostic Interview Schedule (DIS) was used to determine mental disorder according to the criteria of the Diagnostic and Statistical Manual of Mental Disorder (Third Edition; DSM-III, AMA 1980). After controlling for demographic factors such as age and socio-economic status, prevalence of violence was nearly four times higher for those suffering from an Axis I psychiatric diagnosis. However, there were significant effects resulting from co-morbidity, that is, the presence of more than one disorder. When categories were evaluated in the absence of co-morbidity, only schizophrenia and substance misuse were significantly elevated in comparison to the non-disordered community sample.

A more recent community study (Steadman et al 1998) of discharged patients has produced somewhat different results, suggesting that patients with a diagnosis of psychosis were no more dangerous than the 'non-patients' in their neighbourhood. However, the study confirmed Swanson et al's (1990) findings that substance abuse may be an independent risk factor for violence and that its effects were compounded by psychosis (to be discussed later). Therefore, scope remains for alternative interpretations of the literature (Pilgrim and Rogers 2003).

Birth cohort studies

A number of birth cohort studies support the contention that there is a link between mental illness and violence. Hodgins' (1992) report on a large Swedish study, using unselected 'birth cohorts', followed into adulthood, demonstrated that subjects who had been treated for mental disorders such as schizophrenia, psychosis and major affective disorder were 4.2 times more likely to have been convicted of a violent offence than non-disordered subjects. A similar study by Wessely et al (1994) in the United Kingdom found that compared with the general population, women with a major mental disorder had a relative risk of 8.66 times, and men 4.48 times, of committing a violent crime. A number of other studies have reported similar findings (Brennan et al 2000; Rasanen et al 1998).

Methodological issues

There are a number of methodological limitations in research studies investigating the relationship between violence and mental disorder. Among these are the failure of studies to take sufficient account of the criminalization of the mentally ill, the medicalization of deviance, and the confounding differences between comparison groups. (Blumenthal and Lavender 2000: 28).

Criminalization of the mentally ill is a particular problem in such studies because it means that people who are mentally ill are more likely to be arrested for the same offence than their non-mentally ill counterpart (Link and Stueve 1995; Teplin 1984). In contrast, the medicalization of deviance means that deviant behaviours, including violence, are becoming part of psychiatry, and so more violent people are becoming psychiatric patients (Melick et al 1979; Monahan 1973;

Box 4.1 Risk factors for future violence

- ◆ Demographic (age, gender, race and ethnicity, socio-economic status)
- ◆ Historical (previous violence, history of alcohol and drug use, early maladjustment)
- ◆ Clinical
- ◆ Situational factors

Steadman et al 1978). Therefore, studies relying on arrest and conviction rates among psychiatric patients may not represent a relationship between violence and mental disorder, but rather a 'psychiatrizing' of violence (Blumenthal and Lavender 2000: 29). In studies investigating prevalence of violence prior, during and after hospitalization, subjects tend to be those in high-risk groups, who may have been selected for hospitalization because of their high risk of violence. In this case, comparisons with the general population become questionable. Those studies relying on self-report data may be unreliable, owing to their possible provision of socially desirable responses. In addition, most of the studies rely on retrospective data, which does not address the issue of the temporal ordering of violence and mental disorder.

Risk factors for future violence

In the following section, a synoptic overview will be provided regarding the most important factors identified by researchers as predictors of violent behaviour. These can be divided into four categories (see Text Box 4.1).

Demographic factors

Age: Young age is generally associated with risk of violence in both the general and psychiatric population (Swanson et al 1990). A variety of studies have found that assaultative patients are predominately under 40 years of age (Beck et al 1991; Swanson et al 1990) and that the risk of violence diminishes with age (DeJong et al 1992; Klassen and O'Connor 1989). The younger the person is at the time of first violence, the greater the likelihood of recidivism (Harris et al 1991; Lattimore et al 1995).

Gender: General population figures suggest that men are more likely than women to behave violently, and in addition have much higher rates of convictions for violence (Home Office 2002). A variety of research studies have also reported that men are more frequently violent than women (Maxfield and Widom 1996; Monahan 1993). However, inconsistent findings have been reported on the relationship between gender and violence in the general population. For example, the MacArthur research project reported that gender did not play a significant role in the rate of violence (Monahan et al 2001; Steadman et al 1994). According to these researchers, the differences between men and women in the rates of violence were more related to the type of violence and the circumstances in which it occurred. Violent offences committed by men occurred most often in public, whereas women were more inclined to choose family members as targets, and consequently tended to act violently at home rather than in public (Gondolf et al 1991). An anticipated finding was that there is a greater likelihood of serious injury when violence was committed by men compared with women (Monahan 2003).

 The role of gender in prevalence of violence is also less clear in the case of psychiatric patients, with some studies reporting no relationship (James et al 1990), others reporting that women are equally or more frequently violent than men (Nicholls et al 2004; Rasmussen and Lavender 1996), and others suggesting that men are more violent than women (Lee et al 1989). In forensic facilities females tend to be more violent than males (Gudjonsson et al 1999; Larkin et al 1988; Rasmussen and Lavender 1996).

Race and ethnicity: Some studies suggest an increased risk of violence for non-white, discharged psychiatric patients (Klassen and O'Connor 1994; Noble and Rodger 1989). However, further analysis suggests that this association is largely attributable to the prior relationship between socio-economic status and ethnicity. For example, Steadman et al (1994) and Monahan et al (2001) found that the link between race and violent offences becomes insignificant when the crime rate in the offender's residential area is taken into account. It is thus not the population group to which an individual belongs that gives rise to violence but rather the environment in which that person lives.

Socio-economic status: A number of studies suggest that low socio-economic status is associated with increased risk of violence (Swanson et al 1990). Poverty, lack of education and low occupational status have been found to be robust predictors of violence (Monahan 1993; Stueve and Link 1997; Swartz et al 1998; Wessely et al 1994). Swanson et al (1990) suggested that people from lower socio-economic groups may be more inclined to handle conflict with violence than a person from a more affluent socio-economic background. This is attributed to poor socio-economic status giving rise to higher stress levels, compounded by the threatening and dangerous experiences of living in high-crime areas (Stueve and Link 1997).

Historical factors

Previous violence: This has generally been regarded as the most important predictor of future violence, regardless of the context or environment in which the violence occurs (Litwack 1994; Monahan et al 2001; Morrison 1994; Tiihonen and Hakola 1995; Swanson 1993). However, history is a crude predictor of violence. As Gunn (1993) pointed out, the prediction of risk based on previous history of violence correctly identifies 80% of future violence. However, as a predictive tool it has low specificity (35%), and thus two out of three individuals identified as being at risk would be incorrectly identified.

Therefore, it is important to differentiate between those individuals who are likely to be violent in the future from a population of individuals who already have a history of violence. Obviously, more information is required than a simple statement of whether an individual has been violent before, to predict whether they will be in the future. It is necessary to know about the nature of their violence, the type of victim and the contextual and environmental triggers (Doyle and Dolan 2002; Gunn 1993).

History of alcohol and drug abuse

There is general agreement among research studies that the abuse of, or dependency on, alcohol or drugs increases the possibility of violence significantly with the general population (Beck 1994; Hodgins et al 1996; Modestin et al 1996; Pihl and Petersin1993). These indicate that alcohol is implicated in 40% to 60% of assaults and homicides, 30% to 70% of rapes and 40% to 80% of domestic violence. Similarly for drug abuse, the risk of a user committing a violent crime, including homicide, has been reported to be between 10 and 55 times greater than that of the non-drug-abusing population (Steadman et al 1998; Wallace et al 1998).

Substance abuse and major mental disorder co-morbidity has been shown to increase the risk of violence more than substance abuse alone. For example, in the ECA study (Swanson et al 1990), substance abuse was found almost to double the lifetime prevalence of violence in individuals with mental disorder. Crucially, the study found a significant interaction between mental disorder and substance abuse. After controlling for socio-demographic covariates, the odds ratio for violence in a year for this population was 16.8. The importance of substance abuse for violence has also been demonstrated by Steadman et al (1998), who found that compared to non-substance abusing mentally disordered patients, patients with a co-occurring substance abuse disorder reported almost twice the rate of violence (17.9% compared with 31.1%). This was even higher for people with a substance abuse disorder and a diagnosis of personality disorder (43%). Similarly, Rasanen et al's (1998) birth-cohort study involving 11,017 persons in Finland concluded that men with mental disorder who abused alcohol were 25.2 times more likely to commit violent crimes than mentally healthy men, compared with only 3.6 times more for men with mental disorder who did not abuse alcohol. A variety of other studies have reported similar findings (Eronen et al 1996; Hodgins 1992; Wallace et al 1998).

However, other research has found only weak (Harris et al 1993) or no correlation between mental disorder, substance abuse and violence (Cuffel et al 1994; Estroff et al 1994). Other studies suggest that the link between violence and substance abuse is related to a specific diagnosis (i.e. schizophrenia) (Smith and Hucker 1994; Swanson et al 1990), or a combination of specific symptoms (i.e. threat/control/over-ride, TCO) with alcohol or drug disorder (Swanson et al 1997). In contrast, some studies argue that it is the combination of medication non-compliance, substance abuse and severe mental illness that is significantly associated with serious violence (Swartz et al 1998). Yet others have identified a combination of social factors such as low socio-economic status, a delinquent lifestyle and substance abuse to be related to violence among people with mental illness (Gottlieb and Gabreilsen 1992; Lindqvist and Allebeck 1990), suggesting that intoxication at the time of violence may not be relevant (Lindqvist and Allebeck 1990; Steadman et al 1998; Swartz et al 1998).

It appears that the interaction between social, psychological and biological variables in association with psychosis, substance abuse and violence is complex and obscure (Blumenthal and Lavender 2000: 52) and requires considerable research and theory development. It is suggested that risk assessment in relation to alcohol and drug use requires knowledge of the ways in which they relate to violence. For example, this may be due to intoxication or withdrawal or acquisition (Johns 1997) as well as personality, situational and social–cultural factors (Fagan 1990; Pihl and Paterson 1993).

Early maladjustment and violence

A variety of forms of maladjusted behaviour during early childhood years have been correlated with later violence in individuals with mental disorder. These include attention and concentration problems, repeated failure at school, truancy and expulsion from school (Harris et al 1993), early anti-social behaviour (e.g. chronic alcohol/substance abuse and aggressiveness) (Farrington 2001), impulsive, restless and reckless behaviour during adolescence, problems with peer group relationships and hostility towards authority (Melton et al 1997).

Aetiological factors that are associated with early maladjusted behaviour include sexual and physical abuse and neglect (Ferguson and Lynskey 1997; Weiler and Widom 1996; Widom 1989), separation from parents at an early age (younger than 16), parental rejection, low parental involvement, cruel and inconsistent parenting (Muetzell 1995), parental alcoholism (Moffitt 1987; Rydelius 1994; Virkkunen et al 1996) and violence within the family (Blomhoff et al 1990; Fitch and Papantonio 1983; Johnston 1988; Ryan 1989).

Although such factors may not directly cause violent actions, they may structure potential violence and determine triggers to later assaultative behaviour. As Glasser (1996: 273) pointed out, 'It is not psychological malfunctioning per se which causes a schizophrenic to carry out his homicidal act'. In other words, all incidents of violence have a meaning; they represent an attempt to avoid something worse. For example, an individual may kill another to preserve their sanity (Blumenthal and Lavender 2000: 80; Perelberg 1999). Therefore, a thorough risk assessment must pay attention to the meaning of violence to the perpetrator.

Clinical factors

This group of factors play a central role in the evaluation of the risk of violence, and they have been a main focus for research. These factors will be discussed based on psychiatric diagnosis and symptoms.

There has been a great deal of discussion concerning the extent to which mentally disordered offenders have specific risk factors that differentiate them from the general offender population. Bonta et al (1998) conducted a meta-analysis of studies predicting recidivism in mentally disordered offenders and found that broadly similar factors predicted re-offending in mentally disordered and non-mentally disordered offenders. A similar argument has been put forward by Lindqvist and Skipworth (2000), who suggested that predictors of recidivism are largely similar across different offender groups, irrespective of any contribution from mental illness.

However, divergent opinions continue to exist with regard to the role of psychiatric disorders in the occurrence of violence. On one hand, it is generally assumed that violence is significantly increased in people with serious psychiatric disorders (Douglas and Kropp 2002; Douglas and Webster 1999a). On the other hand, research has found that serious psychiatric disorders in themselves do not create an increased risk of violence (Steadman et al 1998), and that violence is lower in the case of serious psychiatric disorder than in the case of personality disorder (Monahan 2001; Steadman et al 1998). It is also lower in the case of schizophrenia compared with depressive and bipolar disorders (Gardner et al 1996; Monahan et al 2001; Quinsey et al 1998).

A diagnosis of anti-social personality disorder is generally regarded as a significant risk factor (Douglas and Webster 1999b; Harris et al 1993). Two meta-analyses of psychopathy indicated a moderate (Hemphill et al 1998) and strong connection (Salekin et al 1996) between violence and psychopathy. Serin and Amos (1995) suggested that the probability of the occurrence of violence is five times greater in the case of psychopathy than in the case of any other mental disorder, and that such people are considerably more likely than others to commit violent acts soon after discharge. Other personality disorders (e.g. paranoid, passive aggressive, borderline) are also associated with violence (Blackburn 2000), although the predictive value of borderline personality disorder is uncertain (Widiger and Trull 1994).

Personality traits other than personality disorder are also associated with violent behaviour (Douglas and Webster 1999b), for example, rage (Novaco 1994), a hostile disposition (Menzies and Webster 1995) and impulsiveness (Barratt 1994; Prentky et al 1995).

Although it is assumed that that there is a link between more serious psychiatric disorder and violent offences, active psychotic symptoms are regarded as being more important predictors of violence than diagnostic category (Monahan 2001: 88–89; Mulvey 1994), and there is some evidence to support the inclusion of the role of psychotic symptoms, for some patients. Particular psychotic symptoms, such as paranoia (Grossman et al 1995) and delusions involving personal targets (Nestor et al 1995), have been associated with violent behaviour. However, there are other studies that do not support such findings (Appelbaum et al 2000).

It has also been suggested that the experience involving loss of self-control (e.g. thought insertion) may lead to loss of constraint on behaviour. Link and Stueve (1994) reported that patients who felt threatened by others and were unable to control their own thoughts were twice as likely to have been violent as those who reported other psychotic symptoms. These have been labelled threat–control–override, or TCO, symptoms. Swanson et al (1997) reported that a combination of substance abuse and TCO symptoms very strongly predicted future violence, leading some to conclude that the real public health issue concerning mental disorder, violence and disturbed behaviour is actually substance abuse (Beck and Wencel 1998).

Command hallucinations are the other major type of symptoms to have been regarded as clinical risk factors. Rogers et al (1990) reported that 43% of forensic referrals with auditory hallucinations also experienced command hallucinations related to their offending. However, in their study of first-episode psychosis, Milton et al (2001) found little evidence to link specific psychotic symptoms with aggression. Some studies regard this relationship as relatively weak, and even uncertain (Douglas et al 2003), whereas some suggest that although command hallucinations in themselves do not increase risk of violence, they do increase risk when they refer to violent behaviour (Monahan et al 2001; Steadman et al 1998).

Situational factors

Situational factors refer to aspects of the environment or to the person–environmental interaction and are thought to be one of the most important factors in the prediction of violence (Monahan 1996). Adequate planning on discharge (Estroff and Zimmer 1994), the availability of supervision and support in the community (Estroff and Zimmer 1994), access to weapons, illicit drugs and victims (Gottleib and Gabrielsen 1992; Lindqvist and Allebeck 1990) and stress factors (e.g. disharmony in the family, breaking up of relationships, family loss, work-related problems) have all been identified as significant violent risk factors (Klassen and O-Connor 1994; Bonta et al 1998). A substantial risk of recidivism has been found to be present where a social support system is lacking (Bonta et al 1998). However, although security of a family may decrease the risk of violence, chronic conflict in a family can actually increase the risk (Estroff and Zimmer 1994).

Lindqvist and Skipworth (2000) suggested that family problems, poor socio-cultural circumstances and therapeutic system dynamics may be additional areas of specific risk in mentally disordered offenders. Clare et al (2000) have also emphasized the role of social and familial factors (such as abuse) in increasing the risk of violence in adolescents. Other risk factors may come from specific management strategies. For example, Swanson et al (2000) reported that outpatient commitment may reduce risk of violence in patients with severe mental illness, and Jamieson et al (2000) suggested that direct discharge into the community from special hospital settings in the United Kingdom may be correlated with increased reconviction rates.

The research suggests that mentally disordered offenders are likely to have a variety of dynamic risk factors, of which some may be implicated in their mental disorder, and others independent of it. These need not be directly associated with mental disorder, and might include attitudes and beliefs surrounding offending, poor anger control and association with criminal peers (Andrews and Bonta 1998).

Assessment of risk for violence

Risk assessment can be defined as the gathering of information and analysis of the potential outcomes of identified behaviour and the identification of specific risk factors relevant to an individual and the context in which they may have occurred. This process requires the linking of historical information to current circumstances to anticipate possible future change (Morgan 2000). This section explores the development of risk assessment approaches over the past decade.

Clinical judgement approach to risk prediction

Historically, the most widely used method of assessing risk of violence in practice is the unstructured, clinical–judgement approach. This approach is based exclusively on the professional expertise of the clinician, where there is complete discretion over which information should be considered, and there are no constraints on the information the assessor can use to reach a decision (Grove and Meehl 1996). However, this approach is plagued with bias and error (Grove and Meehl 1996), as information is highly dependent on interviewing, observation and self-report, and as such its predictive reliability and validity are questionable (Belfrage 1998b; Hart 1998; Monahan 2000; Quinsey et al 1998).

Actuarial approaches to risk prediction

Actuarial risk prediction (defined as the algorithmic, replicable combination of risk factors to arrive at a decision) (Douglas and Ogloff 2003) involves assessors reaching judgements based on statistical information, according to fixed, explicit rules (Doyle and Dolan 2002). A number of statistical instruments have been developed to predict the risk of violence. Among them are the scale for predicting violent recidivism in mentally disordered offenders, the Violence Risk Appraisal Guide, (VRAG; Quinsey et al 1998), the Iterative Classification Trees (Monahan et al 2000) and the Static-99 (Hanson and Thornton 1999). These instruments rely on identified potential predictor variables and possible predictive methods, formulae or techniques. They employ checklists of a number of predictors or factors that have been empirically demonstrated to be associated with violence, which are each allocated a score. The sum of the risk factors is an actuarial, graduated probability measure representing the amount of risk attributed to the individual. Hence decisions are made on specific assessments, which have been coded in a pre-determined manner (Hart 1998; Quinsey et al 1998).

Research suggests that actuarial methods are more accurate in predicting risk of violence than traditional clinical methods. In approximately half of the studies that directly compared actuarial methods with traditional clinical prediction, the former have proved to be more accurate in predicting risk of violence, with increased rates of 11% (Grove et al 2000; Grove and Meehl 1996; Mossman 1994).

However, a number of potential problems with the actuarial method have been highlighted. These include problems of generalizability, the potential inclusion or exclusion of case-specific risk factors, the focus on historical, unmodifiable fixed-risk factors that may lack relevance to treatment, and rigidity in decision-making rules (Douglas and Kropp 2002; Doyle and Dolan 2002; Dvoskin and Heilbrun 2001; Hart 1998; Litwack 2001; Melton et al 1997; Otto 2000). Poor methodology has also been employed in a number of studies that have supported actuarial tools' higher predictive validity (Douglas and Ogloff 2003) and this may limit utility.

Structured clinical approaches to risk prediction

The structured clinical judgement attempts to capture some of the strengths of both actuarial predication (e.g. reliability, relationship outcome, structured assessment procedures) and clinical judgement (e.g. flexibility and relevance to treatment) (Doyle and Dolan 2002) and at the same time minimize their respective weaknesses. This approach utilizes analytically or logically developed guides, intended to structure professional decisions about violence risk through encouraging consideration of key risk factors and the importance they may or may not possess. Clinicians are encouraged to arrive at their own determination of risk level (Douglas and Ogloff 2003). This approach has been reflected in the development of a number of tools, including the Historical Clinical Risk Management Tool (HCR-20; Webster et al 1997).

Research has reported that the omnibus, structured clinical risk rating is predictive of violence and adds incrementally to the predictive validity of the actuarial use of the structured clinical judgement instruments upon which it is based (Douglas and Ogloff 2003; Douglas and Webster 1999a).

However, most research into risk prediction tools are retrospective in design, with only a few prospective studies conducted into the predictive validity (Belfrage et al 2000; Douglas et al 1999). In addition, in most studies data are coded by researchers who through greater familiarity with the prerequisites for attaining good reliability are more likely to produce better results than clinicians, who may lack such knowledge (Philipse et al 2005) and undertake such assessments infrequently. In a study by De Vogel and De Ruiter (2004), clinician inter-rater reliability on risk items in a forensic inpatient setting was found to be substantially lower than that between researchers.

Ethical issues

The process of assessing risk brings with it a plethora of ethical challenges, including custody and accountability. It is expected that health professionals have a moral and legal obligation to predict risk accurately (Monahan 2000). However, to date, no method—clinical, actuarial or combined—has achieved anywhere near 100% predictive power, whether short- or long-term risk is considered. Thus, risk assessment has an inevitable level of error and uncertainty attached, even when the most sophisticated analyses are used (Mossman 1994; Strand et al 1999). The implications are that if a person is predicted to be non-violent and subsequently is violent (false negative), or a person is predicted to be violent and is subsequently not violent (false positive), inappropriate placement, staffing and restrictions could result. Carroll et al (2004) suggested that for forensic patients, the cut-off for decision-making is set so that sensitivity is high and that very few false negatives result. This has the inevitable consequence of low specificity, and therefore many false positives, and as a result patients are detained longer than necessary.

The sources of error and uncertainty in risk assessment warrant consideration. These can be divided into the 'foreseeable' and 'unforeseeable'. As Carroll et al (2004) pointed out, even the most comprehensive risk assessment will incorporate only a small fraction of the intrapersonal and situational factors that will affect patients' future behaviours. They therefore have inherent limitations. The likelihood, for example, of new stressful life events can be estimated, but their actual future occurrence is impossible to know; this is particularly so for events that are independent of the patient's illness. This source of uncertainty cannot be modified but must be acknowledged when estimating confidence limits to risk assessments (Maden 2006).

Knowable sources of uncertainty are theoretically remediable and stem both from the data on which judgements are based, and the inferences drawn from those data. In the present context, the accuracy of risk assessment is contingent on the quality of information used to evaluate risk (Carroll et al 2004; Douglas et al 2003; Doyle and Dolan 2002). Its relevance to the prediction of serious incidents, for example, homicide, has also been questioned (Munro and Rumgay 2000). In practice, uncertainty in risk assessment may be reduced by a service philosophy in which a common and empirically validated language of risk is employed (Maden 2006). This requires the use or development of a practical risk-assessment framework for multi-disciplinary use (see Text Box 4.2; De Vogel and De Ruiter 2004; Doyle and Dolan 2002; Maden 2006).

Box 4.2 Risk: Key considerations

◆ Risk cannot be eliminated. However, it can be reduced through sound clinical approaches that are, as far as possible, multi-disciplinary/multi-agency

◆ Clinicians need to be aware of the benefits and limitations of current risk-assessment strategies in predicting risk

◆ Risk is dynamic, and each case needs to be treated separately with regard to its own particular aspects, including its psychological factors

◆ Unrealistic expectations regarding risk prevention, perpetuated by media misrepresentation, public perceptions and legislative bureaucracy, need to be challenged by mental health practitioners

◆ Continuous effort in research is needed to improve the accuracy of risk-assessment procedures in clinical practice

Conclusion

This chapter has examined the links between violence and mental disorder. These links have been something of a holy grail in the last 20 years for a significant number of researchers. The evidence base has changed and improved, but it still leaves open a number of important questions. These are less to do with the epidemiology of risk and more to do with the application of this hard-won knowledge in clinical practice. The imperative to use this knowledge well comes in no small part from a changing political climate and a risk-averse political system. It remains important to emphasize the continuing uncertainty of violence-risk prediction.

References

American Psychiatric Association 1980 Diagnostic and Statistical Manual of Mental Disorders 3rd Edition. Washington, DC: American Psychiatric Association.

Andrews, D. and Bonta, J. 1998 The Psychology of Criminal Conduct 2nd Edition. Cincinnati OH: Anderson.

Appelbaum, P., Robbins, P. and Monahan, J. 2000 Violence and Delusions: Data from the McArthur Violence Risk Assessment Study. American Journal of Psychiatry 157: 566–572.

Barratt, E. 1994 Impulsiveness and aggression 61–79 in Violence and Mental Disorder: Developments in Risk Assessment (Monahan, J. and Steadman, H. J. Editors) Chicago: Chicago University Press.

Beck, J. 1994 Epidemiology of Mental Disorder and Violence: Beliefs and Research Findings. Harvard Review of Psychiatry 2: 1–6.

Beck, J. and Wencel, H. 1998 Violent Crimes and Axis I Psychopathology 1–27 in Psychopathology and Violent Crime (Skodol, A. Editor) Washington, DC: American Psychiatric Association.

Beck, J. White, K. and Gage, B. 1991 Emergency Psychiatric Assessment of Violence. American Journal of Psychiatry 148: 1562–1565.

Befrage, H. 1998a A Ten Year Follow-up of Criminality in Stockholm Mental Patients: New Evidence for a Relationship between Mental Disorder and Crime. British Journal of Criminology 38: 145– 157.

Belfrage, H. 1998b Making Risk Predictions without an Instrument. The Three Years Experience of the New Swedish Law on Mentally Disordered Offenders. International Journal of Law and Psychiatry 21: 59–64.

Belfrage, H., Fransson, G. and Strand, S. 2000 Prediction of Violence Using the HCR-20: A Prospective Study in Two Maximum Security Correctional Institutions. The Journal of Forensic Psychiatry 11: 167–175.

Binder, R. and McNiel, D. 1988 Effects of Diagnosis and Context on Dangerousness. American Journal of Psychiatry 145: 728–732.

Blackburn, R. 2000 Psychopathy and Personality Disorder in Relation to Violence 195–220 in Clinical Approaches to Violence 2nd Edition (Hollin, C.R. Editor) Chichester: Wiley.

Blomhoff, S., Seim, S. and Friis, S. 1990 Can Prediction of Violence among Psychiatric Inpatients be Improved? Hospital and Community Psychiatry 41: 771–775.

Blumenthal, S., and Lavender, T. 2000 Violence and Mental Disorder: A Critical Aid to the Assessment and Management of Risk. Hereford: Zito Trust.

Bonta, J., Law, M. and Hanson, K. 1998 The Prediction of Criminal and Violence Recidivism among Mentally Disordered Offenders. A Meta-analysis. Psychological Bulletin 123: 123–142.

Brennan, P., Mednick, S. and Hodgins, S. 2000 Major Mental Disorders and Criminal Violence in a Danish Birth Cohort. Archives of General Psychiatry 57: 494–500.

Carroll, A., Lyall, M. and Forrester, A. 2004 Clinical Hopes and Public Fears in Forensic Mental Health. The Journal of Forensic Psychiatry & Psychology 15: 407–425.

Clare, P., Bailey, S. and Clark, A. 2000 Relationship between Psychotic Disorders in Adolescence and Criminally Violent Behaviour. British Journal of Psychiatry 177: 275–279.

Cuffel, B., Shumway, B., Tandy, L. et al 1994 A Longitudinal Study of Substance Use and Community Violence in Schizophrenia. The Journal of Nervous and Mental Disease 812: 704–708.

DeJong, J., Virkkunen, M. and Linnoila, M. 1992 Factors Associated with Recidivism in a Criminal Population. Journal of Nervous and Mental Disease 180: 543–550.

Department of Health 1999 A National Service Framework for Mental Health. London: The Stationary Office.

DeVogel, V. and DeRuiter, C. 2004 Differences between Clinicians and Researchers in Assessing Risk of Violence in Forensic Psychiatric Patients. The Journal of Forensic Psychiatry & Psychology 15: 145–164.

Douglas, K., Cox, D. and Webster, C. 1999 Violence Risk Assessment: Science and Practice. Legal and Criminological Psychology 4: 149–184.

Douglas, K. and Kropp, P. 2002 A Prevention-based Paradigm for Violence Risk Assessment: Clinical and Research Applications. Criminal Justice and Behaviour 29: 617–658.

Douglas, K. and Ogloff, J. 2003 Multiple Facets of Risk for Violence: The Impact of Judgemental Specificity on Structured decisions about Violence Risk. International Journal of Forensic Mental Health 2: 19–34.

Douglas, K., Ogloff, J. and Hart, S. 2003 Evaluation of a Model of Violence Risk Assessment among Forensic Psychiatric Patients. Psychiatric Services 54: 1372–1379.

Douglas, K. and Webster, C. 1999a The HCR-20 Violence Risk Assessment Scheme: Concurrent Validity in a Sample of Incarcerated Offenders. Criminal Justice and Behaviour, 26: 3–19.

Douglas, K. and Webster, C. 1999b Predicting Violence in Mentally and Personality Disordered Individuals 175–239 in Psychology and Law: The State of the Discipline (Roesch, R., Hart S.D. and Ogloff J.R.P. Editors) Plenum: New York.

Doyle, M. and Dolan, M. 2002 Violence Risk Assessment: Combining Actuarial and Clinical Information to Structure Clinical Judgements for the Formulation and Management of Risk. Journal of Psychiatric and Mental Health Nursing 9: 649–657.

Dvoskin, J. and Heilbrun, K. 2001 Risk Assessment and Release Decision-making: Towards Resolving the Great Debate. Journal of the American Academy of Psychiatry and the Law 29: 6–10.

Eronen, M., Hakola, P. and Tiihonen, J. 1996 Mental Disorders and Homicidal Behaviour in Finland. Archives of General Psychiatry 53: 497–501.

Estroff, S. and Zimmer, C. 1994 Social Networks, Social Support, and Violence among Persons with Severe, Persistent Mental Illness 259–95 in, Violence and Mental Disorder: Developments in Risk Assessment (Monahan, J. and Steadman, H. J. Editors) Chicago: Chicago University Press.

Estroff, S., Zimmer, C., Lachicotte, W. and Benoit, J. 1994 The Influence of Social Networks and Social Support on Violence by Persons with Serious Mental Illness. Hospital and Community Psychiatry 45: 669–679.

Fagan, J. 1990 Intoxication and Aggression 241–314 in Crime and Justice: A Review of Research Vol 13 Drugs and Crime (Tonry, M. and Wilson, J.Q. Editors) Chicago: Chicago University Press.

Farrington, D. 2001 Predicting Adult Official and Self-reported Violence 66–87 in Clinical Assessment of Dangerousness—Empirical Contributions (Pinard, G.F. and Pagani, L. Editors) Cambridge: Cambridge University Press.

Ferguson, D. and Lynskey, M. 1997 Physical Punishment/Maltreatment during Childhood and Adjustment in Young Adulthood. Child Abuse and Neglect 21: 617–630.

Fitch, F. and Papantonio, A. 1983 Men Who Batter: Some Pertinent Characteristics. Journal of Nervous and Mental Disease 171: 190–192.

Gardner, W., Lidz, S., Mulvey, E. et al 1996 A Comparison of Actuarial Methods for Identifying Repetitively Violent Patients with Mental Illness. Law and Human Behaviour 20: 35–38.

Glasser, M. 1996 The Assessment and Management of Dangerousness: The Psychological Contribution. Journal of Forensic Psychiatry 7: 271–283.

Gondolf, E., Mulvey, E. and Lidz, C. 1991 Psychiatric Admission of Family Violent versus Non-family Violent Patients. International Journal of Law and Psychiatry 14: 245–254.

Gottleib, P., Gabrielsen, G. and Kramp, P. 1987 Psychotic Homicide in Copenhagen from 1959 to 1983. Acta Psychiatrica Scandanavia 76: 285–292.

Gottleib, P. and Gabrielsen, G. 1992 Alcohol Intoxicated Homicides in Copenhagen, 1959–83. International Journal of Law and Psychiatry 15: 77–87.

Grossman, L. Haywood, T. Cavanaugh, J. et al 1995 State Hospital Patients with Past Arrests for Violent Crime. Psychiatric Services 46: 790–795.

Grove, W. and Meehl, P. 1996 Comparative Efficiency of Informal Subjective, Impressionistic and Formal Mechanical, Algorithmic Prediction Procedures: The Clinical-Statistical Controversy. Psychology, Public Policy and Law 2: 293–434.

Grove, W., Zald, D., Lebow, B. et al 2000 Clinical versus Mechanical Prediction: A Meta-analysis. Psychological Assessment 12: 19–30.

Gudjonsson, G., Rabe-Hesketh, S. and Wilson, C. 1999 Violent Incidents on a Medium Secure Unit over a 17 Year Period. Journal of Forensic Psychiatry 10: 249–263.

Gunn, J. 1977 Criminal Behaviour and Mental Disorder. British Journal of Psychiatry 130: 317–329.

Gunn, J. 1993 Dangerousness in Forensic Psychiatry. Criminal, Legal and Ethical Issues 624–645 (Gunn, J. and Taylor, P.J. Editors) Oxford: Butterworth-Heinemann.

Hafner, H. and Boker, W. 1992 Crimes of Violence by Mentally Abnormal Offenders. Cambridge: Cambridge University Press.

Hanson, R. and Thornton, D. 1999 Static 99: Improving Actuarial Risk Assessments for Sex Offenders. User Report 1999–2002. Department of the Solicitor General of Canada, Ottawa.

Harris, G., Rice, M. and Cormier, C. 1991 Psychopathy and Violent Recidivism. Law and Human Behaviour 15: 625–637.

Harris, G., Rice, M. and Quinsey, V. 1993 Violent Recidivism of Mentally Disordered Offenders: The Development of Statistical Prediction Instrument. Criminal Justice and Behaviour 20: 315–335.

Hart, S. 1998 The Role of Psychopathy in Assessing Risk for Violence: Conceptual and Methodological Issues. Legal and Criminological Psychology 3: 121–137.

Hemphill, J., Hare, R. and Wong, S. 1998 Psychopathy and Recidivism: A Review. Legal and Criminological Psychology 3: 139–170.

Hodgins, S. 1992 Mental Disorder, Intellectual Deficiency and Crime. Evidence from a Birth Cohort. Archives of General Psychiatry 49: 476–483.

Hodgins, S. Mednick, S.A., Brennan, P.A., Schulsinger, F. and Engberg, M. 1996 Mental Disorder and Crime: Evidence from a Danish Birth Cohort. Archives of General Psychiatry 53: 489–496.

Home Office 2002 Criminal Statistics England and Wales 2000. London: HMSO.

James, D., Fineberg, N. and Shah, A. 1990 An Increase in Violence on an Acute Psychiatric Ward. British Journal of Psychiatry 156: 846–852.

Jamieson, E. Davison, S. and Taylor, P. 2000 Reconviction of Special High Security Hospital Patients with Personality Disorder: Its Relationship with Route of Discharge and Time at Risk. Criminal Behaviour and Mental Health 10: 88–99.

Johns, A. 1997 Substance Misuse: A Primary Risk and Major Problem of Co-morbidity. International Review of Psychiatry 9: 2–3.

Johnston, E. Crow, T. Johnston, A. et al 1986 The Northwick Park Study of First Episodes of Schizophrenia 1. Presentations of the Illness and Problems Relating to Admission. British Journal of Psychiatry 149: 51–56.

Johnston, M. 1988 Correlates of Early Violence Experience among Men Who Are Abusive toward Female Mates 192–202 in Family Abuse and Its Consequences: New Directions in Research (Hotaling, G.T. and Finkelhor, D. Editors) Newbury Park, CA: Sage.

Kay, S., Wolkenfeld, F. and Murrill, L. 1988 Profiles of Aggression among Psychiatric Patients: Nature and Prevalence. Journal of Nervous and Mental Disease 176: 539–446.

Klassen, D. and O'Connor, W. 1989 Assessing the Risk of Violence in Released Mental Patients: A Cross Validation Study. Psychological Assessment 1: 75–81.

Klassen, D. and O'Connor, W. 1994 Demographic and Case History Variables in Risk Assessment 229–257 in Violence and Mental Disorder. Developments in Risk Assessment. The John D. and Catherine T. MacArthur Foundation Series on Mental Health and Development (Monahan, J. and Steadman, H.J. Editors) Chicago: Chicago University Press.

Larkin, E., Murtagh, S. and Jones, S. 1988 A Preliminary Study of Violent Incidents in a Special Hospital (Rampton). British Journal of Psychiatry 153: 226–231.

Lattimore, P., Visher, C. and Linster, R. 1995 Predicting Re-arrest for Violence among Serious Youthful Offenders. Journal of Research in Crime and Delinquency 32: 54–83.

Lee, S. Villar, O., Juthani, N. et al 1989 Characteristics and Behaviour of Patients Involved in Psychiatric Ward Incidents. Hospital and Community Psychiatry 40: 1295–1296.

Lindqvist, P. and Allebeck, P. 1990 Schizophrenia and Crime: A Longitudinal Follow Up of 644 Schizophrenics in Stockholm. British Journal of Psychiatry 157: 345–350.

Lindqvist, P. and Skipworth, J. 2000 Evidence Based Rehabilitation in Forensic Psychiatry. The British Journal of Psychiatry 176: 320–323.

Link, B., Andrews, H. and Cullen, F. 1992 The Violent and Illegal Behaviour of Mental Patients Reconsidered. American Sociological Review 57: 275–292.

Link, B. and Stueve, A. 1994 Psychotic Symptoms and the Violent/Illegal Behaviour of Mental Patients Compared to Community Controls 137–160 in Violence and Mental Disorder: Developments in Risk Assessment (Monahan, J. and Steadman, H.J. Editors) Chicago: Chicago University Press.

Link, B. and Stueve, A. 1995 Evidence Bearing on Mental Illness as a Possible Cause of Violent Behaviour. Epidemiologic Reviews 17: 172–181.

Litwack, T. 1994 Assessments of Dangerousness: Legal Research and Clinical Developments. Administration and Policy in Mental health 21: 361–377.

Litwack, T. 2001 Actuarial versus Clinical Assessments of Dangerousness. Psychology, Public Policy, and Law 7: 409–443.

Maden, T. 2006 Review of Homicides by Patients with Severe Mental Illness. London: Imperial College.

Maxfield, M. and Widom, C. 1996 The Cycle of Violence Revisited Six Years Later. Archives of Paediatrics and Adolescent Medicine 150: 390–395.

Melick, M., Steadman, H. and Cocozza, J. 1979 The Medicalisation of Criminal Behaviour among Mental Patients. Journal of Health and Social Behaviour 20: 228–237.

Melton, G., Petrila, J., Poythress, N. et al 1997 Psychological Evaluations for the Courts: A Handbook for Mental Health Professionals and Lawyers 2nd Edition. New York: Guildford.

Menzies, R. and Webster, C. 1995 Construction and Validation of Risk Assessment in a Six Year Follow-up of Forensic Patients: A Tri-dimensional Analysis. Journal of Consulting and Clinical Psychology 63: 766–778.

Milton, J., Amin, S., Singh, S. et al 2001 Aggressive Incidents in First Episode Psychosis. British Journal of Psychiatry 178: 433–440.

Modestin, J., Berger, A. and Ammann, R. 1996 Mental Disorder and Criminality. Male Alcoholism. Journal of Nervous and Mental Disorder 184: 393–402.

Moffitt, T. 1987 Parental Mental Disorder and Offspring Criminal Behaviour: An Adoption Study. Psychiatry: Interpersonal and Biological Processes 50: 346–360.

Monahan, J. 1973 The Psychiatrization of Criminal Behaviour: A Reply. Hospital and Community Psychiatry 24: 105–107.

Monahan, J. 1992 Mental Disorder and Violent Behaviour: Perceptions and Evidence. American Psychologist 47: 511–521.

Monahan, J. 1993 Mental Disorder and Violence: Another Look 287–302 in Mental Disorder and Crime (Hodgins, S. Editor) Newbury Park, CA: Sage.

Monahan, J. 1996 Violence Prediction. Criminal Justice and Behaviour 23: 107–120.

Monahan, J. 2000 Clinical and Actuarial Predictions of Violence 300–318 in Modern Scientific Evidence: The Law and Science of Expert Testimony Vol 1 (Faigman, D., Kaye, D., Saks, M. and Sanders, J. Editors) St Paul MN: West Publishing Company.

Monahan, J. 2001 Major Mental Disorder and Violence: Epidemiology and Risk Assessment 89–99 in Clinical Assessment of Dangerousness—Empirical Contributions (Pinard, G.F. and Pagani, L. Editors) Cambridge: Cambridge University Press.

Monahan, J. 2003 Violence Risk Assessment 527–540 in Hand-book of Psychology Vol 11 (Goldstein, A. Editor) New York: Wiley.

Monahan, J. and Steadman, H. 1983 Crime and Mental Disorder: An Epidemiological Approach 145–189 in Crime and Justice: An Annual Review of Research Vol 4 (Tonry, M. and Morris, N. Editors) Chicago: Chicago University Press.

Monahan, J., Steadman, H., Appelbaum, P. et al 2000 Developing a Clinically Useful Actuarial Tool for Assessing Violence. British Journal of Psychiatry 176: 312–319.

Monahan, J, Steadman, H.J, Silver, E. et al 2001 Rethinking Risk Assessment. The MacArthur Study of Mental Disorder and Violence. Oxford: Oxford University Press.

Morgan, S. 2000 Clinical Risk Management: A Clinical Tool and Practitioner Manual. London: Sainsbury Centre for Mental Health.

Morrison, E. 1994 The Evolution of a Concept: Aggression and Violence in Psychiatric Settings. Archives of Psychiatric Nursing 8: 245–253.

Mossman, D. 1994 Assessing Predictions of Violence: Being Accurate about Accuracy. Journal of Consulting and Clinical Psychology 62: 783–792.

Muetzell, S. 1995 Human Violence in Stockholm County, Sweden. International Journal of Adolescence and Youth 6: 75–88.

Mulvey, E. 1994 Assessing the Evidence of a Link between Mental Illness and Violence. Hospital and Community Psychiatry 45: 663–668.

Munro, E and Rumgay, J. 2000 Role of Risk Assessment in Reducing Homicides by People with Mental Illness. British Journal of Psychiatry 176: 116–120.

National Institute for Mental Health in England 2003 Mental Health Policy Implementation Guide. Developing Positive Practice to Support the Safe and Therapeutic Management of Aggression and Violence in Mental Health In-patient Settings. Worcestershire: NIMHE.

Nestor, P., Haycock, J., Doiron, S. et al 1995 Lethal Violence and Psychosis. Bulletin of the American Academy of Psychiatry and Law 23: 331–341.

Nicholls, T., Ogloff, J. and Douglas, L. 2004 Assessing Risk for Violence among Male and Female Civil Psychiatric Patients: The HCR-20, PCL:SV and McNiel & Binder's Screening Measure. Behavioural Sciences and the Law 22: 127–158.

Noble, P. and Rodger, S. 1989 Violence by Psychiatric Inpatients. British Journal of Psychiatry 155: 384–390.

Novaco, R. 1994 Anger as a Risk Factor for Violence among the Mentally Disordered 21–59 in Violence and Mental Disorder: Developments in Risk Assessment (Monahan, J. and Steadman, H.J. Editors) Chicago: Chicago University Press.

Otto, R. 2000 Assessing and Managing Violence Risk in Outpatient Settings. Journal of Clinical Psychology 56: 1239–1262.

Perelberg, R. 1999 Psychoanalytic Understanding of Violence and Suicide. London: Routledge.

Philipse, M., Koeter, M., Staak, C. et al 2005 Reliability and Discriminant Validity of Dynamic Re-offending Risk Indicators in Forensic Clinical Practice. Criminal Justice and Behaviour 32: 643–664.

Pihl, R. and Peterson, J. 1993 Alcohol/Drug Use and Aggressive Behaviour 263–285 in Mental Disorder and Crime (Hodgins, S. Editor) Newbury Park, CA: Sage.

Pilgrim, D. and Rogers, A. 2003 Mental Disorder and Violence: An Empirical Picture in Context. Journal of Mental Health 12: 7–18.

Prentky, R., Knight, R., Lee, A. et al 1995 Predictive Validity of Lifestyle Impulsivity for Rapists. Criminal Justice and Behaviour 22: 106–128.

Quinsey, V., Harris, G., Rice, M. et al 1998 Violent Offenders: Appraising and Managing Risk. Washington DC: American Psychological Association.

Rasanen, P., Tiihonen, J., Isohanni, M. et al 1998 Schizophrenia, Alcohol Abuse and Violent Behaviour: A 26-Year Follow-up Study. Schizophrenia Bulletin 24: 437–441.

Rasmussen, K. and Levander, S. 1996 Crime and Violence among Psychiatric Patients in a Maximum, Security Psychiatric Hospital. Criminal Justice and Behaviour 23: 455–471.

Rogers, R., Gillis, J., Turner, R. et al 1990 The Clinical Presentation of Command Hallucinations in a Forensic Population. American Journal of Psychiatry 147: 1304–1307.

Rossi, A., Jacobs, M., Monteleone, M. et al 1986 Characteristics of Psychiatric Patients Who Engage in Assaultative Behaviour or Other Fear Inducing Behaviours. Journal of Nervous and Mental Disease 174: 154–160.

Ryan, G. 1989 Victim to Victimiser. Journal of Interpersonal Violence 4: 325–341.

Rydelius, P. 1994 Children of Alcoholic Parents: At Risk to Experience Violence and to Develop Violent Behaviour 72–90 in Children and Violence. The Child in the Family: The Monograph Series of International Association for Child and Adolescent Psychiatry and Allied Professions, Vol 11 (Chiland, C. and Young, J.G. Editors) Northvale, NJ: Jason Aronson.

Sainsbury Centre for Mental Health 2001 The National Service Framework for Mental Health: An Executive Briefing. Briefing 8, London: Sainsbury Centre for Mental Health SCMH.

Salekin, R., Roger, R. and Sewell, K. 1996 A Review and Meta-analysis of the Psychopathy Checklist and Psychopathy Checklist–Revised: Predictive Validity and Dangerousness. Clinical Psychology: Science and Practice 3: 203–215.

Serin, R. and Amos, N. 1995 The Role of Psychopathy in the Assessment of Dangerousness. International Journal of Law and Psychiatry 18: 231–238.

Singleton, N., Meltzer, H., Gatward, R. et al 1998 Psychiatric Morbidity among Prisoners. London: Stationary Office.

Smith, J. and Hucker, S. 1994 Schizophrenia and Substance Abuse. British Journal of Psychiatry 165: 13–21.

Steadman, H., Cocozza, J. and Melick, M. 1978 Explaining the Increased Arrest Rate among Mental Patients: The Changing Clientele of State Hospitals. American Journal of Psychiatry 135: 816–820.

Steadman, H., Monahan, J., Applebaum, P. et al 1994 Designing a New Generation of Risk Assessment Research 101–136 in Violence and Mental Disorder: Developments in Risk Assessment (Monahan, J. and Steadman, H.J. Editors) Chicago: Chicago University Press.

Steadman, H., Mulvey, E. Monahan, J. et al 1998 Violence by People Discharged from Acute Psychiatric Inpatient Facilities and by Others in the Same Neighbourhoods. Archives of General Psychiatry 55: 1–9.

Strand, S., Belfrage, H., Fransson, G., Levander, S. 1999 Clinical and Risk Management Factors in Risk Prediction of Mentally Disordered Offenders—More Important than Historical Data? Legal and Criminological Psychology 4: 67–76.

Stueve, A. and Link, B. 1997 Violence and Psychiatric Disorders: Results from an Epidemiological Study of Young Adults in Israel. Psychiatric Quarterly 68: 327–342.

Swanson, J. 1993 Alcohol Abuse, Mental Disorder, and Violent Behaviour: An Epidemiologic Inquiry. Alcohol Health and Research World 17: 123–132.

Swanson, J., Estroff, D., Swartz, M. et al 1997 Violence and Severe Mental Disorder in Clinical and Community Populations: The Effects of Psychotic Symptoms, Co-morbidity, and Lack of Treatment. Psychiatry: Interpersonal and Biological Processes 60: 1–22.

Swanson, J., Holzer, C., Gunju, V., Jono, R. 1990 Violence and Psychiatric Disorder in the Community: Evidence from the Epidemiological Catchment Area Surveys. Hospital and Community Psychiatry 41: 761–770.

Swanson, J.W., Swartz, M.S., Borum, R., Hiday, V., Wagner, R. and Burns, B. 2000 Involuntary Out-patient Commitment and Reduction of Violent Behaviour in Persons with Severe Mental Illness. British Journal of Psychiatry 176: 324–331.

Swartz, M., Swanson, J., Hiday, V. et al 1998 Violence and Severe Mental Illness: The Effects of Substance Abuse and Non-adherence to Medication. American Journal of Psychiatry 155: 2, 226–231.

Taylor, P. and Gunn, J. 1984 Violence and Psychosis. I. Risk of Violence among Psychotic Men. British Medical Journal 288: 1945–148.

Teplin, L. 1984 Criminalizing Mental Disorder: Comparative Arrest Rate of the Mentally Ill. American Psychologist 39: 794–803.

Tiihonen, J. and Hakola, P. 1995 Homicide and Mental Disorders. Psychiatria Fennica 26: 125–129.

Virkkunen, M., Eggert, M., Rawlings, R. et al 1996 A Prospective Follow-up Study of Alcoholic Violent Offenders and Fire Setters. Archives of General Psychiatry 53: 523 –529.

Wallace, C., Mullen, P., Burgess, P. et al 1998 Serious Criminal Offending and Mental Disorder. British Journal of Psychiatry 172: 477–484.

Webster, C., Douglas, K., Eaves, D. et al 1997 HCR-20: Assessing Risk of Violence to Others version 2. Burnaby, BC: Mental Health Law and Policy Unit, Simon Fraser University.

Weiler, B. and Widom, C. 1996 Psychopathy and Violent Behaviour in Abused and Neglected Young Adults. Criminal Behaviour and Mental Health 6: 253–271.

Wessely, S., Castle, C. and Douglas, A. 1994 The Criminal Careers of Incident Cases of Schizophrenia. Psychological Medicine 24: 483–502.

Wessely, S. 1997 The Epidemiology of Crime, Violence and Schizophrenia. British Journal of Psychiatry 170 suppl. 32: 8–11.

Widiger, T. and Trull, T. 1994 Personality Disorders and Violence 203–226 in Violence and Mental Disorder: Developments in Risk Assessment (Monahan, J. and Steadman, H.J. Editors) Chicago: Chicago University Press.

Widom, C. 1989 Does Violence Beget Violence? A Critical Examination of the Literature. Psychological Bulletin 106: 3–28.

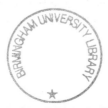

Chapter 5

Gender, crime and violence

Annie Bartlett

Aim

To examine the relationship between gender, crime and violence.

Learning objectives

- To consider concepts of gender
- To describe and analyse patterns of male and female offending
- To critique how the criminal justice system and health and social care incorporate an understanding of the distinctive nature of male and female offending into the systems that manage women's crime and violence

---

Introduction

This chapter first looks at concepts of gender. This can seem a strange starting place, but different understandings of gender challenge what seem to be the self-evident meaning of terms such as men and women, male and female, masculine and feminine. It is important to consider how we arrive at the 'taken for granted' understandings of these words. The purpose of doing it is to be able to think about the relationship of these particular understandings of gender to the bald statistics on men's and women's involvement in crime and violence. The third part of this chapter will look at the different understandings that have been invoked in the last 100 years to explain the startling differences in male and female crime and violence. This will then lead on to a discussion of how these ideas do or do not inform the design of systems to manage women's criminality and dangerousness; systems that have only recently benefited from a gender analysis.

Gender

Gender studies have become fashionable over the last 20 years. Although such studies cover a wide range of academic disciplines, and embrace anthropology, sociology, criminology and economics, to say nothing of physiology and medicine, they share a core interest in the extent to which the categories of male and female are understood in the same way. This in turn covers a range of questions, including the extent to which men and women are different or the same and, if so, in what ways and in what areas of life. The ways in which difference and similarity have been framed include an investigation of the genetics of masculinity and femininity and the physiology of men and women, the extent to which patterns of male and female behaviour are socially learnt or the simple consequence of environmental influences constraining or determining how people live.

As Kessler and McKenna (1978: vii) suggested, 'For the most part, classifying people as women or men is a deceptively easy procedure. For this reason, all theoretical and empirical work in the area of gender has taken this process for granted'. Time has overtaken Kessler and McKenna's work in the sense that there is now a large body of material considering in great detail the extent to which men and women are the same cross-culturally, the extent to which concepts of masculinity and femininity owe their origins to innate characteristics and the extent to which we acquire a veneer, or essence of masculinity or femininity as a consequence of social values and interactions during the course of our lives. It is thus apparent that although there are huge 'within group' differences for both men and for women, there remain important differences in men's and women's upbringing, schooling, school achievement, economic activity, leisure, relationship histories, sexual behaviour, physical and mental health.

More than that, each of us as a gendered individual will also carry around in our heads working models of what men and women are like. These models will be heavily culturally determined, articulated and acknowledged to different degrees and affect both overtly and implicitly our decision making to different degrees and in different circumstances.

Gender may be more or less relevant to social events and to crime and violence. The highly gendered nature of domestic violence (see Bacchus and Aston this volume), where most domestic violence is inflicted by men on women, is a good example of offending where it is impossible to ignore a gender dimension. Other areas of crime, such as fraud, may have gendered components, but they may be harder to see, for example, and more to do with the social opportunities for crime than social attitudes.

Gender is relevant not only to the nature and patterns of crime but also to the response of those in authority, for example, courts and social services. Criminal men and women will find themselves the subject of other, more powerful, people's decision making. It may therefore matter what individuals in positions of authority think about how men and women should behave. This may form at least a component of their decision making in relation to both law and mental health, although teasing this out is difficult. To begin to understand the relationship of gender to violence we need to look both at the criminal and violent actions of both men and women, but also at the way in which society responds to violent actions and the consequences for those individuals.

Images of dangerous people

Gilligan (2000: 34) said, 'No matter how many violent people I have worked with I still find myself amazed by these ordinary looking men, who have actually committed extraordinarily brutal violent, crimes'. Two things are interesting about Gilligan's sentence; the first is that he writes about men, and the second is that he goes on to talk about conflict between his own understanding derived from many face-to-face encounters with men who have committed violent crimes and their representation within mainstream newspapers and other media. In these media, their actions can be subject to sensational as well as serious coverage. We have an interest, and perhaps a very sensible interest, in understanding individuals who have committed acts of serious violence. We may have a special interest in those who stray beyond a notion of simple violence to that which appears to be motivated by sadistic or sexual intent and/or result in multiple deaths. Many working in professional fields know that a lot of media coverage is grossly inaccurate and usually unfair in part to the individuals concerned. It is equally difficult to say what would constitute reasonable reporting to the general public of individuals who have committed serious acts of violence. Coverage by the media of both male and female violent offenders is arbitrary; it can be determined by other world events or their absence, the nearness or otherwise of the crime to metropolitan areas. It runs the risk of becoming disproportionate if the media decide to pursue it either for their own ends or what they believe to be in the public interest. This carries with it risk for the individuals concerned, both of enduring recognition by the public and that they will in part become a personification of evil. This can be a particular risk for women offenders, and images of dangerous women are often created where the woman concerned has offended against conventional female gender roles. 'Normal' women are gentle, caring, nurturing, non-aggressive and law-abiding. The risk for women who kill or seriously injure people close to them, be they lovers, husbands, partners or children, is that they will receive considerable attention in the media, ensuring that their name remains in the public eye. The fact that such crimes are committed considerably more often by men means that the chances of a woman gaining notoriety in this way is considerably greater than it is for any man; thus the names of some women have become infamous, for example, Ruth Ellis, Myra Hindley, Aileen Wuornos and Rosemary West.

Facts and figures on violence

There are a number of ways of assessing the actual extent of men's and women's involvement in crime and violence in England and Wales. Joliffe (this volume pp 21–34) reports on both convictions for violent crime and the self-report of the British Crime Survey and discusses their respective advantages and limitations.

Home Office figures (2006) on those successfully prosecuted show that men are more likely to be convicted of a range of violent offences than women. Women are responsible for only 6% of murders, 1.5% of attempted murders, 16% of manslaughters and 7% of woundings. In 2003, fewer than 200 women were convicted of such serious offences in England and Wales (Home Office 2003). The discrepancy between male and female violence is most obvious in the field of sexual offending; such crimes are almost exclusively committed by men – women are responsible for only 1.3% of sexual offences (Home Office 2006). Sexual offences constitute roughly half of all serious violent offences in any one year.

This is a pattern of violent offending that is consistent over time, and that can be examined in more detail. Home Office statistics also show that the number of women convicted of indictable offences between 1990 and 2000 fluctuated but did not rise. Criminal Justice statistics indicate that men and women are equally likely to be found guilty when they are brought to trial.

Criminal justice processing

Statistics on sentencing show that gender disparities abound. Figures on the prison population show that, overall, women constitute a little more than 6% of the prison population in England and Wales, reflecting their modest contribution to overall rates of offending. In 2006, 4,447 women (5.6%) were imprisoned, while 75,309 men (94.4%) were incarcerated (Home Office 2007b). More than one-third of adult women offenders in prison had no previous conviction, whereas only 15 % of adult men in prison had no previous conviction (Home Office 2005). The total prison population is a combination of both sentenced and remand prisoners. Women awaiting trial or awaiting sentence constitute a higher proportion of the total female prison population than their male counterparts, that is, women appear to be more likely to be remanded in custody than men. Women account for approximately 1 in 10 receptions in prison in the course of the year, but a smaller proportion of the total population at any given time, which is compatible with the idea that they move faster through the prison system than men. Both the male and female total prison populations have risen dramatically since the early 1990s until very recently, although the historical patterns from 1900 are distinct (Home Office 2005). The actual number of women in prison for violent offences has also risen, but the female sentenced prisoner population has risen at three times the rate of the male sentenced prisoner population between 1992 and 2002 (Councell 2003).

The difference between the number of convictions of women and the size of the prison population represents, in part, changes in sentencing practice. Sentencing has become harsher, and individuals who would not previously have been sentenced to a period of imprisonment now are. This has been accompanied by statutory changes in the Criminal Justice Act 2003 that increase the likely length of sentence. These figures warrant careful interpretation, as it is easy to conclude from a superficial glance at the expanding prison population that society is defending itself against a rising tide of antisocial and violent behaviour. Unpicking the difference between convictions for various kinds of offences and the response of the criminal justice system to such convictions is a key task. This is essential to grasp changes in the level of social control and the different philosophies both of government and penal policy.

England and Wales have overall high levels of imprisonment when compared with other countries. Walmsley (2003) noted that England and Wales have the highest rates of imprisonment, per capita, in the old EU, but these are much lower rates than some other jurisdictions, for example, Russia and the United States (Home Office 2005).

Patterns in those subject to community sentences have also altered in the last 15 years, again reflecting, inter alia, adjustments to statute law and to sentencing practice (Home Office 2005: 4). Between 1994 and 2004 there was a 47% rise in females beginning community supervision, compared with only a 17% rise in men. Men are more likely than women to be reconvicted within 2 years of receiving such a sentence.

Mental health issues

There is scope within the criminal justice system to consider the relevance of mental health issues to offending. Commonly, this will be considered at the point of sentence and a key marker of the understanding of male and female violent behaviour will be the number of individuals subject to disposal under the Mental Health Act. Such a disposal, marking the end of a criminal case, is an alternative to a prison or community sentence. Such an outcome affects the rates of admission to secure hospital care and the numbers of men and women so detained.

Figures over time suggest that fewer women than men are on either Hospital Orders or Hospital Orders with Restriction Orders. However, women are more likely than men to be given Section 37 Hospital Orders when convicted of an indictable offence (Home Office 2006). More women are currently detained under Restriction Orders than in earlier years. Home Office figures (Ly and Foster 2005) show that the last 10 years have seen a rise in the total number of restricted patients detained in high secure hospitals and elsewhere; the total for 2004 was 3,282. One in 8 of these were women. Looking at recent admission figures tells a slightly different story. Fewer than 1 in 13 patients admitted in 2004 were women. Fewer than 10 women a year have been admitted to high secure care since 2002. Within the existing cohort of patients under Restriction, women are

---

Box 5.1 Men are more likely than women to

- ◆ Commit crime
- ◆ Commit violent crime
- ◆ Kill someone
- ◆ Be in prison
- ◆ Go to a psychiatric hospital on a Hospital Order with restrictions on the grounds of the risk they pose

more likely to be detained under the legal category of Psychopathic Disorder, which may account for the longer periods of hospitalization.

Both the prison figures and the mental hospital figures begin to suggest that although men's and women's offending seems very different, so too are there differences in the ways in which they are then managed by the criminal justice system and the health service. This needs to be set against a background of changes in statute law, sentencing practices and mental health practice reflecting changes in social policy about antisocial and dangerous behaviour.

Understanding antisocial and dangerous behaviour

Any satisfactory model of criminality must address the enormous disparity in male and female crime described above. The reality is that men and women commit different numbers and types of crime. A model should address why women offend infrequently and usually non-violently, as well as why they offend when they do. It must address why men, in comparison, offend so often, and more often violently than women, as well as why they offend. When applied to violence, the model must explain the fact that women's dangerousness looks very different from men's. Men are more likely to be dangerous to strangers and to their partners, whereas women's violence is almost exclusively confined to their parents and their children. It is rare for women to offend violently for financial gain and very rare for strangers to be victims.

It is also true that any explanatory model must recognize the inadequacies of the available statistics. Violence within the home, both male and female, is liable to underreporting. Child sexual and physical abuse within the family, and domestic violence, are relatively likely to go undetected.

Setting these caveats to one side, it is possible to consider possible contributory factors to differential rates of offending while recognizing that each model has limitations. However, it is important to acknowledge the views of commentators such as Downes and Rock (1995), who observed that the understanding of such different offending profiles in men and women is incomplete and specifically, given women's relative social disadvantage, how it is poor at explaining their small contribution to the overall rate.

Biological theories

Criminology, in particular, is left with an interesting legacy in terms of understanding male and female violence. Early theories relating to female criminality in general, rather than focusing exclusively on female violence, have now largely been discredited. Both Heidensohn (1985) and Klein (1973) provided useful overviews of the work of key figures in early criminology, in particular the work of Lombroso and Thomas, who are easy to criticize on the grounds of poor science.

Much more recent work, particularly in Scandinavia, has led to the conclusion that there is a significant genetic contribution to criminality in men and women (McGuffin and Thapar 1992). Criminality and Antisocial Personality Disorder are linked; much research in this area uses criminality as a reliable measure. The heritable part of criminality appears to be more relevant to minor criminality than to serious violence. A genetic loading is also considered to be more significant in women. The issue of what is genetically transferred is unclear, but there is evidence that an XYY (male but with 3 sex chromosomes) genetic constitution is linked to social deviance more than XY (normal male). Work on molecular genetics is less advanced, but Caspi et al (2002) have made progress at the level of the genotype relevant to the development of antisocial problems; their findings suggest that monoamine oxidase polymorphism may be protective.

Social and cultural theories

There are two ways of considering the relevance of social factors to crime and violence, although these are often considered together. First is the extent to which individual characteristics, or variables, are associated with offender populations rather than community samples. Second is to consider the social processes that lead to involvement in crime and violence, in particular, opportunity and constraint derived from different social arenas. In both cases it is important to be clear that there may be different levels of empirical support for the relationships described. The presence or absence of robust evidence about causation or maintenance (and this may be different) of criminal behaviours will be relevant to the interventions considered in the next section.

There has been extensive work on what are often called criminogenic factors, and the extent to which men and women are similar. Poels (2007) summarized the current situation using the international literature. She wrote that certain factors, that is, substance misuse, family and marital problems, antisocial attitudes and immersion in a social world where such attitudes are frequently found are common to men and women. On the other hand, this commonality is less clear in the domains of education and 'community functioning'. Gelsthorpe et al (2007) commented that even where there is overlap in terms of risk factors the extent to which they are relevant may differ by gender.

In England and Wales, it is recognized that on a range of social variables male and female prisoners are disadvantaged by comparison with the general population. Williamson (2006: 6), citing the Department of Health, noted that prisoners are 13 times more likely to have been in local authority care and to be unemployed. They are 10 times more likely to have truanted from school and to have been excluded. They are more than twice as likely to come from a family where someone else has a criminal conviction. They suffer poor physical and mental health (SCMH 2007), and these problems are compounded by chaotic lives and aspects of social exclusion (Prison Reform Trust 2005; SEU 2002). The psychiatric literature also has something to say in the area of psycho-social variables, most particularly in relation to Antisocial Personality Disorder that is so common in prison populations. It has been clear that behavioural problems in childhood, that amount to Conduct Disorder, predispose to the development of Antisocial Personality Disorder (Robins 1978). Adverse family circumstances contribute to the maintenance of such problems in adult life (see Hill 2003), but so too does childhood hyperactivity (Simonoff et al 2004).

In a range of jurisdictions there has been a recent focus on how women involved, or at risk of being involved, in the criminal justice system are distinct from the men (see Text Box 5.2). Steffansmeier and Allan (cited in Poels 2007) suggested that gender development, including aspects of autonomy and gender role, access to criminal settings, motivations for crime and the detail of offences are importantly different for male and female offenders. Their focus on understanding of female offending stems from the view that insufficient attention has been paid to it. Peugh and Belenko (1999), in a large-scale US study, found that 81% of women in prison were substance involved and, of those, were seven times more likely than similar men to have history of sexual and/ or physical abuse. McClellan et al (1997) found women more likely than men to be unemployed before prison and to have lower educational achievement and different patterns of drug use. Sigurdsson and Gudjonsson (1996) found women in prison more likely to inject drugs than men.

This is echoed in recent reports in the United Kingdom (CSIP 2006; Farrington and Painter 2004; Home Office 2007a). Farrington and Painter (2004) had the opportunity to tease out the correlates of criminality in opposite-sex siblings. For brothers, risk factors related more to their parents, and for sisters in the same family, socio-economic factors and child-rearing practices were more important. The Corston Report (Home Office 2007a: 18–19) highlights different pathways

Box 5.2 Women in prison

- Have high rates of substance misuse
- Have high rates of Post-traumatic Stress Disorder
- Have high rates of personality disorder
- Have high rates of childhood sexual abuse
- Often have basic literacy difficulties
- Are likely to have been unemployed for the 5 years prior to imprisonment
- Are likely to have children at home

into crime for men and women. Specifically, it emphasizes information drawn from the Offender Assessment System in which experience of early abuse, relationship difficulties, coercion by men and addiction are all relevant to female criminal careers and important for reconviction. Women offenders are also much more likely to be single than the general population and they have significant parenting responsibilities. Two-thirds of imprisoned women were living with children beforehand. Women in prison are more likely than men to have accommodation difficulties that affect them both pre- and post-imprisonment. Ten percent of incarcerated women have literacy problems and 40% have no employment in the past 5 years (MoJ/NOMS 2008).

The literature's capacity to distinguish between the needs of male and female prisoners and factors that truly increase the risk of re-offending is limited (Hannah-Moffat 2005). Needs can be relabelled risks. Also, the definition of need is contaminated by the requirement that it can be addressed. The research literature can also be inconsistent when considering factors that predispose individuals to offending (criminogenic factors) as opposed to factors that distinguish offenders from the general population but have no immediate bearing on offending behaviour (non-criminogenic factors). There is also no reason to assume that the status and nature of these factors will hold across different cultural contexts. Given the variation in men's and women's lives across cultures it is unlikely.

Mental health abnormalities

There is little doubt that mental health problems are associated with both criminality and violence at times. This is comprehensively addressed by Burke (this volume pp 35–51). Evidence comes from studies conducted in community and institutional samples. The two issues that concern us here are whether the frequencies of these associations and the mechanisms differ according to gender. In an ideal world there would be robust birth cohorts followed up with good epidemiological and criminological data. This would make it possible to explore both the differential attribution of diagnoses by gender in different populations and the correlation of diagnosis with crime and violence. Detailed examination of this material would then shed light on the motivations for the unwanted behaviour. Unfortunately, data in this area are piecemeal.

Recent robust work on morbidity in prison and secure hospital populations (where most patients are likely to be offenders) indicates differences in the psychiatric profiles of men and women. Maden et al (1994) found sentenced women prisoners had higher rates of personality disorder, drug abuse, neurotic disorder and mental handicap than equivalent men. Singleton et al (1998) found higher rates of psychosis in women prisoners than men, and lower rates and different patterns of personality disorder in women prisoners than in men. Rates of psychiatric morbidity for both men and women prisoners were much higher than in the general population (Meltzer et al 1995). Bartlett et al (2007) examined a large London sample of individuals in secure hospital care. The male and female populations varied both diagnostically and in terms of their offending profiles, although detained in similarly secure services. Both the prison and hospital figures could suggest fundamental gender differences and/or differences in assessment and treatment processes.

Key work also relates to both schizophrenia and to postpartum syndromes where gender differences can be important.

Wessely (1997) considered the relevance to offending of schizophrenia as opposed to other disorders, in both men and women. Schizophrenia was relevant both to offending and violent offending in women, but only to violent offending in men. Hodgkins et al (1996), using a birth cohort in Denmark, found increased rates of crime and violence in women with a range of disorders, including schizophrenia but also including organic disorders, antisocial personality disorder and drug and alcohol use. Bartlett (2001) reviewed a range of Scandinavian studies looking at the relevance of psychiatric morbidity to homicide committed by men and women. Schizophrenia and personality disorder were more highly correlated with homicide in women offenders rather than men. O'Brien et al (2003) found associations between alcohol use and schizophrenia with violence in incarcerated women. Simpson et al (2004) found that of women convicted of homicide, a higher proportion of them than men were mentally abnormal. Depressive disorders were common in the infanticide group of New Zealand homicides (Simpson et al 2004). Infanticide as a legal category relates specifically to women. However, Marks (1996) noted that of children killed under a year old, men are more likely to be responsible than women. She suggested that the mechanisms of child killing require more attention. This is evident in D'Orban's (1979) seminal work on women who kill their own children, where six motivational categories for killing are explored, including mental illness, but no equivalent work exists for men.

Philosophies of systems to deal with crime and violence by women

Workforce issues

Women coming into contact with the criminal justice system encounter a system where men occupy positions of power. Their contact with police, their processing through the courts and the decisions after court are likely to be mediated by men. The police, the CPS, defence solicitors and barristers and judges at different levels of courts are much more likely to be men than women (Fawcett 2007). These professionals will see relatively small numbers of women offenders compared with men during their work. The impact of these gender imbalances need not be negative, but it emphasizes the importance of equipping all staff with a proper understanding of the issues raised by women offenders; to rely on the experience of staff is unlikely to be good enough.

Prisons and hospitals

Institutional care has been widely criticized for providing similar regimes for men and women. Both penal and therapeutic practices have altered and gender-sensitive approaches have been promoted.

Prisons

Most recently, in the United Kingdom, Corston (Home Office 2007a: 23) argued that the gender equality duty, which follows from the Equality Act 2006 and has been applicable since April 2007, applied in the criminal justice system as elsewhere in the public sector; its purpose was to provoke 'equality of outcomes, not necessarily equality of inputs'. Analysis of the different profiles and needs of women offenders has led to concerns about the appropriateness of prison regimes for women. Prisons deal for the most part with men. They are ordered and hierarchical. Female prisons employ significant numbers of male staff, and there is a risk that aspects of the regime can inadvertently echo aspects of early abuse (Benda et al 2005; Henderson et al 1998; Heney and Kristiansen 1997). Corston (Home Office 2007a) drew attention to the failure to design even new prisons with women in mind. Insufficient attention was paid to either the architecture of Peterborough prison or its regime, which was, in essence, the same for men and women. She also criticized particular practices as unsuitable given the overtones of humiliation and degradation, notably widespread use of strip searching. The recent prison service guidance PSO 4800 (HMPS 2008: 1) on women prisoners is explicitly attempting to 'provide regimes and conditions for women prisoners that meet their needs'. This is the first time this has been undertaken, apart from for mothers and babies in prison. It provides very detailed, practical guidance to staff that repeatedly flags up issues that matter more to women in prison, many of whom will be there for the first time. It is written in straightforward language. For instance, it explains the importance of being able to make emergency childcare arrangements following remand into custody. It makes detailed recommendations for the conduct and frequency of child visits. It also provides notes on the risk of previously exploited women being visited by their 'pimps' or other coercive figures from their outside world. It sets out the evidence base for its guidance and audit procedures to benchmark prisons. The simplicity of its language is deceptive; it is very sophisticated in its ability to translate gender-specific insights about women prisoners into operational detail.

Beyond the issue of general prison regimes, the other areas in which prisons have taken forward the gender analysis is in the discussion of gender-specific risk assessments and risk-reduction interventions. Nicholls et al (2001) reviewed the situation in Canada, which has used a mix of jurisdiction-specific and international tools to consider risk in women. Like authors elsewhere (De Vogel and De Ruiter 2005; Odgers 2005; Vitale et al 2002), they are concerned about the validity of such tools when used on women offenders. In the United Kingdom, OASys is used on both male and female offenders.

Gender-specific risk-reduction interventions within North American prisons include those aimed at Post-traumatic Stress Disorder and Substance Misuse Problems (Dowden and Blanchette 2002; Najavits et al 1998; Zlotnick et al 2003). Although these are important initiatives, the size of the studies renders their findings only preliminary. Sorbello et al (2002) suggested that the very absence of an adequate evidence base for interventions with women offenders allows both for the incorporation of a gendered understanding of women's offending and for interventions designed to improve women's abilities and coping mechanisms. This would be a shift away from models of interventions focused exclusively on risk reduction.

In the United Kingdom, the women's prison estate contains four major initiatives, badged differently. Send prison hosts a therapeutic community. Low Newton prison has opened a unit for women construed as having Dangerous and Severe Personality Disorder (DSPD). Holloway prison has commenced the HOST project for women with Borderline Personality Disorder. The prison service has introduced a re-offending package (CARE), informed by developments in the treatment of personality disorder, aimed at high-tariff offenders, but necessarily looking at risk reduction. Both HOST and CARE recognize that women fall through the gaps in the various systems on release, and an explicit part of the programme is continuing contact with workers when women are free. In addition, the IDTS (Integrated Drug Treatment Strategy) allows for the very large number of substance-misusing prisoners to access a range of interventions, but like these other initiatives requires evaluation. Apart from a poorly established evidence base, echoing the situation elsewhere, what all these interventions have in common is a degree of ambiguity about their status; it is hard to see why they could not sit equally well within the mainstream health service.

Hospitals

Just as prisons have absorbed much of the recent thinking both that women's offending has its roots in distress, past and current, and that the current manifestations of that, such as substance misuse, self-harm and personality difficulties, are interconnected, so too have secure hospital services.

'Into the Mainstream' (DH 2002) has been the most influential document in this regard. It recognized the unsuitability of mixed secure-hospital accommodation, that is, vulnerable women with a history of trauma usually inflicted by men having to live with violent and often sexually predatory men in hospital. This was the same point made by Elizabeth Fry in relation to prisons more than 100 years earlier (Zedner 1998: 295–324). It is not always recognized as an issue, either by women so detained or by staff tasked with looking after them (Mezey at al 2005). 'Into the Mainstream' (DH 2002) also made a series of recommendations about holistic care that go beyond diagnosis and that include gender-specific needs. 'Complex needs' has become a short-hand clinical phrase for many women offenders thought to need secure hospital care. The conceptualization of their needs may have changed, but there is little evidence that it has been translated into evidence-based, standard interventions (DH 2003). Standardized treatment regimes are scarcely the hallmark of forensic services (Bartlett 2007, Bartlett et al 2007), but none-theless the absence of robust treatment studies is worrying.

Community

Gelsthorpe et al (2007) laid out the current concerns and initiatives for the care of women offenders in the community. They highlight the recent importance of the Women's Offending Reduction Programme (WORP), the impact of National Offender Management System (NOMS) and the 2006 Equality Act. The WORP has led to the funding of the so-called one stop shops, for example, the Together Women's Programme (TWP), where women offenders' needs can be met in a community setting, in a more normal environment and the complexity of their needs better managed than in prisons. The WORP has at its heart a desire to avoid women, notably non-violent women, ending up in custody. The NOMS was designed to create a single, seamless pathway of support and supervision spanning prison and the community in recognition of discontinuities in this process that jeopardized successful rehabilitation (HMPS 2006). Community funding for similar initiatives was promised (MoJ 2007) in response to the Corston Report (Home Office 2007a). Both these authors and Corston (Home Office 2007a) argued that equality of outcome is supported by the Equality Act, and the ways in which that is achieved may be different for men and women; this must be informed by an understanding of the distinctive origins and contemporary nature of men's and women's difficulties.

The numbers of women involved in CJS community supervision are small by comparison with men, but large when compared with recognized offender women in the care of NHS Trusts. Bartlett et al (2007) found very small numbers of women under the care of community forensic services in the London area, and such women nationally have received scant attention in the research literature. Few women-only community facilities exist, including aftercare hostels, despite pump-priming of projects by the DH. These women are disadvantaged, as elsewhere in the forensic system, by seldom achieving sufficient critical mass to attract the attention of service planners.

Conclusion

A focus on offending women in recent years has gone some way to addressing their historical neglect (Heidensohn 1985; Smart 1976). An understanding of the biological and social basis of gender has allowed for an increasingly sophisticated understanding of the patterns and nature of both male and female offending. Current formulations of offending women in both criminal justice and health arenas substantially overlap. This observation in itself is challenging. There is now much work to be done to flesh out these new formulations with evidence about the utility of interventions designed to improve health and wellbeing, and to reduce the risk of re-offending.

References

Bartlett, A. 2001 NHS Expert Paper: Women for National Programme on Forensic Mental Health Research and Development.

Bartlett, A. 2007 Expert Paper. Social Difference and Division: Women NHS National Programme on Forensic Mental Health Research and Development. www.nfmhp.org.uk/expert paper.htm

Bartlett, A., Johns, A., Fiander, M. and Jhawar, H. 2007 London Secure Units Benchmarking Study. London: NHS London.

Benda, B.B., Harm, N.J. and Toombs, N.J. 2005 Survival Analysis of Male and Female Boot Camp Graduates Using Life Course Theory 87–114 in Rehabilitation Issues, Problems and Prospects in Boot Camp (Benda, B.B. and Pallone, N.J. Editors) New York: Haworth Press.

Caspi, A., McClay, J., Moffit, T.E. et al 2002 Role of Genotype in the Cycle of Violence in Maltreated Children. Science 297: 851–854.

Councell, R. 2003 The Prison Population in 2002: A Statistical Review. Findings 228 London: Home Office.

CSIP (Care Services Improvement Partnership) 2006 Women at Risk: The Mental Health of Women in Contact with the Judicial System. London: DH.

De Vogel, V. and de Ruiter, C. 2005 The HCR-20 in Personality Disordered Female Offenders: A Comparison with a Matched Sample of Males. Clinical Psychology and Psychotherapy 12: 226–240.

DH (Department Of Health) 2002 Women's Mental Health: Into the Mainstream. Strategic Development of Mental Health Care for Women. London: Department Of Health.

DH 2003 Mainstreaming Gender and Women's Mental Health: Implementation Guidance. London: Department Of Health.

D'Orban, P.T. 1979 Women Who Kill Their Children. British Journal of Psychiatry 134: 560–571.

Dowden, C. and Blanchette, K. 2002 An Evaluation of the Effectiveness of Substance Abuse Programming for Female Offenders International Journal of Offender Therapy and Comparative. Criminology 46: 220–230.

Downes, D. and Rock, R. 1995 Understanding Deviance: A Guide to the Sociology of Crime and Rule Breaking. Revised 2nd Edition. Oxford: Oxford University Press.

Farrington, D. and Painter, K. 2004 Gender Differences in Risk Factors for Offending. Findings 196. London: Home Office.

Fawcett Society 2007 Women and the Criminal Justice System: The Facts. www.fawcettsociety.org.uk

Gelsthorpe, L., Sharpe, G. and Roberts, J. 2007 Provision for Women Offenders in the Community. www.fawcettsociety.org.uk

Gilligan, J. 2000 Violence: Reflections on a National Epidemic. London: Jessica Kingsley.

Hannah-Moffat, K. 2005 Criminogenic Needs and the Transformative Risk Subject. Punishment and Society 7: 29–51.

Heidensohn, F. 1985 Women and Crime. London: MacMillan.

Henderson, D. Schaeffer, J. and Brown, L. 1998 Gender Appropriate Mental Health Services for Incarcerated Women: Issues and Challenges. Family and Community Health 21, 3: 42–53.

Heney, J. and Christiansen, C.M. 1997 An Analysis of the Impact of Prison on Women Survivors of Childhood Sexual Abuse. Women and Therapy 20, 4: 29–44.

Hill, J. 2003 Early Identification of Individuals at Risk for Antisocial Personality Disorder. British Journal of Psychiatry 182: 11–14.

HMPS 2006 PSO (Prison Service Order) 3050 Continuity of Health Care for Prisoners. Issue No: 254 10/2/2006.

HMPS 2008 PSO (Prison Service Order) 4800 Women Prisoners Issue No: 297 24/04/08.

Hodgkins, S. Mednick, S.A., Brennan, P.A., Schulsinger, F. and Engberg, M. 1996 Mental Disorder and Crime: Evidence from a Danish Cohort. Archives of General Psychiatry 53: 489–496.

Home Office 2003 Statistics on Women and the Criminal Justice System. A Home Office Publication under Section 95 of the Criminal Justice Act 1991 London: Author.

Home Office 2005 Home Office Statistical Bulletin Offender Management Caseload Statistics 2004 17/05 England and Wales. www.homeoffice.gov.uk/rds

Home Office 2006 Criminal Statistics 2005. www.homeoffice.gov.uk/rds/pdfs06/cs2005vol2pt1.xls

Home Office (2007a) The Corston Report: A Report by Baroness Jean Corston of a Review of Women with Particular Vulnerabilities in the Criminal Justice System. London: Home Office.

Home Office 2007b Population in Custody 2006. www.homeoffice.gov.uk/rds/omcs.html

Kessler, S.J. and McKenna, W. 1978 Gender: An Ethnomethodological Approach. Chicago: University of Chicago Press.

Klein, D. 1973 The Aetiology of Female. Crime Issues in Criminology 8, 2: 3–30.

Ly, L. and Foster, S. 2005 Statistics of Mentally Disordered Offenders 2004 Home Office Statistical Bulletin. www.homeoffice.gov.uk/rds

Maden, T., Swinton, M. and Gunn, J. 1994 Psychiatric Disorder in Women Serving a Prison Sentence. British Journal of Psychiatry 164: 44–54.

Marks, M.N. 1996 Characteristics and Causes of Infanticide in Britain. International Review of Psychiatry 8: 99–106

McClellan, D.S., Farabee, D. And Crouch, B.M. 1997 Early Victimisation, Drug Use and Criminality: A Comparison of Male and Female Prisoners. Criminal Justice and Behaviour 24: 455–476.

McGuffin, P. and Thapar, A. 1992 The Genetics of Personality Disorder. British Journal of Psychiatry 160: 12–23.

Meltzer, D., Gill, B., Pettigrew, M. and Hinds, K. (1995) OPCS Surveys of Psychiatric Morbidity in Great Britain, Report 1: the Prevalence of Psychiatric Morbidity among Adults Living in Private Households. London: HMSO.

Mezey, G., Hassell, Y. and Bartlett, A. 2005 Safety of Women in Mixed Sex and Single-sex Medium Secure Units. British Journal of Psychiatry 187: 579–582.

MoJ (Ministry of Justice) 2007 The Government's Response to the Report by Baroness Corston of a Review of Women with Particular Vulnerabilities in the Criminal Justice System. London: the Stationery Office.

MoJ/NOMS (Ministry of Justice/ National Offender Management System) 2008 National Service Framework for Women Offenders. Web reference, available at www.noms.justice.gov.uk/news-publication.

Najavits, L.M., Weiss, R.D., Shaw, S.R. and Muenz, L. 1998 Seeking Safety Outcome of a New Cognitive Behavioural Psychotherapy for Women with Post-traumatic Stress Disorder and Substance Dependence. Journal of Traumatic Stress 11: 437–456.

Nicholls, T.L., Hemphill, J.F., Boer, D.P., Kropp, P., Randall, Z. and Patricia, A. 2001 The Assessment and Treatment of Offenders and Inmates: Specific Populations 248–282 in Introduction to Psychology and Law: Canadian Perspectives (Schuller, R.A. and Ogloff, J.R.P. Editors) Toronto: University of Toronto Press.

O'Brien, M. Mortimer, N., Singleton, N. and Meltzer, H. 2003 Psychiatric Morbidity among Women Prisoners in England and Wales. International Review of Psychiatry 15: 153–157.

Odgers, C.L. 2005 Violence, Victimisation and Psychopathy among Female Juvenile offenders. Dissertation Abstracts International: Section B: The Sciences and Engineering 66(1-B): 568.

Peugh, J. and Belenko, S. 1999 Substance-involved Women Inmates: Challenges to Providing Effective Treatment. Prison Journal 79, 1: 23–44.

Poels, V. 2007 Risk Assessment of Recidivism of Violent and Sexual Female Offenders. Psychiatry, Psychology and Law 14: 227–250.

PRT 2005 Prison Reform Trust (2005) Bromley Briefings Prison Factfile. London: Prison Reform Trust. www.prisonreformtrust.org.uk

SCMH (2007) Briefing 32 Mental Health Care in Prisons. London: The Sainsbury Centre for Mental Health.

SEU (Social Exclusion Unit) (2002) Reducing Re-offending by Ex-prisoners. London: Social Exclusion Unit.

Sigurdsson, J.F. and Gudjonsson, G.H. 1996 Illicit Drug Use among Icelandic Prisoners prior to their Imprisonment. Criminal Behaviour and Mental Health 6: 98–104.

Simonoff, E., Elander, J., Holmshaw, J., Pickles, A., Murray, R. and Rutter, M. 2004 Predictors of Antisocial Personality Disorder: Continuities from Childhood to Adult Life. British Journal of Psychiatry 184: 118–127.

Simpson, A.I.F., McKenna, B., Moskowitz, Skipworth, J. and Barry-Walsh, J. 2004 Homicide and Mental Illness in New Zealand 1970–2000. British Journal of Psychiatry 185: 394–398.

Singleton, N., Meltzer, H., Gatward, R., Coid, J. and Deasy, D 1998 Psychiatric Morbidity among Prisoners in England and Wales: The Report of a Survey Carried Out in 1997 by the Social Survey Division of the Office of National Statistics on behalf of the Department of Health. London: The Stationery Office.

Smart, C. 1976 Women, Crime and Criminology. London: Routledge Kegan Paul.

Sorbello, L., Eccleston, L., Ward, T. and Jones, R. 2002 Treatment Needs of Female Offenders: A Review. Australian Psychologist 37: 198–205.

Vitale, J.E., Smith, S.S., Brinkley, C.A. and Newman, J.P. 2002 The Reliability and Validity of the Psychopathy Checklist–Revised in a Sample of Female Offenders. Criminal Justice and Behaviour 29: 202–231.

Walmsley, R. 2003 World Prison Population List (4th edition) Findings 188 www.rds.homeoffice.gov.uk/rds/pdfs2/r188.pdf

Wessely, S. 1997 The Epidemiology of Crime, Violence and Schizophrenia. British Journal of Psychiatry 170, 32: 8–11.

Williamson, M. 2006 Improving the health and social outcomes of people recently released from prisons in the UK: A perspective from primary care. www.scmh.org.uk/criminaljustice

Zedner, L. 1998 Wayward Sisters 295–324 in The Oxford History of the Prison: The Practice of Punishment in Western Society (Morris, N. and Rothman, D.J. Editors.) Oxford: Oxford University Press.

Zlotnick, C., Najavits, L.M., Rohsenhow, D.J. and Johnson, D.M. 2003 A Cognitive Behavioural Treatment for Incarcerated Women with Substance Abuse Disorder and Post-traumatic Stress Disorder: Findings from a Pilot Study. Journal of Substance Abuse Treatment 25, 2: 99–105.

Chapter 6

Race and culture: the relationship of complex social variables to the understanding of violence

Sharon Prince

Aim

To explore the relevance of understandings of race and culture to both rates of violence and societal responses to violence.

Learning objectives

+ To understand the differing rates of violence between ethnic groups in the United Kingdom and the propositions advanced to make sense of this phenomenon
+ To comprehend the experience of Black and Minority groups within secure psychiatric services

Introduction

This chapter draws upon a broad range of theories and ideas from the sociological and psychiatric literature to consider what is known about the relationship between violence and aspects of race, ethnicity and culture. This is a complex area of intellectual debate, not least because of the history and contested meaning of key terms, particularly race, culture and ethnicity. This is considered first, followed by examination of statistics relating to violence in particular ethnic groups. This serves to contextualize an understanding of violence both experienced and perpetrated by specific groups.

Definitions of race and culture

The concept and use of the term 'race' can be considered extremely controversial. Historically, it has contributed to the discrimination against and the disadvantage of minority groups. Often, these judgements and evaluations have been based on the most obvious physical difference, that is, skin colour. Certain races, the 'Negroid' in particular, were seen as inferior to the 'Caucasian'. The term 'race' has been taken to refer to biological and physical differences between groups of people, with these differences being determined by the individuals' or groups' 'genetic ancestry'. However, biological and sociological research has questioned the validity of race as a useful concept because the genes which were supposed to differentiate between races actually contribute only a small proportion to the total genetic constitution, that is, when one actually looks at the genetic variations in so-called races, differences are found within each group more often than between groups. According to Fernando et al (1998: 18), 'the myth of race has been exploded', as the assumption that racial groups are biologically distinct is scientifically incorrect.

A more useful concept in the study of the beliefs, behaviours and reactions of different groups of people is to think about 'culture'. Culture is a term used originally by anthropology. Like the term race, its meaning has evolved over the years, and it continues to be used in different ways both within anthropology and in wider society.[1] Originally it was understood as something external to the individual, a social concept, but it is now often conceived in terms of something 'inside' a person – a psychological state. In a broad sense, the term culture can refer to all features of an individual's environment, usually the non-material aspects that the individual holds in common with others forming a social group. For example, it refers to child-rearing habits, language, family systems, beliefs and ethical values (Fernando et al 1998). Culture is a dynamic universal concept, which is influenced by internal and external factors over time and can be considered to be evolving.

It is worth highlighting the concept of ethnicity, which Rack (1982) purported has been used to fill a gap where people have become reluctant to use the word 'race' because of all the associated negative connotations and where the word 'culture' has too broad a meaning. He believes that the term 'ethnicity' captures the notion of a group of people who have a shared ancestry and where genetic factors are not important determinants of behaviour. Fernando et al (1998: 21) appeared to concur with this view:

> Ethnicity is a term that lacks precision but alludes to the definition of both cultural and racial groups. ... The overriding feature of an ethnic group is the sense of belonging together that the individuals within it *feel*; it is basically a psychological matter.

This chapter refers principally to research and observations on Black people, that is, those of African-Caribbean and African origin and South Asians – those of Pakistani, Bangladeshi and Indian origin. It should be noted that within the literature these distinctions are sometimes unclear; however, I have used the terminology adopted by the authors themselves throughout the chapter.

The statistics

According to the 2001 census (Office for National Statistics [ONS] 2008), 7.9% of the population of Britain belonged to an ethnic minority group. As many as 92% were White; 2% were Black (Black Caribbean – 1, Black African – 0.8, Black Other – 0.2); 4% were Asian (Indian – 1.8, Pakistani – 1.3, Bangladeshi – 0.5, Other Asian – 0.4); 1.2% were Mixed; Chinese – 0.4% and Other ethnic groups – 0.4%.

The most reliable figures about the level of violence in Black and Minority Ethnic (BME) groups come from Home Office statistics and incorporate findings from both the British Crime Survey and Police recorded data. However, before outlining a summary of the data it is worth highlighting the difficulties associated with the collection and interpretation of this information. It is only since 2003 that the Criminal Justice System has standardized the recording of race, which is currently based on the self-classification system used in the 2001 census. The efforts to

---

[1] In 'Culture: the Anthropologist's Account', Adam Kuyper (1999) comprehensively rehearses both changing meanings of this key term over time and the ways in which it is invoked in academic and wider discourse. His argument is that the meaning of the word was always contested and it remains so. Anthropology has the advantage over the more parochial literature of the United Kingdom in that it incorporates a profound understanding of the social construction of culture internationally, within and by different peoples.

widen and improve recording was stimulated by the Stephen Lawrence Inquiry (MacPherson 1999), the Race Relations (Amendment) Act 2000 and the 2001 census. Prior to this, collection of data within the different parts of the criminal justice system and within different geographical areas was undertaken using a variety of recording methods, and classification systems were not standardized. The change to self-classification has been welcomed; however, the very broad categorizations fail to take account of the variations within ethnic groups, for example, South Asians. As Britain becomes yet more culturally and ethnically diverse, a state of affairs which has provoked the term 'super diversity', it will be increasingly challenging to capture appropriate self definitions.

The reports of victims in crime surveys and studies of self-reported offending are subject to limitations and biases. For example, surveys exclude or under-represent marginal groups with high levels of victimization or offending; also, there is evidence, which is contested by some, of the systematic differences among ethnic groups in their willingness to admit to offending in self-report questionnaires (Bowling 1990).

In 2007, the prison population of 79,700 (100%) contained 20,900 (26%) prisoners from BME groups. (MoJ 2008). Fifteen percent of male prisoners were Black, 7% Asian, 3% Mixed and 1% Chinese or 'Other'. Twenty-nine percent of women prisoners were Black, 3% Asian, 4% Mixed and 3% Chinese or 'Other'. Foreign nationals accounted for 39% of the BME population. Among male prisoners there has been an increase over recent years in the proportion of Black and Asian prisoners, whereas the White prison population has remained unchanged. Among female prisoners, there has been an increase in Black prisoners, specifically Black Caribbean, and a smaller increase in the Chinese group. The Black prison population increased by 138% between 1993 and 2003; White and Asian prisoners increased by 48% and 73%, respectively (Home Office 2004).

In terms of homicide in England and Wales, in total 2,605 homicides were recorded by the police in the three years 2001/2, 2002/3 and 2003/4. The figures from these years are combined owing to the small number of homicides committed each year. As many as 75% of victims were White, 10% were Black, 6% were Asian, 4% 'Other' and 5% ethnicity unknown. Where known, 92% of White victims were killed by suspects from the same ethnic group. The corresponding proportions, that is, the victims and suspects being from the same ethnic group, were lower for Asian people (66%) and Black people (56%). During this three-year period of study; of the 83% of the identified principal suspects, 46% were acquainted with the victim. Family members were the principal suspects in 30% of the cases for Asian victims, 27% for White and 20% for Black victims. In the three years ending 2006/7, the proportions of homicide victims by ethnic group were similar to the earlier period. Further information included the fact that 27% of Black victims were shot compared with only 8% of Asians and 5% of White victims. Less than 1% of homicides in this period were reported as racially motivated (MoJ 2008).

A higher proportion of Black prisoners (19%) were serving a sentence for robbery than White (13%) and Asian prisoners and those from 'Other' minority ethnic backgrounds (both 12%).

Further exploration of the figures for other violent and sexual offences among BME groups in England and Wales are hard to comment upon reliably, owing to the incomplete data set on ethnicity among Police forces.

Despite the limitations of official statistics, they have reliably indicated over time that people from certain Black and Minority Ethnic groups continue to be disproportionately represented at each stage of the Criminal Justice process. For example, Black people are seven times more likely to be stopped and searched, three times more likely to be arrested and five times more likely to be in prison compared with their White counterparts (MoJ 2008). Hood (1992) found that even after taking into account the nature and circumstances of offences at Crown Courts, there were differences in the outcome between Black and White male offenders. Black men were more likely to plead not guilty and on conviction were dealt with more harshly, but there was also harsher sentencing in general, accounting for approximately 7% of the variation in the proportion of Black men in the general and sentenced prisoner population.

Several theories have been proffered to explain this phenomenon. Criminologists have suggested several factors that might lie at the root of this disproportionate representation, including discrimination on the part of the police, socio-demographic factors or police recording practices. Other authors have suggested that methodological and conceptual issues make it impossible to conclude that people from certain BME groups commit any more or less crime than White people. This chapter aims to explore some of these propositions in understanding the complex relationship between violence and BME groups.

The experience of Black and Minority Ethnic groups in the United Kingdom

BME groups are significantly disadvantaged in social and economic terms compared with the White population, although there is considerable variation within each ethnic group. For example, Chinese and Indian groups tend to suffer little or no economic disadvantage relative to White groups. However, Black Caribbean, Bangladeshi and Pakistani groups suffer a range of severe forms of disadvantage, as do Black African groups, albeit to a lesser degree. This disadvantage relates to factors such as housing, education and employment; factors that are particularly predictive of offending and general involvement in the criminal justice process (Home Office 2005; Kaye 2000).

Given, in the main, this significant disadvantage among some BME groups when compared with their White counterparts, how can we understand the different rates of crime and violence between and within some BME groups, in particular, Black and South Asians?

As previously noted, crime rates among second and subsequent generations of the African and Caribbean population have become substantially elevated compared with their White and Asian counterparts. Smith (1997) and others have argued that social deprivation, including unemployment and poverty, cannot in, and of, themselves explain the rising and elevated crime rate among African Caribbeans, especially when the standard of living for this group has improved more than that of Bangladeshis and Pakistanis, who have not shown elevated rates of offending.

Racial discrimination has also been proposed to explain the elevated rates of crime among Black people and their over-representation in the prison system. However, Smith (1997, 2005) argued that racial discrimination, like social deprivation, on its own, is not enough to explain the elevated rates of crime, as both Black and Asian people encounter similar levels of racial discrimination and prejudice, and Asians have not demonstrated similar elevated levels of crime. However, it is worth highlighting that among the youngest generation of Bangladeshis there has been a recent increase in the crime rate.

Survey results on racial discrimination have consistently shown that prejudice and hostility among the public at large is just as great against South Asians as against Afro-Caribbeans (Brown 1984; Daniel 1968). However, it would seem that South Asians (Daniel 1968) are much less likely than Afro-Caribbeans to say that they had encountered discrimination. Daniel stated that this was because of the different 'survival strategies' adopted by the different groups. In summary, he stated that Black people made more of an effort to adopt a more 'British lifestyle', to assimilate, whereas South Asians would look to their own networks and communities for employment, accommodation and support. Thus, it was argued, the opportunities for experiencing discrimination were fewer among South Asians. However, if individuals were placed in the same situation, the experience of racism and discrimination would be the same. This pattern has continued into the 1970s (Smith 1977) and 1980s (Smith 1989; Brown 1984; Brown and Gay 1986).

Smith (1997) does not dismiss or minimize the effects of racism, but he does highlight a number of issues. First, there are real differences in the rate of offending among Black and White individuals. Second, that the differences in the rate of imprisonment between Blacks and South Asians cannot be explained simply by economic disadvantage and factors associated with migration. Third, that the interaction, if not transaction, between the reality of crime among Black people and the racial hostility, stereotyping and discrimination experienced by Black people serve to further increase the crime rate among this group.

In a more recent paper exploring ethnic variations in crime and antisocial behaviour, Smith (2005) proposed four possible contributory factors to elevated crime rates among African Caribbeans in the second and subsequent generations: first, the long-term consequences of slavery on the relationships between descendants of slaves. Second, African Caribbean migrants' active attempts to assimilate and integrate into British society resulted in them encountering more prejudice and discrimination than South Asians, leading them to compare themselves unfavourably with reference groups in Britain. Third, ongoing conflict between Black people and the police contributed to the perception of Black people as criminals. And finally, Black men's identification with oppositional and confrontational styles of relating. Smith stated that these factors, as hypotheses, require further research. However, he also acknowledged the contribution of racial discrimination within the criminal justice system in the perpetuation of criminality among young Black men.

Black and Minority Groups' experience of violence

In the study of race and violence the literature has tended to focus on the perpetration of violence by BME groups, in particular Black people, and has tended to ignore 'racist violence', that is, violence specifically targeted at ethnic minority communities. All police forces have collected information on racist incidents since 1986. These figures indicate that there has been an increase in racial incidents recorded by the police in England and Wales. However, these figures have to be considered with caution as there has been wide variation in what has been counted and recorded as racially motivated crime. In 2002/03, the risk of being the victim of a racially motivated crime was higher for members of ethnic minority groups than for White people. Four percent of Mixed people, 3% of Asians, 2% of Black people and 2% of those from a 'Chinese or Other' background had experienced a crime they thought was racially motivated in the previous 12 months (Salisbury and Upsom 2004). People from Mixed backgrounds were also at greater risk than other ethnic groups of violence. As many as 11% reported being the victim of a violent crime within the previous 12 months, compared with no more than 5% in any other ethnic group. Subsequent British Crime Surveys (Allen 2006) showed that BME groups were significantly more likely than White people to be worried about violent crime, and in previous studies this has been in relation to fear of violent racism.

Police forces that record the largest number of racially motivated crimes tend to be in urban areas where there are significant ethnic minority communities. However, Maynard and Read (1997) found that three provincial forces in the north of England had the highest rates of victimization: 14 or more per 1,000 Black or Asian population. Although it is difficult to make comparisons over time and place because of differences in recording practices, definitions and other methodological and conceptual problems, this finding is consistent with previous research, which indicates that communities where ethnic minorities make up a small proportion of the local population are at greater risk of victimization than their 'inner-city counterparts' (Bowling 1999; Smith 1989).

A number of theories have been proposed to make sense of racist victimization. A comprehensive overview of these theories and their critique is outside the scope of this chapter; however, in brief, they focus around five main areas. First, that racist attacks are more likely to occur in areas experiencing multiple deprivations, with ethnic minorities becoming scapegoated, that is, they become the focus for the wider community's grievance and disappointment. Second, attacks are more likely to occur where there is a perception in the wider community that the number of people from ethnic minorities is increasing. Third, theories of culture can explain racist violence. Fourth, racist violence is associated with the consumption of alcohol – either as a direct result of intoxication or in the social context of drinking. Finally, the influence and activities of right-wing organizations (see Hawkins 2003).

Black and Minority Ethnic groups and secure psychiatric services

An overview

In a study by Coid et al (2000) investigating ethnic differences in admissions to secure forensic psychiatric services between 1988 and 1994, they found that compared with Whites and Asians, Black patients were more likely to be admitted following charges of, or convictions for, minor crimes of violence (assault occasioning bodily harm, threats to kill, possession of an offensive weapon), major sex offences (rape, buggery and indecent assault), robbery and drug-related offences. These findings are consistent with those of prisoners within England and Wales. There were no differences in types of criminal behaviour such as homicide and more serious violent offences. Asian patients were more likely than Whites to be admitted following homicide offences.

Black patients were more likely to have previous convictions for violent, sexual, acquisitive, drug-related and robbery offences and less likely to have previous convictions for arson and alcohol-related offences than Whites.

Black patients were more likely to be diagnosed as suffering with psychosis and co-morbid drug misuse (Coid et al 2000; Maden et al 1999) and less likely to receive diagnoses of depression, alcoholism, organic brain syndrome and personality disorder than White patients.

Data from their study indicated that between 1988 and 1994, although admissions by White patients to secure services oscillated, there was a continual rise in the number from non-White ethnic groups.

The over-representation of Black people

Data on ethnicity are not systematically or reliably collected with the National Health Service. However, the available data have shown conclusively that, as in the criminal justice system, there is an over-representation of Black people (Cope and N'Degwa 1990; Fernando 1998; Murray 1996) in secure psychiatric hospitals. Black males in England and Wales are six times as likely to be detained in secure forensic psychiatric institutions as White males (Coid et al 2000). This level of over-representation is greater as the level of security increases (Koffman et al 1997; Thornicroft et al 1999). African-Caribbean patients are more likely to be referred from prison while on remand, whereas White patients are more often admitted from NHS and Special Hospitals (Cope and Ndegwa 1990). African-Caribbean and Black African patients are more likely to be compulsorily admitted at first contact with services (Morgan et al 2005). It was recognized by the Reed Report (DH/HO 1994) that 'Black mentally disordered offenders are more likely than white mentally disordered offenders to be: remanded in custody for psychiatric reports; subject to restriction orders; detained in higher degrees of security for longer; be referred from prison to medium secure units or special hospitals'.

A number of factors have been proposed in attempts to make sense of the disproportionate representation of Black people in secure services, such as, greater prevalence of illness, more severe illness, and delayed or inappropriate care and racism (Sharpley et al 2001). Although some of these propositions have some validity, no single factor can account for the phenomena described, and a more complex systemic formulation encompassing some of these factors has to be embraced to account for the ethnic differences observed within secure psychiatric services.

Clinical judgement/risk assessment

Forensic services concern themselves with mentally disordered offenders and ultimately 'dangerous individuals'. Psychiatric assessment is based not solely on the assessment of an individual's mental distress/disorder but also issues of risk. This function of forensic psychiatrists and the European models upon which their understanding of psychiatric disorder is based disadvantages – it is argued – BME clients and, in particular, Black men. Models of distress are conceptualized within a Eurocentric framework, which historically has served to pathologize Black people's distress and more recently failed to be sensitive to the cultural nuances of BME 'patients' (Bhui and Bhugra 2004). Ultimately, psychiatric models of understanding mental disorder serve to pathologize the individual, that is, locate the cause of distress within the individual rather than consider the wider social, political and economic context of the 'patient'. It has been argued that psychiatric practice, like practice within other social systems, for example, the criminal justice system, is inherently racist, and disadvantages clients from BME backgrounds, in particular Black people (Bhui et al 2004).

Black men have been perceived as 'big, bad, aggressive, paranoid, oversensitive and impulsive' (Mercer, 1986). This racial stereotype, it is argued, must pervade, at a conscious or unconscious level, the psyche of psychiatric staff making decisions about patients. This stereotype influences decisions about risk that can be made to the detriment of Black patients, thus increasing the likelihood of the restriction of liberty, whether that is detention in hospital or prison. Spector (2001) concluded that racial stereotyping, and particularly perceptions of dangerousness, influence patient management. However, it is argued that the misdiagnosis of patients, racial bias and stereotyping is not sufficient to account for the elevated numbers of Black people in secure services (McKenzie 2004). Although it is important to advocate for culturally competent practitioners, this in itself is not enough, and is perhaps too simplistic to address the disproportionate numbers of Black people within secure services.

Pathways to care

Rather than focusing on misdiagnosis and racial stereotyping of psychiatric staff, the debate has recently focused on pathways to care. African Caribbean and Black African patients are more likely than their White counterparts to come into contact with mental health services compulsorily via the police and other criminal justice agencies and less likely to be referred by their general practitioner (Bhui et al 2003; Morgan et al 2005).

Unfavourable pathways to care could be a result of differences in service usage and the client's engagement with services at each stage of their illness (Bhui et al 1998; Commander et al 1997); for example, low GP registration and under-utilisation of primary health care (Cole et al 1995; Commander et al 1997), poor case recognition (Commander et al 1997), and the interface between primary and secondary care (Commander et al 1997). It is widely believed that there is a lack of both community and primary care resources for BME groups. Thus it has been found, particularly for African Caribbeans, that they do not receive adequate preventative and supportive care required in the early stages of their illness, and hence there is an increased risk of presentation to services in crisis, often with police involvement (NACRO 1990; Sashidhran 2001).

Adverse experiences of psychiatric services may provoke alienation, poor compliance and loss of contact. These experiences further reinforce the antipathy Black people feel towards mental health services, which they believe to be inappropriate to their needs and oppressive (Francis et al 1989; Parkman et al 1997; Sandamas and Hogman 2000), and they are as a result less likely to approach services when in distress, perpetuating a cycle of crisis admissions.

There is evidence that it is the absence of family or social support and GP involvement that determines adverse pathways (compulsory admission and police involvement), and not ethnicity (Cole at al 1995; Davies et al 1996). Furthermore, Morgan et al (2005) found that the involvement of significant others within a patient's social network in the pathway to care increased the likelihood that a referral to mental health services would be made by a general practitioner, and reduced the likelihood that a referral would be made by a criminal justice agency. However, they concluded that ethnic variations in care pathways were not fully explained by differences in diagnosis, social circumstances and the involvement of others.

Many patients in secure psychiatric facilities demonstrate 'high-risk' patterns of escalating criminal and dangerous behaviour, which is associated with repeated admissions and increasing levels of security (Coid et al 2000). These patterns are more prevalent in Afro-Caribbean patients, suggesting that community-based services may be less successful with this group and may also be one possible reason to explain the disproportionate numbers of admissions of Black patients to secure services (Coid et al 2002). McKenzie (2004) suggested that the increased use of medium security for Black patients could be the long-term consequence of poor early intervention and thus symptom management, with a delay in receiving medication being linked to poor prognosis and symptomatic outcome in positive psychotic symptoms.

Institutional racism

The issues presented above, that is, the epidemiology of mental health, service use, risk assessment and pathways of care, are often discussed alongside and within the concept of institutional racism. As has already been demonstrated, all of these issues contain complex decision making; decision making can be subject to different biases, including the approach of practitioners to different ethnic groups. Institutional racism, when invoked, is often referenced to the MacPherson Report (MacPherson 1999), where it was described as 'the collective failure of an organization to provide an appropriate and professional service to people because of their colour, culture or ethnic origin'. In fact, a rigorous debate has broken out in psychiatry, which has dissected the term, challenged interpretations of statistics on ethnicity in mental health and examined the relevance of cultural awareness to overall practice.

The 'Count me in' census of mental health wards (Healthcare Commission 2005) found that 21% of inpatients were from BME groups although these groups constitute only 7% of the general population. Three groups, Black Caribbean, Black African and White and Black Caribbean were much more likely to be compulsorily admitted. Singh and Burns (2006) argued that this was not necessarily evidence of institutional racism and that such a charge should be empirically tested. They argued that real health inequalities might be missed if commentators and researchers relied upon racism as a complete explanation. McKenzie and Bhui (2007a) argued that the admission figures were further evidence of institutional racism, which, they suggested, was a systemic issue and not an accusation of racism to be laid at the door of clinicians. Singh (2007b: 364) countered that this view of systemic racism was naïve and that the clinical encounter was part of the system and therefore must be understood, in their terms, to be, at times, 'overt, racist discrimination'; to say anything else was sophistry. His solution is sound, scientifically grounded, clinical practice. He cites the Clunis case (Ritchie et al 1994) as a tragic example of poor practice, where individuals failed to diagnose or treat assertively because of an anxiety not to stigmatize a Black patient or

Box 6.1 DRE (delivering race equality) action plan aims

- ◆ Less fear of mental health services among BME communities and service users
- ◆ A reduction in the disproportionate rates of compulsory detention of BME service users in inpatient units
- ◆ A reduction in the use of seclusion in BME groups
- ◆ A reduction in the ethnic disparities found in prison population

indeed to consider him as potentially dangerous. Singh argued that practitioners must be in a robust position to challenge spurious political criticism. McKenzie and Bhui (2007b) considered in more detail how racism might be scientifically examined, in an effort to move it out of pure political argument. They considered how decision making can result in institutionalized health inequality. They saw both individual and structural racism as contributing factors to health inequality, whereas for Singh (2007a: 370) they remain not an empirical reality but 'an ideological position' damaging to patients and practitioners alike, which has allowed psychiatry to be attacked in a way that would not be tolerated in other branches of medicine.

Much energy has gone into this important debate. In tandem, this has been taken up by government in the wake of the David Bennett Inquiry (Norfolk, Suffolk and Cambridgeshire SHA 2003). David 'Rocky' Bennett was a 38-year-old Afro-Caribbean man who died while detained in a secure hospital during an episode of restraint. 'Delivering Race Equality in Mental Health Care' (DH 2005) is a major push by government to create services better able to respond to the diverse needs of BME communities. Part of that initiative is to improve the quality of information about ethnicity in the health service and disseminate knowledge of good practice. Included in the vision of this programme of work is a list of key objectives, including those listed in Text Box 6.1.

McKenzie and Bhui (2007a) broadly support this initiative but are concerned about delays in its implementation. They also contend that the new Mental Health Act will potentially undermine it.

The wider social context

On balance, there is some evidence for racial discrimination within many aspects of the health and criminal justice systems. This racial bias is not enough to account for the over-representation of Black people within these systems, and some argue that the key determinants are social class and age structures. There is substantial evidence that Black people suffer socio-economic disadvantage in terms of wealth, housing, education, employment and services (Brown 1984). Indeed, the relative risk of mental disorder and arrest for offending are increased in deprived areas, where the majority of African-Caribbeans reside. Coid et al (2000) concluded that socio-economic disadvantage was unlikely to account for the variations in ethnic differences within secure psychiatric services. However, there is a widely held belief that deprivation and poverty in the context of racial stereotyping and discrimination is key to understanding the experience of Black service users.

A more complex formulation to understand ethnic differences in the incidence and prevalence of violence and the over-representation of Black people in secure services needs to take into consideration the complex interaction of social, economic and political factors, within a context of institutionalized discrimination.

Acknowledgement

Many thanks to Dr Claire Dimond for her invaluable comments and reflections on this chapter.

References

Allen, J. 2006 Worry about Crime in England and Wales: Findings from the 2003/04 and 2004/05 British Crime Surveys. www.homeoffice.gov.uk/rds/pdfs06/rdsolr1506.pdf

Bhui, K. and Bhugra, D. 2004 Communication with Patients from Other Cultures: The Place of Explanatory Models. Advances in Psychiatric Treatment 10: 474–478.

Bhui, K., McKenzie, K. and Gill, P. 2004 Delivering Mental Health Services for a Diverse Society. British Medical Journal 329: 363–364.

Bhui, K., Stansfeld, S.A., Hull, S., Priebe, S., Mole, S. and Feder, G. 2003 Ethnic Variations in Pathways to Specialist Mental Health Care: A Systematic Review. British Journal of Psychiatry 182: 5–16.

Bowling, B. 1990 Conceptual and Methodological Problems in Measuring 'Race' differences in Delinquency: A Reply to Marianne Junger British Journal of Criminology: 30, 483–492.

Bowling, B. 1999 Violent Racism; Victimisation, Policing and Social Context Revised Edition. Oxford: Oxford University Press.

Brown, C. 1984 Black and White Britain: The Third PSI Survey. London: Heinemann.

Brown, C. and Gay, P. 1986 Racial Discrimination: 17 Years after the Act. London: Policy Studies Institute.

Coid, J., Kahtan, N., Gault, S. et al 2000 Ethnic Differences in Admissions to Secure Forensic Psychiatry Services. British Journal of Psychiatry 175: 528–536.

Coid, J., Petruckevitch, A., Bebbington, P. et al 2002 Ethnic Differences in Prisoners. I: Criminality and Psychiatric Morbidity. British Journal of Psychiatry 181: 473–480.

Cole, E., Leavey, G., King, M., Johnson- Sabine, E. and Hoar, A. 1995 Pathways to Care for Patients with a First Episode of Psychosis: A Comparison of Ethnic Groups. British Journal of Psychiatry 167: 770–776.

Commander, M.J., Dharan, S.P., Odell, S.M. and Surtees, P.G. 1997 Access to Mental Health Care in an Inner City Health District. I: Pathways into and within Specialist Psychiatric Services. British Journal of Psychiatry 170: 312–316.

Cope, R. and N'Degwa, D. 1990 Ethnic Differences in Admissions to a Regional Secure Unit. Journal of Forensic Psychiatry and Psychology 1: 365–378.

Daniel, W.W. 1968 Racial Discrimination in England. Harmondsworth: Penguin.

Davies, S., Thornicroft, G., Leese, M., Higgingbotham, A. and Phelan, M. 1996 Ethnic Differences in Risk of Compulsory Admission among Representative Cases of Psychosis in London. British Medical Journal 312: 533–537.

DH (Department of Health) 2005 Delivering Race Equality in Mental Health Care: An Action Plan for Reform Inside and Outside Services and the Government's Response to the Independent Inquiry into the Death of David Bennett. London: Department of Health.

Department of Health and Home Office (DH/HO) 1994 A Review of Health and Social Services for Mentally Disordered Offenders and Others Requiring Similar Services, Vol 6 Race, Gender and Equal Opportunities, London: HMSO.

Fernando, S. 1988 Race and Culture in Psychiatry. London: Croom Helm. Repr. London: Routledge, 1989.

Fernando, S., Ndegwa, D. and Wilson, M. 1998 Forensic Psychiatry, Race and Culture. London: Routledge.

Francis, E., David, J., Johnson, N. and Sashidharan, S.P. 1989 Black People and Psychiatry in the UK; An Alternative to Institutional Care. Psychiatric Bulletin 13: 482–485.

Goater, N., King, M., Cole, E., Leavey, G., Johnson-Sabine,E., Blizard, R. and Hoar, A. 1999 Ethnicity and Outcome of Psychosis. The British Journal of Psychiatry 175, 1: 34–42.

Hawkins, D.F. 2003 Violent Crime. Assessing Race and Ethnic Differences. Cambridge: Cambridge University Press.

Healthcare Commission 2005 Count Me in Census 2005. London: Healthcare Commission.

Home Office 2005 Race and the Criminal Justice System: An Overview to the Complete Statistics 2003–2004. London: Home Office.

Hood, R. 1992 Race and Sentencing. Oxford: Oxford University Press.

Kaye, C. 2000 Differences Described. In Race, Culture and Ethnicity in Secure Practice: Working with Difference 11–28 (Kaye, C. and Lingiah, T. Editors), London: Jessica Kingsley Publishers.

Koffman, J., Fulop, N.J., Pashley, D. et al. 1997 Ethnicity and Use of Acute Psychiatric Beds: One Day Survey in North and South Thames Regions. British Journal of Psychiatry 171: 238–41.

MacPherson, W. 1999 The Stephen Lawrence Inquiry. Report of an Inquiry by Sir William MacPherson of Cluny. London: The Stationery Office.

Maden, A., Friendship, C., McClintock, T. and Rutter, S. 1999 Outcome of Admission to a Medium Secure Psychiatric Unit: Role of Ethnic Origin. British Journal of Psychiatry 175: 317–321.

Maynard, W. and Read, T. 1997 Policing Racially Motivated Incidents. Police Research Group Crime Detection and Prevention Series, No. 59. London: Home Office.

McKenzie, K. 2004 Commentary: Ethnicity, Race and Forensic Psychiatry–Is Being Unblinded Enough? Journal of the American Academy of Psychiatry and Law, 32: 36–9.

McKenzie, K. and Bhui, K. 2007a Institutional Racism in Mental Health Care. British Medical Journal 334: 649–650.

McKenzie, K. and Bhui, K. 2007b Institutional Racism in Psychiatry. Psychiatric Bulletin 31: 397.

Mercer, K. 1984 Black Communities' Experience of Psychiatric Services. International Journal of Social Psychiatry 30, 1&2: 22–27.

MoJ (Ministry of Justice) 2008 Statistics on Race and the Criminal Justice System 2006/7. www.justice.gov.uk/docs/stats-race-criminal-justice.pdf

Morgan, C., Mallett, R., Hutchinson, G et al 2005 Pathways to Care and Ethnicity. 2. Source of Referral and Helpseeking: Report from the Aesop Study. British Journal of Psychiatry 186: 290–296.

Murray, K. 1996 The Use of Beds in NHS Medium Secure Units in England. Journal of Forensic Psychiatry and Psychology 7: 504–524.

NACRO 1990 Black People, Mental Health and the Courts: An Exploratory Study into the Psychiatric Remand Process as It Affects Black Defendants at Magistrate's Courts. London: NACRO.

Norfolk, Suffolk and Cambridgeshire Strategic Health Authority 2003 Independent Inquiry into the Death of David Bennett. www.nscstha.nhs.uk

ONS 2008 www://statistics.gov.uk/cci/nugget.asp?id=273

Parkman, S., Davies, S., Leese, M., Phelan, M. and Thornicroft, G. 1997 Ethnic Differences in Satisfaction with Mental Health Services among Representative People with Psychosis in South London: PRiSM Study 4. British Journal of Psychiatry 171: 260–264.

Phillips, C. and Bowling, B. 2002 Racism. Ethnicity, Crime and Criminal Justice. 570–619 in The Oxford Textbook of Criminology 3rd Edition (Maguire, M. Morgan, R and Reiner, R. Editors). Oxford: Clarendon Press.

Rack, P. 1982 Race, Culture and Mental Disorder, London: Tavistock.

Ritchie, J., Dick, D. and Lingham, R. 1994 The Report into the Care and Treatment of Christopher Clunis. London: The Stationery Office.

Sainsbury Centre for Mental Health 2002 Breaking the Circles of Fear. A Review of the Relationship between Mental Health Services and African and Caribbean Communities. London: The Sainsbury Centre for Mental Health.

Salisbury, H. and Upsom, A. 2004 Ethnicity, Victimisation and Worry about Crime: Findings from the 2001/02 and 2002/03 British Crime Surveys. London: Home Office.

Sandamas, G. and Hogman, G. 2000 No Change: A Report by the National Schizophrenia Fellowship Comparing Experiences of People from Different Ethnic Groups Who Use Mental Health Services. London: National Schizophrenia Fellowship.

Sashidharan, S.P. 2001 Institutional Racism in British Psychiatry. Psychiatric Bulletin 25: 244–247.

Sharpley, M.S., Hutchinson,G., Murray, R.M. and McKenzie, K. 2001 Understanding the Excess of Psychosis among the Afro-Caribbean Population in England: Review of Current Hypotheses. British Journal of Psychiatry 178, 40: s60–s68.

Singh, S.P. 2007a Institutional Racism in Psychiatry: Author's Response Psychiatric Bulletin 31: 370.

Singh, S.P. 2007b Institutional Racism in Psychiatry: Lessons from Inquiries Psychiatric Bulletin 31: 363–365.

Singh, S.P. and Burns, T. 2006 Race and Mental Health: There is More to Race than Racism. British Medical Journal 333: 648–651.

Smith, D.J. 1977 Racial Disadvantage in Britain. Harmondsworth: Penguin.

Smith, D. 1997 Ethnic Origins, Crime and Criminal Justice 703–759 in The Oxford Textbook of Criminology 2nd Edition (Maguire, M., Morgan, R. and Reiner, R. Editors). Oxford: Clarendon Press.

Smith, D.J. 2005 Explaining Ethnic Variations in Crime and Antisocial Behaviour in the United Kingdom 174–103 in Ethnicity and Causal Mechanisms (Rutter, M. and Tienda, M. Editors). Cambridge: Cambridge University Press.

Smith, S.J. 1989 The Politics of 'Race' and Residence: Citizenship, Segregation and White Supremacy in Britain. Cambridge: Polity.

Spector, R. 2001 Is There a Racial Bias in Clinicians' Perceptions of the Dangerousness of Psychiatric Patients? A Review of the Literature. Journal of Mental Health 10: 5–15.

Thornicroft, G., Davies, S. and Leese, M. 1999 Health Service Research and Forensic Psychiatry: A Black and White Case. International Review of Psychiatry 11: 250–257.

Chapter 7

Domestic violence against women: genesis and perpetuation

Loraine J. Bacchus and Gillian Aston

Aim

To provide a comprehensive account of the origins, nature, frequency and consequences of domestic violence against women

---

Learning objectives

- To understand the social and individual circumstances in which domestic violence is likely to occur
- To account for the different rates of domestic violence
- To understand the physical and mental health problems linked to the experience of domestic violence
- To be aware of the policy and practical responses to domestic violence in the United Kingdom

---

Introduction

Domestic violence is an emotive subject. The available statistics on domestic violence are both astounding and shocking. Despite increasing recognition that domestic violence is a crime and a major threat to public health, the evidence shows that *although* violence against women is a pervasive and universal problem, it is not inevitable and can be eradicated. This chapter will address a range of policy and theoretical perspectives that aim to increase our understanding of violence against women; it utilizes an ecological framework to examine mediating factors that combine to cause interpersonal violence. In addition, the chapter draws on research that has explored the nature and prevalence of domestic violence and the impact it has on women's health. In conclusion, the importance of multi-agency and partnership working between statutory organisations and voluntary sector domestic violence agencies is highlighted. Terms such as 'partner violence', 'men's violence to known women' and 'violence against women' are often used interchangeably with 'domestic violence'. These are all terms that have been used by researchers, seminal writers and health professionals both inside and outside the United Kingdom. It is not our intention to portray women as victims or demonize men as perpetrators, as we acknowledge that many men are engaged in the movement to end violence against women. It is also well recognized that men also experience domestic violence. However, the evidence demonstrates that, globally, women are more likely to be victims and that the nature of this violence tends to be more severe and injurious.

Theories of partner violence

Many researchers have pointed out that no single determinant accounts for partner violence. The evidence itself reminds us how partial our current understanding is about what causes partner violence. Although there is clearly merit in the studies to date, attention has been drawn to methodological deficits, and suggestions have been made that would go some way towards redressing these (Archer 2000; Koss et al 1994; Widom 1989; Worden and Carlson 2005). That said, myths and stereotypes about why men are violent towards women are common. For example, 'She made me do it' . . . 'they enjoy it/want it' . . . 'she needed it' . . . 'I needed to let off steam' . . . 'I just lost control' . . . 'I wasn't myself'. Such ideas and beliefs stand as a narrative of their own, but what is striking are the forms of disavowal or minimization of the violence, denial of responsibility for the violence and beliefs about women's responsibility for the violent behaviour of men. Space constraints make it impossible to give details of every theory and explanation of the causes of men's violence to known women. Instead, three influential theoretical perspectives, that is, biological, psychodynamic and socio-political understandings, are considered below. This leads on to discussion of the ecological model, an attempt to integrate multiple factors into a more comprehensive framework of understanding.

Biological perspective . . . 'That is the way men are'

Probably the commonest explanation that biological factors contribute to the expression and form of violence against women is the fact that men, on average, are larger and physically stronger than women. This implies that violent events (e.g. hitting or shoving) have different meanings, levels of threat and physical consequences for the victim (Dobash and Dobash 1992; Koss et al 1994). Other biological explanations for human behaviour have increasingly made their way into the public domain and have sometimes been used in fairly 'wild' ways in the broadsheet and tabloid press. This is a trend referred to by Hearn (1998: 17), who argued that 'men may be seen as naturally aggressive, and violence may be considered as naturally associated with men. Ideas of "nature" and "the natural", whether as natural rights to do violence or natural explanations of violence, are very persistent both in everyday and professional discourses of violence, frequently underpinned by ideologies of biology.' Not surprisingly, other areas of biological research and explanations have focused on the hormonal or chromosomal differences between men and women. In particular, there has been a burgeoning interest in men convicted of violent crimes and variations in testosterone levels, and chromosome patterns between and among females and males. A link between testosterone levels and aggression has been reported in some animal studies (Hearn 1998).

Psycho-dynamic perspectives . . . 'It is just beyond my will'

Psycho-dynamic approaches to violent men are characterized by common elements. Some stress biochemical, neurological or physical disorder; some rely on notions of intra-psychic conflict; transference of aggression; denial mechanisms; displacement of needs; traumatic childhood; or situational factors such as stress and alcohol abuse. However, there appears to be a consensus that the fundamental cause of violence is faulty personality type or some sort of personality disorder (Dobash et al 2000; Hearn 1998; Koss et al 1994). This has been criticized for negating the agency of men in the choices they make about the way they react to stress. Most important, it makes it impossible for perpetrators to play an active role in transforming their own behaviour (Dobash et al 2000).

Socio-political perspectives . . . 'All the men around here are like that'

Violence against women is embedded in societies worldwide, cutting across class, economic strata and race (WHO 2002). Domestic violence is now recognized by international bodies as one form of violence against women. Many forms of woman abuse occur in most cultures, but some forms are more culturally specific (WHO 2002, 2005). It can be exacerbated by poverty, displacement and previous abuse and is a major health and development issue (Pickup et al 2001). Since the mid-1970s, feminists and women's advocacy groups around the world have been working to draw more attention to the physical, psychological and sexual abuse of women, and to stress the need for action (Kelly and Lovett 2005). Woman abuse has been linked to a web of attitudinal, structural and systemic inequalities that are gender related. Taking a gender approach to violence against women involves engaging in gender divisions, patterns of gender relations and unequal power relations between women and men (Dobash & Dobash 1979; McKie 2005). Feminists have termed this inequality 'patriarchy' (the 'rule of the fathers'). Violence against women has been identified as one of the six structures of patriarchy that ensure men's control and dominance over women (Walby 1990).

The ecological model

Over the past decade there has been a notable growth in the use of an ecological model of violence as a framework to understand the personal, situational and socio-cultural factors that combine to cause interpersonal violence (Heise 1998; McVeigh et al 2005; WHO 2002). Conceptualized as a set of four nested circles (see Figure 1), the ecological model has been used to identify individual factors related to domestic violence (WHO 2002). The ecological model regards violence as the result of interacting and overlapping behavioural influences that operate at four different levels of the social environment.

Individual level. Several factors and characteristics have come to be generally recognized as increasing a woman's chances of being a victim of domestic violence. There is a growing body of research that reveals adolescents and younger mothers are a vulnerable group (Harrykissoon et al 2002; Renker 2006). Witnessing or experiencing violence as a child has also become accepted

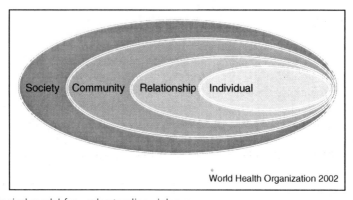

Society Community Relationship Individual

World Health Organization 2002

Fig. 7.1 Ecological model for understanding violence.

as another risk factor (Hosking and Walsh 2005; McVeigh et al 2005). The literature also supports the association between women with low socio-economic status and an increased likelihood of being a victim (DH 2006). Furthermore, mental health problems and a history of domestic violence are known to be linked (Jones et al 2001; Golding 1999; Mezey et al 2005).

Relationship level. The emphasis at this level is on personal and intimate relationships and the immediate context in which violence takes place. This frequently involves the relationships between men and women within the context of the family. Marital conflict and instability are well documented in the literature on domestic violence as primary sources of conflict leading to violent events (Dobash et al 1996, 1979). There is also considerable evidence that male jealousy, possessiveness and proprietary attitudes towards domestic labour, and the disciplining of women by men are strongly predictive of intimate partner violence (Hearn 1998; Dobash et al 1996, 1979; McKie 2005). Some research also links economic deprivation, and male economic and decision-making authority within the family as mediating factors in marital conflict (Heise 1998; Jewkes 2002).

Community level. Several lines of research suggest that the institutions and social structures, both formal and informal, in which relationships are embedded increase the likelihood of violence against women. For example, weak community interventions and sanctions against domestic violence, levels of economic stress and unemployment in the community, poor environmental conditions and housing can 'turn up the volume' of violence (McVeigh et al 2005; WHO 2005). There is also strong consensual agreement that peer-group associations, substance abuse, and poor social and family support networks are considered key factors in promoting violence (McVeigh et al 2005; Hosking and Walsh 2005; WHO 2005).

Societal level. This level refers to the broad set of cultural norms, values and beliefs that influence and inform societies as a whole (Heise 1998; WHO 2005). It involves the influence of social/economic policies and the media. Given the significance of traditional gender norms and societal norms supportive of violence, researchers have argued that violence against women is a marker of inequality between men and women (Heath 2002; Jewkes 2002; McKie 2005). Societies that tend to have higher levels of gender violence are those in which women are economically dependent on men, or where they have little room for manoeuvre either in the home or the political sphere (Heise et al 1999).

What is domestic violence and who is affected?

Domestic violence is one of the most common forms of violence against women globally, and studies have shown that it occurs in all countries regardless of factors such as age, ethnicity, religion and socio-economic group (WHO 2005).

Domestic violence includes a range of behaviours and acts that may be used in isolation or together to control and instil fear in the victim. Physical violence comprises the use of physical force such as hitting, slapping, kicking, punching, the use of weapons or objects as weapons, burning, scalding, choking and hair-pulling in assaults that can result in injury or death. Psychological and emotional abuses include verbal threats, intimidation, constant belittling and humiliation. However, it also encompasses a range of coercive and controlling behaviours, including isolation from potential sources of support such as family and friends, deprivation of basic needs such as food, money, clothing, transportation and health care, and restricting access to information, education, employment and social activities. Sexual violence can refer to coercive or forced sexual contact, rape, being forced to watch or re-enact pornographic material and sexual assault with objects (Bacchus and Bewley 2006).

Box 7.1 Consequences of domestic violence*

	Men	Women
Physical injuries	50%	75%
Mental or emotional problems	10%	37%
Severe physical injuries	2%	8%
Severe bruising	5%	21%

Women are more likely than men to*:

♦ Experience repeat assaults

♦ Live in fear of their partner

♦ Seek medical attention after the assault

♦ Be killed as a consequence of domestic violence**

* Source: Mirlees-Black 1999; Walby & Allen 2004
** Source: Povey 2005

Although it is recognized that domestic violence occurs in the context of same-sex relationships and can also be perpetrated by women against male partners, studies concur that the vast majority of domestic violence is experienced by women and perpetrated by men with whom they have or have had a relationship (Kershaw et al 2000; Walby and Allen 2004).

Criminal statistics for England and Wales 2003–2004 show that 5% of male homicide victims were killed by a current or former partner compared with 38% of female homicide victims (see Text Box 7.1; Povey 2005). Research demonstrates a gender asymmetry in the consequences of domestic violence, and it would appear that the more persistent and injurious type of violence, disproportionately affects women (Mirlees-Black 1999). For the purposes of this chapter, the exploration of domestic violence will focus on violence by men against female partners.

Domestic violence as a human rights issue

Domestic violence is a criminal offence and since the publication of a plethora of guidelines and policy documents from the UK Royal Colleges and health professional governing bodies, it has also received increasing attention as a major public health issue (Bewley et al 1997; British Medical Association 1998; DH 2000, 2006; Royal College of Midwives 1997, 2006). However, more recently policymakers, academics and frontline activists internationally have begun to address domestic violence and other forms of violence against women (e.g. female genital mutilation, exploitation of girls, honour crimes, rape and sexual assault, sexual harassment), as a violation of the human rights of women and girls (Kelly & Lovett 2005; WHO 1997). Placing violence against women within a human rights context highlights the ways in which the multiple forms of abuse experienced by women denies them the most fundamental of human rights: life, liberty, bodily integrity, freedom of movement and dignity of the person (Kelly and Lovett 2005). Violence against women negates women's autonomy, as their daily routines are governed by the threat of violence, surveillance by others and fears about personal safety. This has significant consequences for women because it undermines their potential as individuals and productive members of society (WHO 1997).

Prevalence and nature of domestic violence

The most recent and robust figures on the extent and nature of domestic violence in the United Kingdom can be found in the 2005/2006 British Crime Survey (BCS). The BCS is a large-scale nationally representative sample of 26,214 men and women aged 16 to 59 who are asked to complete a computerized self-completion questionnaire on their experiences of domestic violence, sexual assault and stalking during their lifetime and during the preceding year (Coleman et al 2007). The survey estimates that 29% of women have experienced one or more incidents of partner abuse since the age of 16. This figure includes non-sexual emotional or financial abuse, threats, physical force, sexual assault and stalking by a current or ex-partner. Higher rates of domestic violence have been reported in surveys conducted in community and clinical settings (see Text Box 7.2).

During the 1990s, a number of seminal domestic violence surveys were conducted in community settings. Mooney's (1993) random sample of households in North London found that 30% of women had experienced physical violence by a partner at some point in their lives, and 12% in the past year. Dominy and Radford (1996) conducted a domestic violence survey in shopping centres in Surrey. Thirty-one percent of women reported experiencing 'physical, sexual, psychological or emotional violence, or threats of violence from a known man since the age of 18'. In a national quota sample of 1,007 wives from 10 regions across Britain, 24% of married women and 59% of divorced or separated women reported to have been hit at some time by a husband or ex-husband. Fifty-eight percent of the sample reported having intercourse when 'reluctant or disinclined' and 13% of women had sexual intercourse 'against their will' (Painter and Farrington 1998).

Comparative data from North America

A wide array of data sources have been used to estimate the prevalence and incidence of violence against women in Canada and the United States, although it is recognized that many of these were designed for purposes other than collecting information about violence against women. The National Crime Victimisation Survey (NCVS), funded by the Bureau of Justice Statistics (BJS), is one of the largest ongoing government surveys of victimization experiences in the United States, and it documents violence experienced among those aged 12 and older living in sampled households (Bachman 2000). Other prominent US surveys that estimate the incidence and prevalence of violence against women include the National Family Violence Surveys (NFVS; Straus et al 1988) and the National Violence against Women Survey (NVAWS; Tjaden and

---

Box 7.2 Domestic violence reported by women in GP surgery populations

- ◆ 41% Lifetime prevalence physical or sexual violence
- ◆ 17% Physical or sexual violence in the last year
- ◆ 74% Controlling behaviour by partner (Richardson et al 2002)
- ◆ 39% Partner violence (threats, physical and sexual violence, controlling behaviour (Bradley et al 2002)
- ◆ 60% Some form of violence or abuse
- ◆ 11% Required medical attention in last year (Stanko et al 1998)

Thoennes 1998). The prevalence of past-year partner violence in these surveys ranges from 0.43% (NCVS) to 12% (NFVS). The National Youth Survey, a longitudinal US survey, estimates the past-year prevalence of domestic violence to be approximately 20% (Menard 2002). In a national Canadian survey, 29% of ever-married or cohabiting women reported being assaulted by a spouse or live-in partner, and 25% of all women had experienced violence from a current or former partner since the age of 16. The survey also included questions on emotional abuse such as name-calling or put-downs and controlling behaviours such as limiting contact with other people. Thirty-five percent of ever-married women reported experiencing at least one of these behaviours (Johnson and Sacco 1995).

Measurement issues

These discordant findings demonstrate the challenges of estimating the magnitude of the problem. Factors contributing to variations in estimates are summarized in Text Box 7.3.

Cross-sectional surveys such as the NCVS and the NFVS in the United States only assess violence in a sample at one timepoint, and therefore cannot demonstrate changes in violence over time. The NFVS has produced high estimates of domestic violence, and it is speculated that this can be attributed to the fact that the survey focuses on violence within the context of personal safety, compared with the NCVS, which is conducted within the context of criminal victimization (Moore Parmley 2004). Bachman and Taylor (1994) argued that the focus on crime in surveys such as the NCVS may deter some women from reporting incidents of violence that occur within a domestic setting. A recent review of research on violence against women in the United States acknowledges that although survey research has been influential in setting parameters for the scope of domestic violence, it has been less successful in providing reliable estimates of the prevalence and incidence of domestic violence, an understanding of the context in which violence occurs and how the abuse trajectory develops over time (National Research Council 2004).

In response to the disparate findings and limitations of current national surveys, academics have called for the utilization of a much broader definition of domestic violence in research on violence against women that incorporates a range of controlling and coercive behaviours that constitute non-physical forms of abuse. There is also a need for longitudinal studies that chart the course of violence in intimate relationships. Furthermore, little is known about women's use of violence or domestic violence experienced by lesbian, disabled, homeless and ethnic minority women (Moore Parmley 2004).

Box 7.3 Measurement issues

- Lack of universal definition of domestic violence
- Varied populations making comparison difficult
- Different sampling methods and assessment tools (Moore Parmley 2004; Ferrante et al 1996)
- Exclusion of sexual violence from assessments (Mooney 1993; Walby and Allen 2004)
- Non-response rates
- Recall bias affecting accurate memory of historical events (Ferrante et al 1996)

Understanding the impact of domestic violence on women's health

It is widely recognized that domestic violence is associated with adverse physical and mental health outcomes. Studies demonstrate a correlation between domestic violence and gynaecological problems (Campbell and Alford 1989; Golding et al 1998; Plitchta and Abraham 1996; Schei and Bakketeig 1989), neurological injuries (Diaz-Olavarrieta et al 1999), insomnia, disturbed eating patterns (Sutherland et al 1998) and chronic pain (Haber 1985; Walling et al 1994). Such physical complaints can be symptoms of underlying distress resulting from domestic violence (Newberger et al 1992).

Links between physical and sexual violence. There is an established overlap between physical and sexual violence, and approximately 40% of women who are physically assaulted by their partner also experience sexual violence (Davila and Brackley 1999; John et al 2004). Sexual violence has devastating medical, emotional and mental health consequences. It also has serious implications for women's ability to negotiate contraceptive and condom use to protect themselves from sexually transmitted infections and unwanted pregnancy. El-Bassell et al (1998) found that women who experience partner violence are five times more likely than non-abused women to contract a sexually transmitted infection. A study of 203 women living in rural and urban refuges reported that 55% had been sexually abused and 43% raped by their partner in the previous two months. A third of the women (33%) had acquired at least one sexually transmitted infection, whereas 13% reported contracting multiple sexually transmitted infections. The majority of women (81%) said that their partner never used condoms and 61% said that their abuser had one or more other sexual partners (Wingwood et al 2000). There is also evidence to suggest that domestic violence may occur around the time of disclosure of positive HIV status (Gielen et al 2000). These findings have implications for sexual-health practitioners working with patients living in abusive relationships, as disclosure of a sexually transmitted infection may place a woman at risk of further violence. Therefore, women may need to be assisted in identifying strategies for ensuring their safety prior to disclosing a diagnosis of positive HIV status or other sexually transmitted infection to an abusive partner.

Risks to pregnancy. Unwanted or mistimed pregnancy may be a direct consequence of sexual violence or the abuser's control of contraceptive use in the relationship. Several studies have demonstrated that women who experience domestic violence during pregnancy or in the last year are more likely to describe their pregnancy as unwanted or unplanned (Campbell et al 1995; Cokkinides and Coker 1998; Goodwin et al 2000). Violence experienced during pregnancy has adverse health consequences for the mother and her unborn child, including the delivery of low birth weight babies (Bullock and McFarlane 1989; Fernandez and Kreuger 1999), premature labour, premature rupture of membranes, miscarriage and foetal death (Jejeebhoy 1998; Pak et al 1998; Shumway et al 1999). Studies conducted in UK maternity settings show that between 2.5% and 3.4% of women are abused by a current or former partner during pregnancy (Bacchus et al 2004a, 2004b; Johnson et al 2003) although higher rates of up to 33% have been documented in US studies of pregnant women (Huth-Bocks et al 2002). Domestic violence experienced during pregnancy has also been identified as one of the six risk factors for homicide in an analysis of 56 domestic violence murders that occurred in London between 2001 and 2002. Other factors identified as increasing women's risk of being murdered by their partner include separation, escalation of violence, cultural issues, stalking and sexual assault (Metropolitan Police 2003).

Psychological morbidity. Women affected by domestic violence frequently demonstrate a range of psychological symptoms that are associated with stress and trauma. Studies have found an association between partner violence and mental ill health including anxiety, phobic symptoms, depression, suicide, self-harming, and post-traumatic stress disorder (Astin et al 1995; Bergman et al 1987; Bergman and Brismar 1991; Carmen et al 1984; Gleason 1993; Mullen et al 1988; Stark and Flitcraft 1995). Varying rates of post-traumatic stress disorder have been found in women who have experienced domestic violence (33% Astin et al 1993 to 81% Kemp et al 1995). This is largely due to factors such as sample selection, time elapsed since the last episode of abuse and methods used to assess post-traumatic stress disorder. Higher rates of post-traumatic stress disorder have been found in women affected by more severe violence, forced sex and more injuries compared with women who experience emotional and psychological abuse (Astin et al 1995). Depression in abused women is also higher than in the general population of women. Gleason (1993) found a significantly higher prevalence of major depression, anxiety, post-traumatic stress disorder and simple phobia in a sample of 62 battered women compared with a random sample of 10,953 women taken from a national epidemiological study of mental disorder in the United States. Few studies have assessed for the presence of mental ill health prior to and after the onset of domestic violence. However, there is some evidence to suggest that domestic violence may precede the development of mental ill health. Follow-up studies of women in abusive relationships demonstrate that those no longer abused at follow-up have significantly decreased symptoms of depression compared with women who are still in abusive relationships (Campbell et al 1996; Follingstad et al 1991). Historically, the response of mental health services to victims of domestic violence has been poor. Women living with domestic violence are more likely to be prescribed tranquilizers, antidepressants, pain medication and be admitted for psychiatric illness than women who are not abused by their partners (Stark and Flitcraft 1979; Webster et al 1996).

Practitioners working in mental health settings have a crucial role in supporting women affected by domestic violence, and a council report from the UK Royal College of Psychiatrists (2002) recommends the inclusion of questions about domestic violence in routine clinical assessments. In 2002, the National Women's Aid Federation conducted a survey of a representative sample of community mental health teams in England. The survey found that mental health professionals have a generally low awareness of domestic violence, tend to underestimate the number of patients affected by domestic violence and rarely ask routinely about domestic violence (Barron 2004).

Contextualizing domestic violence: the national policy agenda

There are challenges and barriers to collaborations and partnerships on the issue of domestic violence (Aston 2006; Bacchus and Aston 2005; DH 2005; Health Development Agency 2003; James-Hanman 2000; Kelly 1999; Patel 1999), but these are essential to an effective response.

The Department of Health recently published a handbook for health professionals in which it states, 'All Trusts should be working towards routine enquiry and providing women with information on domestic abuse support services. It is important to take the initiative and be proactive' (DH 2006). Health professionals have been identified as being in a unique position to create safe and confidential environments for routine enquiry and disclosure of domestic violence (Langley 1997: 155). The use of routine enquiry, as opposed to selective enquiry, has the advantage of not stigmatizing women, and it also challenges common stereotypes and myths about 'certain types' of women being affected by domestic violence. Routine enquiry gives women the opportunity to discuss their experiences of domestic violence and be provided with information about sources of support from specialist domestic violence agencies in the community.

It also provides health professionals with the opportunity to empathize, validate women's experiences and offer positive messages to counter harmful ones that women may have received in the past (Bacchus and Aston 2005). However, the introduction of routine enquiry for domestic violence needs to be handled with care. The Department of Health (2006) recommends that any strategy to address domestic violence within the National Health Service must be underpinned by the implementation of clear guidelines and training for practitioners, systems for the confidential documentation of abuse disclosed, referral pathways and information for women, and robust clinical supervision. However, to bring about such fundamental change, commitment is needed from those at a senior and strategic level within the health service to ensure that adequate resources are made available, such as protected time for staff training.

It is also recognized that the National Health Service can best respond to domestic violence by working collaboratively with other statutory and voluntary agencies in multi-agency partnerships. There is a clear expectation from Government that local partnerships be set up under the Crime and Disorder Act 1998 to identify the level of domestic violence in their area and to develop approaches for tackling it as part of a wider crime-reduction strategy. These partnerships are known as Crime and Disorder Reduction Partnerships (CDRPs), and comprise police, local authorities and other statutory and voluntary agencies. Three-hundred-and-seventy-six multi-agency partnerships have been established in England and Wales to implement evidence-based strategies to address the reduction of local crime and disorder (Diamond et al 2004). In April 2004, an amendment to the Crime and Disorder Act 1998 gave Primary Care Trusts a statutory duty to work within Crime and Disorder Reduction Partnerships (DH 2006). This provides an opportunity for the National Health Service to better support women and children affected by domestic violence through joined-up working with organizations such as housing, the police, social services and specialist domestic violence agencies such as Women's Aid. The amendment to the Act also has implications for health services with regard to the documentation of domestic violence for local auditing and the development of protocols for responsible information sharing with other agencies. The need for accurate documentation about abuse disclosed to a health professional is also emphasized in the Domestic Violence Crimes and Victims Act 2004 Part 9 (Establishment and Conduct of Homicide Reviews), whereby a formal review will be conducted for every domestic violence murder. The Secretary of State can direct a specified person or organization, including NHS Trusts, local health boards, Strategic Health Authorities, Primary Care Trusts and other statutory and voluntary agencies, to participate in the review. The reviews will provide recommendations for good practice that may prevent future domestic violence homicides (HO 2006).

The multi-agency approach to addressing domestic violence

No one organization can address domestic violence in isolation, and health services have an important contribution to make in improving effective, integrated responses for survivors of domestic violence. A woman seeking help may need practical assistance from a range of organizations including housing, the police, solicitors, or benefits agencies. She may also need to access emotional support or counselling for herself and her children. Multi-agency work has been recommended as the most effective way to support women and children affected by domestic violence (Hague 1999; Hague and Malos 1997; HO 1995). The multi-agency approach to domestic violence is not a new concept, as refuges and other agencies have been working together for over two decades. However, it is only recently that this approach to working has been formalized. These multi-agency initiatives are commonly known as Borough-based Domestic Violence forums, of which there are approximately 200 in the United Kingdom (Hague and Malos 1997; James-Hanman 2000). Agencies most actively involved in multi-agency domestic violence forums include the police, refuges, social services, and housing authorities. However, the absence of health services and education departments from domestic violence forums has been conspicuous (Hague 1999). A woman may approach many agencies to obtain the help she requires. It is suggested that coordination between agencies can promote a consistent rather than contradictory response, avoid duplication of services, identify gaps in service provision, increase awareness and understanding of domestic violence within agencies and provide a more holistic intervention (James-Hanman 2000). The work of multi-agency forums has included developing publicity campaigns, producing information leaflets, posters and directories of local services, providing training and education to local agencies, improving service responses through the development of policies and good-practice guidelines, and identifying gaps in service provision (Hague 1999). However, authors who have written extensively on the subject of multi-agency approaches to domestic violence have emphasized that the success of these collaborations has varied considerably and that some forums have become nothing more than 'talking shops' (Hague and Malos 1997; James-Hanman 2000).

Potential barriers to effective partnership working

In order to best respond to domestic violence, all those working collaboratively in interdisciplinary partnerships will need to address any misperceptions and false assumptions of one another's roles. Partnerships may be broken without a common meaningful goal, respect for one another's expertise and a willingness to view a problem from a new perspective. Typically, conflicts between local and national priorities, costs in terms of time and resource, and previous failed attempts have all been described as potential barriers to partnership practice (DH 2005).

Although these barriers to effective partnership working make for a sobering read, there is significant consensus in the domestic violence literature on what improves the sustainability and quality of partnership working. First, active commitment and collaboration from senior managers at a policy-making level to multi-agency work to ensure changes at a strategic level (James-Hanman 2000; Moss Kanter 1994). Second, partnership working requires all participants to be sensitive to bridging power differentials between organizations, conflicting organizational philosophies and operational differences. In general, there has been a penchant for statutory agencies to take the lead in partnership working on violence and violence prevention that has contributed to the marginalization of specialist domestic violence agencies such as Women's Aid and the women's refuge sector. Finally, a lack of or finite supply of resources has resulted in competition for resources among advocacy and refuge services. The upshot of this was recognized by Hague and Malos (1997, p 43), who argued, 'Multi-agency working cannot develop beyond the most rudimentary level of networking and information exchange without some form of resourcing'.

Conclusion

Over the past 30 years, great progress has been achieved in addressing violence against women. In the United Kingdom, the National Women's Aid Movement has worked determinedly with local and national government, policymakers, academics and a range of voluntary and statutory agencies to bring about changes in legislation and service provision for women and children affected by domestic violence. This has led to the development of more effective criminal justice and police responses, multi-agency work, children's services and specialist service provision (Harwin 2006). Important research conducted in the past two decades has enhanced our understanding of the prevalence and nature of domestic violence.

More recently there has been greater focus on the development and evaluation of interventions in various settings to reduce the harmful effects of domestic violence. For example, current research is investigating the efficacy of interventions in health settings that involve staff training, routine enquiry or screening for domestic violence and referral to domestic violence advocacy services (Bacchus et al 2007). It is unlikely that women will benefit from a 'one size fits all' approach to intervention. Further research is needed on women's progress through the abuse trajectory and the types of support needed at different stages.

Funding, policies, procedures, managers, frontline implementers and presence or absence of 'champions' shape institutional responses to domestic violence. Differing organizational philosophies can, at times, pose a threat to successful partnership working and interagency cooperation. Achieving greater uniformity and improved coordination in the way that social institutions address domestic violence remains a challenge. Evaluation frameworks that can accommodate the complex and multifaceted nature of current domestic violence intervention programmes hold the most promise.

References

Archer J. 2000 Sex Differences in Aggression between Heterosexual Partners: A Meta-analytic Review. Psychological Bulletin 126: 651–680.

Astin M.C., Lawrence K.J., and Foy D.W. 1993 Posttraumatic Stress Disorder among Battered Women: Risk and Resiliency Factors. Violence and Victims 8: 17–28.

Astin M.C., Ogland-Hand S.M., Coleman E.M., and Foy D.W. 1995 Post-traumatic Stress Disorder and Childhood Abuse in Battered Women: Comparisons with Maritally Distressed Women. Journal of Consulting and Clinical Psychology 63: 308–312.

Aston G. 2006 Domestic Violence and Health Promotion: Midwives Can Make a Difference 176–190 in Health Promotion in Midwifery: Principles and Practice 2nd Edition (Bowden, J. and Manning, V. Editors) London: Hodder Arnold.

Bacchus, L. and Aston, G. 2005 To Screen or not to Screen: That Is the Question . . . or Is It? Asking Routinely about Domestic Violence in Pregnancy. NCT Journal New Digest 31: 8–9.

Bacchus, L. and Bewley, S. 2006 Domestic Violence 1641 in High Risk Pregnancy Management Options (James, D.K., Steer, P.J., Weiner, C.P. and Gonik, B. Editors) Elsevier.

Bacchus, L., Aston, G., Torres Vitolas, C., Jordan, P. and Murray, S. 2007 A Theory-based Evaluation of a Multi-agency Domestic Violence Service Based in Maternity and Genitourinary Medicine Services at Guy's & St. Thomas' NHS Foundation Trust. London: Kings College London. Available online at: www.kcl.ac.uk/nursing/research/violence

Bacchus, L., Mezey, G. and Bewley, S. 2004a Domestic Violence: Prevalence in Pregnant Women and Associations with Physical and Psychological Health. European Journal of Obstetrics, Gynecology and Reproductive Biology 113: 6–11.

Bacchus, L., Mezey, G., Bewley, S. and Haworth, A. 2004b Prevalence of Domestic Violence in Pregnancy when Midwives Routinely Enquire. British Journal of Obstetrics and Gynaecology 111: 441–445.

Bachman, R. 2000 A Comparison of Annual Incidence Rates and Contextual Characteristics of Intimate Partner Violence against Women from the National Crime Victimisation Survey NCVS and the National Violence against Women Survey NVAWS. Violence against Women 6: 815–838.

Bachman, R. and Taylor, B. 1994 The Measurement of Family Violence and Rape by the Redesigned National Crime Victimisation Survey. Justice Quarterly 11: 701–714.

Barron, J. 2004 Challenges for Delivery Services on Mental Health, Substance Misuse and Domestic Violence Report of Findings of Survey 2002–3. Bristol: Women's Aid Federation of England.

Bergman, B. and Brismar, B. 1991 Suicide Attempts by Battered Wives. Acta Psychiatrica Scandinavica 83: 380–384.

Bergman, B., Larsson, G., Brismar, B. and Klang, M. 1987 Psychiatric Morbidity and Personality Characteristics of Battered Women. Acta Psychiatrica Scandinavica 76: 678–683.

Bewley, S., Friend, J. and Mezey, G. 1997 Violence against Women. London: Royal College of Obstetricians and Gynaecologists Press.

Bradley, F., Smith, M., Long, J. and O'Dowd, T. 2002 Reported Frequency of Domestic Violence: Cross Sectional Survey of Women Attending General Practice. British Medical Journal 324: 271–274.

British Medical Association 1998 Domestic Violence: A Health Care Issue? London: BMA.

Bullock, L.F. and Mcfarlane, J. 1989 Birth-Weight/Battering Connection. American Journal of Nursing 89: 1153–1155.

Campbell, J.C. and Alford, P. 1989 The Dark Consequences of Marital Rape. American Journal of Nursing, 89: 946–949.

Campbell, J., Kub, J.E. and Rose, L. 1996 Depression in Battered Women. Journal of The American Women's Medical Association 51: 106–110.

Campbell, J.C., Pugh, L.C., Campbell, D. and Visscher, M. 1995 The Influence of Abuse on Pregnancy Intention. Women's Health Issues 5: 214–223.

Carmen, E.H., Rieker, P.P. and Mills, T. 1984 Victims of Violence and Psychiatric Illness. American Journal of Psychiatry 141: 378–383.

Cokkinides, V.E. and Coker, A.L. 1998 Experiencing Physical Violence during Pregnancy: Prevalence and Correlates. Family and Community Health 20: 19–37.

Coleman, K., Jansson, K., Kaiza, P. and Reed, E. 2007 Homicides, Firearm Offences and Intimate Violence 2005/2006. Supplementary Volume 1 to Crime in England and Wales 2005/2006. 56 Home Office Statistical Bulletin. London: Home Office.

Davila, Y.R., Brackley, M.H. 1999 Mexican and Mexican American Women in a Battered Women's Shelter: Barriers to Condom Negotiation for HIV/AIDS Prevention. Issues in Mental Health Nursing, 20: 333–355.

Department of Health 2000 Domestic Violence: A Resource Manual for Health Care Professionals. London: DoH.

Department of Health 2005 Creating Healthier Communities: A Resource Pack for Local Partnerships. London: DoH.

Department of Health 2006 Responding to Domestic Abuse. A Handbook for Health Professionals. London: DoH.

Diamond, A., Charles, C. and Allen, T. 2004 Domestic Violence and Crime and Disorder Reduction Partnerships: Findings from a Self-Completion Questionnaire. Home Office Online Report 56/04. London: Home Office.

Diaz-Olavarrieta, C., Campbell, J.C., Garcia, De La Cadena, C., Paz, F. and Villa, A. 1999 Domestic Violence against Patients with Chronic Neurological Disorders. Archives of Neurology 56: 681–685.

Dobash, R.E. and Dobash, R.P. 1979 Violence against Wives: A Case against the Patriarchy. New York: The Free Press.

Dobash, R.E. and Dobash, R.P. 1992 Women, Violence and Social Change. London: Routledge.

Dobash, R.E., Dobash, R.P., Cavanagh, K. and Lewis, R. 2000 Changing Violent Men. London: Sage.

Dobash R.P., Dobash, R.E., Cavanagh, K.and Lewis, R. 1996 Research Evaluation of Programmes for Violent Men. Edinburgh: The Scottish Office Central Research Unit.

Dominy, N. and Radford, L. 1996 Domestic Violence 6 in Surrey: Developing an Effective Inter-agency Response. London: Roehampton Institute.

El-Bassel, N., Gilbert, L., Krishnan, S., Schilling, R.F., Gaeta Purpura, S. and Witte, S.S. 1998 Partner Violence and Sexual HIV-Risk Behaviours among Women in AN Inner-city Emergency Department. Violence and Victims 13: 377–393.

Fernandez, F.M. and Krueger, P.M. 1999 Domestic Violence: Effect on Pregnancy Outcome. Journal of the American Osteopathic Association 99: 254–256.

Ferrante, A., Morgan, F., Indermaur, D. and Harding, R. 1996 Measuring the Extent of Domestic Violence. Sydney: Hawkins Press.

Follingstad, D.R., Brennan, A.F., Hause, E.S., Polek, D.S. and Rutledge, L.L. 1991 Factors Moderating Physical and Psychological Symptoms of Battered Women. Journal of Family Violence 6: 81–95.

Gielen, A.C, Mcdonnell, K.A., Burke, J.G. and O'campo, P. 2000 Women's Lives after an HIV-positive Diagnosis: Disclosure and Violence. Maternal and Child Health Journal 4: 111–120.

Gleason, W.J. 1993 Mental Disorders in Battered Women: An Empirical Study. Violence and Victims 8: 53–68.

Golding, J.A., Wilsnack, S.C. and Learman, L.A. 1998 Prevalence of Sexual Assault History among Women with Common Gynaecologic Symptoms. American Journal of Gynaecology and Obstetrics 179: 1013–1019.

Golding, J.M. 1999 Intimate Partner Violence as a Risk Factor for Mental Disorders: A Meta-analysis. Journal of Family Violence, 14: 99–132.

Goodwin, M.M., Gazmararian, J.A., Johnson, C.H., Colley-Gilbert, B. and Saltzman, L.E. 2000 The Prams Working Group 2000 Pregnancy Intendedness and Physical Abuse around the Time of Pregnancy: Findings from the Pregnancy Risk Assessment Monitoring System, 1996–1997. Maternal and Child Health Journal 4: 85–92.

Haber, J.D. 1985 Abused Women and Chronic Pain. American Journal of Nursing, 85: 1010–1112.

Hague, G. 1999 The Multi-agency Approach to Domestic Violence: A Dynamic Way Forward or a Face-Saver and Talking Shop? 10–22 in The Multi-agency Approach to Domestic Violence: New Opportunities, Old Challenges? (Harwin, N., Hague, G. and Malos, E. Editors) London: Whiting and Birch.

Hague, G. and Malos, E. 1997 Inter-agency Initiatives as a Response to Domestic Violence. The Police Journal LXX: 37–45.

Harrykissoon, S.D., Rickert, V.I. and Weimann, C.M. 2002 Prevalence and Patterns of Intimate Partner Violence among Adolescent Mothers during the Postpartum Period. Archives of Pediatric and Adolescent Medicine 156: 325–330.

Harwin, N. 2006 Putting a Stop to Domestic Violence in the United Kingdom: Challenges and Opportunities. Violence against Women 12: 556–567.

Health Development Agency. 2003 The Working Partnership. London: Health Development Agency.

Hearn, J. 1998 The Violences of Men: How Men Talk about and How Agencies Respond to Men's Violence to Women. London: Sage.

Heath, I. 2002 Treating Violence as a Public Health Problem: The Approach Has Advantages but Diminishes the Human Rights Perspective. British Medical Journal 325: 726–727.

Heise, L.L. 1998 Violence against Women: An Integrated Ecological Framework. Violence against Women 4: 262–290.

Heise, L.L., Elleberg, M. and Gottmoeller, M. 2002 A Global Overview of Gender-based Violence. International Journal of Gynecology and Obstetrics 78,Suppl. 1: S5–S14.

Home Office. 1995 Inter-agency Circular: Inter-agency Coordination to Tackle Domestic Violence. London: Home Office.

Home Office. 2006 Guidance for Domestic Homicide Reviews under the Domestic Violence, Crime and Victims Act 2004. London: Home Office.

Hosking, G. and Walsh, I. 2005 The Wave Report 2005: Violence and What to Do about It. Croydon: Wave Trust.

Huth-Bocks, A.C., Levendosky, A.A. and Bogat, G.A. 2002 The Effects of Domestic Violence during Pregnancy on Maternal and Infant Health. Violence and Victims 17: 169–185.

James-Hanman, D.J. 2000 Enhancing Multi-agency Work. 269–286 in Home Truths about Domestic Violence. Feminist Influences on Policy and Practice. A Reader (Hanmer, J., Itzin, C., Quaid, S. and Wigglesworth, D. Editors) London: Routledge.

Jejeebhoy, S.J. 1998 Associations between Wife-beating and Fetal and Infant Death: Impressions from a Survey in Rural India. Studies in Family Planning 29: 300–308.

Jewkes R. 2002 Violence against Women-intimate Partner Violence: Causes and Prevention. The Lancet 359: 1423–1429.

John R., Johnson J.K., Kukreja S., Found M. and Lindow S.W. 2004 Domestic Violence: Prevalence and Associations with Gynaecological Symptoms. British Journal of Obstetrics and Gynaecology, 111: 1128–1132.

Johnson, H. and Sacco, V.F. 1995 Researching Violence against Women: Statistics Canada's National Survey. Canadian Journal of Criminology 37: 281–304.

Johnson, J.K., Haider, F., Ellis, K., Hay, D.M. and Lindow, S.W. 2003 The Prevalence of Domestic Violence in Pregnant Women. British Journal of Obstetrics and Gynaecology 110: 272–275.

Jones, L., Hughes, M., Unterstaller, U. 2001 Post-Traumatic Stress Disorder (PTSD) in Victims of Domestic Violence. Trauma, Violence & Abuse, 2: 99–119.

Kelly, L. and Lovett, J. 2005 What a Waste. The Case for an Integrated Violence against Women Strategy. London: London Metropolitan University.

Kemp, A., Green, B.L., Hovanitz, C.and Rawlings, E.I. 1995 Incidence and Correlates of Posttraumatic Stress Disorder in Battered Women. Shelter and Community Samples. Journal of Interpersonal Violence 10: 43–55.

Kershaw, C., Budd, T., Kinshott, G., Mattinson, J., Mayhew, P. and Mfyhill, S.A. 2000 The 2000 British Crime Survey. England and Wales 36 in Home Office Statistical Bulletin 18/00 London: Home Office.

Koss, M.P., Goodman, L.A., Browne, A., Fitzgerald, L.F., Keita, G.P. and Russo, N.F. 1994 No Safe Haven: Male Violence against Women at Home, Work and in the Community. Washington DC: American Psychological Association.

Langley, H. 1997 The Health Professionals: An Overview 147–155 in. Violence Against Women (Bewley, S., Friend, J. and Mezey, G. Editors) London: RCOG Press.

McKie, L. 2005 Families, Violence and Social Change. Maidenhead: Open University Press.

Mcveigh, C., Hughes, K., Bellis, M.A., Reed, E., Ashton, J.R. and Syed, Q. 2005 Violent Britain: People, Prevention and Public Health. Liverpool: Liverpool John Moores University.

Menard, S. 2002 Short- and Long-term Consequences of Adolescent Victimization. Youth Violence Research Bulletin. Washington, DC: Office of Juvenile Justice and Delinquency Prevention, US Department of Justice.

Metropolitan Police. 2003 Findings from the Multi-agency Domestic Violence Murder Reviews in London. Prepared for the ACPO Homicide Working Group. London: Metropolitan Police.

Mezey, G., Bacchus, L., Bewley, S. and White, S. 2005 Domestic Violence, Lifetime Trauma and Psychological Health of Childbearing Women. BJOG: An International Journal of Obstetrics and Gynaecology 112: 197–204.

Mirlees-Black, C. 1999 Domestic Violence: Findings from a New British Crime Survey Self-completion Questionnaire 22 in Research Study 191. London: Home Office.

Mooney, J. 1993 The Hidden Figure: Domestic Violence in North London. 30 London: Islington Council.

Moore Parmley, A.M. 2004 Violence against Women Research Post VAWA. Violence against Women 10: 1417–1430.

Moss Kanter, R. 1994 Collaborative Advantage: The Art of Alliances. Harvard Business Review 72: 96–108.

Mullen, R.E., Romans-Clarkson, S.E., Walton, V.A. and Herbison, G.P. 1988 Impact of Sexual and Physical Abuse on Women's Mental Health. The Lancet 1: 841–845.

Newberger, E.H., Barkan, S.E., Lieberman, W.S. et al 1992 Abuse of Pregnant Women and Adverse Birth Outcome. Current Knowledge and Implications for Practice. Journal of the American Medical Association 267: 2370–2372.

Painter, K. and Farrington, D. 1998 Marital Violence in Britain and Its Relationship to Marital and Non–marital Rape. International Review of Victimology 5: 257–276.

Pak, L.L., Reece, E.A. and Chan, L. 1998 Is Adverse Pregnancy Outcome Predictable after Blunt Abdominal Trauma? American Journal of Gynaecology and Obstetrics 179: 1140–1144.

Pickup, F., Williams, S. and Sweetman, C. 2001 Ending Violence against Women: A Challenge for Development and Humanitarian Work. Oxford: Oxfam GB.

Plichta, S.B. and Abraham, C. 1996 Violence and Gynecologic Health in Women <50 Years Old. American Journal of Obstetrics and Gynecology 174: 903–907.

Povey, D. 2005 Crime in England and Wales 2003/2004: Supplementary Volume 1: Homicide and Gun Crime. London: Home Office.

Renker, P.R. 2006 Perinatal Violence Assessment: Teenagers' Rationale for Denying Violence when Asked. JOGNN: Journal of Obstetric, Gynecologic and Neonatal Nursing 35: 56–67.

Richardson, J., Coid, J., Petruckevitch, A., Chung, W.S,. Moorey, S. and Feder, G. 2002 Identifying Domestic Violence: Cross Sectional Study in Primary Care. British Medical Journal 324: 274–277.

Royal College of Midwives. 1997 Domestic Abuse in Pregnancy: A Position Paper. London: RCM.

Royal College of Midwives. 2006 Domestic Abuse: Pregnancy, Birth and the Puerperium. Guidance Paper No. 5. London: RCM.

Royal College of Psychiatrists. 2002 Domestic Violence. Council Report Cr102. London: RCP.

Schei, B. and Bakketeig, L.S. 1989 Gynaecological Impact of Sexual and Physical Abuse by Spouse. A Study of a Random Sample of Norwegian Women. British Journal of Obstetrics and Gynecology 94: 1379–1383.

Shumway, J., O'Campo, P., Gielen, A., Witter, F.R., Khouzami, A.N. and Blakemore, K.J. 1999 Preterm Labour, Placental Abruption and Premature Rupture of Membranes in Relation to Maternal Violence or Verbal Abuse. Journal of Maternal–Fetal Medicine 8: 76–80.

Stanko, E.A., Crisp, D., Hale, C. and Lucraft, H. 1998 Counting the Costs: Estimating the Impact of Domestic Violence 21 in The London Borough of Hackney. Wiltshire: Crime Concern.

Stark, E. and Flitcraft, A. 1995 Killing the Beast Within: Woman Battering and Female Suicidality. International Journal of Health Services 25: 43–64.

Stark, E., Flitcraft A. and Frazier, W. 1979 Medicine and Patriarchal Violence: The Social Construction of a 'Private' Event. International Journal of Health Services 9: 461–493.

Straus, M.A., Gelles, R.J. and Steinmetz, S.K. 1988 Behind Closed Doors: Violence in the American Family. Thousand Oaks CA: Sage.

Sutherland, C., Bybee, D. and Sullivan, C. 1998 The Long-term Effects of Battering on Women's Health. Women's Health 4: 41–70.

Tjaden, P. and Thoennes, N. 1998 Prevalence, Incidence and Consequences of Violence against Women: Findings from the National Violence against Women Survey. Research in Brief. Washington DC: National Institute of Justice.

Walby, S. 1990 Theorising Patriarchy. Oxford: Basil Blackwell.

Walby. S. and Allen, J. 2004 Domestic Violence, Sexual Assault and Stalking: Findings from the British Crime Survey 33 in Home Office Research Study 276. London: Home Office Research, Development and Statistics Directorate.

Walling, M.K., Reiter, R.C., O'Hara, M.W., Milburn, A.K., Lilly, G. and Vincent, S.D. 1994 Abuse History and Chronic Pain in Women: I. Prevalences of Sexual Abuse and Physical Abuse. Obstetrics and Gynecology 84: 193–199.

Webster, J., Chandler, J. and Battistutta, D. 1996 Pregnancy Outcomes and Health Care Use: Effects of Abuse. American Journal of Obstetrics and Gynecology 174: 760–767.

Widom, C.S. 1989 Does Violence Beget Violence? A Critical examination of the Literature. Psychological Bulletin 106: 3–28.

Wingwood, G.M., Diclemente, R.J. and Raj, A. 2000 Adverse Consequences of Intimate Partner Abuse among Women in Non-urban Domestic Violence Shelters. American Journal of Preventive Medicine, 19: 270–75.

Worden, A.P. and Carlson, B.E. 2005 Attitudes and Beliefs about Domestic Violence: Results of a Public Opinion Survey. Journal of Interpersonal Violence 20: 1219–1243.

World Health Organization. 1997 Violence against Women Information Pack: A Priority Health Issue. WHO, Geneva.

World Health Organization. 2002 World Report on Violence and Health. WHO, Geneva.

World Health Organization 2005 WHO Multi-country Study on Women's Health and Domestic Violence. WHO, Geneva.

Chapter 8

Sexual offending: understanding motivations*

Julia Houston

Aim

To describe the origins of and motivations for sexual offending against adults and children.

Learning objectives

- To describe the extent of sexual offending
- To outline the biological, developmental, sexual, psychological, interpersonal and cognitive factors that can contribute to sexual offending and examine the relationship between sexual offending and mental disorder
- To explain the different ways of understanding offending against children and offending against adults
- To outline potential treatment interventions with sex offenders

---

Introduction

Sexual offences arouse strong emotional responses in the general public. It can also be difficult for professionals to understand behaviour that appears far removed from one's usual range of experience. For forensic mental health professionals, who will meet individuals who have committed sexual offences in both NHS and Criminal Justice settings, and who need to work effectively with this client group, it is important to know how and why people commit sexual offences.

Society's focus on sexual offending is not new. Soothill (2003) noted that in each of the decades since the Second World War there has been a focus on different aspects of sexual behaviour and offending. In the 1950s, concerns focused on the visibility of prostitution, whereas the 1960s saw the decriminalization of homosexuality. The women's movement in the 1970s highlighted issues in relation to the rape of women, and the extent of child abuse within the family was acknowledged during the 1980s. Concern about the sentencing of rape cases has been a concern since the 1990s, and in the past several years media concern has focused on the issue of convicted 'paedophiles' living in the community, refocusing concern from within the family to the risks posed by 'strangers'.

---

* A previous version of this chapter was published in Houston, J. and Galloway, S. (Editors) Sexual Offending and Mental Health (2008) and is reproduced by permission of Jessica Kingsley Publishers, Copyright © Jessica Kingsley Publishers 2008.

Different terms are often used to describe those individuals whose sexual behaviour causes harm. Strictly speaking, a *sexual offender* is an individual who has been convicted of a sexual offence that is defined in law. However, as outlined below, this term does not reflect the numbers of individuals who engage in sexually assaultative behaviour and are not caught. *Paedophile* is a specific clinical term, defined in the fourth edition of the Diagnostic and Statistical Manual of Mental Disorders (DSM-IV 1994) as a person over the age of 16 years who has engaged in fantasies or behaviours involving children below the age of puberty for six months or more, which have resulted in clinically meaningful difficulties or distress. Clearly, therefore, not all sex offenders are paedophiles, and not all paedophiles are caught or convicted for their behaviour. Other authors use the term *child molester* to distinguish these individuals from others who have offended against adults. The difficulty with all of these terms is that the individual is defined solely on the basis of their behaviour, which is not helpful in a clinical setting, where the aim of understanding motivation is to contribute to treatment and future risk management. This chapter therefore refers to individuals (mostly men, see below) *who have committed sexual offences against children/ adults*, which is taken to include those who have not been caught or convicted.

The chapter focuses on adult male offenders who commit contact (i.e. 'touching') offences against children and adult women, as this cohort make up the greatest proportion of individuals convicted of sexual offences in prison, probation and forensic mental health settings. Women account for about 2% of convicted sex offenders, and although this is generally accepted to be an underestimate, the true figure is probably still less than 10% (see Saradjian and Hanks 1996 for further information about women who abuse).

The extent of sexual offending

It is widely acknowledged that it is difficult to assess the true extent of sexual offending. Official crime statistics can give an indication of different offence *patterns*, such as the fact that more girls are victims of childhood sexual abuse than boys (Home Office recorded crime statistics) but are acknowledged to be grossly under-representative. This is supported by attempts to assess the prevalence of sexual offending by retrospective studies of the experiences of adults, which have their own inherent limitations. Although now more than 20 years old, one of the most reliable UK studies still quoted is that by Baker and Duncan (1985), who found that from a random sample of 2,019 adults, 12% of females and 8% of males reported unwanted sexual contact before the age of 16 years (see Text Box 8.1).

Attempts to more reliably assess rates of sexual offending have been made through the British Crime Surveys (BCS; 1998, 2000). Face-to-face interviews were carried out with 6,944 women aged 16 to 59 and included details of incidents that had not been reported to the police or recorded by them. This found that 4.9% of women reported being raped since the age of 16 years, with 9.7% experiencing some form of sexual victimization (Myhill and Allen 2002). As many as 0.4% of women said they had been raped in the year preceding the 2000 BCS, which represents an estimated 61,000 victims, yet only 18% of these rapes had been reported to the police.

Box 8.1 Sexual offending: Key statistics

- 8% of males and 12 % of females report unwanted sexual contact before the age of 16 years
- 4.9% of females report rape after the age of 16 years
- 6% of reported rapes result in conviction
- Less than 2% of sexual offences against children result in conviction

There are a number of reasons why sexually inappropriate or assaultative behaviour may not lead to a conviction. To become an official crime statistic an offence has to be disclosed, reported to the police and recorded, enough evidence found to successfully investigate, a person charged with the offence and then for prosecution and conviction to occur. There are many obstacles along this process that need to be overcome for the individual to receive a conviction (see also Jolliffe this volume, pp 21-34). A recent UK study across eight police forces found that rape convictions are at an all-time low (HO 2007), with only 6% of reported rape offences resulting in a conviction. Most cases were lost between the reporting of the offence and the charge, with 40% of cases not proceeding owing to insufficient evidence. In 35% of cases the victim withdrew her complaint, not wishing to go through with the investigative or court process and wanting to move on. Only 15% of cases were deemed *not* to be a crime by the police, including 8% where an allegation was established to be false. The report states that improved victim care, better communication and addressing concerns of fear or reprisals, would help to minimize the number of cases which were dropped.

Many men who offend against children in family settings are also never convicted. If the individual denies any inappropriate behaviour and the victim(s) are unwilling to press charges or unable to be a reliable witness, then the police are unable to proceed further. A recent report by Stuart and Baines (2004) estimated that fewer than one in 50 sexual offences against children result in a criminal conviction. It is also recognized that there is a great difference between official reconviction rates and unofficial recidivism (i.e. a lapse into previous offence-related sexual behaviour), with research by Falshaw et al (2003) suggesting that recidivism rates are five times the official figure.

Men with mental health problems who offend are also not always convicted, again because the victim(s) may be women known to them who are unwilling to report this to the police or because offending occurs against mental health professionals who are unwilling to press charges. Alternatively, such individuals may be "diverted' at court with the involvement of a mental health team, and formal charges dropped. This means that many agencies, other than those in the criminal justice system, may be working with men who have behaved in sexually inappropriate or assaultative ways. For example, Lewis (1991) estimated that over two-thirds of patients on some high secure hospital wards presented with a sexual element to their offending.

It is also worth noting that the vast majority of research on sexual offenders has been carried out on those who are identified and/or convicted, and given the above information about conviction rates, could therefore be seen as biased (Brown 2005). However, one consistent feature to be identified from studies of convicted sex offenders is their heterogeneity, with no differences in demographic variables such as age, ethnicity, socio-economic status, level of intelligence and education, from the general population (Wolf 1985). In fact, Marshall (1996: 322) stated that 'the available research suggests greater similarities than differences between sexual offenders and other people', although as Brown (2005) rightly pointed out, this should more accurately be described as 'other men', given that the vast majority of sex offenders are male, as noted above.

Studies of victims of sexual offending indicate that most are known to the offender. In Finkelhor's (1994) review, between 70% and 90% of the abusers were known to the child. Family members accounted for between a third and a half of those who had offended against girls and 10% to 20% of those who had offended against boys. In the recent UK study of rape cases outlined above, one-quarter was carried out by acquaintances and one-fifth by current or ex-partners, with stranger rapes accounting for 14% of cases (HO 2007). When examining *unreported* cases, the figure for assaults being carried out by a current or ex-partner rises to 56%, with 16% by acquaintances, 10% other intimates, 11% by 'dates' and 8% strangers (Myhill and Allen 2002).

Factors contributing to sexual offending

Individuals who sexually offend are a widely heterogeneous group, and it would be presumptuous to believe that the factors outlined below are relevant for every individual. However, these are the key areas that have been studied in populations of men who have sexually offended and have been drawn together to develop aetiological models.

Predispositional and biological vulnerabilities

Early theories of sexual offending attempted to explain this by one predominant factor, such as Goodman's (1987) biological theory, which emphasized the role of genetic and hormonal factors. The limitations of such 'single-factor' theories led to the development of more complex multi-variate theories, such as Marshall and Barbaree's (1990) integrated theory of sexual offending. However, hormonal factors were still viewed as playing a key role. One aspect of this theory is that a critical developmental task for adolescent males involves learning to distinguish between aggressive and sexual impulses, as this has consequences for their ability to control aggressive tendencies during sexual experiences. The authors argue that both types of impulse originate from the same brain structures. Differences in hormonal functioning will make this task more difficult, particularly for vulnerable individuals who have had adverse early developmental experiences.

The role of biological factors was then not predominantly considered throughout the 1990s, as other contributors to sexual offending gained more prominence (see below). However, Smallbone (2006) has proposed an 'attachment-theoretical revision' of Marshall and Barbaree's (1990) integrated theory, in which he argues that the focus on biological influences should be expanded, and it is becoming acknowledged that genetic and environmental factors that cause psychopathology also need to be considered relevant in relation to sexual offending (Ward et al 2006: 331–340).

Childhood and developmental experiences

It is well recognized that negative childhood and developmental experiences can have an important contributory role in the development of later sexual offending, particularly those that impact on the development of secure attachments. Many studies have found that the family backgrounds of sexual offenders are characterized by high levels of disruption, neglect and violence (Craissati et al 2002) and by high rates of childhood disturbances (Craissati and McClurg 1996). Prentky et al (1989) also found that both caregiver inconsistency and sexual deviation and abuse in the family were related to severity of sexual aggression in convicted rapists.

One specific area of focus has been offenders' own experiences of sexual and physical victimization. With regard to physical abuse, rapists have been found to have experienced more physical violence in their families than other types of sex offenders (Marshall et al 1991) and non-sex offenders (Leonard 1993), although high rates (40%) have also been reported among convicted child abusers (Craisatti and McClurg 1996).

There is a wide variation in rates of reported sexual abuse across studies, although a consistent finding is that the rates are higher than for non-sex offenders and non-offenders. In studies of men who have offended against children, rates of victimization have been reported between 46% and 51% (Craissati et al 2002; Craisatti and McClurg 1996; Houston and Scoales 2008). Carter et al (1987) found that 23% of detained rapists had been victims of sexual abuse themselves. However, although it may be an important contributor for some individuals, clearly sexual victimization is neither always necessary nor sufficient for future perpetration of sexual offending.

Sexual development and learning

Another important area of research has been whether men who sexually offend are more aroused by sexually deviant images compared with non-offenders. A meta-analysis of studies using the penile plethysmograph (PPG) suggested that convicted rapists tend to show different sexual preferences to non-offenders and responded more to rape cues than non-sex offenders (Lalumiere and Quinsey 1994). Differences have also been found between men who offend against children within a family setting and non-offenders (Marshall et al 1986). Although about 18% and 19% of both these groups showed some level of sexual arousal to pre-pubescent children, the former group showed lower levels of arousal to adult females. When considering arousal to images of children post-puberty, the rates increased. As many as 32% of non-offending men were aroused by this age group compared to 52% of the intra-familial offenders and 70% of extra-familial offenders. Clearly, being sexually aroused by children is, in itself, not sufficient to explain sexual offending. Similarly, although in some individuals the presence of deviant sexual fantasies are a significant contributor to their offending, the presence of coercive sexual fantasies per se are not sufficient to define a rapist population and are commonly reported by non-offending males (Leitenberg and Henning 1995).

Interpersonal functioning

There is a clear link between childhood experiences and the development of adult attachment styles, and the ability of men who offend sexually to establish and maintain intimate relationships with adults has been extensively studied. Marshall (1989) first observed that there was a link between intimacy deficits and sexual offending and developed this further into one of the most influential earlier theories, the 'integrated' theory of sexual offending (Marshall and Barbaree 1990). Marshall suggested that men who offend sexually against children are likely to have high levels of 'emotional loneliness', difficulties in developing or maintaining close intimate relationships with adults, and insecure attachment styles. A later study by Hudson and Ward (1997) suggested that men who have offended against children tend to be characterized by an anxious, pre-occupied and fearful style of attachment. Convicted rapists have also been found to have intimacy deficits and a limited capacity to form attachments (Seidman et al 1994). They have a greater tendency than both non-offenders and those who have offended against children to have a 'dismissive' style of attachment towards women, in other words to be sceptical of the value of close relationships and blame others for their lack of intimacy.

Underlying beliefs and cognitive factors

Much research has examined the underlying beliefs held by sex offenders, and the ways in which these contribute to the development and maintenance of offending. Over the past 20 years the concept of 'cognitive distortions' has been extremely influential, defined by Abel et al (1989: 137) as 'justifications, perceptions and judgements used by the sex offender to justify his child molestation behaviour'. An example would be something like 'just touching isn't doing any harm'. Identifying and challenging cognitive distortions has been a key part of treatment with offenders against both children and adults. The most recent work in this area has moved on to examine deeper-held beliefs about children and adults. These are more akin to the notion of schemas in cognitive psychology (e.g. Young 1990) and have been described by Ward and colleagues as 'implicit theories'.

Ward and Keenan (1999) proposed that men who offend against children hold implicit theories about the nature of the world that underlie the distorted beliefs used to justify their offending. These are as follows:

1. *Children as sexual beings.* Children are inherently sexual and possess the capacity to make decisions about sexual activity.

2. *Nature of harm.* There are degrees of harm and sexual activity is unlikely to be harmful unless there is physical injury.

3. *Entitlement.* Superior individuals (such as adults) have the right to assert their needs above others (such as children).

4. *Dangerous world.* Other people are likely to behave in an abusive and rejecting manner towards the offender. This can include either both children and adults (in which case children need to be dominated and controlled) or just adults, and children therefore represent a 'safe haven'.

5. *Uncontrollable world.* Events just happen and individuals can do little to control emotions, events or sexual feelings.

Similar work was carried out with rapists (Polaschek and Ward 2002) and the following implicit theories were proposed:

1. *Women are unknowable.* Women are fundamentally different from men and therefore cannot be understood. Encounters with women will therefore be adversarial, and women will be deceptive about what they really want.

2. *Women are sex objects.* Women are constantly sexually receptive to men's needs but not always conscious of this. Their body language is more important than what they say, and women cannot be hurt by sexual activity unless they are physically harmed.

3. *Male sex drive is uncontrollable.* Men's sexual energy can build up to dangerous levels if women do not provide them with sexual opportunities, and once aroused it is difficult not to progress to orgasm.

4. *Entitlement*: Needs (which include sexual needs) should be met on demand, and men should be able to have sex when they want to.

5. *Dangerous world.* Again, the world is a hostile and threatening place, and people need to be on their guard, but there is no safe haven.

Sexual offending and mental disorder

Among general populations of sex offenders, the prevalence of mental illness is low (up to 10%; Sahota and Chesterman 1998b), although that of personality disorders is higher (30%–50%; Ahlmeyer et al 2003; Madsen et al 2006). However, professionals working specifically within mental health settings will clearly see higher rates of this 'co-morbidity'. A common, but errone-ous assumption by some clinicians is that in those with mental health problems, particularly mental illness, any sexual offending is causally related, and the only intervention necessary to reduce further risk is to treat the mental illness. In fact, the relationship is much more complex, as Sahota and Chesterman's (1998b) review of sex offenders with schizophrenia highlighted. They emphasized the importance of not only appraising the role of symptoms in offending behaviour but also the contribution of more specific factors associated with sexual offending, such as those contributing to aetiology and risk. Their work suggests four ways in which the relationship between symptoms of schizophrenia and sexual offending may be manifested. First, a sexual assault may arise directly as a result of delusional beliefs. Second, a sexual assault may be related to less specific features of the illness, such as heightened feelings of arousal and irritability or confused thinking. Third, an assault may be related to 'negative' symptoms of the illness, such as social withdrawal, impaired social performance and blunting of emotional responses, and finally, a sexual assault may be largely unrelated to the schizophrenic illness and more closely related to underlying personality problems and/or deviant sexual interests.

Craissati (2004) noted that determining the temporal aspect of the relationship between the illness and the offending can be difficult. In Craissati and Hodes' (1992) study of 11 mentally ill sex offenders, no evidence of mental illness was found within the prosecution evidence, particularly the transcript of the police interview. However, when assessed shortly afterwards in prison, the majority were found to be floridly psychotic. The authors suggested that, retrospectively, it is likely that although three offences may have occurred as a response to psychotic symptoms, the majority were committed within the context of deteriorating social behaviour and self-care, heightened feelings of anxiety and depression and a degree of sexual pre-occupation, likely to be the 'prodromal phase' of the illness. Further to this, Chesterman and Sahota (1998) found that only 1 of 12 mentally ill sex offenders gave psychotic symptoms as an explanation or motivation for the offence. Six of the seven who admitted to psychotic symptoms at the time gave a range of alternative explanations, involving revenge, sexual frustration, anger and arousal. The authors found similarities between the psychosexual profiles of mentally ill and non-mentally ill sex offenders and suggested that the presence of mental illness alone may provide only a partial explanation of sexual offending in this client group (Sahota and Chesterman 1998a).

Theories of sexual offending

Ward et al (2006: 15) noted that 'Theories are indispensable resources for clinical work with sexual offenders'. Theories should direct the clinician towards areas for assessment, assist with formulation and identify areas for treatment and risk management. The next section outlines the predominant theories which have been, or are, currently influential in this respect. It is perhaps a reflection of the heterogeneity and complexity of sexual offending that most theories have been developed to account for one type of offender.

Theories of sexual offending against children

Finkelhor's four preconditions model

Finkelhor's (1984) model of sexual offending against children was one of the first to take into account its complexity and tried to account for both the factors that contributed to motivation for sexual offending as well as the process by which it occurred. The model has been extremely influential in clinical practice in the United Kingdom, particularly in providing a framework for which many offenders can gain insight into the way their offending occurred.

Finkelhor suggested that there are four factors that are complementary in accounting for the motivation to sexually offend against a child, which make up the first of his preconditions:

I *Motivation.*

1. *Emotional congruence.* This describes the way in which children have a special meaning for many men who abuse children. For such individuals their emotional needs are met by children, who are viewed as safe and accepting, in contrast to adults.

2. *Sexual arousal.* Although the developmental cause may not be clear, some individuals acquire entrenched deviant sexual interests. For other offenders, however, sexual arousal by a child may be more temporary and situational.

3. *Blockage.* This describes the way in which some offenders are 'blocked' in their ability to meet their sexual and emotional needs in adult relationships. This could either be a developmental and persistent blockage (such as fear of intimacy) or situational and temporary (e.g. breakdown in an adult relationship). However, a situational blockage would not in itself be enough to lead to sexual offending without some pre-existing sexual interest.

4. *Overcoming inhibitions.* The above motivational factors therefore make up the first precondition for sexual offending against a child to occur. However, these are unlikely on their own to lead to actual offending behaviour, as further inhibitions need to be overcome. Finkelhor's subsequent preconditions describe the way this occurs.

II *Overcoming internal inhibitions.* Many men who sexually offend against children know at some level that their behaviour is wrong and therefore need to overcome their internal inhibitions. Finkelhor suggested that an individual's capacity for control may be diminished in a number of ways. These could involve internal psychological factors, such as using alcohol or drugs as a disinhibitor, or by failure of the 'incest inhibition mechanism' (i.e. a stepfather not having the usual inhibitions against sexual contact with children). Disinhibiting factors can be temporary or enduring (e.g. distorted beliefs, 'he/she doesn't mind'). Finkelhor also suggested that external societal factors contribute to the overcoming of inhibitions, and a current example of this is the wide availability of child pornography on the internet (Ward et al 2006). Such socio-cultural factors may undermine individuals' attempts to control their behaviour and reinforce their cognitive distortions.

III *Overcoming external inhibitions.* Once an individual has acquired the motivation to sexually offend against a child and overcome their internal inhibitions, the next step is to overcome external obstacles and create an opportunity to offend. Many offenders go to great lengths to set up situations where they can offend, for example, by befriending vulnerable women and children and encouraging the development of trust ('grooming'). There are certain situations that make it easier for an offender to overcome normal external inhibitions (i.e. parental supervision), such as a mother who is absent, ill or emotionally distant, a socially isolated family, or poor familial supervision of a child.

IV *Overcoming the resistance of the child.* The final step is for the offender to overcome any resistance from the child. This may be done in a number of ways, from gradually developing a friendship with the child and offering gifts, or using bribes, overt threats or violence. Often offenders desensitize children to sex by exposing them to pornography, or present their behaviour under the guise of sex education. Children who are emotionally insecure or have previously been abused are particularly vulnerable and may be deliberately targeted by offenders.

There are limitations with the Finkelhor model. Ward et al (2006) noted that it does not really explain how developmental factors contribute to the onset of offending or why emotional congruence and blockage are manifested in a sexual way. There is overlap between the key concepts of developmental blockage and emotional congruence. However, the main limitation is that it assumes that all men who offend against children do so because of a breakdown in their capacity for self-control and self-regulation and need to overcome personal inhibitions. It does not, therefore, account for the men who have no conflict about sexually offending against children and no inhibitions to overcome. Such individuals have clear 'approach goals' (Ward and Hudson 1996), and their problem lies in their choice of harmful goals rather than their lack of self-control. Nonetheless, despite the above theoretical limitations, Ward et al (2006) acknowledged that Finkelhor's preconditions model is useful in clinical practice in helping individuals understand that their offending did not 'just happen', and to identify the processes that preceded this. Areas for intervention, change, and monitoring can then be identified

Wolf's multi-factor model

Wolf (1985) proposed that experience of, or exposure to, early childhood adversity (such as physical, sexual or emotional abuse or neglect) leads to the development of a personality type in which the individual is vulnerable to developing deviant sexual interests. Such individuals are likely to have low self-esteem and a negative self-image, which then leads to an expectation of rejection by others and withdrawal from social contact. Sexual fantasies and masturbation become a way of compensating for a feeling of deprivation and powerlessness, and when those fantasies involve deviant imagery, such as children, they become further reinforced. Wolf argued that these processes operate in a cyclical way, in which following fantasy, a process of grooming a potential victim occurs, accompanied by cognitive distortions to justify their behaviour. Individuals who show this pattern of offending are likely to feel guilty, but alleviate these feelings by further rationalization and minimization. However, at some level, they are aware that what they have done is wrong, which may further lower their self esteem, increasing their vulnerability to start the cycle again.

It is now acknowledged that this model has only limited applicability to a single 'type' of offender, and again, does not account for the range of patterns of offending shown by men who abuse children. However, its focus on how sexual offending can be maintained, and its accessibility to both offenders and professionals, has meant that the model has been extremely influential in treatment programmes in the United Kingdom. Certainly for those individuals for whom the model *does* describe their pattern of offending, it can be extremely useful, first in helping them to identify this and then to guide subsequent interventions and strategies required to break the cycle.

Ward and Siegert's pathways model

The pathways model of child sexual abuse, developed by Ward and Siegert (2002) is the most recent and comprehensive aetiological theory to account for the complexity of contributory factors to sexual offending against children and the heterogeneity of offenders. It was originally constructed by 'theory knitting' the best elements of three previously very influential models (Finkelhor 1984; Hall and Hirschmann 1992; Marshall and Barbaree 1990).

Ward and Siegert observed that there are four clusters of difficulties frequently found in men who offend against children, namely (1) difficulties in identifying and controlling emotional states, such as anxiety or anger; (2) intimacy deficits, social isolation and loneliness; (3) offence-supportive beliefs (cognitive distortions); and (4) deviant sexual fantasies and arousal. These correspond to the four key dynamic (i.e. changing) risk factors identified by Thornton (2002). Vulnerability to these key difficulties will be influenced by biological factors, family environment, social learning and cultural issues. Sexual abuse of children may occur when these varying predispositions interact with situational triggers.

The pathways model suggests that each of the four problem areas and consequent 'implicit theories' (see above) are present to different degrees in men who offend against children. The particular pathway to offending will depending on which cluster provides the primary aetiological mechanism.

Pathway 1: Multiple dysfunctional mechanisms. This pathway represents individuals who have difficulties in all four of the problem areas and are likely to be 'pure paedophiles'. They are likely to have been sexually victimized and acquired a 'sexual script' in which an ideal sexual relationship is one between an older person and a child. They are likely to have an implicit theory of children as sexual beings.

Pathway 2: Deviant sexual scripts. This pathway represents individuals who may have been sexually victimized as a child and subsequently developed 'sexual scripts' in which sex takes place in an impersonal context and as a purely physical means of release. Such individuals may be likely to confuse sexual cues with those of affection and offend against children following periods of rejection by adults.

Pathway 3: Intimacy deficits. The third pathway is developed by individuals who have an insecure attachment style and difficulties with the development of intimate relationships. These individuals will be aroused by adults and generally prefer sexual relationships with adults but treat children as a 'pseudo-partner' in certain situations, for example, if there is a deterioration or break up in an adult relationship.

Pathway 4: Emotional dysregulation. This pathway represents individuals who have enduring problems with emotional regulation. Abuse of a child may be motivated by anger or become associated with a way of managing low mood and self-esteem.

Pathway 5: Antisocial cognitions. The final pathway represents individuals whose sexual offending is just one of a wide range of criminal behaviours. These individuals are unlikely to have enduring deviant arousal to children but hold general antisocial attitudes and disregard all social norms. They are likely to hold implicit theories of entitlement and 'dangerous world', that is, there is often a need to make a 'pre-emptive strike'.

Ward and Siegert acknowledge that the theory still needs refining in some areas and there is not, as yet, a supportive evidence base. The primary strength and subsequent influence of the model is its acknowledgement that there are multiple pathways to offending and that therefore a 'one size fits all' approach to treatment is unlikely to be successful (Ward et al 2006).

Theories of sexual offending against adults

Hall and Hirschmann's quadripartite model (1991)

Hall and Hirschmann's quadripartite model was originally developed to account for sexual aggression towards women and was reformulated to account for child sexual abuse (Hall and Hirschmann 1992). The authors proposed that there are four key vulnerabilities that contribute towards sexual offending: sexual arousal, cognitions justifying sexual aggression, affective dyscontrol (e.g. anger and hostility) and antisocial personality traits. Although each of these factors will contribute to offending, it is likely that one will be prominent, and an offence may occur when a 'critical threshold' is reached, and other situational factors and an opportunity is present. Negative early experiences increase the likelihood of the formation of antisocial attitudes and decrease the probability of adequate socialization. A key component of the model is whether an individual appraises the benefits of sexual aggression to outweigh the costs. This model also leads to a typology of offenders according to which factor is most prominent, and treatment can then be focused accordingly.

Again, this model has been comprehensively critically evaluated by Ward et al (2006), who pointed out the theoretical weaknesses, such as *how* the main components interact to cause sexual offending. However, Ward et al (2006: 59) also noted that the model 'does a marvellous job of identifying the significant clinical phenomena evident in sexual offenders'. The identification of the four clusters of problems are again similar to the four dynamic risk domains later identified by Thornton (2002) and are useful to clinicians in identifying areas of intervention.

Malamuth's confluence model

An important model of understanding sexual aggression towards women, supported by extensive research primarily using college students, has been developed by Malamuth et al (1993). This starts with the concept of 'rape proclivity', which is defined as 'the likelihood that an individual would commit a rape if they were guaranteed to get away with it'. Research to develop the model has focused on the characteristics of coercive men and is therefore particularly useful as a framework to begin to conceptualize men who have behaved in sexually aggressive ways towards women but have not been convicted.

Malamuth and colleagues suggested that childhood experiences lead to individual differences in six variables that have been shown to predict rape proclivity on self-report measures. These are sexual arousal to rape, dominance as a motive for sex, hostility towards women, attitudes facilitating aggression towards women, antisocial personality characteristics and sexual experience. These proclivity factors make up two separate pathways that converge to provide the motivation for sexually aggressive behaviour; *sexual promiscuity* (a preference for impersonal sex) and *hostile masculinity* (hostile, dominating and controlling personality traits). An individual is at high risk of committing a sexually aggressive act when these motivational factors combine with disinhibiting factors and the opportunity to behave in a sexually aggressive way.

Developing this model based on the research with men who have not been convicted of sexual offences is a unique strength. Although it cannot fully inform individual case formulation, the model can suggest useful areas of assessment and draws attention to relevant issues for risk management, such as a continuing preference for consenting impersonal sex (Ward et al 2006).

Treatment of sexual offenders

The last 15 years has seen a rapid expansion in the provision of treatment programmes for individuals convicted of sexual offences, both in the United Kingdom and overseas. In the United Kingdom there is now a comprehensive group treatment programme for convicted contact sexual offenders in the prison system and those on Community Rehabilitation Orders in the community. Mentally disordered sex offenders detained under the Mental Health Act are treated in medium and maximum secure hospitals (Addo 2002; Fisher et al 1998). However, group treatment programmes have been more systematically developed within the prison system than in hospital settings. Although treatment is based on the same theoretical models, treatment delivery in the latter setting is not systematically provided and depends on the availability of suitably trained staff, usually psychologists (see Green 2008; Houston and Scoales 2008 for further accounts of treatment within a forensic mental health service).

Treatment aims to increase the men's insight into their patterns of offending, identify and challenge distorted cognitions and implicit theories, increase victim empathy, address deviant fantasies, increase effective emotional and interpersonal functioning and develop relapse prevention skills and build 'good lives' (see Text Box 8.2; Ward, Yates and Long 2006). Accompanying the development of complex multi-variate models of sexual offending, as outlined earlier, is the

Box 8.2 Treatment focus with sex offenders

- Insight
- Distorted cognitions
- Victim empathy
- Deviant fantasies
- Interpersonal skills
- Relapse prevention
- 'Good lives'

recognition that sexual offenders are a widely heterogeneous group and that a 'one size fits all' approach to treatment is inappropriate (Ward et al 2006). This poses the challenge for group treatment programmes to meet the varying needs of individuals, according to their offence pathways. In particular, it is now acknowledged that the treatments needs of men who have 'avoidance goals' (i.e. those who are aware that their offending is wrong and offend because they use inappropriate coping strategies to deal with high-risk situations) are very different to those who have 'approach goals' (i.e. those whose goals are harmful in the first place and deliberately set out to commit a sexual offence). Treatment should therefore be directly linked with a formulation-based assessment of the individual.

There has been debate in the academic literature about whether treatment outcome studies are robust enough to conclude that the treatment of sex offenders is effective. In an extensive review of the available empirical evidence, including meta-analyses, Marshall (2006) pointed out that such evaluation is no easy task and comments on the difficulties of establishing robust randomized control trials in this area of treatment. He pointed out further that the effect size for sex offender treatment is similar to that for some other forms of psychological treatment and superior to some medical treatments for specified conditions, such as coronary bypass surgery, which despite having poor effect size, is clearly still a treatment worth undertaking. He concluded that the treatments with the greatest empirical support are the ones that have a combination of cognitive–behavioural therapy and relapse prevention, and it is these programmes that have seen the most successful periods of non-recidivism at follow-up.

Gaps in the provision of treatment services still remain for unconvicted offenders, particularly those with mental health problems. Outpatient groups are run by psychologists and colleagues in some forensic mental health services, although this varies around the country. It is unconvicted offenders who pose the greatest challenges to services, as there are no legal obligations on them to attend for treatment and they do not fall under the framework of the Multi-Agency Public Protection Arrangements (MAPPA), the multi-agency panels set up under the Criminal Justice Act 2000 to monitor convicted sex offenders.

Conclusions

Individuals who commit sexual offences clearly make up a widely heterogeneous group, and the aetiology of their behaviour is varied and complex. Information from the research and theories outlined in this chapter underpin approaches to both assessment and treatment. Clearly a range of biological, developmental, sexual, psychological, interpersonal and cognitive factors may be relevant to the development and maintenance of sexual offending. Understanding why and how an individual sexually offends is crucial in making decisions about treatment and future risk management. By being aware of the relevant theoretical background, clinicians are in a more informed position to carry out formulation-based clinical assessments and treatments that are individually focused, and it is encouraging that there is now a move away from the previous manualized 'one-size-fits-all' approach.

Finally, returning to the focus on sexual offending by wider society than just the media, it is clear that the far-reaching consequences for victims means that there is rightly much effort focused on preventing both offending and re-offending. This includes innovative services such as the 'Stop It Now!' telephone help line run by the Lucy Faithful Foundation in the United Kingdom for individuals who are concerned about their sexual behaviour or relatives concerned about that of others. Church organizations are also now addressing the issue of developing contracts with members of the congregation who have a history of sexual offending. It is encouraging that alongside the emotional responses to the fear of the unknown in relation to the 'stranger in our midst', there have developed thoughtful and rational approaches to the identification and management of potential risk posed by individuals who have committed sexual offences.

References

APA 1994 American Psychiatric Association Diagnostic and Statistical Manual 4th Edition. Washington DC: American Psychiatric Association.

Abel, G., Gore, D., Holland, C., Camp, N., Becker, J. and Rathner, J. 1989. The Measurement of the Cognitive Distortions of Child Molesters. Annals of Sex Research 2: 135–153.

Addo, M. 2002 Nursing Interventions and Future Directions with Sex Offenders 165–186 in Therapeutic Interventions for Forensic Mental Health Nurses (Kettles, A.M., Woods, P. and Collins, M. Editors) London: Jessica Kingsley.

Ahlmeyer, S., Kleinsasser, D., Stoner, J., and Retzklaff, P. 2003. Psychopathology of Incarcerated Sex Offenders. Journal of Personality Disorders 17: 306–318.

Baker, A. and Duncan, S. 1985 Child Sexual Abuse: A Study of Prevalence in Great Britain. Child Abuse and Neglect 9: 457–467.

British Crime Survey 1998, 2000 Details can be found at www.homeoffice.gov.uk/rds/bcs1.html.

Brown, S. 2005 Treating Sex Offenders: An Introduction to Sex Offender Treatment Programmes. Devon: Willan Publishing.

Carter, D.L., Prentky, R.A., Knight, R.A., Vanderveer, P.L. and Boucher, R.J. 1987 Use of Pornography in the Criminal and Developmental Histories of Sexual Offenders. Journal of Interpersonal Violence 2: 196–211.

Chesterman, P. and Sahota, K. 1998 Mentally Ill Sex Offenders in a Regional Secure Unit. I: Psychopathology and Motivation. Journal of Forensic Psychiatry 9: 150–160.

Craissati, J. 2004 Managing High Risk Sex Offenders in the Community: A Psychological Approach. Hove, Sussex: Brunner-Routledge.

Craissati, J. and Hodes, P. 1992 Mentally Ill Sex Offenders: The Experience of a Regional Secure Unit. British Journal of Psychiatry 161: 846–849.

Craisatti, J. and McClurg, G. 1996 The Challenge Project: Perpetrators of Child Sexual Abuse in South East London. Child Abuse and Neglect 20: 1067–1077.

Craissati, J., McClurg, G., and Browne, K. 2002 Characteristics of Perpetrators of Child Sexual Abuse Who Have Been Sexually Victimized as Children. Sexual Abuse: A Journal of Research and Treatment 14: 225–238.

Falshaw, L., Friendship, C. and Bates, A. 2003 Sexual Offenders – Measuring Reconviction, Re-offending and Recidivism. Home Office Research Development and Statistics Directorate, Findings No. 183. Available from publications.rds@homeoffice.gsi.gov.uk

Finkelhor, D. 1984 Child Sexual Abuse: New Theory and Research. New York: Free Press.

Finkelhor, D. 1994 Current Information on the Scope and Nature of Child Sexual Abuse. Future of Children 4, 2: 31–53.

Fisher, D., Grubin, D. and Perkins, D. 1998 Working with Sexual Offenders in Psychiatric Settings in England and Wales 191–201 in Source Book of Treatment Programs for Sexual Offenders (Marshall, W.L. Fernandez, Y.M. Hudson, S.M. and Ward, T. Editors) London: Plenum Press.

Goodman, R.E. 1987 Genetic and Hormonal Factors 21–48 in Human Sexuality: Evolutionary and Developmental Perspectives. In Variant Sexuality: Research and Theory (Wilson, G.D. Editor) Baltimore: Johns Hopkins University Press.

Green, T. 2008 Treatment, Relapse Prevention and Building 'Good Lives' 174–194 in Sexual Offending and Mental Health: Multi-disciplinary Risk Management in the Community (Houston, J. and Galloway, S. Editors) London: Jessica Kingsley.

Hall, G.C.N. and Hirschmann, R. 1991 Towards a Theory of Sexual Aggression: A Quadripartite Model. Journal of Consulting and Clinical Psychology 59: 662–669.

Hall, G.C.N. and Hirschmann, R. 1992. Sexual Aggression against Children: A Conceptual Perspective of Etiology. Criminal Justice and Behaviour 19: 8–23.

Home Office – Recorded Crime Statistics 1898–2004/5. Available from Http://www.homeoffice.gov.uk/rds/pdfs/1000years.x1s

Home Office 2007 Rape Conviction Rates. Available from http://www.homeoffice.gov.uk/rds/pdfs07/rdsolrl807.pdf

Houston, J. and Scoales, M. 2008 A Sex Offender Service within a Mental Health Setting. 131–151 in Sexual Offending and Mental Health: Multi-disciplinary Risk Management in the Community (Houston, J. and Galloway, S. Editors) London: Jessica Kingsley.

Hudson, S.M. and Ward, T. 1997 Attachment, Anger and Intimacy in Sexual Offenders. Journal of Interpersonal Violence 12: 13–24.

Lalumiere, M.L. and Quinsey, V.L. 1994 The Discriminability of Rapists from Non-rapists Using Phallometric Measures: A Meta-analysis. Criminal Justice and Behaviour 5: 435–445.

Leitenberg H and Henning K 1995. Sexual fantasy. Psychological Bulletin 117: 469–496.

Leonard, R.A. 1993 The Family Backgrounds of Serial Rapists. Issues in Criminological and Legal Psychology 19: 9–18.

Lewis, P. 1991 The Report of the Working Party on the Assessment and Treatment of Sex Offenders at Broadmoor Hospital. Internal Document.

Madsen, L., Parsons, S. and Grubin, D. 2006 The Relationship between the Five-factor Model and DSM Personality Disorder in a Sample of Child Molesters. Personality and Individual Differences 40: 227–236.

Malamuth, N.M., Heavey, C.L. and Linz, D. 1993 Predicting Men's Antisocial Behaviour against Women: The Interaction Model of Sexual Aggression 63–98 in Sexual Aggression: Issues in Etiology, Assessment and Treatment. (Hall, G.C.N., Hirschmann, R., Graham, J.R. and Zaragoza, M.S. Editors) Washington DC: Taylor & Francis.

Marshall, W.L. 1989 Invited Essay: Intimacy, Loneliness and Sexual Offenders. Behaviour Research and Therapy 27: 491–503.

Marshall, W.L. 1996 The Sexual Offender: Monster, Victim or Everyman? Sexual Abuse: A Journal of Research and Treatment 8: 317–335.

Marshall, W.L. 2006 Diagnostic Problems with Sex Offenders 33–44 in Sexual Offender Treatment: Controversial Issues (Marshall, W.L. Fernandez, Y.M. Marshall, L.E. and Serran, G.A. Editors) Chichester: Wiley.

Marshall, W.L. and Barbaree, H.E. 1990 An Integrated Theory of the Etiology of Sexual Offending 257–275 in Handbook of Sexual Assault: Issues, Theories and Treatment of the Offender (Marshall, W.L., Laws, D.L and Barbaree, H.E. Editors) New York: Plenum Press.

Marshall, W.L., Barbaree, H.E. and Christopher, D. 1986 Sexual Offenders against Female Children: Preferences for Age of Victim and Type of Behaviour. Canadian Journal of Behavioural Science 18: 424–439.

Marshall, W.L., Jones, R.J., Ward, T., Johnston, P.W. and Barbaree, H. 1991 Treatment Outcome with Sex Offenders. Clinical Psychology Review 11: 465–485.

McClurg, G. and Craissati, J. 1999 A Descriptive Study of Alleged Sexual Abusers Known to Social Services. Journal of Sexual Aggression 4: 22–30.

Myhill, A. and Allen, J. 2002 Rape and Sexual Assault on Women: Findings from the British Crime Survey. Home Office Research Development and Statistics Directorate, Findings No. 159. Available from publications.rds@homeoffice.gsi.gov.uk

Polaschek, D.L.L. and Ward, T. 2002 The Implicit Theories of Potential Rapists: What Our Questionnaires Tell Us. Aggression and Violent Behavior 7: 385–406.

Prentky, R.A., Knight, R.A., Sims-Knight, J.E., Straus, H., Rokous, F. and Cerce, D. 1989 Developmental Antecedents of Sexual Aggression. Development and Psychopathology 1: 153–169.

Sahota, K. and Chesterman, P. 1998a Mentally Ill Sex Offenders in a Regional Secure Unit. II: Cognitions, Perceptions and Fantasies. The Journal of Forensic Psychiatry 9: 161–172.

Sahota, K. and Chesterman, P. 1998b Sexual Offending in the Context of Mental Illness. Journal of Forensic Psychiatry 9: 267–280.

Saradjian, J. and Hanks, H. 1996 Women Who Sexually Abuse Their Children: from Research to Practice. Chichester: Wiley.

Seidman, B., Marshall, W.L., Hudson, S.M. and Robertson, P.J. 1994. An Examination of the Intimacy and Loneliness in Sex Offenders. Journal of Interpersonal Violence 13: 555–573.

Smallbone, S.W. 2006 An Attachment – Theoretical Revision of Marshall and Barbaree's Integrated Theory of the Etiology of Sexual Offending 93–107 in Sexual Offender Treatment: Controversial issues (Marshall, W.L. Fernandez, Y.M. Marshall, L.E. and Serran, G.A. Editors) Chichester: John Wiley & Sons.

Soothill, K. 2003 Serious Sexual Assault: Using History and Statistics 29–50 in Sex Offenders in the Community: Managing and Reducing Risks (Matravers, A. Editor) Devon: Willan Publishing.

Stuart, M. and Baines, C. 2004 Progress on Safeguards for Children Living Away from Home: A Review of Action since the People Like Us Report. Available from York Publishing Services, 64 Horefield Road, Layerthrope, York YO31 7ZQ.

Thornton, D. 2002 Constructing and Testing a Framework for Dynamic Risk Assessment. Sexual Abuse: A Journal of Research and Treatment 14: 139–154.

Ward, T. and Hudson, S.M. 1996 Relapse Prevention: A Critical Analysis. Sexual Abuse: A Journal of Research and Treatment 8: 177–200.

Ward, T. and Keenan, T. 1999 Child Molesters' Implicit Theories. Journal of Interpersonal Violence 14: 821–838.

Ward, T. and Siegert, R.J. 2002 Toward a Comprehensive Theory of Child Sexual Abuse: A Theory Knitting Perspective. Psychology Crime and Law 9: 319–351.

Ward, T. Polaschek, D.L.L. and Beech, A.R. 2006 Theories of Sexual Offending. Chichester: Wiley.

Ward, T., Yates, P.M. and Long, C.A. 2006 The Self-regulation Model of the Offense and Relapse Process. A Manual. Volume II: Treatment. Victoria BC: Pacific Psychological Assessment Corporation.

Wolf, F.C.S. 1985 A Multi-factor Model of Deviant Sexuality. Victimology 10: 359–374.

Young, J.E. 1990 Cognitive Therapy for Personality Disorders: A Schema-focused Approach. Sarasota FL: Professional Resource Exchange.

Chapter 9

Responses to violence and trauma: the case of post-traumatic stress disorder

Gwen Adshead, Annie Bartlett and Gillian Mezey

Aim

To describe social and psychiatric models of response to individual and organized violence.

Learning objectives

- To explain how people respond to traumatic events
- To outline the medico-legal significance of Post-traumatic Stress Disorder (PTSD)
- To provide a cross-cultural critique of PTSD
- To understand the possible relevance of PTSD to forensic populations

---

Introduction

Traumatic events can be defined as those that cause intense fear, helplessness and distress in humans (APA 1994). Historically, traumatic events have been understood and reported in religious or dramatic terms: there are reports of the effect of war trauma on soldiers in Homer (Rieu 1957) and Shakespeare described the effects of murder in tragedies such as Macbeth.

> Pluck from the memory a rooted sorrow;
> Raze out the written troubles of the brain;
> And with some sweet oblivious antidote
> Cleanse the stuff'd bosom of that perilous stuff
> Which weighs upon the heart?
>
> Shakespeare: Macbeth (Scene 3, Act 5)

Contemporary writers such as Sebastian Faulks (1984) and Pat Barker (1991) wrote vivid and accessible accounts of war trauma; journalists such as Fergal Keane bear witness to the effects of civil conflict internationally, in this case in Rwanda (1996). Historians such as Anthony Beevor writing about the major European conflicts of the twentieth century (1999, 2003) infuse their factual accounts with an understanding of the human dimension of war. This is emphasized in the personal accounts of writers like Primo Levi (1979) reflecting on the Holocaust or Hanan Al-Shaykh (1996) describing civil war in Beirut. Equally, there are well-known fictional examples of individual trauma, for example, physical abuse of children in Nicholas Nickleby (Dickens 1998) or psychological abuse in 'Oranges Are not the Only Fruit' (Winterson 1991). We have an enduring interest in examining past and present, personal and societal trauma and its consequences. It has not been self-evident that professional understandings of trauma and its consequences carry greater authority than these other ways of reflecting on these issues.

This chapter describes and evaluates the relatively recent mental health models of the impact of trauma. We will discuss the ways that traumatic events affect people, and the political and cultural effects of understanding these consequences as 'disorder', particularly as Post-traumatic Stress Disorder (PTSD). We conclude by looking at the relevance of the concept of PTSD to forensic populations.

It is only in the twentieth century that the psychological effects of trauma have been examined as distinct *psychopathological* phenomena, i.e. as something that is abnormal, diagnosable and requiring treatment, as opposed to understandable and normal responses to stress.[1] The introduction of the railway provided us with the first systematic descriptions of emotional and behavioural responses to trauma, following railway accidents. Symptoms of loss of emotional control, lack of sleep, increased state of alertness and intensification of distress when exposed to reminders, were described, which are very reminiscent of what we would now recognize as PTSD. At the time, the cause of such symptoms was thought to be 'physical', owing to a form of spinal concussion, or 'railway spine', rather than psychological in origin (see Trimble 1981). The second major contributor to our understanding of psychological trauma was World War I, which created a wave of psychological casualties, irrespective of physical injuries, and the first descriptions of 'shellshock' (see Shephard 2000 for history of war trauma). The descriptions of terrified young men, unable to sleep or eat, haunted by images, smells and sounds of battle, incapable of talking or reflecting about the horrors they have witnessed, but appearing to be reliving them, are startlingly similar to modern descriptions of PTSD in both civilian and military causalities.[2]

How people respond to traumatic events

Traumatic events are those that evoke intense feelings of fear or horror and which, in many cases, override the individual's capacity to think or behave in an effective way or to control their emotions. Such events may be very sudden and brief (such as accidents, assaults and natural disasters) or more prolonged and recurring (such as illegal detentions, torture, family and domestic violence). Epidemiological studies indicate that traumatic events are very common in the civilian population. The most frequently reported traumas in Western societies are sexual abuse/assault (for women only), physical assault and road traffic accidents. Only the minority of individuals (about 10%) develop PTSD (Breslau et al 1998) and full psychological recovery from trauma is the norm, even after potentially life-threatening trauma (Kessler et al 1995). Rates of lifetime PTSD in the community are about 7% (Kessler et al 1995), with women being at greater risk of developing PTSD following exposure to a trauma than men (Breslau et al 1997). Although the role of the traumatic event is considered to be crucial in determining post-traumatic responses and recovery, it is also necessary to recognize the role played by other factors, such as personal vulnerability and societal/cultural factors, in the development of PTSD (see Text Box 9.1; MacFarlane 1989).

Although PTSD is probably the most well-known (and controversial) psychiatric disorder following trauma, other psychiatric conditions, in particular depression, anxiety states and alcohol and substance misuse, are equally common responses (Kessler et al 1995). Regardless of

---

[1] This medicalization is therefore not of 'social deviance', the historical critique of the psychiatric enterprise (see Bartlett, this volume), rather it is the medicalization of the 'normal' and their understandable responses to unpleasant things happening to them.

[2] In her war trilogy, Pat Barker brings together fact and fiction, depicting the condition of men rescued from the front in World War I. They receive treatment at Craiglockhart Hospital in Scotland, which did exist and did treat soldiers with shellshock.

Box 9.1 Factors affecting the development of PTSD

+ Pre-trauma – female gender; family or personal psychiatric history; previous trauma or loss; low IQ; low self-esteem; neuroticism

+ Trauma – exposure to death/dying; life threat; intentional harm by others/interpersonal violence; sexual violence; combat; deliberately humiliating experiences, causing intense shame and guilt (such as organized rape, torture, war atrocities, prison abuse)

+ Responses during trauma: perceived life threat, loss of control/helplessness versus effective coping; dissociation

+ Following trauma – cognitions/attributions regarding trauma, including shame/self-blame; stresses resulting from trauma, for example, financial/ housing/occupational/interpersonal; legal proceedings and so on

psychiatric diagnosis, common themes associated with victimization include feelings of loss, betrayal, anger, mistrust, self-blame and a sense of having been fundamentally and (in some cases) irretrievably damaged by the experience (Brewin 2003; Ehlers et al 2000).

This chapter focuses on Post-traumatic Stress Disorder (PTSD) because of the importance it has acquired as the diagnosis 'prima inter pares' for victims, lawyers and psychiatrists (Mezey and Robbins 2001). The diagnosis, which was first introduced in the DSM in 1980 (APA 1980) has subsequently undergone a number of revisions, to reflect changing views and observations about the nature and definition of psychological trauma. Post-traumatic Stress Disorder became incorporated into the ICD classification system for psychiatric disorders only in 1994 (WHO 1994). Both classification systems refer to the pre-existence of a major trauma, which may be life-threatening. The DSM-IV definition of a trauma currently includes indirect exposure, through witnessing or being confronted with a traumatic event as well as directly experienced events. The criteria additionally specify that the individual's subjective responses at the time should include feelings of fear, horror or helplessness. Without a pre-existing traumatic event, no diagnosis of PTSD should be made.

The clinical features of PTSD include symptoms of re-experiencing, such as nightmares, reliving and 'flashbacks' (Criterion B); behavioural and cognitive avoidance of reminders of the trauma (Criterion C) and hyperarousal symptoms, including increased startle response; poor sleep; irritability and hypersensitivity to environmental threat (Criterion D). Symptoms must be present for at least a month and be associated with impaired functioning (social/interpersonal/occupational) or distress. If symptoms have been present for 3 months the condition is described as chronic. Although spontaneous recovery after this point is possible, the longer symptoms persist, the less likely they are to resolve spontaneously without psychological intervention. Studies of PTSD show that the condition may persist unrecognized and untreated over many years (Kessler et al 1995; Kilpatrick et al 1989; Norris 1992).

The bio-neuro-physiology of post-traumatic stress responses is increasingly studied and described, with changes affecting the noradrenergic sympathetic nervous system (the 'fright/flight/fight' response), particularly in the short term; changes in steroid and neurotransmitter production and dysregulation of the hypothalamic–pituitary–adrenal (HPA) axis. The sympathetic nervous system response is designed to be a short-term response only, and it is 'switched off' by the next phase of the fear response, which is mediated by the cortisol parasympathetic response. This cortisol response is regulated by two parts of the brain, the hypothalamus (which controls all hormone production) and the hippocampus (which regulates memory). Cortisol release is a normal response to stress; however, under extreme conditions the production there may be long-lasting hormonal changes, including cortisol production and release which, in turn, may result in damage to brain structures affecting emotional control and memory (Yehuda 2001; Yehuda et al 1993).

If the cortisol response does not activate properly, or is insufficient, then the noradrenergic effects of the sympathetic nervous system will persist, and the effects described above will not resolve spontaneously. Instead, the survivor may continue to experience nightmares and intrusive memories of the event, as if it were happening in the present. In addition, low levels of cortisol, as a result of previous victimization, may make the individual more vulnerable to developing PTSD following subsequent trauma exposure. Resnick and colleagues (1995) found, for example, that rape victims with a previous history of sexual abuse showed an attenuated cortisol response following the rape and also had higher rates of PTSD subsequently than women with no previous sexual-assault history.

It is hypothesized that traumatic events cause such intense emotional responses that they are not easily incorporated into long-term memory in the hippocampus (Brewin 2001; Brewin et al 1996) but continue to manifest themselves, often as partial memories, intrusions or amnesia.

Epidemiological studies have consistently found that certain traumas are more psychologically toxic than others. Victims of interpersonal violence and sexual assault, in particular, and combat veterans appear to be at greater risk of developing PTSD than victims of accidents or 'natural disasters' (Kessler et al 1995; Kilpatrick et al 1989).

The medico-legal significance of PTSD

Since Post-traumatic Stress Disorder was first recognized as a psychiatric diagnosis (APA 1980), it has been used as a basis for a number of different legal actions in England and Wales and elsewhere. Indeed, it has been argued that the diagnosis of PTSD has contributed to and, in many ways, fuelled the growth of a compensation culture because of its legal utility in claiming for psychological damages (Napier and Wheat 1995).

In civil law, people who have experienced traumatic events may claim damages for psychological as well as other injuries suffered. Expert evidence is often required to testify as to whether the individual does have PTSD or other post-traumatic psychiatric illness. Independent experts frequently find themselves giving testimony that is then disputed by the other side. For example, one side may say that the claimant has PTSD, and the other may say they are malingering, or that the psychiatric problem pre-dated the trauma. The psychiatric experts are likely to face cross-examination, the purpose of which is to examine the robustness of the evidence (Mezey 2006).

PTSD has also been used as a basis for a criminal defence, usually to serious charges involving physical violence (Sparr 1996). In the United States, where the insanity defence is used more widely, PTSD has been used as a basis for Not Guilty by Reason of Insanity (Appelbaum et al 1993). In English courts, PTSD has been used as the basis to support both the insanity defence and the diminished responsibility defence in cases of murder (Adshead and Mezey 1997). It has featured most notably in cases involving battered women who have killed abusive partners (Rix 2001). Interestingly, there have also been recent attempts to review historical court martial convictions of cowardice, based on PTSD (Wessely 2006).

In addition to civil and criminal law, PTSD is also important in other legal fora. In the family courts, PTSD may be given as a reason for a mother not allowing her children contact with a father who has allegedly been violent to her. In relation to immigration tribunals, those claiming asylum from persecution in their own country may seek to show that they have PTSD as evidence for having a legitimate fear of returning. This is particularly so in those cases where asylum seekers have been tortured. In employment law cases, PTSD is a recognized sequel to stressful events that an employer should seek to protect employees from under Health and Safety Legislation. There have been a number of cases where employees have sought damages from their employers for failing to prevent them suffering traumatic stress at work, or failing to support them in preventing the development of a post-traumatic psychiatric illness.

Finally, evidence of PTSD may be used to provide corroboration for disputed claims of physical or sexual assault by victims in legal proceedings. This has particularly been tested in cases of rape, domestic violence and child abuse in both criminal and civil settings (Raum 1983).

Given the wide range of uses to which PTSD can be put and the significant judicial and financial incentives associated with a successful claim, it is not surprising that there has been considerable disquiet expressed about the potential for misuse, as well as usefulness, of the diagnosis, in civil claims for psychiatric injury. PTSD, more than any other psychiatric diagnosis, establishes a causal link between the psychological injury and the trauma event. There is thus a perverse incentive for individuals to fabricate or exacerbate symptoms of post-traumatic distress and dysfunction for financial gain. By contrast, individuals who fail to exhibit diagnosable symptoms following the same trauma may be seen to lose out in the compensation lottery. It may be possible to distinguish the genuine from the false claimant by conducting a rigorous clinical examination, cross-referencing across numerous sources of information, checking for consistency and coherence of accounts and applying validated psychological measures of malingering, such as the Structured Interview of Reported Symptoms (SIRS; Mezey 2006; Rogers et al 1992). However, no expert should claim that they are infallible, in the sense of always knowing whether an evaluee's account of their experiences is accurate; evidence given should be appropriately cautious, and experts should qualify any opinion by specifying areas of inconsistency and uncertainty, where they exist.

Over the past few years there have been significant developments in the conceptualization and changes to the diagnostic criteria as well in the management and treatment of PTSD (NICE guidelines 2005). Despite its relatively recent arrival in the list of psychiatric disorders, it is clearly here to stay, although it is likely to be revised for DSM-V (Rosen et al 2008).

The cross-cultural critique of PTSD

Despite the widespread acceptance of the value of the diagnosis, PTSD has its critics. This is evident in the field of cross-cultural psychiatry, where it constitutes the latest battleground between anthropology and psychiatry (Text Box 9.2).

The principal focus of the enduring relationship between anthropology, the study of cultures, and psychiatry has been the problem of illness categories (e.g. Carstairs and Kapur 1976; Littlewood and Lipsedge 1985; Marsella and White 1982; Yap 1965). Anthropology is concerned with the

---

Box 9.2 Critique of PTSD

- A legal construction which persists because of potential financial rewards for lawyers and psychiatrists
- A manifestation of a 'risk-averse' culture, where there are no accidents, and everyone is a victim
- PTSD is insensitive to non-Western responses to stress, and privileges inappropriately psychological frameworks and interventions
- In civil conflict the psychologization of trauma undermines efforts to obtain legal redress

social world and cultural understandings. Psychiatry is necessarily concerned with individuals' mental processes and the ways and extent to which they become pathological, that is, not normal. The two disciplines employ substantially different methods of inquiry and they evaluate data and material by different standards. This has created contested 'knowledge'. The status of trans-cultural psychiatry has been questioned, specifically the value of epidemiological insights and the interventions that might follow from establishing disorders in settings around the world (Leff 1988; Kleinman 1987; Sartorius et al 1986). The charge, in its most generic form, from anthropology is of cultural insensitivity.

The practical consequence of this is that psychiatric classification of a kind found in ICD-10 (WHO 1992) or DSM-IV (APA 1994) is compared, usually unfavourably, with what are presented as sensitive local illness narratives, that is, an alternative, culturally sensitive, set of 'symptoms', classifications and interventions (Fabrega 1982; Good et al 1985). In this sense there is nothing new in suggesting that the international epidemiology of PTSD might be missing the point.

In the field of PTSD, or societal response to trauma, the validity of the category, as a way of capturing responses to traumatic events, is questioned. This critique is based on Kleinman's (1987) category fallacy argument, which observed that indigenous, non-Western illness narratives do not necessarily match those of Western psychiatry, in that crucial symptoms can be left out, or added in and given inappropriate importance. In addition, and linked with this theoretical point, is a debate about appropriate interventions. Psychological treatment is favoured in the NICE guidelines, but that is because of the acceptance of a psychological framework of understanding and evaluated interventions in Northern Europe and North America. The circumstances in which individuals elsewhere might have PTSD may not lend themselves to psychological remedies. This may be because social enterprises, the literal rebuilding of community, may be considered more important. Also, where resources are constrained, difficult decisions may have to be taken as to the best outcome for most people, and psychological intervention may be low down on the list of essential priorities.

The following two case studies of Rwanda and South Africa illustrate how this discussion has taken place in countries suffering recent civil strife.

Rwanda

Rwanda became an independent republic in 1962. Identity cards specifying the ethnicity of the holder, Hutu or Tutsi, had been carried since 1931, and this practice continued until 1994. In 1994, the assassination of the Hutu President Habyarimana sparked widespread massacres of Tutsis (Hatzfeld 2005: xi–xiii). Fergal Keane's account of this civil conflict (Keane 1996: 143–156) describes the aftermath of a massacre in a church in Nyarubuye. The Tutsis in the area had been advised to seek sanctuary in the church by a local Hutu political leader. They rounded themselves up for slaughter. Subsequently, the journalists interviewed survivors, some of whom were troubled by recurrent images of what happened, a classical PTSD 'reliving' experience. But their priorities are practical. They are, if able, caring for survivors who have been physically injured or deprived of food for some time. The Hutu leader has fled his house, leaving his crops rotting and his labourers dead. The presence or absence of psychological symptoms seems to the reader an irrelevance. Food and medical attention for machete wounds are more urgent. Then, the community must deal with the agricultural cycle. Without proper attention to the land, there would be no seeds for the following year and the cattle would die. Then people would starve or become dependent on food aid from Western nations. In Hatzfeld's (2005) account of the perpetrators of the massacre, he documents the return, a decade later, to a semblance of normality in the community of Nyamata, a rural area much affected by the intercommunal violence. Five thousand Tutsis had been killed in a single day in a church and a maternity hospital. By 2003, only six individuals had been executed for these and other homicides. Those who had killed were beginning to emerge from prison on probation. These individuals, he speculates, seem less traumatized than the surviving victims. The survivors suffer recurrent nightmares and great guilt. The killers, if they do have nightmares, dream of their prisons rather than of the horror of their past actions. Now in Nyamata, farming has recommenced. The Tutsis abandoned their isolated housing and opted to live together for safety. The town of Nyamata looks thriving with an influx of new commercial goods and the advent of computers. The humanitarian agencies have left and the town is on its own with its past.

Rwanda attempted to deal with its history of communal strife and violence legally. Only a small number of perpetrators have been brought to justice. The fit between the gravity of the insult to community and the capacity of legal or quasi legal fora to bring either justice or reconciliation is poor.

South Africa

Kaminer et al (2001) reported on the Truth and Reconciliation Commission in South Africa. They argued in support of PTSD. The Commission aired in public, using first-hand testimony, the litany of abuses perpetrated by the apartheid regime. The authors noted that the Commission's final report suggested that it had served a therapeutic function, that is, that it addressed societal and individual trauma using a non-clinical approach. Kaminer et al (2001) found that of 134 participants in the Commission's process, that is, individuals who had suffered major trauma, 42% had a diagnosis of PTSD. Strikingly, none of these individuals had had this diagnosis made previously. The high level of post-Commission morbidity undermines the argument that the Commission was inherently therapeutic. The authors recommended conventional interventions for the symptomatic groups in their sample, despite suggesting that the instruments used to measure PTSD were limited in only having been validated on Western populations. Kagee and Naidoo (2004) argued that Kaminer et al's (2001) study may also have been affected by financial considerations. The study took place at a time when those testifying to the Commission were awaiting financial compensation, a factor that may have affected their reporting of symptoms, albeit not the experience of trauma. Kagee and Naidoo's more general point, in the South African context, was that there are real methodological concerns about the epidemiology of PTSD. First, the quality of the epidemiology is variable, specifically in relation to whether trauma-based symptoms are matched by interference in daily functioning. Second, they question the relevance of PTSD phenomenology to the individual; they suggest the meaning of these symptoms is significantly influenced by the cultural context in which trauma occurred, as has been well documented elsewhere (Jones 2002; Jones and Kafetsios 2002).

This may seem a sterile academic debate about medical model thinking. However, its importance is evident from the scale of international civil conflict. Summerfield (2000) noted 40 active violent conflicts; this has displaced 1% of the world's population. In a series of papers (1999, 2000, 2001, 2002, Bracken et al 1995) Summerfield is sceptical about the value of the concept of PTSD and its applicability to non-Western populations, and fiercely critical of psychological interventions. He stresses the individuality of cultures, the presence of long-term stresses in impoverished communities and seeks to reframe community experience from victimhood to resilience. Social rebuilding, including legal redress, rather than psychological rebuilding is the key. Equally, there is evidence of the apparent utility of PTSD and other psychiatric diagnoses as descriptions of responses to trauma; non-Western populations can use Western-style hospitals alongside indigenous sources of support (Hollifield et al 2008).

Displaced populations in the United Kingdom

The United Kingdom is host to many refugees and asylum seekers. The situation for many of these individuals is very different from that of those able to remain, if not at home, at least in a culturally familiar context. The absence of social support, more likely if one has been uprooted and transplanted many thousands of miles away, may itself cause mental distress (Gorst-Unsworth et al 1998). A proportion of such individuals find themselves arguing for residence in the United Kingdom and some are seen within UK trauma services. Many are victims of state-sponsored torture. Turner and Gorst-Unsworth (1990) suggested that torture can be defined satisfactorily, but responses to it are complex and should incorporate social and political consequences in the framework of understanding. Turner and his colleagues remain wedded to the notion of psychological intervention (McIvor and Turner 1995). They argued that social and community organizations will offer non-clinical support to the majority of individuals; clinic populations have more severe psychiatric problems and warrant explicit treatment. However, later work (Turner et al 2003) showed overall high rates of morbidity using standardized measures in non-clinical samples of refugees; the rate of PTSD is just below 50%. This draws attention to the difficulty, even in a UK context, of allocating resources for treatment and resources for non-clinical interventions and to the resilience of many individuals who have experienced horrific trauma.

In summary, there is an ongoing debate about the value of PTSD as a model to describe people's responses to trauma cross-culturally. Nonetheless, it remains conceptually powerful, not least because it identifies and privileges the cause of an individual's difficulties as well as containing implications for effective intervention.

The relevance of post-traumatic disorders to forensic populations

PTSD and post-traumatic psychiatric illness are frequently encountered in forensic psychiatric practice. Mentally Disordered Offenders (MDOs) have high rates of childhood trauma, particularly physical and sexual abuse, and PTSD often co-exists in these populations with other axis 1 and axis 2 diagnoses (Sarkar et al 2005). Violent offenders may also be traumatized by their own violent behaviour and develop post-traumatic stress reactions, of re-experiencing, avoidance and hyperarousal, not dissimilar to those seen in victims (Evans et al 2007). In addition, forensic practitioners may be required to assess psychological trauma in victims of violent crime, including victims of sexual and domestic violence (King et al 2002; Mezey et al 2005) and family members of homicide victims (Mezey et al 2002). Knowledge of the range of post-traumatic stress reactions may be required for medico-legal purposes, to explain violent or criminal actions and the impact of those acts on the victim, and to comment on treatment approaches and prognosis.

Patients with severe mental illness are more likely to have suffered violent victimization as adults than non-patients (Hodgins et al 2007; Teplin et al 2005; Walsh et al 2003) and have higher rates of lifetime and current PTSD (MacFarlane et al 2001). Patients with pre-existing psychiatric conditions are more likely to develop PTSD after trauma (such as violent assault), and PTSD symptoms, such as irritability, hypervigilance and substance abuse, could increase the risk of violence in such patients, especially those with paranoid psychoses. In psychotic patients, it may be difficult to distinguish hypervigilance from paranoid states (Scott et al 2007). Rates of childhood and adult trauma are even higher in forensic than non-forensic psychiatric populations (Coid 1992; Sarkar et al 2005). Victims of childhood abuse and maltreatment are likely to become aggressive socially excluded adolescents (Dodge et al 1990) who remain at high risk of antisocial behaviour and violence in adulthood (Johnson et al 1999; Luntz and Widom 1994; Widom 1989).

The mechanisms connecting childhood trauma with adult antisocial and violent behaviour are complex and multi-factorial. One possible explanation is that early abuse and neglect produce a chronic fear response in the child, which causes disruption to the cortisol stress response system, which eventually becomes hyporesponsive. The adrenergic system is then comparatively hyperactive, causing chronic irritability, hypervigilance and poor anxiety regulation. Disruption to the serotonergic system has also been implicated as a mediating factor between childhood trauma with increased arousal and impulsivity, early 'personality dysfunction' and delinquency, including substance misuse, often as an attempt to combat symptoms of hypervigilance and hyperarousal (Caspi and Moffitt 2004). Recent research has also identified a functional polymorphism in the gene encoding the neurotransmitter–metabolizing enzyme monoamine oxidase (Caspi et al 2002). Maltreated children with low levels of gene activity are significantly more likely to develop antisocial behaviours in later life than maltreated children with high levels of MAOA expression. These findings suggest a significant gene–environment interaction in determining outcome following maltreatment, and begin to explain why not all abused or maltreated children grow up to behave aggressively or to victimize others.

There has been considerable research interest in whether perpetration of trauma is itself traumatic. There is some limited evidence to support this, mainly from the literature on army veterans (Haley 1974), as well as individual case reports and cohort studies of offenders (prisoners and treatment seekers) who appear to exhibit symptoms of PTSD in relation to their violent actions (Evans et al 2007; Thomas et al 1994). The relatively high rate of claimed amnesia following perpetration of a violent offence has been seen as a possible manifestation of peri-traumatic dissociation at the time of the offence and of post-traumatic avoidance (Pyszora et al 2003). The risk of developing post-traumatic symptoms for violent offenders appears to be highest where there is a pre-existing close relationship with the victim, which creates additional emotional conflict, guilt and complicated grief reactions (Taylor and Kopelman 1984).

It follows that those working in forensic settings need to give some thought to the treatment of post-traumatic psychopathology, especially symptoms of re-experiencing, hyperarousal, hypervigilance and depression. Depression is probably underdiagnosed, especially in male patients, and vigorous treatment with anti-depressants should be considered. Patients who experience post-traumatic imagery may benefit from specific trauma-focused psychological interventions (NICE 2005). Symptoms of hyperarousal may respond to antipsychotic agents in small doses. However, although it is important to acknowledge and validate offenders' accounts of victimization and maltreatment, it is also important to avoid simplistic formulations that assume a deterministic relationship between victimization and offending and remove the individual's responsibility and accountability for their actions.

Conclusion

New ways of conceptualizing and communicating post-traumatic distress are developing. These recognize the possibility of psychiatric illness developing following exposure to trauma, at the same time acknowledging the importance of socio-cultural context and the wide individual variation in post-traumatic responses and recovery. The experience of trauma does not automatically create psychological traumatization. Most people will face disasters and traumatic events of some sort in their lives and most will survive them, even if they are left changed by the experience. Distress, following exposure to a traumatic event, is a normal and self-limiting reaction in the majority of cases; there is little benefit to be had from labelling such distress as a manifestation of 'disease'. On the other hand, the post-traumatic literature, especially in relation to understanding the effects of chronic fear on the brain, has given practitioners and their patients a coherent framework for predicting, assessing and effectively treating individuals who do develop prolonged, and often disabling, post-traumatic psychiatric disorders, including PTSD.

References

Al-Shaykh, H. 1996 Beirut Blues. London: Vintage.

American Psychiatric Association 1980 Diagnostic and Statistical Manual of Mental Disorders 3rd Edition. Washington DC: American Psychiatric Association.

APA (American Psychiatric Association) 1994 Diagnostic and Statistical Manual. Washington DC: American Psychiatric Association.

Appelbaum, P.S., Jick, R.Z., Grisso, T., Givelber, D., Silver, E. and Steadman H.J. 1993 Use of Posttraumatic Stress Disorder to Support an Insanity Defense [See Comments]. American Journal of Psychiatry 150: 229–234.

Barker, P. 1991 The Regeneration Trilogy. London: Viking.

Beevor, A. 1999 Stalingrad. London: Penguin.

Beevor, A. 2003 Berlin: The Downfall 1945. London: Penguin.

Bracken, P., Giller, J. and Summerfield, D. 1995 Psychological Responses to War And Atrocity: The Limitations of Current Concepts. Social Science and Medicine 40: 1073–1082.

Breslau, N., Davis, G.C., Andreski, P., Peterson, E.L. and Schultz, L.R. 1997 Sex Differences in Posttraumatic Stress Disorder. Archives of General Psychiatry 54: 1044–1048.

Brewin C. 2003 Posttraumatic Stress Disorder. Malady or Myths 63–87 in New Haven: Yale University Press.

Brewin, C. R. 2001 A Cognitive Neuroscience Account of Posttraumatic Stress Disorder and Its Treatment. Behaviour, Research and Therapy: 393–393.

Brewin, C. R., Dalgleish, T. and Joseph, S. 1996 A Dual Representation Theory of Posttraumatic Stress Disorder. Psychological Review 103: 670–686.

Carstairs, G.M. and Kapur, R.L. 1976 The Great Universe of Kota: Stress, Change and Mental Disorder in an Indian Village. Berkeley: University of California Press.

Coid, J. 1992 'DSM-III Diagnosis in Criminal Psychopaths: A Way Forward', Criminal Behaviour and Mental Health 2: 78–94.

Dickens, C. 1998 Nicholas Nickleby. Oxford: Oxford University Press.

Dodge, K.A., Bates, J.E. and Pettit, G.S. 1990 Mechanisms in the Cycle of Violence. Science 250: 1678–1683.

Ehlers, A., Maercker, A. and Boos, A. 2000 Posttraumatic Stress Disorder Following Political Imprisonment: The Role of Mental Defeat, Alienation, and Perceived Permanent Change. Journal of Abnormal Psychology 109: 45–55.

Evans, C., Ehlers, A., Mezey, G. and Clark, D. 2007 Intrusive Memories and Ruminations Related to Violent Crime among Young Offenders: Phenomenological Characteristics. Journal of Traumatic Stress 2: 183–196.

Fabrega, H. 1982 Culture and Psychiatric Illness: Biomedical and Ethnomedical Aspects 39–68 in Cultural Conceptions of Mental Health and Therapy (Marsella, A.J and White, G.M. Editors) Dordrecht: D Reidel.

Faulks, S. 1984 Birdsong. London: Vintage.

Good, B.J., Herrerah, H., Good, M.D. and Cooper, J. 1985 Reflexivity, Counter Transference and Clinical Ethnography: A Case from a Psychiatric Cultural Consultation Clinic 193–221 in Physicians of Western Medicine, Anthropological Approaches to Theory And Practice (Hahn, R.A. and Gaines A.D. Editors) Dordrecht, Holland: Reidel.

Gorst-Unsworth C. and Goldenberg, E. 1998 Psychological Sequelae of Torture and Organised Violence Suffered by Refugeees from Iraq: Trauma Related Factors Compared with Social Factors in Exile. British Journal of Psychiatry 172: 90–94.

Haley, S. 1974 When the Patient Reports Atrocities. Archives of General Psychiatry 30: 191–196.

Hatzfeld, J. 2005 A Time for Machetes: The Rwandan Genocide: The Killers Speak (Trans. Coverdale, L.) London: Serpent's Tail.

Heads, T. et al 2002 Patients with SCP and Child Maltreatment.

Heads T., Taylor, P. and Leese, M. 1997 Childhood Experiences of Patients with Schizophrenia and a History of Violence: A Special Hospital Study. Criminal Behaviour and Mental Health 7: 117–130.

Hodgins, S., Alderton, J., Cree, A., Aboud, A. and Mak, T. 2007 Aggressive Behaviour, Victimization and Crime among Severely Mentally Ill Patients Requiring Hospitalisation. British Journal of Psychiatry 191: 343–350.

Hollifield, M., Hewage, C., Gunawardena, C.N., Kodituwakku, P., Bopagoda, K. and Weerarathenege, K. 2008 Symptoms and Coping in Sri Lanka 20–21 Months After the 2004 Tsunami. British Journal of Psychiatry 192: 39–44.

Johnson, J., Cohen, P. Brown, J., Smailes, E. and Bernstein, D. 1999 Childhood Maltreatment Increases Risk for Personality Disorders during Early Adulthood. Archives of General Psychiatry 56: 600–606.

Jones, L. 2002 Adolescent Understandings of Political Violence and Psychological Well-Being: A Qualitative Study from Bosnia Herzogivnia. Social Science and Medicine 55: 1351–1371.

Jones, L. and Kafetsios, K. 2002 Assessing Adolescent Mental Health in War-affected Societies: The Significance of Symptoms. Child Abuse and Neglect 26: 1059–1080.

Kagee, A. and Naidoo, A.V. 2004 Reconceptualising The Sequelae of Political Torture: Limitations of a Psychiatric Paradigm. Transcultural Psychiatry 41: 46–61.

Kaminer, D. Stein, D.J., Mbanga, I. and Zungu-Dirwyi, N. 2001 The Truth and Reconciliation Commission in South Africa: Relation to Psychiatric Status and Forgiveness among Survivors of Human Rights Abuses. 178: 373–377.

Keane, F. 1996 Letter to Daniel: Despatches from the Heart. London: Penguin/BBC.

Kennedy, H. 2005 Eve Was Framed. London: Vintage.

Kessler, R.C., Sonnega, A., Bromet, E., Hughes, M. and Nelson, C.B. 1995 Posttraumatic Stress Disorder in the National Comorbidity Survey. Archives of General Psychiatry 52: 1048–1060.

Kilpatrick, D.G., Saunders, B.E., Amick-Mcmullan, A.A., Best, C.L., Veronen, L.J. and Resnick, H.S. 1989 Victim and Crime Factors Associated with the Development of Crime-Related Posttraumatic Stress Disorder. Behavior Therapy 20: 199–214.

King, M., Coxell, A. and Mezey, G.C. 2002 Sexual Molestation of Males: Associations with Psychological Disturbance. British Journal of Psychiatry 181: 153–157.

Kleinman, A. 1987 Anthropology and Psychiatry: The Role of Culture in Cross-cultural Research on Illness. British Journal of Psychiatry 151: 447–454

Leff, J. 1988 Psychiatry around the Globe: A Transcultural View. London: Gaskell.

Levi, P. 1979 If This Is a Man/the Truce (Trans. Woolf, S.) London: Penguin.

Littlewood, R. And Lipsedge, M. 1985 Culture Bound Syndromes 105–142 in Recent Advances in Clinical Psychiatry 5 (Granville-Grossman, K. Editor) Edinburgh: Churchill Livingstone.

Luntz, B. and Widom, C.S. 1994)Antisocial Personality Disorder in Abused and Neglected Children Grown Up. American Journal of Psychiatry 151: 670–674.

Mcfarlane, A.C., Bookless, C. and Air, T. 2001 Posttraumatic Stress Disorder in a General Psychiatric Inpatient Population. Journal of Traumatic Stress 14: 633–45.

Marsella, A.J. and White, G.M. 1982 Introduction: Cultural Conceptualisation in Mental Health Research and Practice 1–38 in Cultural Conceptions of Mental Health and Therapy (Marsella, A.J and White, G.M. Editors) Dordrecht: D Reidel.

McIvor R.J. and Turner, S. W. 1995 Assessment and Treatment Approaches for Survivors of Torture. British Journal of Psychiatry 166: 705–711.

Mezey, G. 2006 Posttraumatic Stress Disorder and the Law. Psychiatry 5: 243–247.

Mezey, G.C., Bacchus, L.B. and Bewley, S. 2005 Domestic Violence, Lifetime Trauma and Psychological Health of Childbearing Women. British Journal of Obstetrics and Gynaecology 112: 197–204.

Mezey, G.C., Evans, C. E. and Hobdell, K. 2002 Families of Homicide Victims: Psychiatric Responses and Help-Seeking. Psychology and Psychotherapy. Psychotherapy, Research and Practice 75: 65–75.

Mueser, K.T., Goodman, L.B. Trumbetta, S. et al 1998 Trauma and Posttraumatic Stress Disorder etc.

NICE 2005 Posttraumatic Stress Disorder (PTSD): Anxiety: Management of Posttraumatic Stress Disorder in Adults in Primary, Secondary and Community Care. London: National Institute for Clinical Excellence.

Norris, F.H. and Kaniasty, K. 1994 Psychological Distress Following Criminal Victimization in the General Population: Cross-sectional, Longitudinal, and Prospective Analyses. Journal of Consulting and Clinical Psychology 62: 111–123.

Pyszora, N., Barker, A., and Kopelman, M. 2003 Amnesia for Criminal Offences: A Study of Life Sentence Prisoners. The Journal of Forensic Psychiatry and Psychology 14: 475–490.

Rieu, E. 1957. Homer: The Iliad. London: Penguin Books.

Raum, B.A. 1983 Rape Trauma Syndrome as Circumstantial Evidence of Rape. The Journal of Psychiatry & Law: 203–213.

Resnick, H.S., Yehuda, R. Pitman, R.K. and Foy, D.W. 1995 Effect of Previous Trauma on Acute Plasma Cortisol Level Following Rape. American Journal of Psychiatry 152 11: 1675–1677.

Rix K. (2001) Battered Woman Syndrome and the Defence Of Provocation. Journal of Forensic Psychiatry 12: 131–149

Rogers, R., Bagby, R. and Dickens, S. 2002 Structured Interview of Reported Symptoms (SIRS) A Professional Manual. Odessa: Florida.

Rose, S., Bisson, J. and Wessely, S. 2004 Psychological Debriefing for Preventing Posttraumatic Stress Disorder (PTSD). (Cochrane Review) in Cochrane Library, Issue 3. Chichester: John Wiley & Sons.

Rosen, G.M., Spitzer, R.L. and Mchugh, P.R. 2008 Problems with the Posttraumatic Stress Disorder Diagnosis and Its Future in DSM-V. British Journal of Psychiatry 192: 3–4.

Sarkar, J., Mezey, G., Cohen, A., and Olumoroti, O. 2005. Co-morbidity of Posttraumatic Stress Disorder and Paranoid Schizophrenia. Journal of Forensic psychiatry & Psychology 16: 660–670.

Sartorius, N., Jablensky, A., Korten, G. et al 1986 Early Manifestations and First-contact Incidence of Schizophrenia in Different Cultures. Psychological Medicine 16: 909–928.

Scott, J., Chant, D., Andrews, A., Martin, G. and Mcgrath J. 2007 Association between Trauma Exposure and Delusional Experiences in a Large Community Based Sample. British Journal of Psychiatry 190: 339–343.

Shephard, B. 2000 A War of Nerves. London: Jonathan Cape.

Sparr, L. 1996. Mental Defenses and Posttraumatic Stress Disorder: Assessment of Criminal Intent. Journal of Traumatic Stress, 9: 405–425.

Summerfield, D. 1999 A Critique of Seven Assumptions behind Psychological Trauma Programmes in War Affected Areas. Social Science and Medicine 48: 1449–1462.

Summerfield, D. 2000 War and Mental Health: A Brief Overview. British Medical Journal 321: 232–235.

Summerfield, D. 2001 The Invention of Posttraumatic Stress Disorder and the Social Usefulness of a Psychiatric Category. British Medical Journal 322: 95–98.

Summerfield, D. 2002 Effects of War: Moral Knowledge, Revenge, Reconciliation and Medicalised Concepts of "Recovery". British Medical Journal 325: 1105–1107.

Taylor, P.J. and Kopelman, M.D. 1984 Amnesia for Criminal Offences. Psychological Medicine 14: 581–588.

Teplin L.A., Mcclelland, G.M., Abram, K.M. and Weiner, D.A. 2005 Crime Victimization In Adults with Severe Mental Illness: Comparison with the National Crime Victimization Survey. Archives of General Psychiatry 62: 911–921.

Tetreault, P.A. 1989 Rape Myth Acceptance: A Case for Providing Educational Expert Testimony in Rape Jury Trials. Behavioral Sciences and the Law 8: 243–257.

Thomas, C., Adshead, G. and Mezey, G. 1994 Traumatic Responses to Child Murder. Journal of Forensic Psychiatry 5: 168–176.

Turner, S. and Gorst-Unsworth C. 1990 Psychological Sequelae of Torture: A Desriptive Model. British Journal of Psychiatry 157: 475–480.

Turner, S. Bowie, C., Dunn, G., Shapo, L. and Yule, W. 2003 Mental Health of Kosovan Albanian Refugees in the UK. British Journal of Psychiatry 182: 444–448.

Walsh, E., Moran, P. Scott, C. et al 2003 Prevalence of Violent Victimisation in Severe Mental Illness. British Journal of Psychiatry 183: 233–238.

Wessely S. 2006 The Life and Death of Private Harry Farr. Journal of the Royal Society of Medicine 99: 440–443.

WHO (World Health Organisation) 1992 International Classification of Diseases. Classification Of Behavioural And Mental Disorders: Clinical Descriptions And Diagnostic Guidelines. 10th Edition Geneva: WHO.

Widom, C. 1989 Child Abuse, Neglect and Adult Behaviour; Research Design and Findings on Criminality, Violence and Child Abuse. American Journal of Orthopsychiatry 59: 355–367.

Winterson, J. 1991 Oranges Are not the only Fruit. London: Vintage.

Yap, P.M. 1965 Koro – A Culture Bound Depersonalisation Syndrome. British Journal of Psychiatry 111: 43–50.

Yehuda, R. 2001 Are Gluco–Corticoids Responsible for Putative Hippocampal Damage in PTSD? How and when to Decide? Hippocampus 11: 85–89.

Yehuda, R., Resnick, H., Kahana, B. and Giller, E. 1993 Long Lasting Hormonal Alterations to Extreme Stress in Humans: Normative or Maladaptive. Psychosomatic Medicine 55: 287–287.

Forensic psychotherapeutic approaches to mentally disordered offenders

Chapter 10

Introduction: forensic psychotherapeutic approaches and the mentally disordered offender

Gill McGauley

The discussion about what happens to MDOs when they are locked up has often polarized into whether they should be treated or only incarcerated. This section describes one type of treatment: psychotherapy. The authors focus on two of the main types of psychotherapy available to MDOs; psychodynamic and cognitive and their derivatives. Unfortunately, the section could not be all inclusive and these chapters do not comprise a 'how to do it' section; rather we wanted to convey how psychotherapy can contribute to understanding the psychopathology, risk, criminal acts and interpersonal interactions of MDOs.

Psychotherapy in forensic settings encompasses more than the treatment of patients. It can help make sense of how treating and containing MDOs affects both staff and organizations as well as contributing towards understanding how interactions between staff and patients can be pulled off course. The authors emphasize how psychotherapeutically informed supervision and reflective practice can support the therapeutic task by monitoring the dynamics between patients, staff and patients, within the staff team and between the team and the institution.

The introductory chapter describes the key concepts of cognitive and psychodynamic psychotherapies; it then focuses on the particularity of providing psychotherapy in the forensic world. The chapter describes how psychotherapeutic work is influenced by both the nature and the severity of the mental disorders found in forensic patients and the forensic system.

Blumenthal's chapter goes to the heart of the forensic world in its consideration of the index offence. The author illustrates how a psychoanalytic approach can help elucidate the meaning of the offence in the mind of the offender; what drives individuals to act violently and how the therapeutic relationship allows the offender to understand their maladaptive interpersonal relationships. The majority of MDOs in secure health care services suffer from psychotic illnesses, most commonly schizophrenia. van Velsen's chapter adopts a holistic approach, describing the aetiology and phenomenology of schizophrenia before taking a forensic perspective and outlining the relationship between schizophrenia and violence. The chapter describes the contribution of Cognitive Behavioural Psychotherapy (CBT) to the treatment of schizophrenia as well as the way in which a psychodynamic approach aids the management of patients with schizophrenia who are detained.

The following chapter (Adshead and McGauley) covers the other main diagnosis prevalent among MDOs, that is, personality disorder. After discussing the nature of personality disorder in forensic populations, the authors describe how services developed across prison and health care to treat these individuals. With the development of services came the recognition of the problems staff faced while managing individuals with personality disorder, especially in secure settings. The contribution psychotherapeutic work can make to supporting therapeutic and minimizing anti-therapeutic staff–patient interactions is described. The advent of modified cognitive- and psychodynamic-based therapies has led to renewed optimism about the treatability of personality disorder. The chapter concludes with a review of the psychodynamic psychotherapy treatment literature.

The final two chapters focus on the contribution of cognitively based psychotherapies to the treatment of MDOs. Perkins describes how CBT developed differently within the forensic mental health system compared with the prison system. The chapter then complements the previous chapter by reviewing the cognitive psychotherapy treatment literature with respect to offenders with a diagnosis of personality disorder. Finally, Hawes discusses a group of MDOs who have occupied the intersection of the political, psychiatric and legal spotlight in the United Kingdom for the last decade; those with Dangerous and Severe Personality Disorder (DSPD). She charts the social and political background to this initiative, an example of policy driving the development of specific psychological treatment programmes. The chapter ends with a description of the cognitively based programmes developed to treat these high-risk offenders.

There is much that could not be included in this section. However, we hope that the sum of these contributions provides a balanced account of the strengths and limitations of the psychotherapies discussed. The treatment of forensic patients presents fascinating and complex challenges to the discipline of psychotherapy; it is clear that one psychotherapy size does not fit all.

Chapter 11

Introduction to the psychotherapies for mentally disordered offenders

Gill McGauley

Aim

To describe the main modalities of psychotherapy and to outline how the forensic setting influences their application.

Learning objectives

- To outline the main modalities of psychotherapy available to mentally disordered offenders (MDOs)
- To discuss how the delivery of psychotherapy is influenced by both the nature of forensic patients and the forensic setting
- To describe the relevance of systemic thinking to the forensic system
- To describe some of the difficulties in researching psychotherapies in MDOs

---

Introduction

Although psychological explanations for mental disorder were recognized early in the twentieth century, it is only in the last 30 years or so that the range and availability of psychotherapies to treat people with psychiatric and psychological difficulties has increased; however, MDOs have not benefited as much as they might have done from these developments. There are several reasons for this. In the health system, many psychotherapists, both clinicians and researchers, often viewed MDOs as an atypical group who were either too ill or disturbed to benefit from psychotherapy. In the criminal justice system, psychological treatment programmes for offenders frequently excluded those who had mental disorders (mental illness or personality disorder). Forensic patients are highly disturbed and working with them is a disturbing process for staff. Many MDOs have been physically violent to others and themselves. Even if the enactment of this violence is contained, to some extent, by the forensic setting, the capacity of these patients to be violent to their own minds and to the minds of others remains and can evoke feelings of dread and fear in their therapists (Gordon et al 2008; Minne 2008).

As MDOs have often been regarded as unsuitable patients for psychotherapy and have frequently been excluded from offender treatment programmes, they have only a patchy presence in the research literature. The 'What Works' literature on psychological interventions for offenders (McGuire 2000) typically excluded those who had mental disorders and psychotherapy research has often excluded forensic populations (see Roth et al 2005 for a review).

This chapter introduces psychotherapy as applied in the forensic world and signposts areas that are discussed further in this section. The first part of the chapter outlines the theoretical basis and key concepts involved in the main psychotherapy modalities. The section on psychodynamic psychotherapy is necessarily longer as it includes descriptions of terms which, although derived from psychoanalysis, have now spread into forensic clinical work. The second part describes how delivering and researching psychotherapy has been influenced by either the nature of the mental disorder found in forensic populations or the forensic setting. There are other modes of psychotherapy that this chapter cannot do justice to, such as the arts therapies (art, drama, and music), supportive psychotherapy and therapies that integrate theoretical approaches, such as cognitive analytic therapy; all of these contribute to the treatment of MDOs. For a description of psychotherapeutic work delivered in specialist units or institutions that function as Therapeutic Communities (TCs) please see Chapter 14.

Definitions

There are numerous types of psychotherapy; Kazdin (1986) identified more than 400 types. Three of the main divisions are cognitive-behavioural therapy (CBT), psychoanalytic or psychodynamic psychotherapy and systemic psychotherapy that includes family therapy (DH 2001). These therapies can be offered in different formats as individual, group or family therapy and may be provided at different frequencies, normally once or twice a week for forensic patients. They may be offered for different lengths of time; open-ended, through to medium length interventions of 12 to 18 months to relatively short interventions of 3 months or so. In general, the complexity and level of disturbance in MDOs necessitates longer rather than brief courses of psychotherapy.

Whether you are receiving psychotherapy as a patient or providing it as a therapist, both parties are involved in an experiential process. Central to many types of psychotherapy is the therapist–patient relationship and, to a greater or lesser extent, psychotherapies are based on the theory that this interpersonal process will modify disturbed feelings, thoughts, attitudes and behaviours that trouble the patient. Hughes and O'Riordan (2006) provided a generic definition of psychotherapy and its aims as being 'the treatment of emotional, behavioural or personality problems by psychological means'. Psychotherapy aims to relieve symptoms and bring some change to the feelings, thoughts, attitudes and behaviours that are troubling the patient, so that ultimately the

Box 11.1 Common characteristics of all therapies; adapted from Frank 1971

- A confiding relationship with a professionally trained therapist
- A rationale which contains an explanation for the patient's distress or difficulties and how the psychotherapy aims to relieve these
- The provision of new information about the nature and origins of the patient's problems and ways of dealing with them
- The provision of hope for the patient that help can be expected from therapy
- An opportunity for experiencing a sense of mastery during the course of therapy
- The facilitation of appropriate emotional arousal in the patient

person may become more independent and satisfied with his or her life. The common characteristics of all therapies, adapted from Frank (1971), are shown in Text Box 11.1.

Modalities of psychotherapy

Cognitive-behavioural therapy (CBT)

Developments in the cognitive sciences in the latter half of the last century, coupled with the limitations of behavioural therapies, resulted in the development of CBT in the late 1960s. Behaviour therapy had focused on observable behaviour within specific environments, an approach that was subsequently seen to be too narrow to explain human behaviour or effectively assist in managing problem behaviours. In many of the early behaviour therapy treatments, it became evident that the patient's internal thought processes were as important, if not more so, than the behavioural conditioning processes that were thought to be taking place. Consequently, CBT adopted a wider approach that included not only observable behaviour but also took account of internal processes and meanings (see Quayle and Moore 2006 for detailed discussion).

Aims

CBT seeks to reduce dysfunctional behaviours by analysing their symptoms and changing the thoughts that maintain them. Patients are helped to explore and understand the origins of their symptoms, understand the processes and situations that maintain them and rehearse new ways of thinking and behaving. Ultimately, the aim is that the patient understands the model and its application well enough to become their own cognitive therapist.

Theoretical underpinnings and key concepts

The CBT model is based on the concept that a person's thoughts (cognitions) are linked to their feelings and behaviour. Dysfuctionality such as mental health problems and offending behaviour can be ameliorated by analysing and intervening in the interplay between these cognitive, emotional and behavioural systems, so that the individual adapts his or her thinking, emotional responses and behaviours.

In the presence of emotional disturbance the cognitive model states that there will be negative automatic thoughts that can be about oneself (e.g. I am useless), the world (e.g. things always go wrong for me) or the future (e.g. nothing will get better in the future); patterns of regularly occurring errors in thinking in which the way information is perceived and interpreted is distorted (e.g. because my neighbour's daughter smiled at me she likes me and wants to go out with me); and distorted core beliefs, which are beliefs that the person considers true about themselves, others and the world (e.g. people should do what I want). All of these ways of thinking and beliefs affect the way individuals think about themselves and how they relate to others.

Interventions focus on changing cognitions, which in turn change mood and, ultimately, behaviour. Bandura (1977, 1986) found that an individual's perception of their capacity to deal with situations was crucial to allowing behavioural change, and introduced techniques such as 'self-efficacy' and 'self-control' to help patients to think more positively about achieving change. From the early work of Seligman (1975), Beck (1976) and Meichenbaum (1977), techniques were developed to tackle patients' negative automatic thoughts, thinking errors and irrational beliefs. As in other forms of therapy, a detailed history is required, which deals with the origins and maintenance of current patterns of thinking, feeling and behaving.

Schemas are important in the CBT model, especially in the cognitive model of personality disorder. Davidson (Cordess et al 2005) described schemas as stable cognitive structures through which knowledge about the world is gathered, processed and stored; hence they organize experience and guide behaviour. The processing of information through particular schemas generates the individual's core beliefs, behaviour and interpersonal problems. Schemas are often formed by early experiences and are thought to be activated by events similar to those that shaped them (Cordess et al 2005); for example, a person who has been subjected to neglectful and absent parenting may develop a schema that processes external information from the world to mean that they are unlovable. This schema may be reactivated by the threatened breakup of a relationship.

Schema therapy (Padesky 1994; Young et al 2003) combines elements from CBT, attachment theory and psychodynamic psychotherapy. It helps patients more systemically link the ways in which they view the world as a result of early attachments and life experiences, and helps them learn how these schemas affect their current functioning. Schema therapy focuses on the deepest level of cognition, the Early Maladaptive Schema (EMS), and is particularly useful in treating individuals with personality disorder in whom EMS appears to result, in part, from early dysfunctional experiences with parents (Young et al 2003). The behaviours resulting from schemas activated in some types of personality disorder have been linked to the dynamic risk factors described in the offending behaviour literature (Thornton et al 2003). For example, schematic systems active in Antisocial Personality Disorder (ASPD), such as a view of the self that involves the belief 'I should always get my own way', may drive impulsivity and lead to exploitative behaviour. Perkins' chapter (see Chapter 15) further describes cognitive approaches to the treatment and management of MDOs in both the prison and forensic mental health services in the United Kingdom.

Psychodynamic psychotherapy and forensic psychotherapy

Psychodynamic, or psychoanalytic, as it is sometimes called, psychotherapy derives from psychoanalysis and links with other developments in psychotherapy, such as group psychotherapy, TCs and brief dynamic therapies. Its history is linked with periods of human conflict. After the First and Second World Wars army psychiatrists recognized that 'shellshock' could be treated psychotherapeutically and applied psychoanalytic ideas to inpatient settings to treat these cases of war neuroses. The work of NHS doctors from other disciplines, who were also psychoanalysts, established psychoanalytic thought in social, probation and health services. These historical links with the NHS were enhanced by developing training courses and establishing psychotherapy as an independent medical speciality in 1975 (Lockwood 1999).

Within the NHS and prison service cognitively based treatments, often of shorter duration, have seen increasing popularity. However, within forensic mental health services psychodynamic psychotherapy has remained popular. In the UK, the term forensic psychotherapy is used to refer to the application of psychodynamic principles and treatment in the service of understanding and managing MDOs which developed from psychoanalysis, psychodynamic psychotherapy and forensic psychiatry (Welldon 1994). As Blumenthal notes (Chapter 12), one reason why forensic psychotherapy has remained popular is that it embraces a psychoanalytic consideration of the unconscious mind and contributes an additional dimension to understanding the mind, criminal acts and ongoing risk of the offender (Cordess and Williams 1996; Doctor 2003; McGauley 1997; Sohn 1995).

Psychodynamic psychotherapy provides both a type of treatment and a way of thinking about the complexities and dynamics within staff teams and institutions. The contribution forensic psychotherapy makes to thinking about these complexities is described by authors throughout this section (Chapters 12–14). Such an understanding is particularly valuable in forensic institutions and services where the high levels of disturbance in patients can negatively influence the system containing them, either at the level of individual staff members or teams or the institution as a whole (McGauley and Humphrey 2003).

Aims

Psychodynamic psychotherapy aims to help the person understand his or her mind and how he or she might be (or have been) inadvertently contributing to his or her own difficulties. It seeks a personal and specific meaning for the person's symptoms. By helping the patient increase their understanding of their thoughts, feelings and behaviour, both conscious and unconscious, lasting change is possible and symptoms can be reduced by changing the emotional states that have maintained them. Other treatment benefits include an increased capacity to manage frustration and unpalatable affective (emotional) states without resorting to impulsive and destructive behaviour, improved interpersonal relationships, increased capacity for self-understanding and raised self-esteem.

Theoretical underpinnings

Theoretically, psychodynamic psychotherapy has drawn heavily on psychoanalytic thinking as well as incorporating conceptual and theoretical ideas from other psychotherapies. Psychoanalysis aims at a more extensive re-organization of the personality, and as such it is an intensive treatment where the patient sees the analyst four or five times a week as opposed to the one-, or possibly two session-a-week model of psychodynamic treatment.

Two of the central theoretical tenets of psychodynamic psychotherapy are those of the unconscious mind and psychic determinism. To give meaning to mental events such as feelings, symptoms and behaviours Freud further developed the idea of the unconscious mind (Freud 1900). He postulated that much of mental life was unconscious and that the unconscious mind is populated by thoughts, feelings, desires and memories that are often painful or unacceptable (Freud 1910). Painful or unpleasant experiences may be either consciously suppressed, when the person actively chooses not to think about them, or unconsciously repressed, so they cannot be recalled at will but nevertheless affect the conscious mind and the person's behaviour.

Psychic determinism postulates that our feelings, thoughts and behaviours, such as choice of partner or career, are influenced by unconscious forces; they are not random, rather there is some reason and meaning underlying them. Both unconscious and conscious thoughts and feelings that conflict with conscious thoughts and wishes can lead to the development of symptoms. The psychodynamic therapist approaches the patient with the view that conflicts, from a variety of different developmental levels, may converge to produce a symptom or a particular behaviour and that these problems may serve multiple functions.

Psychodynamic theory also stresses the importance of early development as influencing adult interactions. It assumes that personality and behaviour are determined by inherited factors, the early environment and the interaction between them. The genetically based temperament of the child influences the style of interaction with their parents and, in turn, this interaction shapes the child's personality development (Reiss et al 1995). The interaction of nature and nurture leads us to develop internal representations (sometimes called internal objects) or mental pictures of ourselves and others and the relationships between them, which act as templates, guiding our interpersonal interactions as adults (Freud 1917; Hinshelwood 1991). The psychodynamic psychotherapist sees the patient's difficulties as arising from a complex interaction between the child's characteristics, parental interactions and the 'fit' between them (Gabbard 2000), a fit that for forensic patients has, more often than not, been poor.

Key concepts

Although many of the concepts used in psychodynamic psychotherapy derive from psychoanalysis, many of them have developed a more general meaning and have spread into the clinical vocabulary of forensic settings, as seen from the following example.

Therapeutic alliance: The original use of this term referred to the patient's conscious and unconscious co-operation with psychoanalysis. It is now more broadly used across psychotherapies to denote the working agreement between the therapist and the patient. The therapist's capacity for empathy and containment will aid the development of a strong therapeutic alliance; however, as forensic patients find therapeutic engagement difficult, the therapeutic alliance takes longer to develop. The term has developed an even wider meaning beyond psychotherapy and is used by forensic staff to refer to the relationship between the patient and the treating team. The following terms do not constitute an all-inclusive list but are some of the most relevant concepts with respect to forensic work.

Psychological containment: This refers to a state of mind where the person is not overwhelmed and threatened by internal psychological anxieties. The capacity for containment is fostered in infancy by attentive care that provides the infant with the appropriate balance between nurturing and frustrating experiences. This allows the infant to develop an internal security which, in turn, allows the child to explore the world and other relationships without experiencing unmanageable separation anxiety (Bowlby 1973). The terms containment and security take on different meanings in forensic work. Forensic patients, often as a result of neglectful and or abusive parenting, have been unable to develop adequate self-containment, especially in emotionally stressful situations; for example, when faced with situations of real or anticipated abandonment. In forensic patients, failures of containment often manifest as aggressive and destructive behaviours to others as well as the self. Consequently, forensic institutions have to provide containment by concrete, physical security, whereas professionals, particularly therapists, try to increase the patients' capacity for self-containment through both relational security and therapeutic work.

Relational security arises from a therapeutic understanding of the relationship between staff and patients and involves fostering a robust therapeutic alliance (Kinsley 1998). Good relational security allows patients to explore alternative approaches to stressful situations before containment fails and they are propelled to aggressive action. Robust relational security also allows staff to monitor the patients' psychological state and provide extra support during vulnerable periods.

Repetition compulsion, enactment and acting out: Since Blumenthal (Chapter 12) discusses them in detail, only a brief description of these concepts is provided here. Repetition compulsion refers to the patient's tendency to repeat behavioural patterns rather than remembering. Blumenthal makes the point that it is a peculiar feature of forensic work that what is not remembered is repeated in action.

Enactment is a term that specifically describes a process in therapy where the patient's thoughts and ways of relating are played out in the therapeutic setting, rather than verbally described to the therapist and then thought about; for example, the patient who habitually comes late to sessions rather than acknowledge the mixed feelings about both wanting to come while resenting needing to have treatment. The term acting out (Freud 1914) originally applied to people who were in therapy, and was used to describe an enactment that took place outside the therapy session, arising as a result of unconscious conflicts. For example, the patient who is unable to contain the feelings stirred up in therapy until they can be thought about in the next session, and acts them out in another setting by, for example, trying to dissolve their feelings with alcohol. Acting out has come to have a more general meaning, and although it still refers to maladaptive behaviour arising from unconscious conflicts, it now describes behaviour in other therapeutic relationships, for example the patient who self harms when her primary nurse goes on leave.

Transference and countertransference: Transference is the transferring of feelings and aspects of relating that belong to a past relationship, most often with a parental figure, onto a present relationship, most often with the therapist. The feelings and attributions are inappropriate to the present relationship. Transference is a universal phenomenon that happens in all relationships, but it is intensified by the psychoanalytic process, where it is used in a restrictive sense to refer to the patient's relationship with the psychoanalyst or psychodynamic therapist (Sandler et al 1987). It is a live process that happens out of the conscious awareness of the patient but allows the therapist and ultimately the patient access to and understanding of how their current interpersonal relationships are driven by previous early relationships. The legacy of the often disturbed and cruel upbringings experienced by forensic patients is that aspects of these experiences have been internalized; aggressive, frightening or sexualized aspects of their internal psychological world are often transferred onto those working with them.

In its original usage, countertransference referred to the psychoanalyst's unconscious view of the patient, coloured by figures in the analyst's past, which impeded the analyst treating the patient (Freud 1910). In other words, it paralleled the transference from the patient. Countertransference has now developed a broader usage and refers to the feelings, thoughts and behaviour that the therapist has towards the patient. The countertransference is a valuable therapeutic tool as it allows the therapist access to the feelings and reactions the patient activates in their other relationships.

Working with forensic patients evokes pronounced countertransferential responses in staff (Gordon and Kirtchuk 2008), including fear that the patients' aggression and violence will harm or destroy them or feelings of horror and repulsion about what the patient has done. Both of these reactions may lead staff to protectively withdraw and distance themselves from the patient. Another dynamic is that patients may treat staff as if they are dangerous and persecuting figures; such transference may result in staff wishing to dominate, control and, at the extreme, inflict suffering on the patients. If this countertransference reaction is acted upon devastating consequences for the patient, the professional and the institution or service can result (see Chapter 14 for a fuller discussion).

Resistance: One of the paradoxes of psychotherapy is that patients are motivated to embark on therapy because they have a problem for which they want help. However, asking for help activates a degree of resistance. Freud (1914) observed that patients were ambivalent about getting better and unconsciously, as well as consciously, opposed attempts to help them. The prospect of change inherent in the process of getting better is anxiety provoking and resistance may be viewed as the way in which patients defend themselves from changing, consequently maintaining their problems or illness. For example, resistance may manifest itself by 'forgetting' what happens in, or coming late to, therapy sessions. For forensic patients, the change involved in getting better is particularly frightening, as it involves owning and thinking about their aggressive and violent actions towards themselves and others. Originally thought of as an obstacle to treatment, helping the patient understand their resistance is now seen as a central task of psychodynamic psychotherapy, as it can reveal information about the transference and the patient's interactions with others.

Example. A female patient who felt that her female therapist's interpretations were critical and aimed at 'putting her down' often 'forgot' what happened in the sessions. This view of her therapist was eventually understood as being characteristic of her relationship with her mother and other adults who offered her help.

Psychological defence mechanisms: Everyone uses psychological defence mechanisms in everyday life, as they have a protective function in reducing anxiety or other painful affective states and protect us from wishes that conflict with rational and moral standards. They can be both conscious and unconscious; the common ones are listed in Table 14.3. For a more extensive list and description please see Gabbard (2005). As strategies they can be adaptive or maladaptive, pathological or helpful. Psychological defence mechanisms keep disturbing experiences out of conscious awareness; however, as they influence the person's pattern of behaviour they colour the person's interpersonal relationships. They are considered maladaptive if they restrict a person's life or lead to primitive patterns of coping in the face of anxiety. Forensic patients frequently employ primitive, unconscious defence mechanisms. Over-reliance on these ways of interacting has a personal cost as it distorts the person's perception of reality and, if acted upon, incongruous or dangerous behaviour may result (Bateman 1996). Some of the common psychological defence mechanisms used by forensic patients are described in the following paragraphs.

Splitting occurs when a person separates his or her experience of self and how he or she mentally represents his or her experience of others into rigid and separate mental compartments. In this state of mind, the components of experience, such as thoughts, affect and behaviour, remain unintegrated and separated in the person's mind. In its simplest form, aspects of the self and others are divided into good or bad. Symptomatically, contradictions are observed between the person's behaviour, affect and thoughts. However, if attention is drawn to these, the person might react with indifference, denial, surprise or indignant outrage (Gabbard 2005). The splitting off of aspects of experience is a defensive solution, protecting the person from the conflict generated if two polarized aspects of self or others converge. Treatment needs to consider both aspects of the patient. In forensic populations, this polarization or splitting of aspects of the self is often seen in patients' descriptions of their offending, or rather what is left out of their description.

Example. A patient with a long history of interpersonal violence, culminating in a homicide, described himself as a gentle, non-violent man who wouldn't harm a fly. He couldn't understand why he was in a secure unit and felt deeply resentful about his detention. In this man's mind, knowledge and experience of his aggression and violence had been split off, allowing the patient to present himself as 'the victim' without reference to 'him' as 'the perpetrator'. He could not see the contradiction between his behaviour and his description of himself.

Splitting can be observed in the incongruity of affect and cognition that can be seen in the communications of psychotic patients.

Example. When asked if he had any thoughts of harming himself, a young man with a diagnosis of schizophrenia gave a detailed description of how he had tried to hang himself while on unescorted leave. With the same rather monotonous tone of voice and with the same lack of facial expression he then asked the nurse if he could have an extra portion of pudding with his meal.

Sometimes split-off aspects of the self are projected. Projection involves perceiving unacceptable feelings and impulses in oneself as if they were outside the self; most often these impulses are lodged in other people. Forensic patients often project their split-off aggressive, violent or what they consider shameful aspects of themselves, which can lead to the patient feeling paranoid, as they then believe that the other person is feeling aggressive and will attack or intrude upon them. These projective processes can often underpin seemingly random stranger attacks (Sohn 1995).

Example. A young man, unaware of the conflicting feelings his homosexuality aroused in him, split off and projected his homosexual wishes and impulses and so developed the paranoid belief that the man sitting opposite him on an empty bus was sexually interested in him in a predatory way. When the man passed close by to get off the bus he stabbed him, believing the man was making an intrusive homosexual advance.

In psychosis, split-off aspects of the patient's experience may be projected into non-human objects as well as people and the patient's own thoughts are experienced projectively as the 'voices' of auditory hallucinations, for example, the man who heard his dog telling him to kill his mother. These phenomena as they relate to psychosis are discussed further in Chapter 13.

When the recipient of the projection is identified as and reacted to by the patient as if they were really feeling and thinking in this way, the phenomenon is called projective identification, originally described by Melanie Klein (1946). Projective identification takes place at an unconscious level and also involves the patient exerting subtle interpersonal pressure on the recipient of the projection to take on the aspects of the self that are being projected. The person who is the recipient of the projection often begins to think, feel and sometimes behave in keeping with what has been projected. If staff succumb to this pressure and behave in line with the split-off and projected aspects of their patients, there is an increased risk of boundary violations.

Example. A male patient with a long history of aggression to others severely self-harms on a regular basis on the ward. Despite all the help the staff provide, the patient says he is frightened to tell staff when he feels like harming, but after the event he accuses them of not caring for him. After a cluster of episodes of self-harm, the ward is so disrupted that the patient's primary nurse alters his shifts to provide nursing support for the patient. When the patient, once again, tells his primary nurse that he is not looking after him properly, the nurse uncharacteristically finds himself shouting angrily at the patient that he is 'sick and tired of him'.

This patient has split off and projected the aggressive aspects of himself into the nursing staff, which he then identifies with as being in them, and feels frightened that they will be aggressive towards him. In addition, he unconsciously pressurizes the nurse to behave in line with what he has projected.

Another variation underpinned by splitting is when split-off aspects of the patient's experiences are projected into teams. Particular groups of staff may regard the patient as vulnerable and needy, whereas others may see the patient as manipulative and aggressive. These are merely the projected and conflicting aspects of the patient's experience and, if understood as such, can help the team understand their patient. If members or sub-groups in the team take up and act on these projections, the team can become split and the patient's conflicts become acted out by the team, leaving the patient as an observer, freed of conflict. Poorly functioning teams where there is weak communication, or rivalry and division between members, are especially vulnerable to splitting. At times, teams who are split blame this dynamic entirely on the patient; however, at a less conscious level teams have to 'want' to be split.

Idealization is also a common psychological defence mechanism used by forensic patients. Patients attribute perfect or near-perfect qualities to others to avoid negative or hostile feelings. Forensic patients have often endured cruelty and neglect from parental figures that have failed them. In adult life, the patient may idealize the parent to protect themselves from the rage, shame and sense of loss that a more accurate representation of the parent might stimulate.

Example. A patient described his mother as always 'being there for him' and as 'a diamond of a mother'. In reality, his mother was alcohol dependent and her neglectful mothering resulted in him being taken into care at the age of four.

Treatment principles and model

Psychodynamic psychotherapy accesses unconscious as well as conscious thoughts and feelings. It has structured sessional boundaries, with respect to time and place, but is relatively unstructured within the session to encourage access to unconscious processes by allowing the patient to free associate; to tell his or her therapist whatever comes into his or her mind in an uncensored way.

The regularity and continuity of the therapeutic relationship means that the patient develops a particular attachment to the therapist. It is an unusual relationship as it is both intimate and professional. The often-held view that the therapist functions as a silent blank screen is misleading, as the therapist is actively engaged in what is happening. The nature of the therapist's stance, which is one of interest in the patient's story and difficulties but both non-judgemental and non-directive, allows the patient to tell the psychotherapist intimate information about his or her thoughts and feelings. As the psychotherapist reveals little personal information in return, this imbalance facilitates the development of the transference, as it allows the patient to imagine and assume what they choose about the therapist. The psychotherapist is then able to analyse the patient's associations and the therapeutic relationship in terms of the transference and countertransference and help the patient see this by interpreting what is happening. Table 11.1 compares aspects of CBT and psychodynamic psychotherapy.

Systemic and family therapy

Aims

A systemic approach aims to understand individual problems by considering them in the context of family relationships and the impact of the wider social and economic context on people's lives, their well-being and mental health. Human systems can involve an individual, a couple, a family or larger groups such as institutions; consequently, the systemic approach includes family therapy, as family therapy aims to explore and understand how the identified patient's problems are maintained by the needs of the family system.

Key concepts

Systemic and family therapeutic approaches have their roots in General Systems Theory (von Bertalanffy 1962). The concepts underpinning systems theory were developed as an alternative approach to a cause and effect model of understanding events (Bentovim 1996); for example, to the propensity of psychodynamic models to see past events as predicting future ways of relating.

Table 11.1 Comparison between CBT and psychodynamic psychotherapy

CBT	Psychodynamic psychotherapy
Often time limited with a short to medium time frame.	Has a medium to longer-term time frame but may be open-ended.
Emphasis on changing thoughts to effect symptom change.	Emphasis on changing emotions to effect symptom change.
Works on conscious rational thought process.	Works on conscious and unconscious thought processes, emotions and impulses.
Often used for specific conditions such as anxiety or depression or for a specific focus, for example, offence-related.	Tends to be used as a treatment when the person recognizes problematic patterns in their interpersonal interactions.
Uses techniques such as clarification, guided questioning, challenging, homework.	Uses free association, interpretation both within and outside of the transference as well as clarification and challenging.
The therapeutic relationship is important but is not used as an active part of treatment.	Attends to and uses the therapeutic relationship as an active part of treatment in the transference and countertransference.

Systemic thinking addresses complex human systems and their interactions. One principle of human systems is that personal beliefs, actions and relationships are all interrelated and influence the beliefs, behaviours and relationships of others, and will likewise be influenced by those of others.

Forensic considerations

Many of the contributors to this book have referred to systemic thinking, although these references may not have been explicit. The editors have described how MDOs are caught in a spider's web of a system where they are often in contact with many parts of the system (all systems in their own right) at once, for example, health, criminal justice, social care, legal and voluntary sectors (see Introduction). The following paragraphs draw together how a systemic approach and thinking relates to the forensic world.

First, although the offence is the responsibility of the person committing the act, their offending behaviour occurs in a context. It can be viewed as the product of a complex set of interactions that affect the individual and arise from their family and the person's wider social network (Bentovim 1996). Understanding the interrelationships and interactions between the individual, family system and society allows for a more comprehensive understanding of offending behaviour and the possibility of more effective interventions. For example, Minuchin (1974) realized that delinquent behaviour in children was sometimes associated more with social stressors such as poverty and immigration rather than with their parents' early history. Systemic thinking can make a valuable contribution in terms of understanding the allocated role of the patient within the family system and how this may link with their offending behaviour. Such information aids risk assessment, as the patient may often re-enact family dynamics with staff, especially in secure institutions.

A second and linked concept is that offending behaviour is seen as the symptom which affects the individual, family and social system. This symptom can be maintained by the system and the symptom may also stabilize the system. This systemic view links with a psychoanalytic view of the offence being a symptom, which has a personal meaning to the individual and is acted out (Chapter 12). In her critique of the medical model, Bartlett (Chapter 2) describes how strict adherence to this model risks losing the meaning of psychiatric symptoms to the individual and their context; likewise the meaning of the offence if it is decontextualized. Viewing the offence as a symptom allows an exploration of developmental, family and social factors that are associated with criminality as well as the factors in systems that may be protective (Chapter 3 and Chapter 8).

Third, MDOs remain in systems which care for and also incarcerate them for many years. Systemic thinking makes a valuable contribution to seeing how others in the system may influence the MDO in maintaining dysfunctional patterns of relating and how the MDO influences the system containing them at a team, or ward level, or at the level of the service or institution. Systematic therapy has an important role to play in helping teams; services and institutions think about their boundaries, hierarchical systems, subsystems and rules. The ethical considerations of how staff relate to the patient and each other, within and across systems, are discussed in Chapter 25.

The index offence may have taken place within the family system. In addition, forensic patients and their families have often suffered abusive experiences, one consequence of which is distorted family boundaries and hierarchies. The family systems of MDOs often exhibit higher than average levels of dysfunctional interrelationships. For other MDOs, the family system may have broken down, resulting in early and prolonged separation from the family in institutionalized care. For all of these reasons, careful consideration must be given as to whether to embark on formal family therapy involving both the forensic patient and their family. However, family therapy can be undertaken with part of the family unit and the designated patient need not necessarily be in the room. Families may well benefit from therapy to help them deal with issues of bereavement, either for a relative who was the victim or for the loss of their relative who has been incarcerated.

Overarching forensic variations

The following section describes how the delivery of psychotherapy, irrespective of modality, is influenced by both the nature of the forensic patients and the setting.

The patients and their interactions

Generic psychotherapy aims to help the patient change feelings, thoughts and behaviours that have been troubling them. One of the distinguishing characteristics of MDOs is that they have troubled others by virtue of their aggressive and offending behaviour. Many forensic patients are troubled by either psychotic symptoms, such as hallucinations and delusions; neurotic symptoms, such as anxiety and depression; or symptoms arising from developmental processes that have affected their personality structure, resulting in personality disorder with its concomitant symptoms of impulsivity, poor affective (emotional) control, abnormal processing of aggression and failure to respond to the distress of others. Many patients have multiple psychiatric diagnoses; for some the primary diagnosis may be difficult to establish.

Many patients will have suffered deprived and abusive childhoods within the context of dysfunctional families or care systems where parenting has been at best inadequate and at worst neglectful and cruel. Consequently, they have little expectation of receiving proper care or treatment. If selection kept strictly to the qualities therapists look for when assessing non-forensic patients' suitability for psychotherapy (see Text Box 11.2), the majority of forensic patients would not qualify.

The nature and degree of psychological disturbance in forensic patients means that these patients frequently act out aspects of their disturbance in their offence and in the context of their

---

Box 11.2 Suitability for psychotherapy

The person

+ Is psychologically minded and aware that he or she has a problem
+ Recognizes that the problem has a mental or emotional component as opposed to, for example, a physical cause
+ Has an appropriate sense of responsibility and ownership with respect to his or her difficulties
+ Is curious about their problems and has the capacity to self-question and reflect
+ Is motivated to understand his or her problems and change his or her behaviour
+ Has staying power in other areas of his or her life and does not abandon tasks, especially when personal effort is required
+ Has the capacity to relate to another person. This is more important in therapies where the nature of the therapist-patient interaction is emphasized
+ Has an adequate capacity for self-containment and can tolerate some degree of emotional discomfort without acting destructively

interpersonal relationships. Crucially, within a psychotherapy context, when faced with areas of painful psychological difficulty, these people may continue to use impulsive acts of violence or aggression to reduce the anxiety therapy may engender, consequently putting the therapist at risk.

Example. A patient who developed a delusional attachment to a member of staff was convinced that she loved him and would marry him. His anger and feelings of rejection when the staff member did not reciprocate his affection led to him threatening to kill her.

This propensity, coupled with the strength and nature of the reactions that can be evoked in staff, highlights the need for supervision to be available for staff, irrespective of seniority. The response of the institution to acting out is also important, as particular responses may perpetuate such behaviour (Norton and Dolan 1995); throughout this section, authors repeatedly describe how working with patients who are violent, sexually perverse, mentally ill, or personality-disordered can affect staff. Supervision, reflective practice groups and consultation work (Ruszczynski 2008) can attend to and help staff understand the psychodynamic processes in the forensic setting that arise from the effects of managing and treating such patients. At low levels of security, or in non-secure community forensic settings, the psychotherapist may well see patients whose compulsion to act out dangerously is less; however, their psychopathology may be no less complex.

A common and over-riding characteristic of forensic patients is to split off and locate their difficulties as existing outside their own minds, often locating them in others. The forensic clinician frequently hears phases such as, 'I killed him because the voices told me to'.

Example. When asked what he was thinking after a violent and unprovoked attack on a woman, for which he was convicted of attempted murder, a patient, who had developed some awareness of his capacity to split his mind, replied, 'I think I was trying to actually blame her for what I had done like, you know, look what she's made me do'.

The difficulty forensic patients have in taking an appropriate level of responsibility and agency for their involvement in their aggressive and offending behaviour often necessitates their continued detention. The systems and nature of the institutions that provide for this detention affect the process and delivery of psychotherapy.

The offence

In psychotherapy with MDOs, the therapist has the additional consideration of the offence. Offence-related work is core to psychotherapeutic work with forensic patients. The therapist aims to help the patient understand and change his or her feelings, thoughts and attitudes connected with the offending and aggressive behaviour, and ultimately to modify it, reducing future risk. Through this process psychotherapy provides information relevant to several areas of risk management, for example, how patients currently view their past offences and the degree to which they can take responsibility for their offending. The contribution of psychodynamic and cognitive behavioural psychotherapies to offence-related work is further explored in subsequent chapters (Chapters 13, 15 and 16). Psychotherapeutic work with MDOs needs to consider the role of trauma in these patients' experiences. Many forensic patients have suffered traumatizing backgrounds. Their offences have traumatized others and may contain replayed, but unacknowledged, aspects of their own childhood trauma. However, the traumatizing nature of the awareness a patient may develop, through psychotherapy, of the effect of their offence on others is often underestimated.

The triangular relationship

The fact that there has been an offence and a victim means that, unlike generic psychotherapy, a third party, the Criminal Justice System, representing society, is involved. Psychotherapy with forensic patients involves a tripartite relationship, with the therapist working at the interface of these three interacting systems—the psychotherapist, the patient and the Criminal Justice System (de Smit 1992). The extent to which this triangular relationship influences therapy will vary depending on the setting. For example, the Criminal Justice System contributes to determining when the patient is transferred, which may either prematurely interrupt therapy or, at the very least, introduce discontinuity into the therapeutic process.

The security treatment tension

For psychotherapists working with forensic patients the issue of security is omnipresent, however it takes on an additional meaning in forensic compared to generic work. In both, 'security' denotes the development of a positive quality in the therapeutic alliance, allowing the patient to feel free to confide and trust in their relationship with a therapist. In addition, because of the tendency of forensic patients to act out aggressively to others, 'security' in forensic settings also refers to the physical security of the walls, locks and surveillance equipment, as well as procedural security measures such as spot checks and searches. Undoubtedly, these security measures alter the environment in which therapy is delivered. Some would argue that as patients are not 'free' to choose to come to therapy, the nature of the therapeutic alliance in secure conditions is so fundamentally altered as to be quantitatively different from that in generic psychotherapy. Although elements of security conflict and affect the process and content of psychotherapy, even secure hospital patients have some choice, and a productive therapeutic alliance can be established (Campbell and McGauley 2005).

Confidentiality

As issues of confidentiality which arise when caring for MDOs in security are discussed throughout the ethics section (Chapter 24), they will only be touched on here. Confidentiality is a fluid concept and is influenced by the context the therapist is working in and the therapist's professional code of conduct. If working in a multidisciplinary team the therapist needs to determine the level to which they can discuss the therapeutic work within the team while preserving the strength of the therapeutic alliance with their patient. Without regular sharing of the therapeutic work with the team the therapist remains at risk of being pulled off a straight therapeutic course and may be unwittingly drawn into, at best, an unhelpful, and at worst, a toxic relationship with the patient. Working without careful multidisciplinary sharing may also expose the therapist to risk as, no matter how well you know your patient, there are, as Stanton and Swartz pointed out (1954), the other '23 hours'. Scant communication also carries the risk that therapy will become marginalized and its contribution to the patient's treatment and risk will be diminished. However, reporting clinical work in too much detail may damage the therapeutic relationship if the institution reacts punitively.

The double-bind that Fullford describes to both disclose and keep secret is felt particularly by those working in forensic mental health (Fullford 2000; Hale 2006). With the organization of mental health care into multi-agency teams, once disclosed it is difficult to control the spread of confidential information, especially as there is an increasing expectation that information will be shared across different agencies; for example, with Multi-Agency Public Protection Panels that may have different functions and duties with respect to the MDO.

A note on groups in forensic settings

In forensic settings, group psychotherapy that focuses on providing insight, rather than education and teaching, is predominantly analytic in nature. Group analysis, as described by Foulkes (1948), has been developed in forensic inpatient and outpatient populations respectively by the work of Cox (1976) and Welldon (1993). Group analytic psychotherapy aims to make patients more aware of themselves in their relationships to others. Foulkes postulated that the healing power of the group came from the fact that, collectively, individuals in the group 'constitute the very norm from which, individually, they deviate' (Foulkes 1948: 29). As a result, the stronger, healthier group can wear down and correct the abnormal responses of its individual members and reinforce healthy reactions. Individual psychopathology is diminished by articulating and understanding the unconscious destructive aspects of the individual, and the deeper disturbance underlying the person's symptom or offending behaviour can be understood within a social context as represented by the group. In forensic settings, group work can contain and modify violent affect and allow patients to become aware of the consequences of their actions on others through the reactions and challenges of group members. However, this process can happen only if the group is functioning well, and therapists need to pay close attention to group members' attempts to subvert the group process.

Researching psychotherapies in forensic populations

There are particular challenges associated with conducting well-run research trials in MDO populations that have resulted in a less robust evidence base for psychotherapy for MDOs compared with that for their non-forensic counterparts. These difficulties fall roughly into three groups: patient-centred problems, research-centred difficulties and service- or institutional-centred problems. The following section flags only a few of these.

MDOs are often hard to engage in the treatment process. Many have psychotic illnesses, the symptoms of which, such as paranoid states of mind, mean that they may not be able to provide informed consent to participate in research trials. Others, particularly those detained against their will, understandably may not want to participate in extra research-driven contact with staff. Consequently, recruiting and sustaining patients' engagement throughout lengthy research projects has particular difficulties in forensic populations. In addition, patients often have more than one psychiatric diagnosis, complicating those research projects that aim to select a homogeneous diagnostic group; for example, to assess the outcome of a particular psychotherapy treatment.

MDOs in the health system are often detained for several years; admission rates and patient throughput are liable to be slow. Consequently, it can be a lengthy process to recruit enough individuals to adequately power quantitative research studies. Small sub-groups of MDOs, such as women and black and ethnic minority patients, may be less likely to be involved in quantitative research to look at the effectiveness of psychological interventions. In the prison system, the rapid throughput of many MDOs and the difficulty of following up these individuals may mean that studies have high attrition rates, potentially limiting the interpretation of their results.

A crucial question for researchers interested in quantitative psychotherapy outcome research is how to define the outcome? There are two approaches. The first of these is to take the primary outcome measure as risk-related and examine whether a particular psychotherapy intervention decreases risk. Risk is often assessed by the degree and severity of recidivism or wider proxy measures of risk, such as frequency and severity of aggressive incidents. Difficulties in this approach can arise because recidivism has a low base rate so a large number of MDOs need to be followed up for a long time, post-release. Gathering accurate data on proxy measures of risk can also be difficult, as the researcher may have to rely on incomplete records. The longer the follow-up, the greater the number of variables that may intervene, so it can become increasingly difficult to establish whether the treatment reduced the risk.

The second approach is to examine whether a particular treatment improved the patients' psychiatric symptoms or behaviours. Outcome measures include change in the diagnostic frequency of personality disorder, in personality characteristics such as impulsivity, in psychotic symptoms, in mood or in suicidal or self-harming behaviour. As a rule, methodology that allows the outcome of a psychotherapy intervention to be examined across risk, psychological and psychiatric variables is to be recommended. A common problem with the evidence base to date is that often studies have used different instruments to measure outcome, making it almost impossible to compare studies or combine data meta-analytically.

The effective delivery of psychotherapy requires the consistent availability of a core of staff to both deliver the intervention and attend training and supervision to ensure fidelity to the intervention being researched. Institutional and service pressures work against achieving this. Many treatment initiatives in secure care fail, fizzle out or cannot be evaluated effectively because operational pressures impinge upon staff consistency and availability. Service and financial pressures, tight staffing levels and redeployment of ward staff at short notice to risk manage patient situations are common in secure environments.

More detailed accounts of the research findings can be found in the subsequent chapters in this section. Please see Chapter 13 for a discussion of the evidence base for psychodynamic therapy and CBT in psychosis; Chapter 14 for an account of psychodynamic and derived approaches, such as mentalization-based treatment (MBT) in personality disorder; and Chapter 15 for a discussion of CBT and modified cognitive approaches such as Dialectic Behavioural Therapy (DBT) in personality disorder.

Conclusion

The context in which psychotherapy takes place with MDOs differs from that of generic psychotherapy. Those working psychotherapeutically with MDOs need to keep in mind both their work with their patients and their responsibilities to society. Although there is diversity among the branches of psychotherapy, there are commonalities too, and in forensic work the shared aims of treatment are to decrease the patients' symptoms and risk, help patients become aware of how their mind works, what they have done and how their actions have affected others. To help the man who said, 'I don't know, I don't think about it I don't worry about it I only think, the only time I think, I think about the offence really is when you lot talk to me about it. Apart from that it doesn't really cross my mind' begin the traumatic process of working towards an understanding of his actions, as has been partially achieved by the man who said, 'I had no idea of the amount of injuries that I had inflicted upon . . . , not until I saw the pathologist's report several months later. I couldn't understand, even months afterwards. I'm still trying to understand why.'

In other words, to help patients progress from unthinking states of mind, which preclude them from being able to take responsibility for their actions, towards making reparation and changing, psychotherapy is undertaken alongside pharmacological treatments, occupational therapy and educational and skills-based interventions all aimed at improving the mental health, reducing the risk and aiding the rehabilitation of MDOs.

The provision of psychotherapy for MDOs is patchy. Resource issues and the nature of the forensic systems mean that many MDOs cannot access psychotherapeutic help. Even if more were available, some MDOs are too disturbed to be able to really benefit from psychotherapy. However, caring for MDOs is a disturbing process and psychotherapeutic principles can help staff to think about their work.

Key points

◆ Psychotherapy is one of the main treatment modalities for MDOs

◆ Providing psychotherapy in forensic settings requires additional considerations compared with generic settings

◆ Although different types of psychotherapy are provided for MDOs, they share a common aim of reducing the patients' symptoms and risk

◆ The contribution of psychotherapy in forensic settings is more than providing treatment. Its principles and techniques can be used to provide supervision and reflective practice for staff and to aid systemic understanding

References

Bandura, A. 1977 Self-efficacy: Toward a Unifying Theory of Behavioral Change, Psychological Review 84: 191–215.

Bandura, A. 1986 Social Foundations of Thought and Action: A Social Cognitive Theory. Englewood Cliffs NJ: Prentice-Hall.

Bateman, A. 1996 Defence Mechanisms: General and Forensic Aspects 41–51 in Forensic Psychotherapy: Crime, Psychodynamics and the Offender Patient (Cordess, C. and Cox, M. Editors) London: Jessica Kingsley.

Beck, A.T. 1976 Cognitive Therapy and the Emotional Disorders. New York: International Universities Press.

Bentovim, A. 1996 Systems Theory 107–115 in Forensic Psychotherapy: Crime, Psychodynamics and the Offender Patient (Cordess, C. and Cox, M. Editors) London: Jessica Kingsley.

Bowlby, J. 1973 Attachment and Loss Vol II: Separation. Basic Books: New York.

Campbell, C. and McGauley, G. 2005 Doctor–Patient Relationships in Chronic Illness: Insights from Forensic Psychiatry. BMJ 330: 667–670.

Cordess, C., Davidson, K., Morris, M. and Norton, K. 2005 Cluster B Antisocial Personality Disorders 269–278 in Oxford Textbook of Psychotherapy (Holmes, J. Beck, J. and Gabbard, G. Editors) Oxford: Oxford University Press.

Cordess, C. and Williams, A. H. 1996 The Criminal Act and Acting Out 13–21 in Forensic Psychotherapy, Crime, Psychodynamics and the Offender Patient (C. Cordess and Cox, M. Editors) London: Jessica Kingsley.

Cox, M. 1976 Group Psychotherapy in a Secure Setting. Proceedings of the Royal Society of Medicine 69: 215–220.

de Smit, B. 1992 The End of the Beginning is the Beginning of the End: The Structure of the Initial Interview in Forensic Psychiatry, Proceedings of the 17th International Congress of the International Academy of Law and Mental Health, Leuven, Belgium.

Department of Health. 2001 Treatment Choice in Psychological Therapies and Counselling. Evidence Based Clinical Practice Guideline.

Doctor, R. 2003 Introduction 1–6 in Dangerous Patients, A Psychodynamic Approach to Risk Assessment and Management (Doctor, R. Editor) London: Karnac.

Foulkes, S. H. 1948 Introduction to Group Analytic Psychotherapy. London: Heineman.

Frank, J. 1971 Therapeutic Factors in Psychotherapy, American Journal of Psychotherapy 25: 350–361.

Freud, S. 1900 The Interpretation of Dreams in The Standard Edition of the Complete Works of Sigmund Freud (Strachey, J. Editor) London: Hogarth Press.

Freud, S. 1910 The Future Prospect of Psychoanalytic Therapy in The Standard Edition of the Complete Works of Sigmund Freud (Strachey, J. Editor) London: Hogarth Press.

Freud, S. 1914 Remembering, Repeating and Working-Through 147–156 in Standard Edition, XII, London: Hogarth Press.

Freud, S. 1917 Mourning and Melancholia 147–156 in The Standard Edition of the Complete Works of Sigmund Freud, (Strachey, J. Editor) London: Hogarth Press.

Fullford, K.W.M. 2000 The Paradoxes of Confidentiality. A Philosophical Introduction 7–25 in Confidentiality and Mental Health (Cordess, C. Editor) London: Jessica Kingsley.

Gabbard, G.O. 2000 Psychodynamic Psychiatry in Clinical Practice 3rd Edition. Washington DC: American Psychiatric Press.

Gabbard, G.O. 2005 Major Modalities: Psychoanalytic/Psychodynamic 3–13 in Oxford Textbook of Psychotherapy (Gabbard, G. Beck, J.S. and Holmes, J. Editors) Oxford: Oxford University Press.

Gordon, J., Harding, S., Miller, C. and Xenitidis, K. 2008 X-treme Group Analysis: On the Countertransference Edge in Inpatient Work with Forensic Patients 41–61 in Psychic Assaults and Frightened Clinicians, Countertransference in Forensic Settings (Gordon, J. and Kirtchuk, G. Editors) London: Karnac.

Gordon, J. and Kirtchuk, G. 2008 Introduction 1–9 in Psychic Assaults and Frightened Clinicians, Countertransference in Forensic Settings (Gordon, J. and Kirtchuk, G. Editors) London: Karnac.

Hale, R. 2006 Confidentiality 289–291 in Personality Disorder and Serious Offending, Hospital Treatment Models (Newrith, C., Meux, C. and Taylor, P.J. Editors) London: Arnold Hodder.

Hinshelwood, R.D. 1991 A Dictionary of Kleinian Thought. London: Free Association Books.

Hughes, P. and Riordan, D. 2006 Dynamic Psychotherapy Explained 2nd Edition. London: Radcliffe Medical Press.

Kazdin, A.E. 1986 Comparative Outcome Studies of Psychotherapy: Methodological Issues and Strategies. Journal of Consulting and Clinical Psychology 54: 95–105.

Kinsley, J. 1998 Security and Therapy 75–84 in Managing High Security Psychiatry Care (Kaye C. and Franey, A. Editors) London: Jessica Kingsley.

Klein, M. 1946 Notes on Some Schizoid Mechanisms 1–24 in The Writings of Melanie Klein Vol 3; Envy, Gratitude and Some Other Works. London: Hogarth Press 1975.

Lockwood, K. 1999 Psychodynamic Psychotherapy 134–154 in Essentials of Psychotherapy (Stein S. M., Haigh, R. and Stein, J. Editors) Oxford: Butterworth Heinemann.

McGauley, G.A. 1997 The Actor, the Act and the Environment: Forensic Psychotherapy and Risk. The International Review of Psychiatry: Special Edition on Risk Assessment and Management in Psychiatric Practice 9: 257–264.

McGauley, G.A. and Humphrey, M. 2003 The Contribution of Forensic Psychotherapy to the Care of the Forensic Patient. Advances in Psychiatric Treatment 9: 117–124.

McGuire, J. 2000 Offender Rehabilitation and Treatment: Effective Programmes and Policies to Reduce Offending. Chichester: Wiley.

Meichenbaum, D. 1977 Cognitive Behavioral Modification: An Integrative Approach. New York: Plenum Press.

Minne, C. 2008 The Dreaded and Dreading Patient 27–40 in Psychic Assaults and Frightened Clinicians, Countertransference in Forensic Settings (Gordon, J. and Kirtchuk, G. Editors) London: Karnac.

Minuchin, S. 1974 Families and Family therapy. London: Tavistock.

Norton, K. and Dolan, B. 1995 Acting Out and the Institutional Response. Journal of Forensic Psychiatry 6: 317–332.

Padesky, C. 1994 Schema Change Processes in Cognitive Therapy. Clinical Psychology and Psychotherapy 1: 267–278.

Quayle, M. and Moore, E. 2006 Maladaptive Learning? Cognitive-behavioural Therapy and Beyond 134–145 in Personality Disorder and Serious Offending, Hospital Treatment Models (Newrith, C. Meux, C. and Taylor, P.J. Editors) London: Arnold Hodder.

Reiss, D., Hetherington, E. M., Plomin, R. et al 1995 Genetic Questions for Environmental Studies. Differential Parenting and Psychopathology in Adolescence. Archives of General Psychiatry 52: 925–936.

Roth, A., Fonagy, P. and Parry, G. 2005 What Works for Whom? A Critical Review of Psychotherapy Research 2nd Edition New York: The Guilford Press.

Ruszczynski, S. 2008 Thoughts from Consulting in Secure Settings 85–95 in Psychic Assaults and Frightened Clinicians, Countertransference in Forensic Settings (Gordon, J. and Kirtchuk, G. Editors) London: Karnac.

Sandler, J., Holder, A. and Kawenoker-Berger, M. 1987 Theoretical and Clinical Aspects of Transference 264–284 in From Safety to Superego (Sandler, J. Editor) London: Karnac.

Seligman, M.E.P. 1975 Helplessness: On Depression Development and Death. San Francisco CA: W.H. Freeman.

Sohn, L. 1995 Unprovoked Assaults-Making Sense of Apparently Random Violence. International Journal of Psychoanalysis 76: 565–575.

Stanton, A.H. and Schwartz, M.S. 1954 The Mental Hospital. A Study of Institutional Participation in Psychiatric Illness and Treatment. New York: Basic Books.

Thornton, D., Mann, R., Webster, S. et al 2003 Distinguishing and Combining Risks for Sexual and Violent Recidivisim Annals of The New York Academy of Sciences 989: 225–235.

von Bertalanffy, L. 1962 General Systems Theory: A Critical Review. General Systems 7: 1–20.

Welldon, E. 1993 Forensic Psychotherapy and Group Analysis. Group Analysis 26: 487–502.

Welldon, E. 1994 Forensic Psychotherapy 470–493 in The Handbook of Psychotherapy (Clarkson, P. and Pokorny, M. Editors) London: Routledge.

Young, J.E., Klosko, J.S. and Weishaar, M.E. 2003 Schema Therapy – A Practitioner's Guide New York: Guilford Press.

Chapter 12

A psychodynamic approach to working with offenders: an alternative to moral orthopaedics

Stephen Blumenthal

> "I and the public know
> What all school children learn,
> Those to whom evil is done
> Do evil in return"
> *(W H Auden)*

Aim

To describe how a knowledge of unconscious processes contributes to an increased understanding of the psychopathology and criminal actions of offenders as well as the impact they can have on those working with them.

Learning objectives

- To describe how an understanding of psychodynamic concepts can contribute to an understanding of the criminal act
- To describe how a psychodynamic approach conceptualizes violence
- To discuss how developmental factors and concepts from attachment theory are relevant to Mentally Disordered Offenders (MDOs) and their treatment
- To outline how the safety of the therapeutic relationship allows the offender to understand their maladaptive interpersonal relationships
- To describe the impact on mental health professionals and organizations of working with offender patients

Introduction

In 'Discipline and Punish', Foucault (1977: 10) described the evolution of criminal justice from the marking of the body physically to the marking of the mind and the will. He wrote that with the diminished role of physical punishment 'psychologists and minor civil servants of moral orthopaedics proliferated on the wound it left'.

Psychoanalysis has had a presence in mental health services since the inception of the National Health Service and the development of psychodynamic psychotherapy in the NHS represents an important application of these ideas. The influence of psychoanalytic ideas has waxed and waned over the years, yet a conception of the unconscious is critical to understanding normal and pathological processes in individuals and in groups. In 1933, Edward Glover and others pioneered the treatment of delinquent and criminal patients with psychodynamic psychotherapy, and this led to the opening of the Portman Clinic (Fishman and Ruszczynski 2007). However, it is only in recent years that forensic psychotherapy has become a discipline in its own right (Norton and McGauley 2000; Welldon 1994).

A notion of the unconscious is particularly important when working with offenders. It is fundamental to understanding the mind of the offender, the impact their complicated psychopathology has upon those who manage and care for them and the complex nature of change within the therapeutic context. Forensic mental health workers deal with some of the most complex and disturbed patients, who arouse complicated responses. The law of the talion, an eye for an eye, is deeply embedded in all of us. A psychodynamic approach tries to make sense of our impulse to respond to violence with violence, or Foucault's sanitized equivalent, 'moral orthopaedics'. A psychoanalytic understanding sheds light on the question of what drives particular individuals to act violently and the impact they have on those working with them.

This chapter discusses what the author considers to be the hallmarks of the psychoanalytic approach with respect to offenders. It begins by addressing the meaning of the criminal act and its developmental roots and then considers the particular nature of the therapeutic relationship and the impact on staff of working with offender patients. The final section of the chapter briefly discusses institutional and organizational issues arising from treating and managing these individuals. Wherever possible, heavily disguised and anonymized case material is provided to illustrate the concepts discussed.

Meaning in action: repetition, compulsion and enactment

In generic treatment settings, the focus of psychodynamic psychotherapy is on the patient's psychic reality, whereas in the forensic field we are confronted each day with actuality; acts that have taken place often with devastating consequences. From a psychodynamic point of view the act has a meaning. It is not some random tragic event but is the outcome of comprehensible precursors. The act itself is usually understandable in the context of the actor's mental state, their relationships and their history. Psychodynamic psychotherapy is concerned with elucidating the meaning of symptoms. In a forensic context, the offence is considered to have an equivalent status or role. It is, in effect, the symptom which we attempt to understand. One of the tasks of therapy is to help the patient to understand their actions.

Clinical vignette

A 25-year-old man began attending psychodynamic therapy after receiving a number of convictions for exhibitionism. He worked as an actor and during treatment, the therapist and the patient arrived at the formulation that his work provided the opportunity of satisfying an impulse to exhibit himself in a socially acceptable way. It gradually emerged during treatment that he had felt ignored by his parents, although this was not evident in a conscious form at the beginning of his therapy. He recalled attempts to shock his parents into taking notice of him, but these tended to go unnoticed. He was surprised by the length of time it took to be arrested for his habitual offences. It seemed that no one noticed or took seriously his attempts to be seen.

Freud (1914) originally conceived of the term 'acting out' in the context of the therapeutic relationship. In the course of treatment, the patient compulsively repeats certain actions rather than remembering and acknowledging them. These actions relive unconscious wishes and fantasies from early life in relation to the person of the analyst or therapist. Therefore 'acting out' is understood as a dimension of the unacknowledged aspect of the transference relationship between the patient and analyst. This meaning of the term has particular relevance in the forensic field, where patients frequently relate to members of the multidisciplinary team in a way that evokes their early relationships, particularly those with parental care-givers. Some of the patient's actions in the present may be understood in the context of the patient's conflicts that cannot be articulated and which relate to the past.

Since Freud's time, the term 'acting out' has been adopted in a more colloquial way to signify the repetition of unconscious conflicts in action in a more general manner, outside of the context of the therapeutic relationship. Despite the dilution of the term, there are a number of important features that remain, which are particularly applicable to a forensic context. A theoretical tenet of the psychoanalytic approach, adopted by psychodynamic psychotherapy and forensic psychotherapy, is that action represents an extension of the mind, so that what is not consciously remembered is repeated in action or in symptoms. It is a peculiar feature of the forensic context that what is not remembered is repeated in action. What is unconscious has to find a different form of expression. Almost always, the criminal actions that an individual involves himself or herself in bear an important relationship with that person's character. From a psychodynamic point of view, the act is a marker, a symptom, which carries with it a meaning about the overall personality of the actor. For Freud, symptoms or actions were mnemic symbols. They reproduce, in a repetitive way and in a more or less disguised form, elements of past conflicts in the present: 'A thing which has not been understood inevitably reappears; like an unlaid ghost, it cannot rest until the mystery has been solved and the spell broken'. (Freud 1909).

The tragedy of criminality is that there has typically been a chronic failure of understanding, and it is when issues cannot be understood mentally that they are often acted out, bodily. If the principle task of parenting is to provide an emotional container in which the infant is understood and can develop, there has been a failure; a lack and often complete absence of this parental function in the early life of offenders. For Hobson (2002), the quality of emotional connectedness between mother and infant is the cradle for the development of an apparatus for thinking. Similarly, understanding other minds or the capacity to 'mentalize', defined as the ability to interpret the actions of oneself and others as meaningful based on intentional mental states – that is, based on of an understanding of the feelings, beliefs, thoughts and intentions of oneself and others (Baron-Cohen 2000) – is not a given. This capacity develops through a process of having experienced oneself in the mind of another during childhood, in the context of a secure attachment relationship (Fonagy and Target 1997). Symbolization refers to the mental capacity to allow one thing to stand for another in a representative way. For some offenders the capacity to symbolize has broken down completely, revealing a striking concreteness in the criminal mind and the criminal act. This is most evident in the case of offenders with severe mental illness where delusions may be understood as having meaning, although they have lost their 'as if' quality and are believed to be real by the patient.

Clinical vignette

A schizophrenic man was interviewed in prison following the near fatal assault on his father. He believed himself to have been provoked by his father's refusal to accept that he was not his son. Despite being unmistakably oriental in origin, he believed himself to be the long lost son of Prince Charles and Camilla Parker-Bowles. This delusion seemed to be an isolated phenomenon; in other respects he was a functioning, capable and intelligent man. Rational challenges to this belief, such as on the basis of genetics or his date of birth, were met with thoroughly researched arguments to the contrary.

There are no simple rules about the meaning of a symptom or act, and psychodynamic work with offenders involves a painstaking process of elucidating this meaning. Nevertheless, there are some general principles that can guide the therapist towards an understanding of the criminal act.

As already outlined, the offence represents the malignant emergence of mental conflict. The offence involves a repetition, but it often also involves an inversion; where once the person was a victim, they are now in the position of perpetrator. At one level the action may be a repetition of a childhood trauma but, at another level, it can be an exact reversal of that trauma. Consequently, the individual is spared the painful memory and his or her actions represent a mastery of the early experiences he or she suffered passively (Campbell and Hale 1991). For example, the boy who felt humiliated by a bullying father may, in adulthood, reverse the experience and bully and intimidate others. Identification with the aggressor shifts the individual from a sense of weakness to one of power, the passive experience being turned into an active one.

Risk assessment and meaning

Contemporary approaches to risk assessment have tended to forgo an interest in the meaning of the act. Glasser (1996b) pointed out the importance of establishing the meaning of the violent action. He suggested two fundamental types of violence. The first is driven by a biological urge to survive and is aimed at eliminating danger or threat. It may be characterized as 'self-preservative'. The second, according to Glasser's typology, has the aim of inflicting physical and or emotional pain on the victim and may be characterised as 'sadistic'. Glasser illustrated how these two types of violence are interrelated, in that sadistic violence has its roots in the self-preservative instinct: 'The intention to destroy is converted into a wish to hurt and control' (Glasser 1996a: 287). From this perspective, violence exists on a continuum. At one end lies ordinary teasing, shading into sadomasochistic relationships in which individuals play destructive games with one another, sexual crimes, rape, bodily harm and, at the extreme end of the continuum, homicide. To determine an individual's potential dangerousness, understanding both the meaning of the act to the perpetrator and the quality of the violence are essential pieces of information.

Psychotic violence is most frequently of the self-preservative kind, whereas relatively more psychologically integrated individuals generally perpetrate malicious acts. For example, a homicide may result from a paranoid delusion that there was a real and immediate danger from the victim. The consequence of this conceptual scheme is that decisions about risk, treatability and management are fundamentally different. Those whose violence is self-preservative are generally safe as long as they remain out of contact with the trigger for their violence and the 'stimulus conditions' in which the violence occurred. Glasser (1996b) proposed that a primary task of risk assessment, in this context, is a microscopically detailed discernment of the trigger. Treatment should aim to diminish vulnerability associated with the trigger and management should assist the perpetrator to avoid contact with the trigger until it no longer has the power to act as such. On the other hand, the maliciously motivated offender presents more difficult and complex problems in that the act is associated more with characterological features of the individual that are difficult to change. Glasser (1996b) recommended the careful building of a relationship in which the offender feels able to trust. This relationship may extend to a psychotherapeutic one where the basis for the violence can be identified and addressed.

Childhood narratives: attachment, separation and loss

Research on developmental pathways to criminality indicate that children who are neglected or abused are more likely to be arrested later in life for delinquency, adult criminality and violence (Dodge et al 1990; Farrington 1978; Widom 1989). Indeed, in the vast majority of cases offending behaviour is a fairly predictable aspect of the developmental trajectory rather than a departure from it. Hale (personal communication) states, when a person goes on trial for their crimes they are really on trial for their childhood. An important first step is to establish an individual's history before attempting to understand it. Patients' histories are lost in secure settings with surprising regularity. Doubtless this is, in part, owing to the wish not to know about the extremes of pain and suffering that many of these individuals have endured. There also seems to be an institutional repetition of a childhood situation in which history and origin are regarded as unimportant and are lost.

Clinical vignette

A traumatized young man who was prone to serious interpersonal violence was asked what he knew about his birth. He told the interviewer that he had asked his mother this very question but she had replied that she had forgotten. It emerged that he was her forgotten child in many other respects too. He was neglected as a child and placed in care for periods. At these times, his mother's contact with him was erratic. He was never sure whether he was in her mind.

One of the most striking characteristics of working with forensic patients is the extent to which their early development is characterized by neglectful and abusive parenting, often with separations from or loss of parental figures. The life histories of many offenders, with their numerous disruptions to attachment processes, evidence of failed parental sensitivity and their difficulties in forming mature interpersonal relationships, strongly suggest the relevance of attachment theory to aid our understanding of this population (McGauley and Rubitel 2006). Bowlby (1977: 207) formulated attachment theory as a body of explanations concerned with 'conceptualizing the propensity of human beings to make strong affectional bonds to particular others and of explaining the many forms of emotional distress and personality disturbances, including anxiety, anger, depression and emotional detachment to which unwilling separation and loss give rise'.

The formation of an attachment bond between the human infant and its primary caregiver, most often the mother, is necessary to protect the vulnerable infant and promote its security and survival. Bowlby postulated that this bond forms during the first year of life and continues as part of the normal repertoire of child and adult behaviour. Attachment behaviour is activated when there is a threat, real or perceived, to this attachment bond. In these situations the child, distressed on the withdrawal of the attachment figure, shows a strong tendency to seek proximity with the attachment figure, especially when in pain or frightened (Bowlby 1982). Disruption, or the threat of disruption, of these bonds through separation, deprivation or bereavement stimulates painful affective states and in some cases leads to the development of psychopathology.

A key concept in attachment theory is that of internal working models (Bowlby 1973). Bowlby used this term to describe an individual's representation of the world, of their attachment figures, of themselves and the relationships between these representations. Internal working models are acquired in infancy through internalization of the characteristic interpersonal interactions of the child's major attachment figures. If the attachment figure has been sensitive to the infant's needs, the child is likely to develop an internal working model of the self as valued. If, however, the parent has been rejecting or neglecting of the child's attempts to elicit comfort or to explore the world, Bowlby postulated that the child is likely to construct an internal working model of the self as unworthy or incompetent (Bretherton 1995). The type of internal working models a child constructs is therefore of great importance. These structures not only integrate past experiences but also regulate the child's behaviour with attachment figures and come to organize and predict behaviour in future adult attachment relationships.

Bowlby (1944) also conceptualized some forms of violence arising as a result of a disorder of the attachment and care-giving systems. Although threats to the attachment system through trauma, separation and loss stand out in the early experiences of offenders, it is notable that many individuals dismiss the significance of these relationships and events in their attachment narratives of their early experiences. It is only relatively recently that researchers have studied attachment in forensic populations (Frodi et al 2001; Levinson and Fonagy 2004; Van IJzendoorn et al 1997). McGauley and Rubitel (2006) summarized the research to date and discussed the relevance of attachment theory, with particular reference to forensic patients with personality disorder. Compared to both normal and clinical psychiatric populations, forensic patients have higher levels of insecure attachment status as measured by the Adult Attachment Interview (AAI) (George et al 1996; Main and Goldwyn 1994). The AAI is a semi-structured interview, consisting of a series of questions and probes, which elicits a narrative about the individual's childhood attachment experiences and assesses their mental representation of attachment as an adult.

In particular, a 'dismissing' attachment status was over-represented in these forensic groups (Frodi et al 2001; Levinson and Fonagy 2004; Van IJzendoorn et al 1997). In other words, individuals who are dismissing with respect to their attachment status are individuals who typically negate and disavow the significance of attachment relationships in both childhood and adulthood while claiming self-sufficiency. Clinically, these are patients who characteristically do not see themselves as having any difficulties and therefore do not feel in need of help or treatment; consequently, they are difficult to engage.

Levinson and Fonagy (2004) also reported a low level of reflective function in their sample of prisoners with mental health problems, signalling an underlying deficit in their capacity to mentalize. They proposed a model that conceptualizes some interpersonal violence as resulting from disorganization of the attachment system (Fonagy 2003; Levinson and Fonagy 2004). They suggested that severe early trauma, in the context of attachment experiences, leads to a developmental line of psychopathology characterized by both a disavowal of attachment experiences and the capacity to think about them resulting in a deficit in reflective functioning and the capacity to mentalize. In the context of high levels of arousal, non-mentalizing cognitive processes increase and predominate; the individual is then more prone to misperceive their own experience and the mental states of others. Levinson and Fonagy proposed that such a failure of mentalization predisposes the person towards committing violent acts. Such acts may occur as either a response to misperceiving the world, including the actions or intentions of others, or to evacuate intolerable mental affects or bodily sensations that cannot be thought about. In addition, the institution may come to stand for the secure attachment relationships which were previously lacking.

Clinical vignette

A patient in a medium secure unit said that he thought the term 'secure unit' referred not to the protection of the public from him, but rather as a place of safety and security for him.

One patient who had been discharged from a secure unit to more independent living in a pre-discharge house absconded. He telephoned a couple of days later saying that he wanted to come 'home'. Upon his return he was placed in a more secure ward.

Levinson and Fonagy's (2004) findings fit well with clinical experience; working with offenders who have a poor mentalizing capacity and who are insecure with respect to their attachment relationships is one of the challenges of working psychotherapeutically with forensic patients. Forensically the patients' deficit in mentalization means that they frequently find it difficult to think about their offending behaviour with respect to understanding their feelings, beliefs, thoughts and intentions at the time, the impact of these on their victim and what their victim was experiencing and thinking during the offence. The sequelae of having an insecure attachment mean that the temporal boundaries of treatment can be difficult to establish with this patient group. Entering into a therapeutic relationship is complex, as is negotiating the separation at a treatment break. Breaks in treatment are often a time of concern for forensic psychotherapists because it is understood that, despite the patient's frequent disavowal of the importance of the relationship with the therapist, the break is experienced at a very primitive level, often as abandonment, but frequently this cannot be thought about or mentalized. This is one of the reasons why brief psychotherapy can pose particular difficulties for forensic patients.

Glasser (1996a) helpfully outlined this dynamic in his concept of the 'core complex', in which he described how the offender manages their intense fears of abandonment and merger by establishing 'contact at a distance'. Therapists may have to work painstakingly hard to resist the patient's unconscious pressure to join in with a core complex enactment in which this 'contact at a distance' is perpetuated. Unfortunately, this patient characteristic can, at times, be exacerbated by service demands to decrease the pressure on waiting lists or move patients to less secure provision because of bed-pressure and service targets, creating a situation in which patients' treatment needs are never fully addressed.

Clinical vignette

A patient had a 10-year history of contact with a forensic outpatient service. He was difficult to engage in assessment, constantly suggesting times when he could be seen that he knew could not possibly be offered. He disappeared and reappeared on a number of occasions and eventually agreed to treatment. When offered treatment, he said that he could not start immediately. He had compelling reasons to go to live in another town for six months because he had recently resolved a complicated relationship with his estranged parents. However, it seemed no coincidence that, yet again, he had found a reason to evade engagement in psychotherapy.

These types of difficulties are common in a forensic setting. The other town seemed to be as much a place in the patient's mind as it was an external one. The patient appeared to need to take refuge from the treatment and, while he was not consciously aware of any anxiety, at a behavioural level his conflicts were expressed in the only language that the patient could speak; in action. It was in action that he could express his need for a psychic retreat (Steiner 1993) from the pain and anxiety that emotional contact with his therapist, and consequently with a part of himself, would entail. Of course, such situations can be professionally and personally corrosive to those working with such patients. This is because it is difficult to establish a working alliance and the therapist's natural aspirations for an engagement with the patient can easily be dashed. Consequently, it is of the utmost importance to make sense of the impact of the work in the context of good regular supervision.

The impact of the work: the offence, transference and countertransference

Professionals working directly with patients, clients, probationers or prisoners within a mental health or criminal justice setting have a dynamic relationship with those they work with. Such a relationship holds both therapeutic possibility as well as potential pitfalls. Whatever one's theoretical persuasion, a dynamic relationship exists and it is safer and therapeutically advantageous if this relationship is acknowledged and understood. There are a number of features of this relationship that are peculiar to working in a forensic setting. Principally, there is an abnormal act that has taken place often involving the transgression of other people's boundaries. In itself, this has a profound impact on those who work with this group. There is also the repetition within the therapeutic relationship of often malignant patterns of relating based in childhood as well as repetition of aspects of the criminal act itself.

Freud's notion of the repetition of the unremembered past within the context of the therapeutic relationship was one of his most profound insights (Freud 1914). Infantile prototypes of relating to important others, which reflect our developmental histories, form the basis of the person's internal working models of relating, which are as individual and distinct as our DNA. As described earlier, the infant forms internal working models through internalizing aspects of parental figures and the way in which they relate to the infant. In the course of our interaction with others these are externalized once more, both in our choice of relationships and in the nature of our interpersonal interactions. We create situations, in the context of our relationships, that are organized by these internal working models. These then become actualized in the treatment, where the therapeutic frame allows for their close examination. The reliving of the patient's internal working models in the context of the therapeutic relationship is similar to the psychoanalytic process of the transference described earlier (Chapter 11). There is also considerable pressure brought to bear on the therapist to join in the replaying of an internal set of object relations in the therapy. Through the unconscious processes of projection (the locating of parts of the self in the person of the therapist) and projective identification (where the person who is the target of the projection then begins to feel, think and behave in keeping with what is being projected, confirming to the person projecting that the unwanted parts of the self are really aspects belonging to the other person; Chapter 11) the patient's subtle assumptions about their therapist, and the way in which the psychotherapist feels drawn into responding, provide the window for understanding the patient.

Glasser's (1996a) notion of the 'core complex' is an important conceptual tool in understanding the therapeutic relationship in the forensic context. The 'victim-perpetrator' or sadomasochistic dynamic is a typical feature of the transference in a forensic context. This is understood as a means of managing the fear of merger and abandonment by maintaining contact but at a safe distance. Through projection and projective identification a relationship is set up in which therapist and patient inevitably occupy these positions through reciprocal role relationships (Sandler 1976). Whatever one's therapeutic persuasion, this dynamic is important to understand as it often underpins the pull into overt or covert punishment of the patient. Paradoxically, this inadvertently gratifies perverse wishes in the offender. Examples of the above situation abound in secure settings, particularly in prisons, where there is often the mistaken belief that the aversive experience of harsh punishment will reduce the likelihood of criminal behaviour in the future. If anything, a cruel response to cruelty tends to fuel the conditions that led to the offending in the first place.

Sohn (Browne et al 1993) pointed out that treating a patient who has assaulted or abused another individual cannot take place without recognizing how the crime or aspects of the crime appear in the transference relationship. One of the difficulties is that these aspects do not reoccur in the transference as exact likenesses of the previous forensic actions; they may occur overtly, but more often their appearance is covert. Clinical experience shows that when there is work taking place in the transference, that is, that the crime and the person's character are metabolized within the transference relationship, enactment, and consequently risk, are reduced. Working in the transference helps the patient to begin to symbolize and as a result increases their tendency to express their pathology in vivo rather than in action.

Clinical vignette

A man, who had a long history of fraudulent behaviour, came for treatment. He was talented but repeatedly spoiled his chances of success in work by committing fraud just when he might achieve success, such as being promoted. His presentation in treatment was complex. At times he was engaged and gained insight, but at these points of connection he would typically react negatively to the therapy and all the work that had painstakingly taken place would be undone. He described how his parents had always been ambitious for him. As a child he was a talented musician, and they bought him a music synthesizer. His music was received with some acclaim but when this happened, much to his parents' dismay, he stopped playing. In the therapeutic relationship, the therapist could not help but have some ambition for him, but the more he made use of therapy the less he attended and eventually he dropped out of treatment. Despite addressing the way in which the therapy itself was being defrauded, the therapist was left with the feeling of having been cheated.

This man epitomized what Freud (1916) described in his paper 'Criminals from a Sense of Guilt'. The crime was a real-ization, a 'making real' of an internal sense of guilt relating to a much earlier phase of life for which he sought punishment. Indeed the therapy itself became caught up in a re-enactment of this to the extent that the patient saw the therapist as a parental figure whose wishes for him had to be thwarted. The offence was certainly relived in the therapeutic relationship, and it was worked with, but the re-enactment obliterated the therapy itself. The man did, however, return to the clinic some years later and sought further help.

One defining feature of forensic psychotherapy is the importance of the presence of 'a third object', in addition to the dyad of patient and therapist. This 'third object' takes the form of the criminal justice system or other outside agency. It is increasingly the case that psychotherapy within the NHS requires reporting to a third party, but this process is more pronounced in the case of psychotherapy with offenders. This intrusion into the therapist–patient dyad is clearly necessary, but the presence of a powerful agency or institution has important transference implications which need to be carefully considered.

Institutional and organizational issues

When treating forensic patients, the 'third object' often takes the form of the institution that frequently functions as the container in which psychopathology is played out. Individuals who cause injury to others also have the capacity to inflict emotional harm on those working with them. This can, in turn, have a caustic effect on the organization itself. The boundary violations that have occurred in many secure institutions that care for and incarcerate offenders are testament to this. The second Ashworth Inquiry (Fallon et al 1999; Chapters 14 and 24) details the collusion of staff in the most disturbing corruption of personality-disordered patients. However, even in 'healthy' units or services there will always be a degree of 'infection'.

Clinical vignette

Staff in a supported-living housing project accepted a 53-year-old man who was on release from prison on licence. He had a string of convictions for many different offences, including motor vehicle offences, assault, sexual assault, burglary and breaking the conditions of his licence. He used a variety of pseudonyms. He had failed at a previous hostel because the staff had not been able to manage him. He was charming and likeable, and the staff had found themselves inadvertently drawn into some rather compromising situations. They had then felt stung by his response, which was to quote policy and procedure and use the rules to prove that they had been in the wrong, rather than him.

The housing project staff had some misgivings about accepting him but felt that they had substantial expertise in understanding and managing such clients. The client tended to stir things up in the hostel and whip up dissatisfaction among the resident group, skilfully playing one person off against another. However, despite these management problems, overall his stay went well. After a year, despite predictable difficulties, the staff team felt satisfied with their work in managing a man who presented complex challenges to the service. Just as a planned discharge approached, with the help of the cleaner in the hostel, he stole a new computer and absconded.

Systemic issues are important because for many offenders individual psychodynamic psychotherapy is not a viable option; what is required is sensitive and thoughtful management. Winnicott (1956: 125) described how the antisocial tendency compels the environment to be important:

> The child provokes total environmental reactions, as if seeking an ever-widening frame, a circle which had as its first example the mother's arms or the mother's body. One can discern a series – the mother's body, the mother's arms, the parental relationship, the home, the family including cousins and near relatives, the school, the locality with its police-stations, the country with its laws.

Psychotherapists often consider themselves to have a particularly significant contribution to make in helping the system think about itself. For example, Cox (1986: 163) stated, 'It is within the "inner world" of the hospital itself that the psychotherapist may, in the long run, assume his most important role.'

Therapeutically, group or milieu therapy is often a treatment option and, even when individual therapy is indicated, the milieu is still vitally important. The reasons for this are alluded to by Winnicott (1956). The healthy milieu or group provides the necessary level of containment to the forensic patients at an intensity of emotional contact that they can manage. Working closely with such disturbed individuals can take its toll and requires good supervision and a context in which to make sense of the work, such as in reflective practice groups. Without these fora the tendency is for staff to become overwhelmed and burnt out, to become emotionally unavailable or for the organization to become excessively punitive and hostile.

Conclusion

This chapter has discussed how a psychodynamic approach informs an understanding of the MDO and their aggressive acts (see Key points). The offender, through their antisocial behaviour, speaks the language of action, often with devastating consequences. An ordinary human impulse is to reply to the offender in the same mode of expression and to retaliate. Psychodynamic sspsychotherapy attempts to interpret this language and so help the offender and those working with them discover a different idiom. The offence is a primitive and concrete expression of adversity which has a profound impact on those working with offenders. An understanding of unconscious processes promotes thinking and reduces the need to resort to action both in the offender and in ourselves.

Key points

- Criminality is the behavioural representation of a complex psychological situation
- Consideration of unconscious as well as conscious processes provides a fuller understanding of the thinking and behaviour of the offender
- Consideration of developmental and attachment experiences can inform the therapeutic approach to MDOs
- The application of psychodynamic concepts can help both the individual and organizations avoid toxic dynamics, harmful to both parties, arising from the offenders' psychopathology

References

Baron-Cohen, S. 2000 Theory of Mind And Autism: A Fifteen Year Review 3–20 in Understanding Other Minds: Perspectives from Developmental Cognitive Neuroscience (Baron-Cohen, S. Tager-Flusberg H. and Cohen, D.J. Editors) Oxford: Oxford University Press.

Bowlby, J. 1944 Forty-four Juvenile Thieves: Their Characters and Home-life. International Journal of Psycho-analysis 25: 19–52.

Bowlby, J. 1973 Attachment and Loss, Vol II: Separation. New York: Basic Books.

Bowlby, J. 1977 The Making and Breaking of Affectional Bonds. I. Aetiology and Psychopathology in the Light of Attachment Theory. An Expanded Version of the Fiftieth Maudsley Lecture, Delivered Before the Royal College of Psychiatrists, 19 November 1976. British Journal of Psychiatry 130: 201–210.

Bowlby, J. 1982 Attachment and Loss, Vol I: Attachment. New York: Basic Books.

Bretherton, I. 1995 The Origins of Attachment Theory 45–84 in Attachment Theory, Social, Developmental and Clinical Perspectives (Goldberg, S., Muir, R. and Kerr, J. Editors) Hillsdale NJ: The Analytic Press.

Browne, F., Gudjonsson, G., Gunn, J., et al 1993 Principles of Treatment for the Mentally Disordered Offender 646–690 in Forensic Psychiatry: Clinical, Legal and Ethical Issues (Gunn, J. and Taylor, P. Editors) Oxford: Butterworth Heinemann.

Campbell, D. and Hale, R. 1991 Suicidal Acts 287–306 in Textbook of Psychotherapy in Psychiatric Practice (Holmes, J. Editor) London: Churchill Livingstone.

Cox, M. 1986 The 'Holding Function' of Dynamic Psychotherapy in a Custodial Setting: A Review. Journal of the Royal Society of Medicine 79: 162–164.

Dodge, K. A., Bates, J. E. and Pettit, G. S. 1990 Mechanisms in the cycle of violence. Science, 250, 1678–1683.

Fallon, P., Bluglass, R., Edwards, B. and Daniels, G. 1999 Report of the Committee of Inquiry into the Personality Disorder Unit, Ashworth Special Hospital. Cm 4194-ii. London, The Stationery Office.

Farrington, D. 1978 The Family Backgrounds of Aggressive Youths 73–93 in Aggression and Antisocial Behaviour in Children and Adolescence (Hersov, L., Berger, M. and Shaffer, D. Editors) Oxford: Pergamon.

Fishman, C. and Ruszczynski, S. 2007 The Portman Clinic: A Historical Sketch 15–21 in Lectures on Violence, Perversion and Delinquency (Morgan, D. and Ruszczynski, S. Editors) London: Karnac.

Fonagy, P. 2003 Towards a Developmental Understanding of Violence. British Journal of Psychiatry 183: 190–192.

Fonagy, P. and Target, M. 1997 Attachment and Reflective Function: Their Role in Self-organization. Development and Psychopathology 9: 679–700.

Foucault, M. 1977 Discipline and Punish. London: Allen Lane.

Freud, S. 1909 Analysis of a Phobia in a Five Year Old Boy 101–147 in Standard Edition, X. London: Hogarth Press.

Freud, S. 1914 Remembering, Repeating and Working-Through 147–156 in Standard Edition, XII. London: Hogarth Press.

Freud, S. 1916 Criminals from a sense of guilt 332–333 in Standard Edition, XIV. London: Hogarth Press.

Frodi, A., Dernevik, M., Sepa, A. et al 2001 Current Attachment Representations of Incarcerated Offenders Varying in Degree of Psychopathy. Attachment and Human Development 3: 269–283.

George, C., Kaplan, N. and Main, M. 1996 The Adult Attachment Interview 3rd Edition. Berkeley CA: Department of Psychology, University of California at Berkeley.

Glasser, M. 1996a Aggression and Sadism in the Perversions 279–299 in Sexual Deviation (Rosen, I. Editor) Oxford: Oxford University Press.

Glasser, M. 1996b The Assessment and Management of Dangerousness: The Psychoanalytical Contribution. Journal of Forensic Psychiatry 7: 271–283.

Hobson, P. 2002 The Cradle of Thought. Basingstoke: Macmillan.

Levinson, A. and Fonagy, P. 2004 Offending and Attachment: The Relationship between Interpersonal Awareness and Offending in a Prison Population with Psychiatric Disorder. Canadian Journal of Psychoanalysis 12: 225–251.

Main, M. and Goldwyn, R. 1994 Adult Attachment Scoring and Classification System. version 6. Berkeley CA: Department of Psychology, University of California at Berkeley.

McGauley, G. and Rubitel, A. 2006 The Contribution of Attachment Theory and Personality Disordered Patients 69–80 in Personality Disorder and Serious Offending (Newrith, C. Meux, C. and Taylor, P. Editors) London: Hodder Arnold.

Norton, K. and McGauley, G. 2000 Forensic Psychotherapy in Britain: Its Role in Assessment, Treatment and Training. Criminal Behaviour and Mental Health 10: S82–S90.

Sandler, J. 1976 Countertransference and Role-responsiveness. International Review of Psycho-analysis 3: 43–47.

Steiner, J. 1993 Psychic Retreats. Pathological Organizations in Psychotic, Neurotic and Borderline Patients. London: Routledge.

van IJzendoorn, M.H., Feldbrugge, J.T., Derks, F.C. et al 1997 Attachment Representations of Personality-Disordered Criminal Offenders. American Journal of Orthopsychiatry 67: 449–459.

Welldon, E. 1994 Forensic Psychotherapy 470–493 in The Handbook of Psychotherapy (Clarkson, P. and Pokorny, M. Editors) London: Routledge.

Widom, C. S. 1989 The Cycle of Violence. Science 244: 160–166.

Winnicott, D. 1956 The Antisocial Tendency 120–31 in Deprivation and Delinquency (Winnicott, C., Shepherd, R. and Davis, M. Editors). London: Routledge.

Chapter 13

Psychotherapeutic understanding and approach to psychosis in mentally disordered offenders

Cleo Van Velsen

Aim

This chapter describes a psychodynamic perspective of schizophrenia and the frequently encountered dynamics of treating such patients in secure forensic institutions.

Learning objectives

- To outline the aetiology and phenomenology of schizophrenia
- To understand the relationship between schizophrenia and violence
- To describe how psychoanalytic thinking contributes to an understanding of psychosis
- To outline the psychological approaches to the treatment of schizophrenia
- To describe how a psychodynamic approach contributes to the management of patients with schizophrenia detained in security

---

Introduction

Psychosis is defined in the Collins English Dictionary (1979) as 'any form of severe mental disorder in which the individual's contact with reality becomes highly distorted'. To be blunt, when people talk about 'madness' they are referring to psychosis. Psychosis, in itself, is not the diagnosis but a descriptive term denoting symptoms and signs associated with certain disorders that are designated as severe mental illness. Psychotic illnesses essentially affect the person's thinking, and as these conditions often entail loss of insight, the sufferer may be unaware that their thinking has become distorted. The individual's capacity to distinguish between subjective experience and external reality is impaired to a greater or lesser degree, and the person can construct a 'false' environment based on their misperceptions and symptoms such as delusions and hallucinations.

The majority of the patients in both general and forensic psychiatric services in the United Kingdom suffer from 'severe and enduring mental illness', which usually means psychosis. In particular, most of the patients in medium and high secure NHS forensic units are men suffering from schizophrenia, a psychotic illness. There are other psychotic disorders, for example, schizoaffective disorders, delusional disorders and psychotic mood disorders which, although they resemble schizophrenia, do not meet all the criteria required to make this diagnosis. Although some people can be offensive as a result of these disorders, these individuals constitute a minority of detained forensic patients; thus schizophrenia will be used as an exemplar of a psychotic illness for this chapter.

There are two main classification systems for diagnosing mental disorder: The International Classification of Diseases (WHO 1992) and the Diagnostic and Statistical Manual of Mental Disorders (DSM-IV) (American Psychiatric Association 1994). To avoid confusion this chapter will refer to the DSM-IV system.

The chapter begins with a brief description of the aetiology, epidemiology, descriptive pathology and treatment approaches to schizophrenia. Throughout the chapter the particularity of the patient suffering from schizophrenia who has committed a violent act against others will be highlighted. It is important to remember that the minority of people with schizophrenia are violent but, by definition, those who have committed a violent act against others form the majority of the patients within forensic settings. The second part of the chapter explores, from a psychodynamic view, the impact such patients have upon the institution in which they are contained and vice versa. Using a medium secure unit based within a deprived inner-city area as an example this chapter will examine the various divisions and conflicts that emerge in the thinking, management and treatment of these patients in their institutions.

Schizophrenia accounts for the majority of the burden of chronic psychiatric disability. It is diagnosed by the identification of specific symptoms and signs, rather than by any biological markers. This has led to a long-standing discussion of the validity of the diagnosis, with one strand of the 'anti-psychiatry' movement, particularly associated with the radicalism of the 1960s, disputing the value of psychiatric diagnosis per se (Cooper 1967; Szasz 1961; see Chapter 1 for a fuller discussion). Although the perspective that schizophrenia is present in all countries and all cultures with a lifetime risk of approximately 1% has gained wide acceptance (Leff 1988; Murray et al 2004), the value of both the diagnostic approach and the diagnosis itself is still disputed (Kleinman 1987).

Aetiology of schizophrenia

Although the precise aetiology is unknown, it is clear that both genetic and environmental factors are important. Having a first-degree relative who suffers from schizophrenia greatly increases the risk of developing the illness; between 10% and 15% in siblings and children where one parent has schizophrenia, and up to 40% for the children of two schizophrenic parents. The concordance rate in identical twins is approximately 40%, illustrating not only that there is a genetic effect but that environmental factors are operating as well. However, no single gene is responsible, and the proposed model is polygenetic, with several additive genes each having a small individual effect. Genetic linkage and association studies have identified some of these genes, the presence of which increases the vulnerability of the individual to developing schizophrenia. The overarching aetiological model is therefore a multi-factorial one, in which genetic predisposition interacts with various environmental, psychological, familial and social factors. Environmental risk factors include various neurological insults occurring early in life, such as those arising from obstetric complications, or childhood head injuries that can slightly increase the risk of developing the illness in adulthood. For a fuller discussion of these factors the reader is referred to Wright et al (2000) and Murray et al (2004).

Epidemiology of schizophrenia

The annual incidence of schizophrenia is between 10 and 20 individuals per 100,000 of the population. Both men and women are equally affected by the illness, although the age of onset differs; for most men it is between the ages of 15 and 25 years, whereas in women between 25 and 35 years. Schizophrenia is a young person's disease, which often becomes a chronic illness; both have risk and management implications for a forensic population. It is also important to note that the lifetime suicide risk for schizophrenia is 10%, as this can sometimes be forgotten in the concern about violence to others.

As it is a chronic disorder, the prevalence of schizophrenia is much higher than the incidence, about 4 people per 1,000. There is an increased prevalence of schizophrenia in certain groups; urban populations, lower socio-economic classes and prison populations. In the United Kingdom, men of Afro-Caribbean origin and first-generation immigrants are over-represented in psychiatric hospitals and forensic units, particularly in the population detained under the Mental Health Act (HMSO 2007; see Chapters 2 and 6).

Phenomenology of schizophrenia

There are a multitude of symptoms associated with schizophrenia but most patients do not suffer from all of them; so a certain number of symptoms, over a certain period, are necessary to make the diagnosis. All of these symptoms are well described in the major psychiatric textbooks such as The Shorter Oxford Textbook of Psychiatry (Gelder et al 2006). They are briefly referred to here to provide background for the later discussion illustrating how these phenomena are conceptualized from a psychodynamic perspective.

The most dramatic symptoms of schizophrenia, sometimes referred to as the 'positive symptoms', occur in the acute or active phase and were described by Schneider (1959) as the 'first rank' symptoms (see table 13.1). These were seen as important in differentiating schizophrenia from other disorders.

The passivity phenomena include 'thought insertion', where a patient believes that thoughts are being inserted into his or her mind by external agencies; 'thought withdrawal', where the patient experiences an abrupt cessation in thinking, leading to a belief that his or her thoughts have been completely removed by something or someone and 'thought broadcast', where a patient believes that others have access to his or her thoughts. Patients can also experience thought echo, when they hear a voice repeating what they are about to say or have just been thinking. Another group of passivity symptoms occur when the patient's feelings, impulses and actions are experienced as having been caused or controlled by an agency or person outside of him or herself; for example, radio waves that are 'making' his eyes close.

A hallucination is defined as a perception experienced in the absence of an external stimulus to the corresponding sense organ; for example, hearing a voice when no one is speaking. To qualify as a hallucination the perception must be experienced as a true perception and appear to emanate from outside of the person's head or mind. Auditory hallucinations are commonly called 'voices'. These are psychoanalytically understood as unacceptable, bizarre and frightening

Table 13.1 Schneider's 'first rank' symptoms of schizophrenia

Thought insertion or withdrawal
Thought broadcast
Thought echo
Made feelings, thoughts or actions
Third-person auditory hallucinations
Running commentary auditory hallucinations
Somatic hallucinations
Delusional perception

thoughts and experiences that the patient has projected, that is, forcibly expelled from his or her mind so that they are experienced as external to the self. They often refer to the patient in the third person, which can be in the form of a 'running commentary', referring to him or her as 'he or she', or a discussion between voices about the patient. What is said can be derogatory but can also, on occasions, be positive. Voices can also be experienced in the second person, that is, directly addressing the person. More rarely auditory hallucinations take the form of 'command hallucinations', which tell a patient to commit an action. These are particularly relevant in the forensic population as they are a risk factor for violent offending. Somatic hallucinations, although one of Schneider's 'first rank' symptoms, are relatively uncommon. They may be experienced as physical sensations, for example, a feeling of insects crawling on the person's skin.

Delusions are defined as false, unshakeable ideas or beliefs, out of keeping with the patient's social and cultural background. They are held with conviction and certainty, are not open to argument and their content is 'impossible', although this is complex, as there is a range of beliefs between unlikely and impossible. In delusional perception, the person misinterprets the significance of something they perceive normally. For example, a patient may become convinced that on hearing a particular piece of music, they are destined to save the world. A key point is that delusions arise from abnormal thought processes.

Clinical vignettes

A male patient with schizophrenia described being unable to leave his room because whenever he did he was followed by small blue elves.

This is an example of a bizarre delusion. The following delusion is most unlikely but not impossible.

A male patient with schizophrenia described his conviction that his room had been bugged by the Special Branch.

Therefore, to establish whether a belief is a delusion, it is necessary to seek other abnormal mental state phenomena as well as a collateral history from the patient's friends and family. When considering a patient's beliefs, it is important to contextualize them culturally and consider diversity; for example, to decide that a belief about the 'spirits of the ancestors' is delusional without considering the patient's cultural background can lead to misdiagnosis.

Of note, with regard to delusions, is the way in which one patient on a ward can have a fixed delusional system while 'happily' living alongside a patient with a different, but just as fixed, delusional system. Such a situation illustrates that a core symptom of psychosis is isolation, which is linked to impairment in the patient's capacity to place himself or herself into the mind of another. A delusion can be understood as a psychological response to unbearable feelings or affect, and this does not require others to share in the sufferer's 'world view'. Delusions are, to a greater or lesser extent, linked with anxiety, a connection that will be discussed later.

Schizophrenia is also associated with 'formal thought disorder', in which there are recognizable disruptions to the form and flow of thought. This is a complex phenomenon, which can be hard to diagnose, but is important to recognize when working with patients with schizophrenia, as it can significantly affect the patient's capacity to communicate and to be understood. One example of a disorder in the form of thinking is when a patient finds abstract ideas problematic and displays 'concrete thinking'. Psychodynamically, this difficulty is described as impairment in the capacity to symbolize. In other words, an inability to let an image or a word stand for anything other than what it is. For example, patients with schizophrenia are often unable to understand proverbs, such as 'a watched pot never boils'; indeed, asking about proverbs forms part of the mental state examination. Instead they will interpret the proverb literally and may say something like 'the power was not switched on'. Recognizing the presence of deficits in symbolization is important, as it helps the clinician to make sense (meaning) of their patients' communications.

Clinical vignette

A patient was asked whether her appearance in a Mental Health Review Tribunal went 'all right', her reply was, 'No, it went all left'.

At one level this is a concrete non-symbolic response to a question but, from a dynamic view, it can also be understood as a communication about her experience which the clinician can, hopefully, use his or her capacity to symbolize and thus make meaningful.

As important as the active or positive symptoms of schizophrenia, such as delusions, hallucinations and thought disorder, are the 'negative symptoms' that 'subtract' from normal functioning. They are often the hardest to treat in the long term and include symptoms such as social withdrawal, poverty of thought, flattened affect (reduced emotional responsiveness), amotivation, apathy and anhedonia (not being able to take pleasure from activities that previously provided enjoyment).

Psychodynamic thinking proposes that all of these symptoms share the commonality of loss: loss of aspects of personality functioning, loss of role, loss of relationships, loss of a sense of self, loss of a capacity to face reality and insight into these losses. The treatment of someone suffering from schizophrenia can be a fraught process as it necessitates helping the patient face the damage the illness has caused to himself or herself and his or her life. The 'forensic' patient with schizophrenia also has to face the damage he or she has done to others.

Schizophrenia and violence

The relationship between mental disorder and violence has commanded much debate and research over the last two decades and has been reviewed together with its methodological limitations by Burke (see Chapter 4). With respect to schizophrenia, a major study is Swanson's (Swanson et al 1990) Epidemiological Catchment Area Survey of 10,000 individuals living in the community. Over a 12-month period, violence was reported by 2% of individuals, compared with 8% of people with schizophrenia, and 13% of individuals whose schizophrenia was complicated by substance misuse or personality disorder. These findings do not imply causality, that is, that schizophrenia causes violence, but that patients with schizophrenia are at an increased risk of behaving violently compared with individuals with no psychiatric diagnosis. Although the increased risk is not great, it is statistically significant (Maden 2007). Maden asserts that 'in scientific terms, the existence of a link between psychotic mental illness and violence in the community is of a similar magnitude to the association between smoking and lung cancer' (Maden 2004: 23).

Taking another methodological approach, one that examined the frequency of mental illness among those who had exhibited violent behaviour, and using homicide as a specific form of violence, Shaw et al (2006) showed that, in England and Wales, schizophrenia had a prevalence of 5% in homicide perpetrators compared with 1% in the general population.

The current cultural preoccupation with violence and those suffering from schizophrenia has been well critiqued by Taylor and Gunn (1999), who demonstrated that the actual number of homicides committed by mentally ill people in the United Kingdom, since the introduction of community care, has not significantly increased, contrary to popular belief. However, although homicides by mentally ill people are rare, each is a tragedy and is properly the concern of psychiatry.

Psychosis frightens people and the fear of 'psycho-killers' reflects a general fear of madness and breakdown; a contributory factor in the stigma associated with mental illness. In particular, apparently random and unprovoked attacks appear motiveless, generating further fear. Sohn (1999) has described how, in some cases, a psychodynamic understanding of the patient's mind can shed light on what appears to be this random violence. Sohn links the victim and the attacker, in the mind of the attacker, showing how the victim fits the 'need' of the attacker's paranoid fantasy at a particular time.

The large epidemiological studies into the link between mental disorder and violence emerging from The MacArthur Study in the United States (Monahan et al 2001) demonstrated that, in mental health settings, the contribution of criminogenic factors to violence had been under-emphasized; for example, co-morbid substance misuse and personality structure plus broader social and cultural causes of antisocial behaviour such as poverty, deprivation, translocation, immigration and family problems.

Howells et al (2004: 394) argued that mental health training is often based on a 'medical model' that favours an analysis based on an individual being 'ill', experiencing subjective distress and functioning poorly. The authors suggest that 'exclusive interpersonal and disorder-based explanations for violent crime are likely to be of limited utility given the range of interpersonal and social factors that we know are related to committing a violent offence'. The result is a polarized situation where the 'mad' are seen as located within mental health and the 'bad' are located in the criminal justice system. Each system can only partially address a person's needs and moral judgements can parade as clinical ones.

These findings are of importance, not only from the point of view of risk assessment but also because they relate to the difficulty staff in mental health settings have managing their patients' behaviour if it is viewed as non-psychotic, that is, 'bad'. For example, a patient with schizophrenia may be deemed to have been 'treated' but if difficult behaviour persists they may then be described as no longer belonging in a mental health setting, by virtue, for example, of having a 'personality disorder', which is then perceived as being untreatable (DH 2003).

Psychoanalysis, psychodynamic theory and schizophrenia

Freud was pessimistic about the ability to treat patients suffering from a psychotic illness. He famously analysed Judge Schreber's autobiographical account of his own breakdown into psychosis (Freud 1911) and, in summary, concluded that one important mechanism in psychosis was a regression to a 'primitive state of narcissism'. By this he meant a psychological retreat to the state of mind associated with the earliest developmental phase of childhood in which, Freud theorized, the infant was aware only of itself and its needs. He also described projection (or expulsion) of the inner world into the external environment, including other people. In Freud's view, treating psychosis by psychoanalysis was not possible because the psychic mechanisms involved mitigated against the formation of a transference relationship with the analyst; a relationship that implies the capacity to acknowledge the separateness of another person and their mind (see Bateman and Holmes 1995 for a further discussion).

This view has since been challenged by psychoanalysts, in particular those influenced by Melanie Klein, an Austrian psychoanalyst who settled in the United Kingdom and became the pivotal figure for the development of 'Kleinian' psychoanalysis, which places a particular emphasis on the understanding of primitive and destructive states of mind.

Freud did helpfully describe delusions as being a 'patch over a rent in the ego', that is, they develop secondarily to overwhelming or annihilatory anxiety to 'explain' it, so that a feeling of unknown dread is replaced by a rationale. As Freud (1911: 70–71) elegantly said:

> The end of the world is a projection of this internal catastrophe: his, i.e. the paranoiac's subjective world has come to an end since his withdrawal of love for it . . ., the paranoiac builds it again, not more splendid it is true, but at least so that he can once more live in it. He builds it up by the work of his delusions. The delusional formation, which we take to be the pathological product, is in reality an attempt at recovery, a process of reconstruction.

Although the conceptualization that delusional beliefs arise from the mind's attempts to recover some state of psychic equilibrium may seem counter-intuitive, the following example illustrates the formation of a delusion that 'made sense' of an inchoate feeling of dread; the patient killed out of overwhelming fear and believed he had acted in self-defence.

Clinical vignette

A man was seen in a police station having just been arrested for a frenzied attack on his father; he was extremely agitated and unable to describe what had happened. The next morning he was calmer and stated that his father was the devil, and the patient had to defend himself against damnation.

Hinshelwood (2004) has helpfully summarized the various contributions of psychoanalytic thinking to psychosis. Of particular importance, in the view of this author, are the contributions of Bion (1967), who described the psychotic and non-psychotic parts of the mind that can coexist; the bizarre objects formed in the internal world and the 'attacks on linking', all of which are associated with psychosis. This phenomenological approach is helpful as it illuminates clinical findings, allowing them to be less impervious to understanding.

Clinical vignette

A patient in a medium secure unit who was suffering from schizophrenia said in a group, 'Doctor, you and the nurses do good work, but people still die of broken thoughts.'

The above is a clear illustration of the capacity of the non-psychotic part of the patient to understand something of the process he is undergoing. It demonstrates insight, although the language used is not that imposed on patients by the prevailing psychiatric discourse. Patients may not accept that they suffer from an illness called 'schizophrenia', but they may be able to describe the way that their thoughts don't work.

The ultimate aim of treatment is always going to be to attempt to communicate with the non-psychotic part of the patient about his or her psychosis. Hannah Segal (1957) wrote about the breakdown in symbolic thinking, describing the importance of symbolic equations where, instead of an ability to distinguish between the symbol and what is symbolized, there is no distinction. This leads to a difficulty in recognizing reality but does not necessarily lead to meaninglessness.

Clinical vignette

A patient called Miranda was asked why she had absconded. She replied, 'Well it's obvious, it's in my name: Mi-ran-da.'

This vignette illustrates how the patient's name, a symbol of her, became her actions.

Developing psychological theories to illuminate the symptoms of schizophrenia is important. It helps mental health professionals avoid mirroring what their patients do, that is, avoid seeing the sufferers of schizophrenia as bodies with symptoms rather than people with disordered minds, who can be understood, albeit partially. People with schizophrenia are often reluctant to face the psychic pain of thinking about themselves, and it is all too easy for mental health professionals to collude with this.

Psychoanalysts have not always differentiated between the explanation and understanding of symptoms in schizophrenia and positing an alternative aetiology. This approach has, unfortunately, left significant suspicion on the part of psychiatry that psychoanalysts have disregarded the important and compelling research on the biological aspects of schizophrenia. Turkington et al (2005) have described how one unhelpful consequence of the early aetiological theories of psychosis, posited by psychoanalysts, was the perception that these theories attributed blame to family members, for example, the idea of a 'schizophrenogenic' mother (Fromm-Reichmann 1948). These misunderstandings have resulted in a long-standing hostility from psychiatrists, patients and carers towards psychoanalysis (Milton et al 2004).

Psychoanalysts recognize that 'pure' psychoanalytic technique cannot be used directly with schizophrenic patients because it leads to an increase in anxiety which, although useful for the neurotic patient, can lead to decompensation or 'breakdown' in somebody who has the fragile sense of self associated with psychosis. Patients may literally feel they are fragmenting. However, modified psychoanalytic technique, such as that used in psychodynamic psychotherapy, can help clarify and explain not only the phenomena of the symptoms but also their impact on the patient's interpersonal relationships with family, staff and others.

An example of a beneficial contribution from psychoanalytic theory to forensic practice is the analysis of affect as an important factor in understanding the relationship between delusions and violence. In the vignette that described a man killing his father, whom he believed was the devil, the relationship between the delusion and the violence appears obvious. However, many sufferers of schizophrenia have paranoid delusions that are not acted upon. Why is this? A psychodynamic view is that the affect associated with the delusion is key, namely the anxiety and distress associated with the belief. Maden (2007) summarized the psychiatric research that supports the importance of emotions such as distress, fear and anger as factors in those patients who act on delusions. This is also an example of concordance between psychodynamic and empirical research, a potentially more creative situation than the frequent polarization of views leading to an adversarial stalemate.

The feelings aroused in a patient by a therapist, conscious and unconscious, and vice versa, are called, respectively, the transference and countertransference. Such feelings emerge from a mixture of inherent personality characteristics plus experience, not only of early relationships but later events, for example, the trauma of being a victim of crime or indeed the trauma of developing a mental illness such as schizophrenia. Psychoanalytic theory suggests that the inevitable consequence is the impossibility of any therapeutic relationship being neutral and therefore such feelings need to be made explicit. If unacknowledged, these powerful emotions, which in forensic settings can commonly involve a spectrum ranging from dislike to hatred as well as fear, can lead to unhelpful and anti-therapeutic interactions. Naming these interactions is a contribution specific to the psychodynamic model.

Psychological treatment of schizophrenia

Psychodynamic psychotherapy

The National Institute for Health and Clinical Excellence (NICE) is an NHS-funded body that evaluates the research evidence for the treatment of physical and mental illness and disorder.

Pharmacological treatment, in the form of anti-psychotic medication, is the mainstay of psychiatric treatment for schizophrenia, and NICE (2002) recommends the use of atypical anti-psychotic medication as first-line treatment. The NICE guidelines also address psychological treatments and they emphasize the importance of forming a therapeutic alliance with patients in which supportive counselling is a part. Although they state that there is insufficient evidence to recommend the use of psychoanalytic or psychodynamic therapy in the routine treatment of schizophrenia, they do recommend that the principles of such an approach may help health professionals 'understand the experience of individual service users and their interpersonal relationships' (NICE 2002). In residential settings this would also include understanding the impact of schizophrenia on the relationship between those suffering from schizophrenia and those working with them.

Turkington et al (2005) reviewed the few studies that have researched using psychodynamic approaches in treating schizophrenia. They argued for the 'needs adapted approach' akin to that practised in Scandinavia, where 'a range of interventions are used according to a comprehensive ongoing evaluation, including a psychodynamic understanding of each patient's specific situation'.

The place of psychodynamic psychotherapy within forensic settings will always be as one of a range of treatment options rather than as the main treatment intervention.

Systemic theory and schizophrenia

Research, documented in the NICE guidelines (2002), demonstrates that psycho-educational family therapy can reduce the relapse rate following the first episode of psychosis. The guidelines recommend that mental health trusts provide family therapy where indicated. Unfortunately, this has not happened in clinical practice and Leff (2000) has suggested that family therapy is not being delivered to patients with schizophrenia, owing to mental health professionals having high caseloads, lack of appropriate supervision and the need for crisis work.

An additional explanation, favoured by this author, is that the lack of comprehensive and effective delivery of family therapy to patients with schizophrenia cannot simply be explained on pragmatic grounds but is a paradigm of the way that treating institutions can 'collude' unconsciously with the psychotic part of the patient's mind, which is invested in a denial of reality. Lack of compliance, the need for detention under the Mental Health Act (HMSO 2007), lack of insight and difficulty in managing and facing the reality of mental illness are all related to this phenomenon. Treatment systems and institutions are much better at ensuring compliance with medication than compliance with psychological interventions, such as family and other psychological therapies; concentrating on the former allows avoidance of the psychic pain necessarily involved in engaging in psychological work.

Cognitive-behavioural therapy

Although cognitive-behavioural therapy (CBT) is probably best known as a treatment for depression, there has been an accumulating body of research relating to its application in psychosis, dating from classic papers by Aaron Beck, the founder of cognitive therapy, on the treatment with CBT of a chronic schizophrenic patient (Beck 1952). There have been several well-conducted trials of CBT that have established it as an evidence-based treatment for psychosis (Turkington et al 2006). The NICE guidelines now recommend CBT for psychosis to 'reduce psychotic symptoms, increase insight and promote medication adherence' (NICE 2002).

CBT attempts to challenge schizophrenic symptoms in a structured and focused way. Turkington and Siddle (1998) emphasized the importance of establishing trust and the need to avoid both confrontation and collusion with the psychotic symptoms. A cognitive approach involves developing the individual's understanding of the illness and its symptoms, helping the patient recognize environmental stressors as precipitants of symptom relapse and developing the person's coping skills. Normalization techniques are also used to decrease isolation and increase the therapeutic alliance.

Cognitive strategies can involve using distraction- or attention-narrowing techniques to decrease the impact of persistent auditory hallucinations and reduce the arousal associated with them. Hallucinations may be treated as 'automatic negative thoughts', and delusions are written down and questioned to challenge them, in a way manageable by the patient. Behavioural techniques may include altering the level of social engagement and increasing activity levels. At present there are no high-level methodological trials of CBT in forensic or offender patients with psychosis. It will be interesting and important to see if the effectiveness of CBT transfers to this population whose frequent co-morbid pathologies and complex clinical needs present additional treatment challenges.

Summary

Although psychological interventions do not offer a cure for schizophrenia, policy guidelines stress the importance of psychological treatments for patients and their families, in the effort to promote recovery. CBT and family interventions, together with psycho-educational approaches, can be used to prevent relapse, reduce positive symptoms, increase insight and self-esteem and promote adherence to medication.

Psychodynamic psychotherapy is not recommended for patients who are acutely psychotic, as their often disordered and concretized thinking means that they find this treatment too stressful. A psychodynamic approach, however, involves seeking to understand the personal meaning of an individual's symptoms and behaviour, especially those aspects that do not make rational sense. Applying psychodynamic understanding can therefore help the patient, carers and professionals understand the more bizarre or frightening aspects of a psychotic patient's behaviour. Helping carers or relatives who understand the patient's symptoms can help the patient feel more understood, minimize the chances of anti-therapeutic reactions towards the patient on the part of staff and the institution, and improve treatment concordance.

The contribution of forensic psychotherapy

Schizophrenia is a complex illness that can have devastating effects on the patient and their associates. Research has led to a better understanding of both its aetiology and treatment. The development of the atypical anti-psychotic drugs have aided the treatment of both negative and positive symptoms and led to a reduction in unwanted side-effects. The setting of a medium secure unit, where the patients generally remain for more than 2 years, allows an opportunity to fine-tune the medication so that maximum benefit is obtained. However, the provision and fine-tuning of psychological therapies is less certain, and appears to be a much more random process. In reality, many patients still do not receive family therapy or other psychological therapies and, even if provided, often patients are hard to engage. Research studies have frequently sampled 'pure' cultures of patients, for example, those with only a psychotic illness and no other co-morbidity such as co-existent personality disorder or substance abuse, namely the group of patients more representative of psychotic forensic patients. The actual day-to-day management of patients with co-morbid conditions as well as schizophrenia is demanding and difficult.

Other interventions are, of course, essential to the management of forensic patients with schizophrenia, for example, occupational therapy, arts therapies, social work and, most obviously, good nursing care; nurses have the most exposure to the patients in medium secure settings.

It is important to stress that, although the brief of this chapter has been to address psycho-therapeutic approaches to understanding and treating mentally disordered offenders, providing optimum care for these patients involves close multidisciplinary and inter-professional working.

Hinshelwood (2004) argued that one of the essential and most helpful features of psychoanalysis is that it does not place rationality at a higher level than irrationality and that it is important to consider the painful aspects of the treatment of psychosis. Bearing this in mind, the final section of this chapter describes certain observations regarding management and treatment of patients in a medium secure unit and forensic psychiatry service.

Psychiatry, psychology, occupational therapy and nursing are all based on a positivistic model and rational view of the world. There is an assumption that a patient is 'ill' and he or she comes into a medium secure unit to be treated and to get 'well'. In reality, therapeutic efforts are often 'sabotaged' by patients in the form of negative therapeutic reactions. This is when progress is made, only for disruption to occur, for example, a patient who, within a week of being discharged, overstays his leave from the unit, gets drunk and thus stops his discharge. Linked to this positivistic model is the implicit assumption that staff and the institution are not only 'well', but are caring and compassionate, that is, lacking forensic features. As can be frequently observed in forensic workplaces, delinquency, aggression and destructiveness are not located solely in patients.

There are also occasional 'catastrophic' events, for example, homicide leading to inquiries, experiences of persecution, risk avoidance and significant changes in policy from 'top-down'. Interestingly, these are often based on a 'single case model'; a paradox in a culture where the randomized controlled trial is frequently valued above all other research methodologies.

A common theme in homicide inquiries has been criticism of communication processes (Sheppard 1996) and what appears, in retrospect, to be bizarre decisions of omission or co-omission.

Clinical vignette

A community psychiatric nurse was presenting a recently seen community patient to the psychodynamic psychotherapist. The man was suffering from schizophrenia and, at the time of being seen, was naked, covered in his own faeces, kneeling on the floor and barking like a dog. When it was suggested that the patient needed to be in hospital, the psychotherapist was told that it could not be justified because the patient was 'not a risk to others'.

This above vignette illustrates an objectification of the patient. In this case, 'objectification' due to an over-arching model of risk to others that prevents recognition of the patient's suffering. Hinshelwood (2004) linked this to a consequence of the 'scientifization' of psychiatry, leading to a tendency to objectify a patient, neglecting the human aspects.

In clinical practice there is a concentration on what is explicitly observed and stated by a patient, with little reference to a model for the 'unsaid' and other forms of communication, such as the transference and countertransference. For example, there is little acknowledgement of the paradoxical situation in which a forensic inpatient can be placed. The patient is encouraged to say what is on his or her mind, though he or she knows that what he or she says can be used 'against' him or her, so to speak, in reports, which will ultimately determine the future detention. If the patient does not say anything, this can also be used 'against' him or her. This dynamic can be described as a classic double-bind situation, in which there is no correct response for the patient, leading to helplessness, despair and an increase in the feeling of being trapped.

Judgements appear to be made about morality and responsibility. A patient who is clearly psychotic and commits a violent act can be perceived and treated as 'ill'. However, if the patient resists treatment and is troublesome, then there is a tendency to apply a moral judgement: 'badness'. This is often reflected in the language used about patients who have been causing problems for staff, such as 'manipulative', 'attention seeking' and 'behavioural'. A professional conclusion may be that, in fact, the patient has a personality disorder and therefore is not the responsibility of mental health services. Consequently, the diagnosis is changed from schizophrenia to personality disorder. The label 'personality disorder' is applied sometimes, not in order to understand and explain the patient but to sanction a moral judgement. This process is also related to the lack of treatment directed towards criminogenic behaviour discussed earlier, as it leads staff into the realm of 'bad' behaviour, where they often feel less comfortable, rather than 'mad' behaviour.

The question that could be more helpfully asked of mental health professionals is: 'What is the patient trying to manipulate?' In other words, 'What has not been understood?' And similarly, 'What is the patient drawing attention to?' The word 'behavioural' implies the patient has no mind at all.

Clinical vignette

A young man with a history of assaults on others plus deliberate self-harm in the form of lacerating his body, conceals razors in his room and cuts himself. The staff suggest that all items be taken from his room in order to protect him from harming himself. The psychotherapist suggests that staff feel attacked by and angry with the patient and that the idea of creating a strip cell is driven by unconscious punitive wishes.

The above vignette illustrates how clinical decisions may be based on unacknowledged countertransferential feelings that are acted out rather than understood. Thus the psychodynamic model, which examines subjective responses to the patient, can paradoxically lead to a more objective view.

Isabel Menzies-Lyth (1959), in her classic paper, suggested that social systems organize themselves to defend against anxiety. She studied nursing staff and process in a general hospital and described the institutional defences that are established against illness and death. Hinshelwood (1987) has further developed this to describe institutional defences against 'madness' and 'breakdown' in psychiatric settings. Similar defences exist in a forensic unit where the feared outcome is that of madness and violence. This means that the prevailing atmosphere on many wards is that of lethargy and lack of activity, that is, 'deadness', not overt disturbance. Although staff find this 'deadness' difficult, it appears to result from a joint, unconscious collaboration with the patients to create a space where there will be no risk of liveliness, as this could lead to madness and violence.

Stanton and Schwarz (1954) described the way in which the internal dynamics of the patient can be externalized into the institution. In other words, through projection and projective identification, there is a mirroring of the patients' psychopathology by the system.

Clinical vignette

A surprise night time visit to a ward in a medium secure unit by the nursing manager revealed one member of nursing staff stretched out asleep on the sofa, ignored by the other staff member who was reading a newspaper. The patients had been told not to disturb them.

This illustrates the creation, via projection identification, of delinquent and neglectful parents, characteristic of many of the patients in their own lives and their own early experiences. Thus the assessment of any patient within an institution, such as a medium secure unit, needs to take into account the patient's impact on the system and the system's impact on them, as well as individual observations regarding the patients' diagnosis and behaviour.

Patients are often described as 'well' when they are not floridly psychotic, but this can be unhelpful because a patient suffering from chronic schizophrenia, who has been detained for several years, is not 'well' in the way that term implies; the patient is just not actively psychotic. This is important, as a patient needs to own his or her illness and not see it as a visitation from elsewhere, that comes and goes without rhyme or reason. It is by helping patients to become interested in their own minds and how they work (or not) that insight is developed. Another description used about patients within the discourse of the ward is that of being 'settled', as if a lack of overtly disturbed behaviour indicates a settled mind, when in fact the opposite can be true. Patients who occupy staff time, because of their acting out behaviour on a ward, are often the subject of discussion but, just as important, are the patients who are never discussed or always last on the ward round list and often forgotten.

The ideal clinical service would consist of a coherent, well-resourced, needs-led treatment service, which is multi-disciplinary and multi-modality. However, this is rarely available. Instead there are significant divisions or 'splits' between professionals, disciplines and the theoretical models individuals embrace. The term 'split' is used here to denote a tendency to see the world in a polarized way (characteristic of the paranoid mental state of schizophrenia). Disciplines and professionals differentiate themselves from each other by seeing their model of work or thinking as 'right' and the other as 'wrong'. This mitigates against a more creative state of mind available when 'right' and 'wrong' are integrated. There can be splits between psychiatry and psychodynamic thinking and between biology and psychology. There are those who believe that all patients are victims of circumstance and the institution, leading to a sentimental view of the patient. In contrast, others are quick to see a patient only in terms of a mental illness, rather than in terms of the person having individual characteristics and needs.

Conclusion

There is no clear evidence, for example, randomized controlled trials, for the use of psychoanalytic or psychodynamic treatment in patients with schizophrenia. However, it is clear from research into homicide inquiries and clinical observation that problems with communication and a full understanding of an individual's mental state are common. Much evidence-based research is conducted, by definition, on collections of individuals, and there is always a difficulty in translating such research findings to render them useful for the care of the individual patient. This chapter argues that forensic patients suffering from psychosis are unusual. They are already outside the norm, and it is essential to pay attention to both the psychotic and non-psychotic parts of the patient's mind and functioning to aid the individual's recovery. It is proposed that a psychodynamic model can aid the therapeutic alliance with, and comprehension of, an individual suffering from schizophrenia.

The role of forensic psychotherapy in secure forensic settings encompasses more than the treatment of individual patients. The internal dynamics of the patients evoke reactions in the staff and the institution that arise either from the staff's unconscious response to the aspects of their patients' internal world or from mobilization of the staff and institution's unconscious defence mechanisms to reduce anxiety (McGauley and Humphrey 2003). If unattended these processes at best diminish the therapeutic potential of the environment while at worst result in boundary violations that necessitate inquiries (DO 1992; Department of Health and Social Security 1980).

One way of increasing staff's immunity against such toxic practices is to ensure that they attend reflective practice groups that provide a forum for keeping a psychodynamic eye on the dynamics between patients, staff and patients, within the staff team and between the team and the institution. This culture is more established within forensic services treating patients with personality disorder (see Chapter 14). Although the majority of medium secure units see themselves as predominantly treating mental illness, their patients are severely disturbed and often have co-morbid personality psychopathology. The discourse of psychotherapy may appear alien to staff on such units. However, within the current climate of expansion in medium secure services, such units may be wise to utilize the contribution forensic psychotherapy can provide to aid the risk assessment and management of psychotic patients.

References

American Psychiatric Association 1994 Diagnostic and statistical manual of mental disorders 4th Edition DSM-IV. Washington DC: APA.

Bateman, A. and Holmes, J. 1995 Introduction to Psychoanalysis: Contemporary Theory and Practice. London and New York: Routledge.

Beck, A.T. 1952 Successful Outpatient Psychotherapy of a Chronic Schizophrenic with a Delusion Based on Borrowed Guilt. Psychiatry 15: 305–312.

Bion, W.R. 1967 Second Thoughts. London: Heinemann.

Collins English Dictionary. 1979 Collins: London and Glasgow.

Cooper, D. 1967 Psychiatry and Anti Psychiatry. Tavistock: London.

Department of Health. 1992 Report of the Committee of Inquiry into Complaints about Ashworth Hospital Vol I and II. London: HMSO.

Department of Health. 2003 Personality Disorder: No Longer a Diagnosis for Exclusion. Policy Implementation Guidance for Development of Services for People with Personality Disorder. London: Department of Health.

Department of Health and Social Security. 1980. Report on the Review of Rampton Hospital Boynton Report. London: HMSO.

Freud, S. 1911 Psychoanalytic Notes on an Autobiographical Account of a Case of Paranoia. Standard Edition, Vol 12. London: Hogarth.

Fromm-Reichmann, F. 1948 Notes on the Development of Schizophrenia by Psychoanalysis and Psychotherapy. Psychiatry V 11: 263–273.

Gelder M.G., Cowen P. and Harrison P.J. 2006 Schizophrenia and Related Disorders 119–136 in Shorter Oxford Textbook of Psychiatry. OUP: Oxford.

Hinshelwood, R.D. 1987 The Psychotherapist's Role in a Large Mental Institution. Psychoanalytic Psychotherapy 2: 207–215.

Hinshelwood, R.D. 2004 Suffering Insanity: Psychoanalytic Essays on Psychosis. Brunner-Routledge.

HMSO. 2007 The Mental Health Act 2007 HMSO, London, c12.

Howells, K., Day, A., Thomas-Peter, B. 2004 Changing Violent Behaviour: Forensic Mental Health and Criminological Models Compared. Journal of Forensic Psychiatry and Psychology 15: 391–406.

Kleinman A. 1987 Anthropology and Psychiatry: The Role of Culture in Cross-cultural Research on Illness. British Journal of Psychiatry 151: 447–454.

Leff, J. 1988 Psychiatry around the Globe: A Transcultural View. London: Gaskell.

Leff J.P. 2000 Role of the Community Psychiatric Nurse in the Management of Schizophrenia. Commentary. Advances in Psychiatric Treatment 6: 250–251.

Maden, A. 2004 Violence, Mental Disorder and Public Protection. Psychiatry 3, 11: 1–4.

Maden, A. 2007 Treating Violence: A Guide to Risk Management in Mental Health. Oxford University Press: Oxford.

McGauley, G.A. and Humphrey, M. 2003 The Contribution of Forensic Psychotherapy to the Care of the Forensic Patient. Advances in Psychiatric Treatment 9: 117–124.

Menzies-Lyth I. 1959 A Case Study in the Functioning of Social Systems in the Defence Against Anxiety. Human Relations 13: 95–121. Republished in I Menzies Lyth (1988) Containing Anxiety in Institutions. London: Free Association Books.

Milton, J., Polmear, C. and Fabricius, J. 2004 Critiques of Psychoanalysis 79–98 in A Short Introduction to Psychoanalysiso. London: Sage.

Monahan, J., Steadman, H.J., Silver, E. et al 2001 Rethinking Risk Assessment. The MacArthur Study of Mental Disorder and Violence. Oxford: Oxford University Press.

Murray, R.M., Jones, P. B., Susser, E., Van Os, J., Cannon, M. (Editors) 2004 The Epidemiology of Schizophrenia. Cambridge: Cambridge University Press.

National Institute for Clinical Excellence. 2002 Clinical Guideline 1: Schizophrenia Core Interventions and the Treatment and Management of Schizophrenia in Primary and Secondary Care. London: Author.

Schneider, K. 1959 Clinical Psychopathology Trans. Hamilton, B.W. New York: Grune and Stratton.

Segal, H. 1957 Notes on Symbol Formation. International Journal of Psychoanalysis 38: 391–397. Republished 1981 in The Work of Hanna Segal. New York: Jason Aaronson.

Shaw, J., Hunt, I. M., Flynn, S. et al 2006 Rates of Mental Disorder in People Convicted of Homicide: A National Clinical Survey. British Journal of Psychiatry 188: 143–147.

Sheppard, D. 1996 Learning the Lessons 2nd Edition. London: Zito Trust.

Sohn, L. 1999 Psychosis and Violence 13–26 in Psychosis Madness (Williams, P. Editor) London: The Institute of Psychoanalysis.

Stanton, A.H. and Schwartz, M.S. 1954 The Mental Hospital. A Study of Institutional Participation in Psychiatric Illness and Treatment. New York: Basic Books.

Swanson J W, Holzer C E, Ganju V K, Jonjo R T 1990 Violence and Psychiatric disorder in the community: evidence from the Epidemiological Catchment Area surveys. Hospital and Community Psychiatry 41: 761–770.

Szasz, T.E. 1961 The myth of mental illness. Hoeber-Harper, New York.

Taylor, P.J. and Gunn J. 1999 Homicides by people with mental illness: myth and reality. British Journal of Psychiatry 174: 9–14

Turkington, D and Siddle, R. 1998 Cognitive therapy for the treatment of delusions. Advances in Psychiatric Treatment 4: 235–242

Turkington, D., Martin-Dale, B. and Bloch-Thorsen, G.R. 2005 Schizophrenia 163–176 in Oxford Textbook of Psychotherapy (Gabbard, G.O., Beck, J.S. and Holmes, J. Editors) New York: Oxford University Press.

Turkington, D., Kingdon, D. and Weiden, P.J. 2006 Cognitive Behaviour Therapy for Schizophrenia. American Journal of Psychiatry 163: 365–372.

World Health Organisation (WHO). 1992 International Classification of Diseases 10th Edition. Classification of Behavioural and Mental Disorders: Clinical Descriptions and Diagnostic Guidelines. Geneva: WHO.

Wright, P. 2000 Schizophrenia and Related Disorders in Core Psychiatry (Wright, P., Stern, J. and Phelan, M., Editors) Livingstone: Saunders W.B. Churchill.

Chapter 14

Caring for individuals with personality disorder in secure settings

Gwen Adshead and Gill McGauley

Aim

This chapter outlines the nature and extent of personality disorder in Mentally Disordered Offenders (MDOs) and describes the problems faced by staff caring for these people in secure settings.

Learning objectives

- To describe aspects of personality disorder with respect to MDOs
- To describe the problems that staff face managing individuals with personality disorder in secure settings
- To understand the impact of these problems on staff
- To describe the psychological approaches to the treatment of MDOs with personality disorder

Introduction

MDOs with personality disorder have a propensity to act violently to others. Engaging them in treatment and maintaining an appropriate therapeutic framework presents many challenges. This chapter reviews the nature and extent of personality disorder in forensic populations, some of the problems that these patients experience, discusses the therapeutic challenges they pose in residential care and explores some of the interventions and structures that can be put in place to address the complex needs of this difficult group.

The nature of the problem: personality and its disorder

Defining 'personality', let alone what constitutes a 'healthy personality', is problematic. Quantifying the extent to which components of an individual's personality need to vary from the 'norm' to fall into the range of personality 'disorder' or 'pathology' is difficult, not least as these are abstract concepts. There appears to be some consensus in the psychiatric and psychological literature that the concept of personality refers to the persistent and enduring characteristics and attitudes of an individual, which include the person's way of thinking (cognition), feeling (affectivity) and behaving (ways of relating to others) across a wide range of circumstances.

Personality development occurs from infancy through to adolescence and early adulthood, after which the individual's personality characteristics become less malleable; this is reflected in the psychiatric definition of personality disorder as an 'enduring' pattern of experience and behaviour (American Psychiatric Association 2000). It is more accurate to say that, although personality characteristics (traits) can and do change in adulthood, change may be limited.

Personality traits are consistent patterns of actions, thoughts or feelings that both distinguish between people and denote a disposition for people to behave in certain ways under relevant conditions, for example, someone can be described as impulsive or sociable (see Appendix 14.1 for the diagnostic criteria for personality disorder). Personality traits, unlike the symptoms of mental illness, are seen as being on a continuum so that, in trait terms, personality and personality disorder are inseparable concepts. In this dimensional model, the difference between personality and personality pathology or disorder is seen as quantitative rather than qualitative (Blackburn 2006). There is considerable debate as to whether personality disorders are best described as dimensions in the trait approach or by categories or types. Both approaches have their advantages and disadvantages (the reader is referred to Blackburn 2006; Moore 2006 as a fuller discussion is beyond the remit of this chapter).

The idea that personality characteristics were inflexible is important within the context of the development of services for and the treatment of people with personality disorder. This idea held sway for a long time and legitimized the view held by some mental health professionals that adults with personality disorder were 'untreatable' (Adshead 2001). However, the last decade has seen a growing empirical evidence base demonstrating both symptom improvement in various personality-disordered patient populations (inpatient and community) (Lenzenweger 1999; Zanarini et al 2003) and positive responses to psychological treatment interventions that are inconsistent with the stability hypothesis (Bateman and Fonagy 1999; Linehan et al 1991).

The magnitude of the problem in secure settings

The prevalence of personality disorder increases from the community through inpatient to secure settings. In the community, the estimated prevalence of personality disorder is in the region of 4% (Coid et al 2006; Singleton et al 2003). When diagnostic instruments are used it is estimated that 20% to 40% of psychiatric outpatients and approximately 50% of psychiatric inpatients meet the criteria for personality disorder (de Girolamo and Reich 1993; Dowson and Grounds 1995). However, the prevalence of personality disorder in secure settings is much higher. Singleton's study estimated that 78% of male remand prisoners, 64% of male sentenced prisoners and 50% of female prisoners in England and Wales had a personality disorder (Singleton et al 1998). Fazel and Danesh's (2002) systematic review of 23,000 prisoners across Western countries, including the United States, revealed that 65% of male prisoners and 42% of female prisoners had a person-ality disorder, with little difference in proportion depending on whether they were on remand or sentenced. Looking at the type of personality disorder, 47% of male prisoners and 21% of the women prisoners with personality disorder had antisocial personality disorder (ASPD). In other words, prisoners were about 10 times more likely to have ASPD than individuals in the general population.

The situation is similar in high secure hospital settings. Sixty-six percent of Blackburn's sample of MDOs detained in a high secure hospital met the criteria for at least one personality disorder (Blackburn et al 1990, 2003). The main classification systems for medical and psychiatric disorders, the International Classification of Diseases (WHO 1992) and the DSM-IV-TR (American Psychiatric Association 2000) include behavioural criteria as part of the diagnostic criteria for personality disorder. In MDO populations most individuals with personality disorder have acted in ways that are frightening and disturbing to others and continue to have the propen-sity for impulsive and aggressive behaviour towards others and themselves.

The breadth and complexity of the problem

There are two strands of research evidence that need to be kept in mind to have an accurate picture of the level and type of psychopathology present in MDOs with a diagnosis of personality disorder. First, many personality-disordered MDOs also have high rates of mental illness as diagnosed on Axis I of the DSM-IV-TR (American Psychiatric Association 2000). Coid (1992) found high rates of depression (40%) and schizophrenia (23%) in his series of male patients. Blackburn (Blackburn et al 2003) reported high levels of mood and anxiety disorders and alcohol and drug misuse in 53 patients legally detained as suffering from Psychopathic Disorder as defined under the 1983 Mental Health Act. Personality-disordered individuals frequently have difficulty in appropriately seeking help, complying with treatment, coping with illness and establishing a therapeutic alliance. Consequently, the clinical significance of coexisting mental illness and personality disorder is that personality dysfunction adversely affects the prognosis, management and treatment of mental (and also many physical) illnesses.

Second, many MDOs satisfy the criteria for a diagnosis of more than one personality disorder as assessed by DSM criteria. Coid reported a mean of 2.7 personality-disorder diagnoses for male and 3.7 for female patients detained under the 1983 Mental Health Act classification of Psychopathic Disorder (Coid 1992). ASPD was the most frequent, followed by borderline personality disorder (BPD) and then narcissistic and paranoid personality disorder (Coid et al 1999). As discussed above this degree of 'co-morbidity' raises a question about the validity of a categorical approach to diagnosing personality disorder. An alternative viewpoint is that the person does not have two or three separate disorders but that the degree of overlap between the individual categories of personality disorder is such that the individual has one disorder that is inadequately defined (Tyrer 2006). In an attempt to address the issue of co-morbidity, personality variation has been grouped into three major clusters and the individual DSM personality disorders grouped within them. The personality disorders found in MDOs mainly fall into the DSM Cluster B group of personality disorders (antisocial, borderline, narcissistic and histrionic, see Table 14.1 and Appendix 14.1 for further descriptors); sometimes referred to as the 'dramatic' or 'flamboyant' group. Individuals with these disorders relate to the world in a way that makes other people notice them; as the term 'flamboyant' suggests, they draw attention to themselves.

ASPD is the commonest type of personality disorder seen in forensic practice. However, there is a particular sub-group of antisocial people who demonstrate extreme lack of care for others and act in cruel and exploitative ways. These people are thought to have a particular type of personality trait called 'psychopathy', which is probably caused by a mixture of genes and poor rearing (Blair et al 2005; Hare 1991). About 30% of the prison and forensic population score highly for psychopathy (Hare 1991) and they present a particular danger in terms of recidivism. Such patients may be referred to as 'psychopaths'. However, this term should not be confused with the category of 'Psychopathic Disorder' which existed in the 1983 Mental Health Act. Although colloquially patients who were detained under the legal category of psychopathic disorder were and may still be referred to as 'psychopaths', this is misleading, as only a minority of these patients will score highly on the Psychopathy Checklist-Revised (PCL-R; Hare 1991, 2003) and satisfy Hare's concept of psychopathy.

Personality disorder as a developmental disorder

One way of conceptualizing personality disorder is as a developmental disorder arising from an interaction between a genetically determined predisposition and the environment. Genes have powerful interactive effects with environmental influences. Likewise, the environment can both activate and inhibit genes. These gene/environment interactions are operational at all

Table 14.1 DSM-IV-TR classification of personality disorders commonly found in MDOs

DSM-IV classification	Description
Antisocial (Cluster B)	Failure to conform to social norms. A pervasive pattern of disregard for and violation of the rights of others occurring since the age of 15. Deceitfulness, impulsivity and lack of remorse
Borderline (Cluster B)	Pervasive instability of mood, interpersonal relationships and self image associated with marked impulsivity, fear of abandonment, identity disturbance and recurrent suicidal behaviour
Narcissistic (Cluster B)	Pervasive grandiosity, lack of empathy, arrogance and requirement for excessive admiration and a sense of entitlement
Histrionic (Cluster B)	Excessive emotionality and attention seeking. A labile mood with dramatic behaviour and global impressionistic and superficial reasoning
Paranoid (Cluster A)	Pervasive distrust and suspicion of others. Interpretation of people's motives and actions as deliberately demeaning or malevolent and threatening. Quick to react angrily and counterattack

developmental stages. Early in the lifecycle they operate between the child and the parent or main caregivers where environmental factors such as disrupted attachments, trauma and abuse in combination with genetic vulnerabilities, predispose to the development of personality disorder. Later in the lifecycle, these environmental influences are broader and encompass the direct effects of the social environment, including factors such as poverty and deprivation as well as factors that lead to other types of adversity. Although, by no means the only model, this biopsychosocial developmental model has gained widespread acceptance under the general framework of developmental psychopathology that sees development as an active, dynamic process with individuals adding meaning to experience and biology shaping and being shaped by these experiences (Fonagy, personal communication).

The internal world: disorganization

Adding meaning to experience requires the person to organize the various components of their experience, specifically the capacity to organize:

1. Thoughts; including the capacity to integrate and evaluate new information.

2. Feelings; through regulating and modulating emotions (also known as affects), especially negative ones, such as fear, anxiety, anger and sadness. As emotions can be experienced physically as well as mentally, the capacity to organize feelings includes the capacity to recognize and name the experience of having emotions. Emotional organization also includes the capacity to soothe one-self when distressed, or to seek out ways of being soothed.

3. Memory; which is vital for both assessing and integrating information. It is also involved in mood regulation by identifying experience chronologically. Healthy psychological functioning includes the capacity to recognize when an experience is in the past and when it is in the present.

4. A sense of reality; monitoring what is real and what is not is an everyday part of human experience. A well-organized awareness of reality is so essential to everyday thinking that we hardly notice it, although we may notice its absence. For example, we may 'drift' out of full conscious awareness while driving long distances, without any risk at all, and then 'come to' as soon as some increased attention is needed.

5. A sense of self that allows the individual to integrate all these capacities, thoughts, memories and feelings, into a coherent sense of 'I-ness' that continues over time and place. The more organized our sense of self, the more we are able to reflect on that experience, so that we can think about thinking or think about feelings. An individual's sense of self needs to be both flexible enough to adapt to external stressors but sufficiently consistent to provide the person with a secure base for their interpersonal relationships. A well-integrated sense of self is also essential in organizing our perception of others. Some authors have referred to this capacity as 'self-reflective function' or 'mentalization' (Fonagy and Target 1997).

Anything that causes disorganization of these capacities can result in some degree of personality dysfunction. Particular types of personality disorder can signal which of these underlying capacities has been affected. People with highly disorganized affect regulation tend to present with borderline personality disorder (Sarkar and Adshead 2006), as well as depression and other types of mood disorder (Kramer 1993). People with little sense of self tend to present as unempathic and antisocial or narcissistic, whereas people with very poor fear regulation tend to present as having paranoid personality disorder and sometimes with an increased capacity for cruelty (American Psychiatric Association 2000; Akhtar and Samuel 1996; Kernberg 1998; Kramer 1993).

The external world: defences and distortions

Disorganizing experiences have most impact if they occur whilst personality is most rapidly developing, in childhood. Children (and adults) use psychological defences to minimize the effect of these experiences and to help them manage the conflict that occurs between internal wishes and external disorganizing stressors. Psychological defences are configurations of cognitions (thoughts) and affects (feelings) that help reduce anxiety and other painful affective states, regulate self-esteem and maintain an intra-psychic balance (Vaillant 1994, 1995; see also Chapter 11). These defences are largely unconscious and healthy people use a mixture of mature, average and immature defences (Vaillant 1995). Defence systems are important as they influence the individual's pattern of behaviour and colour the person's interpersonal relationships and the way that they interact with others. Psychological development and growth during the life span is associated with changes in the types of defence that people use and the way they use them (Vaillant 1995, 1997).

Failure to develop and use more mature defences is associated with poor psychological and interpersonal function (Vaillant 1994). Table 14.2 lists some of the psychological defences commonly found in individuals with personality disorder. If too many immature defences are used repeatedly and excessively, they can, over time, become part of the person's sense of self and personality structure; a part that is inherently unstable. The case example (Text Box 14.1) describes how immature defences may be used by a traumatized child and then become an inflexible part of personality, putting the young man at risk of developing both a personality disorder and mental illness (Johnson et al 1999).

It is likely that people with personality disorders, especially in forensic settings, have developed an immature and pathological defence style partly because of their insecure attachment experiences in childhood (Frodi et al 2001; Van IJzendoorn et al 1997). People with personality disorders either make intrusive, unrealistic and unstable attachments or are highly avoidant of relating to others. Sadly, these toxic attachment patterns tend to be repeated with health care professionals (Adshead 1998, 2002).

The most important aspect of our external world is our relationships with others. It is part of our mammalian heritage to live in groups; those who live socially isolated lives are at risk of a premature death from illness, neglect and violence. Our personalities are an essential component

Table 14.2 Examples of psychological defence mechanisms

Immature defences (common in personality disorder)	Higher level defences (less common in personality disorder)	Mature defences (largely absent in personality disorder)
Acting out	Displacement	Altruism
Denial	Externalization	Anticipation
Distortion	Identification	Humour
Dissociation	Intellectualization	Sublimation
Idealization	Isolation of affect	Suppression
Projection	Rationalization	
Projective identification	Reaction formation	
Regression	Repression	
Somatization	Sexualization	
Splitting		

of our capacity to make and maintain good quality relationships with others. Poor-quality relationships may lead to isolation from others, or exclusion from social groups in ways that are potentially risky. In particular, we need to relate to others when we are in distress, when we are ill, frightened, weakened or in pain. At these times, it is important that vulnerable individuals can effectively elicit care from others and not alienate others who can help them.

Box 14.1 Case example: the problem and the defence against the problem

Jim suffered overwhelming fear experiences in childhood when he was the victim of repeated physical abuse by his father and grandmother. As a child he used immature defences to cope with his stress, such as dissociation, denial, projection and magical thinking. However, his stress levels were not soothed by these defences and he is left with poor emotional regulation. He now has two problems; his poor fear regulation means that he is still constantly assailed by fearful feelings, which he is still using immature defences to cope with.

◆ He somatizes so he is constantly seeking help from physicians for his unexplained physical symptoms

◆ He displaces his fear externally and misuses substances to soothe himself

◆ He projects his fear into others, which allows him to blame others for making him feel frightened

◆ His magical thinking has increased in intensity so that it has reached a delusional level ('I am the Prince of Darkness')

Over time, these defences become so much a part of his sense of self that he perceives others as a threat and acts aggressively to keep them at bay. It is not long before he is diagnosed as having a 'paranoid personality disorder'. He is also intermittently psychotic. His magical thinking and dissociation along with his substance misuse mean that his reality-testing capacity is severely impaired.

Most people belong to some sort of group, even if it is only their family group. Many belong to multiple groups; work groups, social groups and hobby groups. In all these groups they have to relate to other people. The experience of projectively seeing characteristics or attributes of ourselves in other people and understanding our own emotional response to this experience through engaging with others in a group is called 'mirroring' and is an important part of our social experience. People with personality disorder often have a poorly developed sense of self; they are not good at knowing where they end and others begin. Consequently, individuals with personality disorder may experience 'malignant mirroring' (Zinkin 1983); that involves projectively seeing unwelcome characteristics of oneself in another and consequently regarding these as being unacceptable in the other.

As people with personality disorder can be either intrusive, avoidant or fearful of others they frequently fail to register the group rules that connect people. They are therefore often regular social rule breakers, which results in their further alienation. A sub-group of people with personality disorders regularly break the group rules that society has designated to be 'the criminal law', which leads to their exclusion from the wider community. It is therefore not surprising that people with personality disorder are over-represented in groups of people who are rejected by others and that there is a high prevalence of people with ASPD in prisons.

The development of residential services for people with personality disorder

Historically, people with personality disorder have been excluded from mental health services (DH 2003); however, there has been a recent impetus to develop non-forensic and forensic services dedicated to treating people with personality disorder. Traditionally, patients with personality disorder were most often seen in psychotherapy services, which sometimes offered residential treatment. In the 1950s and 1960s, the emergence of an understanding of the social context of psychiatry led to the idea that environments could be therapeutic and, importantly, anti-therapeutic. Jones (1982) described how a residential psychiatric treatment service became a therapeutic community (TC), that is, a place where the total environment was therapeutic. Subsequently, several therapeutic communities have been developed as treatment resources for patients with personality disorder, and there is evidence that they are effective for mild to moderate degrees of personality disorder (Lees et al 1999; Warren et al 2003).

However, residential TCs, such as the Henderson or Cassel Hospitals, necessarily excluded the more antisocial patients, who were found in prisons or on probation and were not free to join regular TCs. Modified TCs were set up for some of these people within the prison system with some success, such as in Grendon prison (Hobson et al 2000). The Reed Review of Health and Social Services for Mentally Disordered Offenders (Department of Health and Home Office Working Group on Psychopathic Disorder 1994) supported the development of specialist Personality Disorder Units (PDU) in forensic psychiatric settings; previously, patients with personality disorder were managed together with patients with mental illness.

Although the modified TCs set up in prisons have been moderately successful, there have often been doubts about whether residential treatment can be helpful for forensic patients with severe personality disorder. An effective admission to a therapeutic community probably requires that the resident has some pro-social attitudes, will not be rejected by the group and has the capacity to use care that is offered by others (Dolan 1998). Many forensic personality-disordered patients lack these psychological attributes and there has been concern that they exploit them in others (Rice et al 1992). The public inquiry into the PDU in Ashworth Hospital (Fallon et al 1999) showed that patients either exploited staff trust or were vulnerable to exploitation, which suggests a lack of the basic capacity for interpersonal relating that is necessary for a TC to function well.

However, the data from the Grendon TC do suggest that people with ASPDs can benefit from a structured TC model within a secure setting. It suggests that residential services for forensic personality-disordered patients need to have properly trained staff and a consistently delivered, highly structured model of care that emphasizes autonomy and personal responsibility (McMurran and Duggan 2005). In the United Kingdom, the Home Office and Department of Health have jointly initiated the Dangerous and Severe Personality Disorder (DSPD) services for individuals whose personality disorder is both severe and presents a high risk to others (DH, HO, HM Prison Service, 2005; see Chapter 16). The secure treatment facilities for this group have been developed both in prisons and secure NHS hospitals. These units and their treatment programmes are still in their infancy, and the results of their evaluation are awaited over the next few years.

Life in secure settings: problems for staff and patients

People with personality disorder are detained in conditions of security not solely because they have a personality disorder but because they have acted dangerously towards others within the context of this condition and are thought to be at risk of so doing again. As discussed previously, MDOs with personality disorder who are detained in secure care have in common particular developmental histories and psychopathological profiles.

It is rare to find a patient with personality disorder in forensic settings who has not experienced either severe abuse or neglect as a child (Bland et al 1999; Coid 1992). Following the biopsychosocial developmental model, trauma and abuse in combination with genetic vulnerabilities predispose to the development of personality disorder (Leckman 1999). There is now robust evidence that child abuse, especially physical abuse and neglect, significantly increases the risk of developing a personality disorder in adulthood (Battle et al 2004; Johnson et al 1999; Macmillan et al 2001). Childhood sexual abuse increases the risk of developing suicidal behaviours and depression in adulthood (Soloff et al 2002); so individuals who have suffered both physical and sexual abuse and neglect are at increased risk of developing a wide range of psychological problems. Trusting professional carers and authority figures is a particular problem for this patient group because many MDOs with a personality disorder will have been abused by people who have claimed to be both their carer and trustworthy. It is therefore hardly surprising that people with personality disorder frequently expect professional carers to 'let them down', test them to see if they are trustworthy, engage cautiously in psychological therapies and require long periods of treatment.

With respect to psychopathology, MDOs have a wide range of personality difficulties that often span several DSM categories, and they frequently have additional Axis I disorders such as substance misuse or depressive disorders. However, the symptoms and signs of personality disorder most obviously manifest in the individual's social functioning and interpersonal relationships. This characteristic, when combined with the physical and procedural constraints of a secure environment, means that individuals with personality disorder will struggle in residential secure settings. However, paradoxically, the presence of many other people with personality disorder offers opportunities for learning.

Hinshelwood (1999) had described people with severe personality disorder as having relationships that are suffused with feelings, often very unpleasant ones. As most forensic patients have aspects of antisocial, borderline, narcissistic and paranoid personality disorders, they find it hard to trust others and are frequently overwhelmed by feelings of rage and fear, which they cannot modulate themselves. To rid themselves of these feelings they act them out physically, usually in the form of impulsive physical assaults, either on others or on themselves (as acts of deliberate self-harm or suicide). Those with more borderline symptoms may struggle with feelings of emptiness, sadness and hopelessness, which greatly increase their risk of suicidal behaviour. Many personality-disordered forensic patients have a diminished capacity for an accurate and empathic understanding for others. This is most usually seen in their inability to perspective take, their lack of curiosity about themselves and others and a tendency to intellectualize feelings and emotional states.

As MDOs with personality disorder have difficulty modulating and tolerating their feelings these are often discharged onto other patients or staff. Patients both consciously and unconsciously interfere with their carers' feelings so that staff often feel intruded upon, manipulated and pressurized to react in a certain way towards the patient (Hinshelwood 1999). This dynamic can result in staff feeling resentful and result in them having hostile interactions with patients, or withdrawing and becoming distant, with all the risks either position brings. If unattended to, these processes diminish the therapeutic potential of the environment and decrease the effectiveness of the particular therapeutic task, whether that be primarily one of containment or treatment.

It is the testing of the staff–patient relationship that evokes most problems in residential settings. Patients with personality disorder test staff by breaking or challenging group boundaries and rules, by attempting to split the care team so that staff become disorganized and fight between themselves or by attempting to seduce carers into giving them 'special' care which is actually unhelpful (Main 1957; Norton 1996). Patients may seek help, rejecting it when it is offered and often express contempt for staff members' capacities to both empathize and effect change. Sometimes the patients' behaviour will be conscious and overt; sometimes it will be much less conscious or much more covert.

One approach to working with personality disorder is to consider the difficulties, not only from the perspective of the individual but also from the perspective of the groups, communities and institutions to which the person relates, usually in a negative way. The diagnostic criteria for personality disorder reflect these two perspectives; the symptoms personality-disordered patients suffer reflect the way they construe and experience their world from the *inside*, their behaviours reflect the way they experience and impact on others *outside* themselves. It is useful to hold both these perspectives in mind.

Case example: the Ashworth inquiries

The less conscious and more covert challenges to the staff–patient relationship are by far the most dangerous for all concerned. Ashworth Hospital in the north of England was the subject of two public inquiries because of concerns about staff behaviour towards patients (DH 1992; Fallon et al 1999). The first Ashworth Inquiry found evidence that some staff had been physically abusive to some patients, many of whom were mentally ill, but some of whom, as research would suggest, almost certainly had personality disorders as well. The second inquiry found evidence that staff had either colluded with patients with personality disorder in rule breaking behaviour, turned a blind eye to it, or 'not noticed' it.

These problems may appear different but there are commonalities. They are sad examples of how staff can get caught up by the challenges patients' present and by the emotions and reactions that patients, with both mental illness and personality disorder, unconsciously evoke in others. Staff have conscious reactions to their patients, such as hostility, rage, contempt and fear, of which they can be aware. However, they will almost certainly have unconscious reactions as well when the relationship triggers reminders of their past relationships.

Part of the remit of the first Ashworth Inquiry was to investigate allegations of ill-treatment and improper care of patients. It could be assumed that some staff perceived the patients as especially provocative and frightening to have reached the point of using 'a good deal of harassment' and 'some physical bullying' towards them (DH 1992, Vol I). As the Inquiry found that there was an uncaring and demeaning attitude to patients and an overstrict, rigid and punitive regime in parts of the hospital, it may be that the patients unconsciously triggered fears in staff about their own capacity to become disorganized and anxiety about their capacity to contain the patients.

Many patients with personality disorder find it difficult to contain their unpalatable feelings and may experience conscious anxiety about this deficit; for others, their anxiety is still there but unconscious and split off from their awareness; either way, these patients often rely on others to ensure they will not be overwhelmed by their affects. This anxiety is then mirrored by the staff, who may behave in an over-controlling and harsh way to patients in response to their own sense of panic that they are not in control. If, in reality, staff numbers are decreased or the ward is particularly stressed, then the likelihood of staff feeling helpless and panicky rises which, in turn, can increase the risk of staff acting in a hostile way to patients. This explanation is not offered to excuse unprofessional behaviour but rather to provide a framework for understanding what happened in the hope of preventing repetition.

Similarly, in the second Ashworth Inquiry it is possible that the staff also felt overwhelmed and helpless by the patients' cruelty and hopelessness. It is possible that they failed to notice what was going on and/or failed to take action because they felt there was no point in either noticing or acting. In this way, they may have unconsciously identified with their patients' victims as well as the victim part of each patient's history. Victims of violence characteristically 'freeze' and become passive in the face of danger; they can also experience overwhelming hopelessness and helplessness, which further increases passivity (Seligman 1973).

Staff may have also identified with the cruel and delinquent part of each patient's mind. Both cruelty and successful rule-breaking can lead to a (usually brief) sense of triumph that may have contributed to a 'superficially' positive atmosphere on the ward, where both staff and patients were able to convince themselves that everything was well. It is a human characteristic to not wish to disturb what appears to be working well, even when there are underlying problems, especially if this means confronting people who have been violent and cruel. Rule-breaking patients, who wanted to deceive staff, may have gone out of their way to be pleasant and engaging in a way that can be seductive in secure settings that are often otherwise so turbulent. The sad truth is also that staff members may have failed to see the patients as patients: a situation that can lead to collusion. One speculative possibility is that any such collusion with rule breaking may also have been more likely in staff who themselves had a history of rule breaking in their own childhoods; or who had also had insecure attachment experiences themselves. Given the prevalence of insecure attachments in the general population (Van IJzendoorn and Bakermans-Kranenburg 1996), it would be surprising if some people with an insecure attachment style did not become health care professionals; indeed, Bowlby himself suggested that one way to cope with having had an insecure childhood is to become a professional carer in adulthood (Bowlby 1980).

Psychological treatment: generic and specific

Personality disorders are conditions that result in functional impairment and psychological distress; in forensic populations, personality disorder has often driven offending. The mainstay of treatment is psychological.

Psychological treatment may be conceptualized as comprising both a generic and a specific limb; the former needs to be embedded in the patients' mental health care and can be delivered by all mental health staff; the specific refers to particular psychological treatment interventions. The generic component includes the team, as well as individual staff members, forming and sustaining a healthy therapeutic relationship with their patients – one that can resist or quickly repair the ruptures that frequently beset the therapeutic alliance when working with MDOs with personality disorder. As such, the generic component of treatment includes attention to staff patient interactions and how they might become anti-therapeutic.

Professional boundaries and their violation in secure care

What happened in Ashworth were rather extreme examples of violations and the erosion of professional boundaries. Boundaries are those beliefs, insignia and behaviours that help define our identities and roles. They literally mark out the territory of our identity; on one side of the boundary I am this person, on the other I am that. Boundary violations are those responses by staff to patients that take them out of their professional role. The next section discusses boundary violations with respect to personality-disordered patients and offers some suggestions for management, for a discussion of the ethical aspects of boundary violations (see Adshead, this volume: pp 303–312). For most staff in forensic settings the boundary of professional identity will be marked out by both non-verbal and verbal signs.

Mental health professionals, especially those working in long-stay residential settings, are at increased risk of professional boundary violations (Sarkar 2004). In forensic settings, staff have to manage their personal boundaries more carefully because the patients often have very little experience of boundary keeping. Staff have to be able to keep boundaries in a reasonably consistent way, but more important, they need to be alert to the ways in which boundaries can regularly be broken. In an ideal world no staff member would ever cross professional boundaries but the reality is that they do, especially with personality-disordered patients. The commonest types of boundary violation are listed in Table 14.3.

By far the commonest type of boundary violation is inappropriate self-disclosure, which may arise as a result of poor communication skills and is discussed below. Sexual boundary violations can and do occur in secure settings; interestingly, they frequently involve female staff and male patients (Garrett 1998).

Although there is well-established literature on boundary violations, it is often a difficult topic to discuss. It is much easier to hiss with disbelief at other people's boundary violations than it is to think about how we might commit minor boundary misdemeanours (Gutheil and

Table 14.3 Common professional boundary violations by staff working with individuals with personality disorder

◆ Inappropriate self-disclosure to a patient
◆ Excessive advocacy for or criticism of a patient
◆ Inappropriate involvement in a patient's care, for example, taking on cases outside of one's remit or expertise
◆ Inappropriate physical touching with a patient which may be hostile or seductive and sexualized
◆ Inappropriate dependence and emotional involvement with patients
◆ Inappropriate bartering or financial involvement with patients
◆ Lying to patients or lying to colleagues about patients

Gabbard 1993). The issue is further complicated by the fact that some minor boundary misdemeanours can have reportedly good effects on the therapeutic relationship and major boundary violations can sometimes be experienced positively in the short term (Jehu et al 1988). One example of this is in relation to the 'no touch' approach frequently seen in forensic settings (Ramsden et al 2006). However, staff often find themselves touching patients when they have to search or restrain them, if they are reassuring them or sometimes when they give hugs to patients who seem in need of comfort. Unfortunately, although both parties may appear to enjoy and value physical exchanges, such as hugging, the problem is that it often sets up expectations that then cannot be met professionally or emotionally.

It is only by accepting that boundary violations can and do happen that it becomes possible to talk about them and manage them better. If they are denied, especially when they involve senior staff, then little can be done to prevent them happening again and the risk of repetition may increase. This is particularly true with respect to those patients with personality disorder who have little sense of personal boundaries and who often act in ways that encourage staff to also break boundaries. MDOs with personality disorder may act aggressively, causing staff to get angry or abusive; they may act in seductive ways, inviting staff to break rules or to go against policies for their particular benefit; they may use superficial charm to encourage the staff to 'trust' them so they can then exploit staff. In addition, they may tell conflicting stories about their experiences or symptoms and act in different ways with different staff members, increasing the possibility of staff arguing with each other, which can cause splits within the team and increase the chance that staff will take 'sides' either for or against the patient.

Often these behaviours are symptoms of the patient's personality disorder that become manifest in their interpersonal interactions with staff and other patients. As such, they are available for the staff team to observe, think about and put in place the appropriate therapeutic intervention with the patient. It is when these processes fail to happen and staff 'react' to such patient behaviours that the problematic dynamics outlined above are more likely to become established. However, it is important to remember that boundary violations are likely to be a regular occurrence in forensic psychiatric settings and when they occur it is essential that they be thought about and monitored.

Professional boundaries: maintenance and management

The structure and context in which individuals with personality disorder are cared for can contribute to boundary violations. They are more likely to occur when staff and patients have to engage in long-term relationships of medium and high dependency i.e. where patients are dependent on staff for intimate care and staff are dependent on patients to behave. They are also more likely when the relationship involves some sort of psychological intimacy and mutuality, which increases over time. The following are offered as guidelines to help teams make and maintain good boundaries.

1. *Conceptual model*: Ensure that the staff have a model for understanding personality disorder and boundary violations. If the entire team shares the conceptual model, they will form a strong professional group (Bateman and Tyrer, 2004b). The model can be taught on induction and refreshed through professional development. The model does not have to be followed slavishly but there needs to be enough agreement that staff feel identified with and supportive of it.

2. *Acknowledgment that boundary violations happen*: Staff who feel defensive and anxious about their actions will not talk about them. In this climate small boundary misdemeanours will not be discussed. It is well established that most serious boundary violations begin with small

ones (Sarkar 2004), so there need to be safe and containing spaces where boundary violations can be discussed in a non-judgmental way.

3. *Creating of a culture of enquiry*: This term was first used by Tom Main (Main 1983) to describe a climate in democratic TCs aimed at understanding the meaning that underpins behaviour. It is used here to both denote this and to emphasize that a culture that helps people to be curious about each other aids empathic understanding and pro-social attitudes. Staff need a way to communicate and reflect on their interactions with patients and with each other, preferably in groups, so that multiple and dissenting opinions can be heard. The way in which staff manage conflict and anger with each other is crucial for boundary maintenance. Such a culture requires good communication skills in all members of staff, especially the senior staff. This is an important training issue because many senior staff, may not have had any training in communication skills, and new staff may need additional training to deal with the types of complex communications that happen in personality-disorder units.

4. *Mandatory supervision and reflective practice*: The term 'mandatory' is used to emphasize the expectation that the staff group attend both clinical supervision and reflective practice sessions. It is not envisaged that failure to do so would be a disciplinary issue for staff, although it could be. To some extent, if the first three guidelines are established the fourth follows naturally. Given the nature and difficulty of the work it is the *duty* of each mental health professional to ensure they have supervision to both assist and support them. Hopefully the culture would be such that the staff *want* to attend because they know that the work is tough.

5. *A structured day*: Evidence regarding the effectiveness of therapies for personality disorder suggests that highly structured programmes assist in containing distress and supporting interpersonal boundaries. The most effective services for personality disorder have highly structured daily programmes (Bateman and Fonagy 1999, 2001; Lees et al 1999; McMurran 2002).

6. *Reflective groups for patients*: Within the structured day there need to be spaces for reflection on behaviour and feeling, where the expectation is that people take responsibility for what they say and feel. If it is accepted that one of the main features of the ASPD is a tendency for the patient to blame others for their own unpalatable feelings and thoughts, then it becomes crucial that sessions be factored into the structured programme where individuals can be helped to take responsibility for their own psychological experience. Traditionally psychodynamic groups do this best and also have the advantage of reinforcing social boundaries, promoting acceptance and tolerance and reducing shame (Welldon 1993). Such groups can also promote a capacity for mentalizing; for having 'mind in mind' (Allen and Fonagy, 2006). Mentalization-based treatment (MBT) has been shown to be effective with borderline personality disorder (Bateman and Fonagy 1999, 2001, 2008) and may be effective in antisocial personality disorder (Bateman and Fonagy 2003).

Specific treatment: are psychological interventions effective?

Part of the historical prejudice against people with personality disorder was that they were thought to be 'untreatable', an odd concept that used to be applied to diseases like cancer or to the physically disabled (Adshead 2001). The advent of new theoretically driven psychological treatments over the last decade has increased therapeutic optimism with respect to the treatability of non-forensic patients with personality disorder. However, the application of these treatments to forensic patients has been patchy and to date there are no high-quality treatment trials, such as randomized control trials (RCTs) in inpatient forensic populations (Duggan et al 2007;

McMurran 2002). This section briefly reviews some of the research findings with respect to psychological treatment interventions for MDOs with personality disorder. The research evidence relating to cognitively based treatment interventions is described in both Perkins's and Hawes's chapters (see Chapters 15 and 16).

There are particular challenges, both practical and methodological, in conducting research studies in secure units with personality-disordered patients. These difficulties have often affected the quality of the outcome research and researchers' attempts to address these difficulties have resulted in a disparate body of literature that makes it difficult to compare the efficacy and effectiveness of psychological treatment interventions. Practical difficulties include gaining institutional access; engaging and sustaining the engagement of patients and staff who may be sceptical about the research process; involving busy and often overstretched staff in research and gaining access to routinely collected data. Methodological difficulties that have hampered the process of comparing studies and using meta-analytical approaches to look across the data have included the wide range of study designs; differing criteria for identification and selection of participants; high attrition rates; descriptions of treatment interventions that lack adequate detail; a wide choice of outcome measures and variable follow-up periods. For example, in MDOs with personality disorder there is debate about the areas interventions should primarily target; criminogenic factors such as impulsivity, victim empathy, offence- related work, enhanced thinking skills or psychiatric factors such as personality structure, mental disorder and psychological distress. Consequently, a wide array of outcome measures have been used, ranging from behavioural measures such as recidivism to measures of personality change and psychological functioning.

A key question is whether people who feel better actually behave better. For treatment to be effective follow-up research needs to establish if improved pro-social behaviour in secure care generalizes to the community. It may also be misleading only to target behaviours, as this can lead to compliance not change. Changing values and attitudes in those with ASPD may be a more effective treatment aim but harder to evaluate in terms of success.

ASPD and psychopathy

Assessing the evidence base for the effectiveness of treatment interventions for individuals diagnosed as having ASPD or 'psychopathic disorder' has been hampered by the tendency for different jurisdictions and practitioners to use similar concepts in different ways. For example, in the United Kingdom, the term 'psychopathic disorder' was a legal not a diagnostic construct as it was one of the four categories of mental disorder in the Mental Health Act (HMSO 1983) under which an individual could be legally detained. The *concept* of psychopathy refers to the combination of interpersonal, affective, lifestyle and antisocial traits that make up the Psychopathy Checklist-Revised (PCL-R; Hare 1991, 2003). The checklist was derived from the work of Cleckley (1941). Those who score 30 (25 in UK) or more meet criteria for psychopathy (see Chapter 15 and 16). Neither Hare 'psychopathy' nor the old UK legal category of 'psychopathic disorder' are synonymous with ASPD as defined by DSM-IV-TR (American Psychiatric Association 2000). Although they overlap symptomatically, ASPD is a broader category and emphasizes antisocial and criminal behaviours rather than personality traits (McGauley et al 2008).

Although there is a recognized need for effective psychological treatments for forensic patients with personality disorder, especially ASPD, the two systematic treatment reviews (Duggan et al 2007; Warren et al 2003) highlight the lack of methodological rigour in many of the published studies. Considering only RCTs, Warren did not find any RCTs of treatment interventions for ASPD, irrespective of setting. Duggan identified two studies (Brooner et al 1998; Messina et al 2003) that met Cochrane inclusion criteria (Khan et al 2003), both involving individuals with a dual diagnosis of substance misuse or dependency as well as ASPD, and the study subjects were not detained in forensic settings. The findings of the Duggan review confirmed those of earlier reviews (Warren et al 2003; Bateman and Tyrer 2004a) that the evidence base for psychological treatment interventions in ASPD is weak. They stress the importance of conducting further treatment trials in this group and the need to fund properly designed and powered randomized trials of treatment intervention in those with ASPD if the evidence base is to be strengthened.

In order to address some of the limitations of previous reviews the draft guidelines from the National Institute for Health and Clinical Excellence (NICE 2008a) adopted a wide approach to reviewing treatment interventions for people with ASPD in so much as they both reviewed treatment for specific components of ASPD, such as impulsivity and aggression, and included interventions aimed at reducing re-offending in offender populations. With respect to the treatment of ASPD the draft NICE review did not identify any studies meeting their rigorous quality criteria for inclusion. The guideline group also concluded that the evidence for the treatment of constructs of ASPD was so limited that no recommendations could be drawn. There was modest evidence for the effectiveness of group based cognitive behavioral skills interventions delivered to adult offenders in criminal justice settings such as prison or probation and parole. However, the effect sizes were small and not all of the offenders in these study groups had a diagnosis of ASPD.

With respect to the concept of psychopathy opinion has oscillated regarding the extent to which individuals who have high scores on the PCL-R are treatable (see Chapter 16). Dolan and Coid's (1993) review of treatments concluded that there was no convincing evidence that individuals with pronounced psychopathic traits could or could not be successfully treated and that the prevailing therapeutic pessimism was unjustified. However, a series of papers in the 1990s (Rice et al 1992; Harris et al 1994) concluded that 'psychopaths' simply exploited the trust and vulnerability of others and raised concerns that some forms of group psychotherapeutic approaches made psychopathic traits worse. There have been similar concerns that sex offenders with ASPD who attend therapeutic programmes might simply learn better ways to groom or otherwise exploit potential victims. D'Silva (D'Silva et al 2004) examined the research evidence that psychopaths were untreatable and may even be made worse by treatment. They reviewed ten studies and found that although four studies suggested that Hare 'psychopaths' had a negative response to treatment, another four suggested the opposite.

Salekin's systematic review and meta-analysis (Salekin 2002) specifically addressed the treatment of individuals with psychopathic traits. His review of 42 treatment studies concluded that there was little scientific basis for the view that 'psychopathy' was untreatable, and he suggested that previous therapeutic pessimism was both unwarranted and premature because some psychopathic traits such as lying, lack of remorse, lack of empathy and interpersonal dysfunctional relationships may in fact be amenable to treatment. A key question is which traits might be amenable to change and how may these be monitored in incarcerated populations? (Hobson et al 2000).

BPD

The evidence base for the efficacy of psychological interventions in BPD is stronger and more consistent (Bateman and Tyrer 2004a), although this evidence base is from non-forensic populations. With respect to specific psychological treatments, the most promising interventions to emerge in the last decade can be grouped into cognitive behavioural therapy (CBT), therapies using modified CBT such as Dialectic Behaviour therapy (DBT) and modified psychodynamic therapies such as mentalization-based therapy (MBT). Duggan's (Duggan et al 2007) review of the psychological treatments for people with BPD identified seven RCTs, six of which used DBT as a treatment intervention and the other, MBT (Bateman and Fonagy 1999). Duggan concluded that, although the studies were small and of moderate quality, according to Cochrane criteria, problems such as self-harm, suicidality and depressive symptoms in people with BPD are amenable to treatment with either DBT or MBT. Clarkin's (Clarkin et al 2007) subsequent paper reports that patients who received transference-focused psychotherapy improved across more outcome domains than those who received either DBT or supportive treatment. For a more detailed description of DBT see Chapter 15.

In the longest follow-up to date, patients with BPD who received MBT have been shown to maintain their clinical improvement 5 years post-treatment termination compared to the patient group who received treatment as usual (Bateman & Fonagy 2008). Mentalization refers to the ability to implicitly and explicitly interpret the actions of oneself and others as meaningful on the basis of intentional mental states, e.g. on the basis of an understanding of the feelings, beliefs, thoughts, desires, intentions and needs of oneself and others. Mentalization is a normal ability which refers to the capacity to ascribe meaning to human behaviour and shapes our understanding of others and ourselves. In this attachment-mentalization model, BPD is seen as a developmental disorder resulting from an early disorganization of primary attachment relationships, leading to diminished social-cognitive capacities which in turn decrease the individual's capacity to form secure relationships with caregivers. Early disorganized attachment relationships coupled with maltreatment also result in disorganization of the self structure and decreased ability to mentalize, especially when affect is aroused and attachment activated. In this model of BPD (Bateman & Fonagy, 2006), the failure of mentalization means that subjective emotional states cannot be represented or tolerated by the individual, and this results in the common symptoms of BPD, such as self harm, suicidality and impulsive acts of violence. The aim of MBT is to increase the patient's capacity to understand their own mental states and the mental states of others.

In 2008, NICE issued guidelines which reviewed the evidence base for psychological treatment interventions for BPD, but only in non-MDO populations (NICE 2008a). They differentiate two classes of psychological intervention: complex interventions, which combine more than one modality of treatment, for example, individual therapy plus group therapy, and are delivered by more than one therapist, as in DBT and MBT; and single modality psychological therapies, either individual or group therapies, usually offered weekly in an outpatient setting. They advise that, if psychological therapy is recommended for an individual with BPD, the therapy offered should be in at least two modalities, have a well-structured programme, a coherent theory of practice, and that therapist supervision should be included within the framework of the service. Although the guidelines do not discuss MDOs with BPD, many of these recommendations would seem to apply. Furthermore, since most of the patients with personality disorder in forensic psychiatric care will fall into the Cluster B group, and have a mixture of BPD and ASPD, it seems reasonable that they have access to treatment for their BPD traits. Better mood regulation may encourage therapeutic engagement, which in turn may make it easier to recruit for the RCTs of psychological treatment in ASPD that are so badly needed.

Therapeutic communities

There is evidence that mild to moderate degrees of personality disorder are effectively treated in TCs (Lees et al 1999; Warren et al 2003). Lees' systematic review of outcome research of TCs' effectiveness in treating people with personality disorder in secure, non-secure psychiatric and other settings, generally found TCs to be beneficial for personality disorder, although which aspects of the treatment programme were the most effective for specific patient groups remained unclear. Unfortunately, none of the randomized trials were conducted on personality-disordered offenders. The Grendon literature suggests that a prison TC can contribute to reducing recidivism in men with ASPD and degrees of psychopathy (Hobson et al 2000). The difficulty with TCs is that they do not lend themselves to evaluation by RCT, since self-selection is a crucial aspect of patient admission.

Conclusion

Perhaps the most obvious question raised in this chapter is, 'Why would anyone want to work with people with personality disorder?' It is human to be interested in other people's disasters (as anyone who has slowed down to look at a motorway pile-up might agree). It is also true that for some people, working in a forensic setting with very disturbed people may be the only job available. However, for many people, working with personality-disordered patients in secure settings is, in part, determined by unconscious factors that have real emotional meaning and significance.

Secure settings concretely provide containing environments into which staff can project unwelcome aspects of themselves. Problems arise if these dynamics are kept out of the individual's and the organization's awareness. Evacuation of these aspects allows them to be seen as entirely lodged within patients and frees staff from taking responsibility for their own aggressive feelings and violent impulses. It is easy to see how, in such a climate, a rigid 'them and us' culture can develop, with the risk of staff cruelly dealing with those they are there to contain and treat. Alternatively, the raw affects and the knowledge of how many MDOs have acted on these and inflicted suffering on others can, at times, become too powerful for staff to process. If this becomes the norm and the institution does not provide a process to support staff in this task, it affects and the concomitant anxieties they arouse in staff can become disavowed, leading to a situation where staff can over-identify with those they are there to treat, seeing them solely as misunderstood victims. Either distortion can foster boundary violations and result in the patient receiving poor care and treatment. One of the most taxing tasks of working with personality-disordered individuals in secure settings is to maintain an accurate empathic stance; one of being able to project oneself into the other while retaining the capacity to think about them with one's own mind.

Acknowledgements

The authors have learnt much about personality disorder from both their patients and peers. They would like to thank members of the Broadmoor Wednesday Group (a multidisciplinary supervision group), Anne Aiyegbusi, Jude Deacon and Sameer Sarkar and all the members of the forensic psychotherapy service at Broadmoor Hospital.

References

Adshead, G. 1998 Psychiatric staff as Attachment Figures. British Journal of Psychiatry 172: 64–69.

Adshead, G. 2001 Murmurs of Discontent: Treatability and Personality Disorder. Advances in Psychiatric Treatment 7: 407–416.

Adshead, G. 2002 Three Degrees of Security: Attachment and Forensic Institutions. Criminal Behaviour and Mental Health 12: S31–S45.

Akhtar, S. and Samuel, S. 1996 The Concept of Identity: Developmental Orgins, Phenomenology, Clinical Relevance, and Measurement. Harvard review of Psychiatry 3: 254–267.

Allen, J. and Fonagy, P. 2006 Handbook of Mentalization-Based Treatment. Chichester: John Wiley.

American Psychiatric Association. 2000 Diagnostic and Statistical Manual of Mental Disorders 4th Edition, Text Revision DSM-IV-TR. Washington: American Psychiatric Association.

Bateman, A.W. and Fonagy, P. 1999 The Effectiveness of Partial Hospitalization in the Treatment of Borderline Personality Disorder – A Randomised Controlled Trial. American Journal of Psychiatry 156: 1563–1569.

Bateman, A.W. and Fonagy, P. 2001 Treatment of Borderline Personality Disorder with Psychoanalytically Oriented Partial Hospitalization: An 18-Month Follow-up. American Journal of Psychiatry 158(1): 36–42.

Bateman A.W. and Fonagy, P. 2003 Advances in Treatment of Personality Disorder International Society for the Study of Personality Disorders Annual Conference. Munich.

Bateman, A.W. and Fonagy, P. 2006 Using the Mentalization Model to Understand Severe Personality Disorder. 11–28 in Mentalization-Based Treatment for Borderline Personality Disorder, A Practical Guide (Bateman, A and Fonagy, P Editors) Oxford: Oxford University Press.

Bateman, A.W. and Fonagy, P. 2008 8-Year Follow-up of Patients Treated for Borderline Personality Disorder: Mentalization-based Treatment versus Treatment as Usual. The American Journal of Psychiatry 165(May): 631–638.

Bateman, A.W. and Tyrer, P. 2004a Psychological Treatment of Personality Disorders. Advances in Psychiatric Treatment 10: 378–388.

Bateman, A.W. and Tyrer, P. 2004b Services for Personality Disorder: Organisation for Inclusion. Advances in Psychiatric Treatment, 10: 425–433.

Battle, C.L., Shea, T., and Johnson, D.M. et al 2004 Childhood Maltreatment Associated with Adults Personality Disorders: Findings From the Collaborative Longitudinal Personality Disorders Study. Journal of Personality Disorders 18: 193–211.

Blackburn R. 2006 Describing Personality and its Abnormal Deviations. 32-37 in Personality Disorder and Serious Offending, Hospital Treatment Models (Newrith, C., Meux, C. and Taylor, P.J. Editors) London: Hodder Arnold.

Blackburn R., Clare Crellin M., Morgan E.M. and Tulloch R.M.B. 1990 Prevalence of Personality Disorders in a Special Hospital Population. Journal of Forensic Psychiatry 1: 43–52.

Blackburn R., Logan C., Donnelly J. and Renwick S. 2003 Personality Disorders, Psychopathy and Other Mental Disorders: Co-morbidity among Patients at English and Scottish High-security Hospitals. The Journal of Forensic Psychiatry and Psychology 14: 111–137.

Blair, K., Mitchell, D. and Blair, J. 2005 The Psychopath, Emotion and the Brain. Oxford: Blackwell.

Bland, J., Mezey, G. and Dolan, B. 1999 Special Women, Special Needs: A Descriptive Study of Female Special Hospital Patients. Journal of Forensic Psychiatry 10: 34–45.

Bowlby, J. 1980 Attachment and Loss Vol. III: Loss: Sadness and Depression. London: Basic Books. P206.

Brooner, R.K., Kidorf, M., King, V.I. and Stoller, K. 1998. Preliminary Evidence of Good Treatment Response in Antisocial Drug Abusers. Drug and Alcohol Dependence 49: 249–60.

Cleckley, H. 1941 The Mask of Sanity. 1st Edition. St Louis: Mosby.

Coid, J. 1992 DSM-III Diagnosis in Criminal Psychopaths: A Way Forward. Criminal Behaviour and Mental Health 2: 78–94.

Coid, J., Kahtan, N., Gault, S. and Jarman, B. 1999 Patients with Personality Disorder Admitted to Secure Forensic Psychiatry Services. British Journal of Psychiatry 175: 528–536.

Coid, J., Yang, M., Tyrer, P., Roberts, A. and Ullrich, S. 2006 Prevalence and Correlates of Personality Disorder in Great Britain. British Journal of Psychiatry 188: 423–431.

Department of Health. Report of the Committee of Inquiry into Complaints about Ashworth Hospital 1992 Blom-Cooper, L., Brown, M., Dolan, R. and Murphy, E. London, HMSO, Volume I and II. Cm 2028-I and II.

Department of Health and Home Office Working Group on Psychopathic Disorder. 1994 Review of Health and Social Services for Mentally Disordered Offenders and Others Requiring Similar Services the Reed Report. London: HMSO.

Department of Health. 2003 Personality Disorder: No Longer a Diagnosis for Exclusion. Policy Implementation Guidance for Development of Services for People with Personality Disorder. London: Department of Health.

Department of Health, Home Office, HM Prison Service. 2005 Dangerous and Severe Personality Disorder DSPD High Secure Services for Men: Planning and Delivery Guide, DSPD Programme.

D'Silva, K., Duggan, C. and McCarthy, L. 2004. Does Treatment Really Make Psychopaths Worse? A Review of the Evidence. Journal of Personality Disorders 18(2): 163–177.

de Girolamo, G. and Reich, J.H. 1993 Epidemiology of Mental Disorders and Psychosocial Problems: Personality Disorders. Geneva: World Health Organization.

Dolan, B. 1998 Therapeutic Community Treatment for Severe Personality Disorders 407–430 in Psychopathy: antisocial, criminal and violent behaviour (Millon, T., Simonsen, E., Birkett Smith, M. and Davis, R.D. Editors) New York: Guilford.

Dolan, B. and Coid, J. 1993. Summary of Findings and Recommendations for Future Research Chapter 12 in Psychopathic and Antisocial Personality Disorders: Treatment and Research Issues. (Dolan, B. and Coid, J. Editors) London: Gaskell.

Dowson, J.H. and Grounds, A.T. (Editors) 1995 Personality Disorders, Recognition and Clinical Management. Cambridge: Cambridge University Press.

Duggan, C., Adams, A., McCarthy, L. et al 2007 A Systematic Review of the Effectiveness of Pharmacological and Psychological Treatments for those with Personality Disorder. NHS National R & D Programme in Forensic Mental Health available at: www.nfmhp.org.uk/MRD%2012%2033%20Final%20Report.pdf (last accessed June 2008).

Duggan, C., Huband, N., Smailagic, N., Ferriter, M. and Adams, C. 2007 The Use of Psychological Treatments for People with Personality Disorder: A Systematic Review of Randomized Controlled Trials. Personality and Mental Health 1: 95–125. Published online in Wiley InterScience www.interscience.wiley.com

Fallon, P., Bluglass, R., Edwards, B. and Daniels. G. 1999 Report of the Committee of Inquiry into the Personality Disorder Unit, Ashworth Special Hospital Vol 1 Cm 4194-II. London: Stationery Office.

Fazel, S. and Danesh, J. 2002 Serious Mental Disorder in 23000 Prisoners: A Systematic Review of 62 Surveys. The Lancet 359: 545–550.

Fonagy, P. and Target, M. 1997 Attachment and Reflective Function: Their Role in Self-organisation. Development and Psychopathology 9: 679–700.

Frodi, A., Dernevik, M., Sepa, A., Philipson, J. and Bragesjo, M. 2001 Current Attachment Representations in Incarcerated Offenders Varying in Degrees of Psychopathology. Attachment and Human development 3: 269–283.

Garrett, T. 1998 The Prevalence of Sexual Contact between British Clinical Psychologists and Their Patients. Clinical Psychology and Psychotherapy 5: 253–263.

Gutheil, T. and Gabbard, G. 1993 The Concept of Boundaries in Clinical Practice: Theoretical and Risk Management Dimensions. American Journal of Psychiatry 150: 188–196.

Hare, R.D. 1991 The Hare Psychopathy Checklist-Revised. Toronto, Ontario, Multi-health Systems.

Hare, R.D. 2003 Manual for the Hare Psychopathy Checklist–Revised 2nd Edition. Toronto: Multi-health Systems.

Harris, G.T., Rice, M.E. and Cormier, C.A. 1994 Psychopaths: Is a Therapeutic Community Therapeutic? Therapeutic Communities 15(4): 283–299.

HMSO 1983, The Mental Health Act 1983, HMSO, London, c12.

HMSO 2007, The Mental Health Act 2007, HMSO, London, c12.

Hinshelwood, D. 1999 The Difficult Patient. British Journal of Psychiatry 174: 187–190.

Hobson, J., Shine, J. and Roberts, R. 2000. How Do Psychopaths Behave in a Prison Therapeutic Community? Psychology, Crime and the Law 6: 139–154.

Jehu, D. Gazan, M. Klassen, C. 1988 Beyond sexual abuse: Therapy with women who were childhood victims. Oxford, England. John Wiley and Sons.

Johnson, J., Cohen, P., Brown, J., Smailes, E.M. and Bernstein, D. 1999 Childhood Maltreatment Increase Risk for Personality Disorder in Early Adulthood. Archives of General Psychiatry 56: 600–606.

Jones, M. 1982 The Process of Change. London: Routledge and Kegan Paul.

Kernberg, O. 1998 The Psychotherapeutic Management of Psychopathic, Narcissistic and Paranoid Transferences 372–392 in Psychopathy: Antisocial, Criminal and Violent Behaviour (Millon, T., Simonsen, E., Birkett Smith, M. and Davis, R.D. Editors) New York: Guilford.

Khan, K.S., Kunz, R., Kleijnen, J. and Antes, G. 2003 Systematic Reviews to Support Evidence-based Medicine: How to Review and Apply Research Findings of Healthcare Research. London: Royal Society of Medicine Press.

Kramer, P. 1993 Listening to Prozac. New York: Viking Books.

Leckman, J. 1999 Incremental Progress in Developmental Psychopathology: Simply Complex. American Journal of Psychiatry 156: 1495–1498.

Lees, J., Manning, N. and Rawlings, B. 1999 Therapeutic Effectiveness. A Systematic International Review of Therapeutic Community Treatment for People with Personality Disorders and Mentally Disordered Offenders CRD Report 17: The University of York. NHS Centre for Reviews and Dissemination.

Linehan, M.M., Armstrong, H.E., Suarez, A., Allmon, D. and Heard, H.L. 1991 Cognitive-behavioural Treatment of Chronically Parasuicidal Borderline Patients. Archives of General Psychiatry 48: 1060–1064.

Lenzenweger, M.F. 1999 Stability and Change in Personality Disorder Features: Findings from a Longitudinal Study of Personality Disorders. Archives of General Psychiatry 56: 1009–1015.

Macmillan, H., Fleming, J., Streiner, D. et al 2001 Childhood Abuse and Lifetime Psychopathology in a Community Sample. American Journal of Psychiatry 158: 1878–1883.

Main, T.F. 1957 The Ailment. British Journal of Medical Psychology 30: 129–145.

Main, T.F. 1983 The Concept of the Therapeutic Community: Variations and Vicissitudes 197–217 in The Evolution of Group Analysis (Pines, M. Editor) London: Routledge and Kegan Paul.

McGauley, G.A., Adshead, G. and Sarkar, S. 2008 Psychotherapy for Psychopathic Disorders 449–466 in The International Handbook on Psychopathic Disorders and the Law (Felthous, A.R. and SaB, H. Editors) John Wiley and Sons.

McMurran, M. 2002 Personality Disorders. Expert Paper for the NHS National Programme on Forensic Mental Health Research and Development.

McMurran, M. and Duggan, C. 2005 The Manualisation of a Therapy Programme for Personality Disorder. Criminal Behaviour and Mental Health 95: 17–27.

Messina, N., Farabee, D. and Rawson, R. 2003. Treatment Responsivity of Cocaine-dependent Patients with Antisocial Personality Disorder to Cognitive-behavioral and Contingency Management Interventions. Journal of Consulting and Clinical Psychology 71(2): 320–329.

Moore, E. 2006 Clinical Assessment of Individuals with Personality Disorder in the Secure Hospital. 40–57 in Personality Disorder and Serious Offending, Hospital Treatment Models (Newrith, C., Meux, C. and Taylor, P.J. Editors) London: Hodder Arnold.

National Institute for Health and Clinical Excellence (NICE) 2008a. Antisocial personality disorder: Treatment, Management and Prevention. National Clinical Practice Guideline. National Collaborating Centre for Mental Health, Commissioned by the National Institute for Health and Clinical Excellence, chapter 7, pp. 165–203. Full Guideline Draft.

National Institute for Health and Clinical Excellence (NICE) 2008b. Borderline personality disorder: Treatment and Management. National Clinical Practice Guideline. National Collaborating Centre for

Mental Health, Commissioned by the National Institute for Health and Clinical Excellence. Full Guideline Draft.

Norton, K. 1996 Management of Difficult Personality Disorder Patients. Advances in Psychiatric Treatment 2: 202–210.

Ramsden, E., Pryor, A., Bose, S., Charles, S. and Adshead, G. 2006 Something Dangerous: Touch in Forensic Practice 163–178 in Touch Papers: Dialogues on Touch in the Psychoanalytic Space (Galton, G. Editor) London: Karnac.

Rice, M.E., Harris, G.T. and Cormier, C.A. 1992 An Evaluation of a Maximum Secure Therapeutic Community for Psychopaths and Other Mentally Disordered Offenders. Law and Human Behavior 16: 399–412.

Salekin, R.T. 2002. Psychopathy and Therapeutic Pessimism. Clinical Lore or Clinical Reality? Clinical Psychology Review 22: 79–112.

Sarkar, S.P. 2004 Boundary Violations and Sexual Exploitation in Psychiatry and Psychotherapy: A Review. Advances in Psychiatric Treatment 10: 312–320.

Sarkar, J. and Adshead, G. 2006 Personality Disorder as Disorganisation of Attachment and Affect Regulation. Advances in Psychiatric Treatment 12: 299–305.

Seligman, M.E.P. 1975 Helplessness: On Depression, Development and Death. San Francisco CA: W.H. Freeman.

Singleton, N., Bumpstead, R., O'Brien, M., Lee, A. and Meltzer, H. 2003 Psychiatric Morbidity among Adults Living in Private Households 2000. International Review of Psychiatry 15: 65–73.

Singleton, N., Meltzer, H. and Gatward, R. 1998 Office of National Statistics Survey of Psychiatric Morbidity among Prisoners in England and Wales. London: HMSO.

Soloff, P., Lynch, K.G. and Kelly, T.M. 2002 Childhood Abuse as a Risk Factor for Suicidal Behaviour in Borderline Personality Disorder. Journal of Personality Disorders 16: 201–214.

Tyrer, P. 2006 Diagnostic Categories of Personality Disorder 19–31 in Personality Disorder and Serious Offending, Hospital Treatment Models (Newrith, C., Meux, C. and Taylor, P.J. Editors) London: Hodder Arnold.

Vaillant, G.E. 1994 Ego Mechanisms of Defense and Personality Psychopathology. Journal of Abnormal Psychology 103: 44–50.

Vaillant, G.E. 1995 The Wisdom of the Ego. New York: Basic Books.

Vaillant, L.M. 1997 Changing Character: Short-term Anxiety-regulating Psychotherapy for Restructuring Defenses, Affects and Attachment. New York: Basic Books.

Van IJzendoorn, M.H. and Bakermans-Kranenburg, M.J. 1996 Attachment Representations in Mothers, Fathers, Adolescents and Clinical Groups: A Meta-analytic Search for Normative Data. Journal of Consulting and Clinical Psychology 64: 8–21.

Van IJzendoorn, M.H., Feldbrugge, J.T., Derks, F.C. et al 1997 Attachment Representations of Personality-disordered Criminal Offenders. American Journal of Orthopsychiatry 67: 449–459.

Warren, F., McGauley, G.A., Norton, K. et al 2003 Review of Treatments for Severe Personality Disorder. Online report 30/03. www.homeoffice.gov.uk/rds/pdfs2/rdsolr3003.pdf London: Home Office.

Welldon, E. 1993 Forensic Psychotherapy and Group Analysis. Group Analysis 26: 487–502.

World Health Organisation 1992 ICD-10; Classification of Mental and Behavioural Disorder. Geneva: WHO.

Zanarini, M.C., Frankenburg, F.R., Hennen, J. and Silk, K.R. 2003 The Longitudinal Course of Borderline Psychopathology: 6 Year Prospective Follow-up of the Phenomenon of Borderline Personality Disorder. American Journal of Psychiatry 160: 274–283.

Zinkin, L. 1983 Malignant Mirroring. Group Analysis 16:113–126.

Appendix 14.1: Definition and classification of personality disorders

The importance of traits is recognized in both of the main diagnostic systems for personality disorder, which describe this condition as being a recognizable "pattern of symptoms and behaviours which are associated with poor interpersonal and social functioning" (International Classification of Diseases, WHO 1992) and an "enduring pattern of inner experience and behaviour that deviates markedly from the expectations of the culture of the individual who exhibits it" (DSM–IV-TR), American Psychiatric Association 2000; see Table A 14.1 for full criteria). However, the DSM and WHO-ICD classifications then identify 10 and 8 individual personality disorders respectively, using a categorical model, which suggests qualitative distinctions between normal and abnormal functioning and clear boundaries between categories. This categorical, as opposed to dimensional, approach to classifying personality disorder has commanded considerable debate about the validity and reliability of these categories, however the medical tradition has preferred a categorical approach.

Table A 14.1 Definition and general criteria for diagnosing personality disorder according to DSM-IV-TR

"An enduring pattern of inner experience and behaviour that deviates markedly from the expectations of the culture of the individual who exhibits it". This pattern is manifest in two or more of the following areas;

- ◆ Cognition; ways of perception and interpretation of the self, others and events
- ◆ Affect; the range, intensity, lability and appropriateness of feelings and emotional responses
- ◆ Interpersonal functioning; the style of relating to others
- ◆ Impulse control

The following general criteria also need to be met in addition to the specific criteria which are listed for each of the 10 personality disorders recognized in DSM-IV-TR. The pattern;

- ◆ Is inflexible and pervasive across a broad range of social and personal situations.
- ◆ Leads to clinically significant distress or impairment in social, occupational or other important areas of functioning
- ◆ Is stable and of long duration and its onset can be traced back at least to adolescence or early adulthood
- ◆ Is not better accounted for as a manifestation or consequence of another mental disorder
- ◆ Is not due to the direct physiological effects of a substance or a general medical condition, such as the neurological sequelae of a head injury

---

Chapter 15

Cognitive approaches to working with mentally disordered offenders

Derek Perkins

Aim

This chapter describes cognitive approaches to the treatment and management of Mentally Disordered Offenders (MDOs).

Learning objectives

- To understand the history of the development of Cognitive Behavioural Therapy (CBT) in the United Kingdom prison and forensic mental health services
- To describe some of the theoretical and practical considerations relating to the cognitive treatment of MDOs, especially those with personality disorder

---

Introduction

The application of cognitive-based therapies to the treatment of MDOs has developed differently within the forensic mental health system compared to the prison system. In both systems, attitudes to and conceptualizations of offending and the treatment of mental disorder have meant that interest in the application of cognitively based psychotherapies, as for other modalities of psychotherapy, has been cyclical. This chapter describes the development of cognitive approaches to working with offenders in the prison system and MDOs in the forensic mental health system. The chapter then describes the application of CBT and its derivatives to offenders who have a diagnosis of personality disorder.

Although the personality disordered group is differentiated in the forensic mental health literature, the tradition in the prison literature has been to apply cognitive interventions to offenders based either on their criminogenic profile (e.g. sex offender) or on their offender status, as opposed to their psychiatric diagnosis. Although, based on the high rates of personality disorder in prisoners, many of these offenders will have a personality disorder (Fazel and Danesh 2002; Singleton et al 1998), the offender literature does not often describe them in these terms. The chapter concludes with a description of an integrated programme available to MDOs in high security. It illustrates the fact that psychological treatment programmes need to combine interventions from different modalities in a sequenced way across the care pathway to optimize patient motivation and to allow patients to build on their therapeutic work.

CBT and its derivatives: a brief background

Cognitive-behavioural therapy emerged from the learning theory literature of the post-war period of the last century through the observation that maladaptive patterns of behaviours and their related thoughts and emotions can be relearnt and reinforced. Although there are many varieties of CBT, a common principle is the degree to which cognitive and behavioural change are the focus of treatment. The approach is based on a collaboration between the therapist and client (patient, offender etc) in developing an understanding of how maladaptive behaviours are maintained by both their triggering events, either within the environment or internal to the individual, and by their effects (positive or negative) on the individual within specific settings. Through a shared analysis of these antecedents and consequences of maladaptive behaviours, strategies are developed to help the individual embark on a process of understanding and change through challenging dysfunctional beliefs and thoughts, and relearning, so that previous dysfunctional behaviours become functional.

Early approaches focused on observable behaviours, such as phobic avoidance, angry violence, and counter-productive social behaviours, and aimed to help the individual learn alternative behavioural responses through techniques including gradual exposure to feared situations so as to counteract anxiety and avoidance of feared situations; aversion therapy, to counteract pleasurable but illegal impulses; and social skills training to improve forming and maintaining relationships.

The cognitive-behavioural and cognitive therapies that followed these behavioural approaches focused on helping a person make connections between their thoughts, feelings and behaviour, and specifically the interactions between the individual's maladaptive behaviours and their related thought processes. Many of these thoughts or cognitions are 'loaded' with emotions such as fear, anger, and dejection; for example: 'I will never overcome my fears'; 'everyone is picking on me'; 'I deserve to have whatever I want'. The individual attempts to cope with these negative thoughts by repeating a cycle of maladaptive responses such as avoidance, violence, social isolation.

Using CBT techniques it became apparent that many of the dysfunctional thought processes occurred automatically and were linked to underlying 'schemas'; ways of seeing the world that relate to early life experiences, including early attachment and trauma experiences. Consequently, modifying maladaptive patterns of behaviour, thinking and feelings required interventions that helped the individual understand and resolve the connections between early life experiences and related schemas. As these schemas are not typically held within conscious experience, innovative therapies such as work involving 'life maps', 'learning from the past', 'role playing' and 'dramatherapy' were needed to access them and help the individual reappraise and modify unhelpful core beliefs that underpin the maladaptive behaviours, thoughts and feelings.

CBT has been used to treat Axis I disorders, such as psychosis (see Chapter 13) as well as Axis II personality disorders (American Psychiatric Association 2000). The aim of CBT for personality disorder is to identify and modify core beliefs and associated overdeveloped behavioural patterns that are maladaptive and interfere with healthy functioning (Davidson 2000). As difficulties are long-standing, treating personality disorder with CBT requires a prolonged course of treatment (over a year), as opposed to the shorter treatment courses that can be used for the treatment of psychosis.

A number of variations of CBT have been developed over recent years to address particular problems and needs. One of the strongest evidence bases is for Dialectical Behaviour Therapy (DBT) (Brazier et al 2006; Linehan 1993), a manualized, derived cognitive behavioural treatment, originally designed for women with borderline personality disorder (BPD) who self-harmed, but which has since been applied to other populations (Linehan et al 1991, 1994). Linehan postulated that the principles of traditional CBT alone, which are effective in changing problematic behaviours, would be insufficient to effect change in individuals with BPD, as CBT's continuous focus on change would be destabilizing for people with affective instability, poor impulse control and limited problem-solving skills. To balance the emphasis on change, Linehan combined elements of

Zen practices of mindfulness and acceptance with CBT approaches. The tensions between the CBT principles of change and those of Zen practice are held together and integrated within the framework of dialectic philosophy, which allows for the synthesizing of oppositions (Heard et al 2005).

DBT is multi-modal and delivered both in individual sessions, which target motivational issues, and in groups, which attend to skills training. Core strategies in sessions comprise problem solving and validation with attention to processes, conflicts and behaviours (such as self-destructive acts) that impede therapeutic progress. Five stages of treatment are described: pre-treatment, achieving behavioural control, emotionally processing the past, resolving ordinary problems in living and capacity to experience sustained joy. However, service users are unlikely to obtain treatment in the last two stages in most generic health care settings (National Institute for Health and Clinical Excellence [NICE] 2008b).

Research in DBT has focused on stage one, achieving behavioural control, which aims to help the individual develop and sustain motivation for treatment while reducing suicidal behaviours, non-suicidal self-injury and other impulsive behaviours, for example, substance misuse, binge eating (NICE 2008b). Research conducted to date suggests that complex interventions, such as DBT and the psychodynamically derived mentalization-based treatment (MBT), may benefit people with borderline personality disorder. However, trials conducted to date have been small, have often excluded men and have generally examined interventions delivered in centres of excellence. Randomized controlled trials in non-forensic patients have shown a decrease in the frequency and intensity of parasuicidal behaviour, fewer psychiatric inpatient days and higher global and social functioning in the DBT-treated group (Linehan 1993; Linehan et al 1991, 1994). The application of DBT in offender and forensic populations is reviewed below.

Schema-focused therapy is another variant of CBT which, like other CBT-based therapies, has integrated a number of ideas and techniques from other theoretical models. Research by Young (Young and Flannagan 1998; Young and Glukoski 1996) indicated that many intractable psychological problems are mediated through 'early maladaptive schema', that is, ways in which individuals regard themselves and their relationships, which result in stable patterns of dysfunctional thinking and behaviour. These maladapative schemas are thought to develop during childhood when the child begins to internalize, for example, punitive, critical or self-justifying comments of parents into their own beliefs and perceptions. Schemas relate closely to notions of personality functioning, in that the stable traits of interpersonal functioning are seen to be underpinned by the person's underlying schema. The person may not be consciously aware that this is the case, and schema-focused therapy was developed by Young and others to help individuals gain insight into their schemas, understand the connections between schemas and typical modes of behaving and relating to others and to take steps towards more functional behaviour.

Schemas identified within this approach have been seen to fall into five general categories: 'disconnection and rejection' (schemas of abandonment, mistrust, defensiveness); 'impaired autonomy and performance' (schemas of failure, dependence, vulnerability); 'impaired limits' (schemas of low-frustration threshold, overindulgence, low self-control); 'other directedness' (schemas of approval-seeking, self-sacrifice, subjugation); and 'over-vigilance and inhibition' (schemas of emotional inhibition, unrelenting standards, punitiveness). A range of intervention strategies for working with maladaptive schemas have been developed (Young et al 2003), and these have been used in both prison treatment programmes and in forensic mental health services.

Cognitive programmes in the prison service

Use of psychological therapies in the prison service has fluctuated over time. Optimism that interventions, ranging from occupational and educational to individual and group psychotherapy, could help offenders lead better lives after release gave way in the 1970s and 1980s to a therapeutic pessimism that 'nothing works' (Martinson 1974). For a time the formal ethos of the prison service was limited to 'humane containment'; there was no formally recognized expectation that imprisonment could do anything other than serve as a deterrent, keep offenders out of society for a while and mark society's disapproval of their offences. Psychologists who had previously been involved in individual and group therapies, albeit not coordinated in a comprehensive or consistent way, were deployed onto other tasks, such as research, staff training and management consultancy, although some therapeutic work did continue in pockets during this period.

During the 1980s, however, evidence from a range of treatment evaluation studies suggested that some types of interventions might work for some offenders to some degree, even though effect sizes were small (Blackburn 1980; Gendreau and Ross 1987). There was also interest in whether even modest changes in offending could be cost-effective in terms of societal harm and the economics of the criminal justice system, as well as providing a means to enhance staff motivation and job satisfaction. The prison service set up a central 'Behaviour Modification Committee' that oversaw and sponsored the development of behavioural and cognitive-behavioural therapies in a number of prisons. A combination of this resurgence of interest in and evidence for the effectiveness of some psychological interventions, along with some high-profile cases of sexual and violent re-offending, brought about a reappraisal of the role of psychological therapy in the Prison Service. In 1990, the then Home Secretary set the direction for national treatment programmes for violent and sexual offending, to be followed later by a wide range of other treatment programmes. A central advisory panel with international experts was set up to steer these developments. This was later superseded by the Joint Accreditation Panel and then the Correctional Services Accreditation Panel (CSAP).

Much of the early emphasis in the prison treatment programmes was to (1) design treatment interventions that targeted empirically derived risk factors associated with serious offending behaviour (criminogenic factors); (2) utilize evidence from the international literature on 'what works' in treating offending behaviour; which was at that stage primarily cognitive-behavioural approaches and (3) utilize group programmes that could be 'manualized' and delivered by a range of staff with limited training, with the aim of providing an appropriate service to as many high-risk offenders as possible, that is, maximizing the cost-effectiveness of the interventions. This led some critics to highlight the lack of individualization in the programmes. However, given the limited resources available, compared with forensic mental health services, programmes were successfully developed. Each programme had a built-in accreditation and evaluation component (see Text Box 15.1) to demonstrate to the prison service that the investments were justified by the outcomes. The UK Offending Behaviour Programmes (see Text Box 15.2) became some of the largest and most systematic in the world, providing large samples for evaluative research that have demonstrated their positive effects on reducing re-offending (Friendship et al 2002; Lipton et al 2002).

Cognitive programmes in forensic mental health

Over the last century, the treatment of MDOs in forensic mental health services has predominantly taken place in high secure hospitals (previously known as the special hospitals). A medium secure level of service was developed as a result of the Butler Committee (Butler Committee 1975) to bridge the gap in managing risk that existed between high security and ordinary psychiatry provision. Delivery of psychological interventions in the high secure hospitals began in the 1960s through small numbers of psychotherapists, generally from a psychoanalytic tradition, and psychologists, generally from a behavioural tradition, the latter initially being employed to provide

Box 15.1 Accreditation criteria for CBT used in the criminal justice system by CSAP

- A clear model of change
- Selection of offenders
- Targeting a range of dynamic risk factors
- Effective methods
- Skills oriented
- Sequencing, intensity and duration
- Engagement and motivation
- Continuity of programmes and services
- Maintaining integrity
- Ongoing evaluation

Box 15.2 CBT-orientated programmes offered by the offending behaviour programme unit

Enhanced Thinking Skills (ETS) is a relatively short programme that addresses the thinking and behaviour associated with offending. It includes impulse control, flexible thinking, social perspective taking, values and moral reasoning, reasoning and interpersonal problem solving.

Cognitive Skills Booster Programme is run by both the Prison and Probation Service and is designed to reinforce learning from general offending programmes (such as ETS) through skills rehearsal and relapse prevention.

Controlling Anger and Learning to Manage It (CALM) is a course for offending associated with poor emotional control. It aims to enable participants to reduce the intensity, frequency and duration of negative emotions such as anger, anxiety and jealousy, which are associated with their offending.

Cognitive Self Change Programme (CSCP) targets high-risk violent offenders and includes group and individual sessions. It equips prisoners with skills to help them control their violence and avoid reconviction. It is aimed at offenders with a history of violent behaviour and is suitable for those whose violence is either reactive or instrumental.

Sex Offender Treatment Programmes (SOTP) is a range of group programmes available for sexual offenders. A menu of options is offered according to the level of risk and need of the offender.

Chromis is an intensive programme that aims to reduce violence in high-risk offenders whose psychopathic traits disrupt their ability to accept treatment and change. It provides participants with the skills to reduce and manage their risk of reoffending (see Chapter 16).

an assessment and research service. Over time, the level of these provisions increased and, as in the prison service, there was a rapid growth in the 1980s and 1990s in behavioural and cognitive-behavioural treatments to complement the psychodynamic therapies provided by the psychotherapists.

Whereas the prison service developed its treatment programmes from a central unit focused on (1) driving treatments from evidence of criminogenic needs and known risk factors for re-offending and (2) maximizing the cost-effective use of staff resources to meet the needs of the maximum numbers of offenders, the approach of forensic mental health services was characterized by focusing on the specific needs of the individual patient. These services had less clearly coordinated pathways of treatment for their detained patients. Treatments were sometimes not sequenced logically or delivered in a timely way. Group interventions were often set up on an ad hoc basis with little possibility of coordinating these intervention with the most appropriate patients at the optimum time in their care pathway. It was not until the 1990s that systematic group work provision began to be developed through aggregating patients' needs into themed groups informed by a range of theoretical underpinnings (psychodynamic, cognitive-behavioural, systemic) and styles of delivery (discussion, practical exercises, roleplay and the use of arts, music and drama therapies).

Over the last few years, both prison and mental health services have learned from each other's strengths, and prison programmes now typically integrate life history material and individualized approaches with their group work programmes. Equally, forensic mental health services have developed more themed and integrated group work services to complement individual therapies in addressing patients' needs for 'therapeutic engagement', 'mental health restoration' and 'risk reduction'. Within forensic mental health services, a wide range of other group-based and individual psychological therapies are now provided; however, more trained therapists are needed if patients are to receive adequate and sustained psychological treatment. Many CBT interventions are delivered in group format to capitalize on the benefits of shared experience, group support and sometimes group challenge, but most of these groups will be complemented by a wide range of other individual and group-based psychological interventions. Assessing motivation and readiness for treatment are key issues that are managed through the multidisciplinary team and through close collaboration with patients.

An MDO within forensic mental health services will typically take part in a series of individual and group work CBT interventions covering such themes as ETS; reasoning and rehabilitation (R&R); understanding mental illness and/or personality disorder; interventions aimed at reducing specific symptoms of mental illness and personality disorder and, usually in the latter stage of the care pathway, interventions to reduce risk and offending behaviour, such as violence, sex offending, substance misuse and fire setting.

Typically, sessions are structured around agreed therapeutic goals, for example, to become more comfortable in social situations or to reduce the risk of violent offending. Analysis of typical patterns of behaviour and related thoughts and feelings complements a detailed history of how problems have developed. Interviews, questionnaires, collateral information, roleplays and other practical exercises are used to explore patients' repertoire of functional and dysfunctional behaviour. Functional analysis of problem behaviours forms a focus for understanding and working on the factors that maintain the dysfunctional behaviour, as well as helping look for new ways of behaving and relating. Diaries of current behaviour, thoughts and feelings are used to encourage patients to both try out new ways of thinking and relating to others and to monitor the feedback they receive.

The effective delivery of the prison service programmes required that there were a number of exclusion criteria; consequently, offenders with mental health problems, including those with personality disorder, were either excluded or were unable to integrate successfully into the programmes' structures. Prisoners who have 'failed' prison treatment programmes, because of mental health issues, frequently become involved in forensic mental health treatment programmes that are more flexible in their application and responsive to these mental health issues. A sense of having 'failed' previous therapies can be an important barrier for patients to overcome in remaining motivated, and forensic mental health therapies often combine individual and group therapies in ways that are not feasible in the prison service. Quayle (Quayle and Moore 2006) noted the relevance of patients' experiences of abuse and trauma that are often linked to personality disorder and require complex combinations of therapy interventions. Within the Broadmoor Centralized Group Work Service, most patients undertake individual and group therapies in parallel. An analysis of patients' needs at Broadmoor Hospital carried out by Dr Emily Glorney and colleagues (to be published shortly) highlights the need for psychological interventions in three broad areas: engagement and motivation; mental health restoration and risk reduction/criminogenic need.

Evaluation and meta-analysis of treatment outcomes for both offenders and MDOs have found that interventions that address specific needs rather than generic causes of offending demonstrated positive and promising results and that cognitive-behavioural, skill-orientated and multi-modal programmes provide the most promising results (McGuire 1995, 2000).

Within secure forensic mental health services the secure psychological services network has developed a number of principles that underpin the delivery of psychological interventions:

1. *Responsivity*: Users of secure services should have access to psychological interventions that are appropriate to and address the needs and problems that contributed to their admission. These should be delivered in a manner that is meaningful to the individual and appropriate to his or her learning style and profile of strengths and difficulties.

2. *Treatment pathways*: Psychological interventions should be provided on the basis of a timely and logically sequenced assessment of patients' needs and capacities. The pathway starts with supportive and motivational work to facilitate engagement, including socialization into a therapeutic culture in which active participation in treatment is expected, followed by work on different areas of need through more focused and potentially challenging interventions. The aim is to help patients move to the lowest appropriate level of security and support this transition through further work that includes their involvement and engagement in their care pathway. Progress is not linear and opportunities should be available for revisiting and refreshing previous work as necessary.

3. *Assessment and treatment approaches*: Psychological interventions should be based on careful assessment of patients' needs and capacities and, as far as possible, should be evidence-based. Where good-quality evidence exists for a particular intervention, the therapy should be faithful to this model. It is recognized that the effectiveness of most 'evidence-based' treatments has been demonstrated with different populations from those in secure mental health services. The delivery of these interventions should therefore be flexible and responsive to service users' individual circumstances. All developments, innovations and adaptations should be based on sound psychological theory and knowledge and allow for the emergence of practice-based evidence.

4. *Treatment effectiveness*: The effectiveness of psychological interventions should be evaluated by a range of measures, including self-reports, relevant observer reports, behavioural observations, psychometric data and other specialized assessments as required. Evaluations should be carried out involving individual service users, therapeutic programmes, groups and ward communities, so that practice can improve on the basis of evidence of clinical effectiveness

and risk reduction. The most rigorous evaluation methods, notably randomized controlled trials, should be incorporated wherever possible into psychological therapy evaluations with research collaboration between clinicians and researchers and in line with Research and Development systems and ethics procedures.

5. *Holistic approach*: Psychological understanding of service users' needs, difficulties and behaviour is integral to both effective therapeutic work and risk management throughout the whole care pathway. Much of the therapeutic work that is essential to users' progress takes place in the day-to-day environment of the ward, outside structured individual and group treatment sessions. Psychological interventions designed to support a therapeutic ward milieu include the following:

   a. Staff consultation, reflective practice, structured discussion and formal training to increase teams' understanding of the emotional and behavioural challenges that service users present as well as face during their day-to-day life on the ward.

   b. Community meetings that enhance service users' ability to manage their social and interpersonal environment.

   c. Supervision and support for nursing staff to reinforce and facilitate service users' generalization of specific skills learned in psychological therapy sessions.

   d. Structured sessions for both ward staff and service users to address specific needs of the ward community, for example, in relation to bullying and harassment.

   e. Integration of all psychological interventions into services users' care plans.

   f. Consideration of the impact and management of change with respect to service users, staff and ward communities.

6. *Supporting psychological therapies*: Effective psychological interventions require systems for selection, training and supervision of therapy staff, as well as planning and reviewing the delivery of the therapy. Attention needs to be paid to the resource balance between training, supervision and delivery. Effective therapy requires full and active coordination between therapy providers and multidisciplinary clinical teams. The needs and skill mix of staff involved in psychological therapies should be planned and coordinated to make the most effective and cost-effective use of multidisciplinary resources. All staff who work closely with patients, irrespective of whether they are delivering formal psychotherapy, need to attend regular supervision and reflective practice groups.

CBT and DBT for MDOs with personality disorder

Most patients in forensic psychiatric services display features of personality disorder (Blackburn et al 1990, 2003), even though they may have been legally detained under the old Mental Health Act category of mental illness (HMSO 1983), and will continue to be detained under the broader category of mental disorder (HMSO 2007). Livesley (Livesley and Jang 2000) suggested that interventions for those displaying the core features of personality disorder, such as impulsivity, empathy deficits, egocentricity (which apply to most of these patients and are also implicated as risk factors in offending behaviours) need to deal with the patients' core beliefs that others will be hostile towards them, for example, 'It's better to attack others before they attack me'. It is suggested that empathic interventions that seek to create and maintain a consistent therapeutic process and collaborative treatment alliance are needed to create self-validating styles of thinking, the promotion of autonomy, the building of new skills and competencies and the maintenance of motivation to change. This is consistent with Prochaska's (Prochaska et al 1992) 'stages of change' model, with its emphasis on providing interventions relevant to the stage of change which the individual has reached.

Livesley suggested a four-stage therapeutic process for treating personality disorder, namely (1) problem recognition, in which the therapist creates a safe atmosphere for the individual to begin exploring how personality problems affect other aspects of his or her life; (2) exploration, in which the individual is helped to recognize connections between different aspects of thinking, feeling and behaviour, to reframe negative thoughts more adaptively and to observe and monitor his or her behaviour; (3) acquisition of alternative behaviours, through a process of developing new skills and inhibiting maladaptive patterns of behaviour and (4) consolidation and generalization, through the application of new skills to everyday behaviours. Livesley and Jang emphasize that the goal of treatment is to enhance the patient's adaptation by building competence. (Livesley and Jang 2000). Livesely's approach acknowledges that there are different 'brands' of CBT that contribute to the treatment of personality disorders. Preliminary findings suggest that both CBT and DBT show promise (Bateman and Tyrer 2004).

It has been proposed that DBT is well-suited to the treatment of aggression and poor impulse control (Evershed et al 2003) and therefore should benefit patients in forensic settings (Berzins et al 2004). To date, DBT studies in MDO populations have been small, have excluded men and are in need of more robust methodological design. Studies report a reduction in self-harm and a general improvement in borderline symptoms in women in both forensic mental health settings (Low et al 2001) and female juvenile offenders (Trupin et al 2002). Nee and Farman's review paper (Nee and Farman 2005) examined five pilot studies of DBT in women with BPD in three British prisons. As the sample size was small and the attrition rate high, with only 16 of the 30 women enrolled in the 5 pilots completing their therapy, the results must be interpreted with caution. The authors report improvements in the women's impulsivity, self-esteem, levels of dissociation and self-harm during the therapy. Although there was a slight increase in the rate of self-harm on discontinuation, this did not return to its pre-treatment level.

The development and application of CBT for offenders with psychopathy, as measured by the Psychopathy Checklist-Revised (Hare 1991, 2003), Antisocial Personality Disorder (ASPD) or who meet the criteria for Dangerous and Severe Personality Disorder (DSPD) is described in the following chapter (Chapter 16). CBT for individuals with ASPD focuses on developing and strengthening adaptive behavioural strategies aimed at improving interpersonal relationships and managing conflict by promoting perspective-taking. Negative thoughts about others such as 'I must get them before they get me' are loosened as they underpin low self-esteem. MDOs with ASPD tend to interpret interpersonal situations as being more threatening than they are in reality. As these individuals often cannot tolerate ambiguity, they tend to rapidly attribute negative intentions to the motivations and actions of others and react accordingly with impulsive and aggressive behaviour. Cognitive techniques such as learning to 'stop and think' before acting can help these individuals tolerate uncertainty, as long as they are able to acquire some capacity for perspective-taking (Cordess et al 2005). Recent guidelines recommend that cognitively based interventions such as R&R and ETS groups, which focus on reducing offending and other antisocial behaviour, should be offered to MDOs with ASPD (NICE 2008a).

Modes of delivery: an integrated approach

Delivering a psychological treatment programme requires an integrated approach at a range of levels, such as mode of delivery, the provision of groups with differing theoretical underpinnings and the integration of groups that address mental health and criminogenic need across the MDO care pathway. There is now a comparable set of individual and group treatment programmes running across the high secure psychiatric services. Individual and group-based CBT programmes run alongside therapies using different models and modalities, although the CBT stream is the most common approach. Broadmoor High Secure Hospital (like its sister hospitals) runs an integrated group work programme described by Perkins (Perkins et al 2007). The range and description of the groups available is shown in Text Box 15.3.

Box 15.3 Range and description of groups provided by the group work programme at Broadmoor high secure hospital

Groups to promote mental health

Aims: To reduce distress, disablement, reliance on medication and promote emotion regulation, relationship maintenance skills, self-esteem

Short courses or training sessions:

Understanding Mental Illness (UMI): A psycho-educational group providing information about a range of diagnoses

Understanding Personality Disorder (UPD): A module informed by the cognitive model to assist participants in understanding the personal, clinical-diagnostic, legal and developmental aspects of the diagnosis

Semi-structured modular group sessions:

Dialectical Behaviour Therapy (DBT): Offered in conjunction with individual sessions, this integrative cognitive approach targets serious self-harm and self-sabotaging behaviour

*Mentalization-Based Therapy (MBT): Aims to develop mentalization, namely the capacity to understand one's own and others' mental states, via group dialogue; MBT promotes empathy, agency and perspective-taking

Cognitive-Behavioural Therapy (CBT) for psychosis: A group for patients with a diagnosis of schizophrenia which targets symptomatic and emotional recovery via coping and relapse-prevention skills

Anger management: Explores cognitive, physiological and behavioural domains of anger, promotes problem-solving and assertiveness skills as alternatives to aggression

Substance misuse: Helps participants develop the ability to name and monitor feelings via group dialogue. It also promotes empathy, agency and perspective-taking

Long-term, slow-open group therapy:

Family awareness: Provides participants with an opportunity to think about their early relationships and experiences and how these might impact on their current interpersonal relationships and their choices in the here-and-now

Stigma and discrimination: A psycho-educational and supportive group for any patient in high security. The group provides an opportunity to discuss the impact of social exclusion with peers who have had similar experiences

Groups to reduce offending

Aims: To reduce risk, to target offence related thinking, to reduce impulsivity and promote problem-solving, perspective-taking, moral reasoning and awareness

Short courses or training sessions:

Enhanced Thinking Skills (ETS): A cognitive skills course designed to reduce pro-criminal thinking styles

Reasoning and Rehabilitation (R&R): A cognitive-behavioural programme used to teach social and cognitive skills to offenders

> **Box 15.3** *(Continued)* **Range and description of groups provided by the group work programme at Broadmoor high secure hospital**
>
> **Long-term, slow-open group therapy:**
> *Homicide group: A group run on psychodynamic lines for men who have killed a family member or partner to allow them to think about, understand and process their offence
> **Semi-structured, closed group work (9–18 months):**
> Violent offenders group (VOG): A group offered to men with several convictions for interpersonal violence and those who have committed 'one-off' fatal attacks on others. The group aims to eliminate violent and abusive behaviour
> **Sex offenders group (SOG):** Using a cognitive-behavioural focus this group targets antecedents to sex offending, relationship skills, fantasies and deviant arousal and risk reduction via a relapse-prevention model
> **Fire-setting:** A group for patients with a history of arson which aims to increase awareness of the danger of fire
>
> *Denotes groups whose theoretical underpinning and modus operandi is psychodynamic.

A combination of both individual and group psychotherapy is offered according to need. Some forms of CBT are provided by both groups and individual therapy, for example, schema-focused therapy and DBT to address mental health needs and violence reduction and sex offending reduction work to address criminogenic need. Many patients have reservations about entering group therapy programmes for a variety of reasons; previous experiences of being let down, lack of trust, low self-esteem and shame about their discussing their offending behaviour in front of others. Consequently, many individuals will require preparatory work before entering into group work related to mental health restoration or risk reduction. This can be achieved either through individual work in which trust and understanding of the need for other therapies is built up, or through groups that are more educational in nature, such as understanding mental illness or understanding personality disorder, or are aimed at strengthening generic thinking and problem-solving skills (ETS and R&R).

The current programme, as developed by Dr Estelle Moore and her colleagues at Broadmoor Hospital (see Perkins et al 2007), is illustrated in Table 15.1. Following work on motivation and readiness for group work, patients generally progress from the generic groups (ETS and R&R) and psycho-educational groups to groups that target mental health restoration for mental illness and personality disorder, as well as groups for a range of 'risk reduction' themes, namely violence, homicide, sex offending and fire setting.

Conclusion

Cognitive-behavioural therapy for MDOs has developed over time to embrace the complex interactions between patients' thoughts, feelings and behaviours and to link early life experiences, including attachment and trauma experiences (previously a focus of psychodynamic therapies but neglected by CBT therapies) to issues of mental health and offending behaviour. CBT and its variations such as DBT and schema-focused therapy are a key part of patients' therapy within forensic mental health services, in terms of engagement and motivation, mental health restoration and risk reduction. Pathways of treatment are becoming more sophisticated to enable interventions to be sequenced in a logical and timely way that both engages and motivates patients and

Table 15.1 Options for group work provided by the Broadmoor Centralized Group Work Service as part of the clinical pathway for treatment in high security (Perkins et al 2007)

Therapeutic engagement: early stages. Emphasis on psycho-education and enhancing coping skills	Active treatment phase		Consolidation and rehearsal of relapse prevention skills and preparation for leaving high security
	Mental health restoration	Specific risk reduction: targeting offending behaviour	
Introduction to groups: Why do group work?	*Family awareness (open group)*	Fire-Setting (6–12 months)	*Art and drama therapy (post-offence group) (open; reviewed regularly)
Understanding mental illness (15–20 sessions)	*CBT for psychosis (12 months)*	Violent offenders group (12–18 months)	Stigma and discrimination (open; reviewed by patients as to usefulness)
Understanding personality disorder (20 sessions)	*Dialectical behavioural therapy (12 months plus option to review)*	*Homicide group (open; reviewed annually)	**Leavers' group (open; available to all)**
Enhanced thinking skills (20–25 sessions)	*Mentalization-based therapy (12–18 Months)*	Sexual offenders group (12–18 months)	Substance misuse (12–18 months)
Reasoning and Rehabilitation (16 sessions)	Anger management (9–12 months)		Relapse prevention workshops and psychodrama (currently in planning)

* Denotes groups whose theoretical underpinning and modus operandi is either psychodynamic or integrated.

Italicized text denotes groups primarily aimed at promoting mental health restoration.

Normal text denotes groups primarily targeting criminogenic need and risk reduction.

builds sequentially on the therapeutic work. Groups with different theoretical underpinnings are now being integrated into CBT-based group work programmes. Pathways may need to be varied for particular patients; some patients may require individual motivational work prior to group work; others may prefer and be suitable for introductory group work before individual therapy; some types of CBT, such as DBT, are offered using both group and individual sessions together. Evidence to date suggests cautious optimism that combinations of individual and group-based CBT programmes operated within a well-supervised and supported therapeutic regime can be helpful to most forensic patients.

Key points

- Attitudes to and conceptualizations of offending and the treatment of mental disorder have meant that CBT has developed differently in the UK prison and forensic mental health services
- Integrated programmes are now being developed that address the four main areas of need: therapeutic engagement, mental health restoration, criminogenic need and risk reduction and relapse prevention
- There is a growing evidence base for CBT and in particular for its derivative therapy DBT. However, better methodological studies are needed in MDO populations

References

American Psychiatric Association. Diagnostic and Statistical Manual of Mental Disorders 2000 4th Edition Text Revision (DSM-IV-TR). Washington DC: American Psychiatric Association.

Bateman, A. W. and Tyrer, P. 2004 Psychological Treatment for Personality Disorders. Advances in Psychiatric Treatment 10: 378–388.

Berzins, L.G. and Trestman, R.L. 2004 The Development and Implementation of Dialectical Behavior Therapy in Forensic Settings. International Journal of Forensic Mental Health 3: 93–103.

Blackburn, R. 1980 Still not Working? A Look at Recent Outcomes in Offender Rehabilitation. Paper Presented at the Scottish Branch of the British Psychological Society's conference on Deviance, University of Stirling.

Blackburn, R., Clare Crellin, M., Morgan, E.M. and Tulloch, R.M.B. 1990 Prevalence of Personality Disorders in a Special Hospital Population. Journal of Forensic Psychiatry 1: 43–52.

Blackburn, R., Logan, C., Donnelly, J. and Renwick, S. 2003 Personality disorders, psychopathy and other mental disorders: co-morbidity among patients at English and Scottish high-security hospitals. The Journal of Forensic Psychiatry and Psychology 14: 111–137.

Brazier, J., Tumur, I., Holmes, M. et al 2006 Psychological Therapies Including Dialectical Behaviour Therapy for Borderline Personality Disorder: A Systematic Review and Preliminary Economic Evaluation. Health Technology Assessment 10: 117.

Butler Committee. 1975 The Butler Committee on Mentally Abnormal Offenders. Cmnd 6244. London: HMSO.

Cordess, C., Davidson, K., Morris, M. and Norton, K. 2005. Cluster B antisocial Personality Disorders 269–278 in Oxford Textbook of Psychotherapy (Holmes, J., Beck, J. and Gabbard, G. Editors) Oxford: Oxford University Press.

Davidson, K.M. 2000 Cognitive Therapy for Personality Disorders: A Guide for Clinicians. London: Arnold Hodder.

Evershed, S., Tennant, A., Boomer, D., Rees, A., Barkham, M. and Watsons, A. 2003 Practice-based Outcomes of Dialectical Behaviour Therapy DBT Targeting Anger and Violence, with Male Forensic Patients: A Pragmatic and Non-contemporaneous Comparison. Criminal Behaviour and Mental Health 13: 198–213.

Fazel, S. and Danesh, J. 2002 Serious mental disorder in 23000 prisoners: a systematic review of 62 surveys. Lancet 359: 545–550.

Friendship, C., Blud, L., Eriksson, M. and Travers, R. 2002 An evaluation of cognitive-behavioural treatment for prisoners. Findings 161. London: Home Office.

Gendreau, P. and Ross, R.R. 1987 Revivication of rehabilitation. Evidence from the 1980s. Justice Quarterly 4: 349–407.

Hare, R.D. 1991 The Hare Psychopathy Checklist-Revised. Toronto, Ontario: Multi-Health Systems.

Hare, R.D. 2003 Manual for the Hare Psychopathy Checklist–Revised 2nd Edition. Toronto, Ontario: Multi-Health Systems.

Heard, H.L., Linehan, M.M., Norcross, J.C. and Goldfried, M.R. 2005 Integrative therapy for borderline personality disorder 299–320 in Handbook of Psychotherapy Integration (Norcross, J.C. and Goldfried, M.R. Editiors). London: Oxford University Press .

HMSO. 1983 Mental Health Act 1983, HMSO, London, c12.

HMSO. 2007 Mental Health Act 2007, HMSO, London, c12.

Linehan, M. 1993 Cognitive-behavioural Treatment of Borderline Personality Disorder. Washington DC: Guilford Press.

Linehan, M. M., Armstrong, H.E., Suarez, A., Allmon, D., and Heard, H.L. 1991 Cognitive-behavioral Treatment of Chronically Parasuicidal Borderline Patients. Archives of General Psychiatry 48: 1060–1064.

Linehan, M.M., Tutek, D.A., Heard, H.L. and Armstrong, H.E. 1994 Interpersonal Outcome of Cognitive Behavioral Treatment for Chronically Suicidal Borderline Patients. The American Journal of Psychiatry 151: 1771–1776.

Lipton, D.S., Pearson, F.S., Cleland, C.M. and Yee, D. 2002 The effectiveness of cognitive-behavioural treatment methods on offender recidivisim 75–112 in Offender Rehabilitation and Treatment: Effective Programmes to Reduce Re-Offending (McGuire, J. Editor) Chichester: Wiley.

Livesley, W.J. and Jang, K.L. 2000 Toward an empirically based classification of personality disorder. J Personal Disord 14: 137–151.

Low, G., Jones, D., Duggan, C., Power, M. and Macleod, A. 2001 The Treatment of Deliberate Self-harm in Borderline Personality Disorder Using Dialectical Behaviour Therapy: A Pilot Study in a High Security Hospital. Behavioural and Cognitive Psychotherapy 29: 85–92.

Martinson, R. 1974 What Works? Questions and Answers about Prison Reform. The Public Interest 35: 22–54.

McGuire, J. 1995 Reviewing What Works: Reducing Re-offending: Guidelines from Research and Practice. Chichester: Wiley.

McGuire, J. (Editor) 2000 Offender Rehabilitation and Treatment: Effective Programmes and Policies to Reduce Offending. Chichester: Wiley.

National Institute for Health and Clinical Excellence (NICE) 2008a Antisocial Personality Disorder: Treatment, Management and Prevention. National Clinical Practice Guideline. National Collaborating Centre for Mental Health, Commissioned by the National Institute for Health and Clinical Excellence. Full Guideline Draft.

National Institute for Health and Clinical Excellence (NICE) 2008b Borderline Personality Disorder: Treatment and Management. National Clinical Practice Guideline. National Collaborating Centre for Mental Health, Commissioned by the National Institute for Health and Clinical Excellence. Full Guideline Draft.

Nee, C. and Farman, S. 2005 Female prisoners with borderline personality disorder: some promising treatment developments. Criminal Behaviour and Mental Health 15: 2–16.

Perkins, D.E., Moore, E. and Dudley, A. 2007 Developing a Centralised Group Work Service at Broadmoor Hospital. Mental Health Review – Brighton 12: 16–20.

Prochaska, J.O., DiClemente, C.C., and Norcross, J.C. 1992 In search of how people change. Applications to addictive behaviors. American Psychologist 47: 1102–1114.

Quayle, M. and Moore, E. 2006. Maladaptive Learning: Cognitive-behavioural Treatment and Beyond 134–145 in Personality Disorder and Serious Offending. Hospital Treatment Models (Newrith, C., Meux, C. and Taylor, P.J. Editors) London: Hodder Arnold.

Singleton, N., Meltzer, H., Gatward, R., Coid, J. and Deasy, D. 1998 Office of National Statistics Survey of Psychiatric Morbidity among Prisoners in England and Wales Stationery Office. London

Trupin, E.W., Stewart, D.G., Beach, B. and Boesky, L. 2002 Effectiveness of Dialectical Behaviour Therapy Program for Incarcerated Female Juvenile Offenders, Child and Adolescent Mental Health 7: 121–127.

Young, J.E. and Flannagan, C. 1998 Schema Focused Therapy for Narcissistic Patients 239–268 in Disorders of narcissism: Diagnosis and Clinical Implications (Ronningstam, E. Editor)Washington DC: American Psychiatric Press.

Young, J.E. and Glukoski, V.L. 1996 Schema-focused diagnosis for personality disorders 300–321 in Handbook of Relational Diagnosis and Dysfunctional Family Patterns (Kaslow, F.W. Editor) New York: Wiley.

Young, J.E., Klosko, J.S. and Weishaar, M. 2003 Schema Therapy: A Practitioner's Guide. New York: Guildford.

Chapter 16

Treating high-risk mentally disordered offenders: the dangerous and severe personality disorder initiative

Val Hawes

Aim

This chapter discusses the social and policy background to the development of the dangerous and severe personality disorder initiative in the United Kingdom and describes some of the cognitively based programmes developed to treat these high-risk mentally disordered offenders (MDOs).

Learning objectives

- To outline the background to and debate surrounding the development of dangerous and severe personality disorder (DSPD) services in the United Kingdom
- To discuss the concept of severe personality disorder and psychopathy
- To describe some of the cognitively based therapeutic programmes available in the DSPD programme

Introduction

As described in Chapter 15, the application of cognitive-based therapies to the treatment of MDOs developed differently within the forensic mental health system compared with the prison system. However, the DSPD programme, which spans both mental health and the criminal justice systems, has resulted in the development and adaptation of cognitively based treatment programmes that have been implemented in both prison and health settings. This chapter focuses on cognitive therapeutic approaches to the treatment of high-risk offenders, particularly those meeting the inclusion criteria for the DSPD programme. Pendulum swings in attitudes towards individuals who fall into this category are described together with a summary of the policy developments that resulted in the DSPD programme in the United Kingdom.

Some of the controversy surrounding the legislative developments relating to the treatment and control of this offender group will be summarized. A brief account of the clinical issues relating to 'severe personality disorder' will be given, followed by a description of three of the main cognitive treatment approaches in use in the programme. The chapter will close with consideration of the impact on staff and participants of these service developments.

Attitudes and policies concerning psychopathic offenders and the birth of the DSPD programme

Following the introduction of the 1957 Homicide Act (HMSO 1957), with its defence of diminished responsibility in cases of homicide, and the 1959 Mental Health Act (HMSO 1959), which included the category of psychopathic disorder, there was a rise in the number of homicide perpetrators detained in high secure hospitals for treatment (Dell 1984). During this period, positive treatment outcomes were being reported from the therapeutic community treatment at Grendon Underwood Prison (Gunn et al 1978; Hobson et al 2000). However, by the time the Butler Committee reported (Butler Committee 1975), there was considerable concern about the treatment of individuals who were detained in secure hospitals under the legal category of psychopathic disorder and the Committee recommended that specialized treatment units should be set up in prisons.

Among the subsequent developments relating to offenders detained under the category of psychopathic disorder there were the serious concerns that led to the Fallon Inquiry into the Personality Disorder Unit at Ashworth Hospital (Fallon et al 1999). Among the report's conclusions was the recommendation that hospital treatment should be reserved for compliant patients and that non-compliant and treatment-resistant individuals with personality disorder should be managed in prison.

By this stage, a significant factor driving policy development in the United Kingdom and elsewhere was the increasing public, media and political concern about public protection in relation to homicides committed by MDOs. The tragedy of each of these deaths was further highlighted in the inquiry reports that listed failures of communication between professionals (Jewesbury and McCulloch 2002). Although some of the focus was on homicides committed by mentally ill offenders such as Christopher Clunis (Ritchie 1994), there was increasing attention on those committed by individuals diagnosed as having a personality disorder. In the public domain, these concerns came to a head through reactions to the conviction in 1999 of Michael Stone for the attack on Lin Russell and her daughters, Megan and Josie (Freedland 2002), although the report of the inquiry into his care and treatment was not published until 2006 (NHS South East Coast 2006). However, prior to Stone's conviction, a working party from the Department of Health and Home Office (now the Ministry of Justice) was already considering how to better manage high-risk offenders. The convergence of this work and the high-profile case led to the DSPD policy initiative (DH 2005; HO and DH 1999, 2002).

These proposals were greeted with dismay by some forensic psychiatrists (Eastman 1999; Mullen 1999), mental health professionals, service users and civil rights organizations. The main concern was the over-emphasis on public protection with the proposed introduction of orders that would allow 'preventive detention' of both the convicted and the unconvicted, as well as both the treatable and the untreatable. The wording in the proposals implied that that the proposals 'would allow indefinite detention of people who had not committed any offence and were not suffering from a treatable mental disorder' (Jewesbury and McCulloch 2002). Concern about the implications of preventive detention was further fuelled by Buchanan's (Buchanan and Leese 2001) review of 21 studies, which concluded that six people would need to be detained to prevent one violent act.

Opponents of the proposals were clear that there was a real need for mental health services for severely personality disordered individuals. However, they objected to proposals that appeared to take little account of the civil liberties of the unconvicted and those designated untreatable, and the ethical dilemmas that these proposals presented for health professionals (Mullen 1999). As the proposals were seen to emphasize management and public protection rather than treatment, and as many of the 'patients' were thought to be untreatable, it was argued that, for many detainees, health professionals would be operating more as public protectors rather than treating clinicians (Eastman 1999). The initial reaction of the Royal College of Psychiatrists (1999) was generally negative, although the British Psychological Society (1999) expressed caution but recognized that such services would develop multidisciplinary teamwork skills and enhanced training.

Although Michael Stone's conviction was perceived by many to catalyse the DSPD proposals, it is argued they were motivated not only by this single tragic event but also by the long-standing frustration within government at what it saw as the refusal of psychiatrists to address the problem of high-risk offenders with personality disorder (Maden 2007). Part of the impetus for the DSPD initiative was that some psychiatrists had used the term 'personality disorder' in a flexible and perhaps questionable way to decide which patients they would and, importantly, which they would not have within their services (Gunn 2000). In support of this 'flexible' approach, psychiatrists could call on the concept of 'untreatability', with its firm link to the old Mental Health Act's (HMSO 1983) concept of psychopathic disorder. This was because in the 1983 Act the 'treatability' test (see Box 16.3) had to be applied before compulsory admission could be effected for someone deemed to be suffering from psychopathic disorder. Gunn and Felthous (2000) argued that this meant that patients who presented serious management problems in terms of either chronicity of problems, or more particularly their associated aggression and violent behaviour, were likely to be pronounced 'untreatable'.

The UK Government set out further proposals on changes to mental health legislation in the White Paper 'Reforming the Mental Health Act' (DH 2001), part II of which focused on the management of high-risk offenders. This drew a further negative reaction from mental health professionals and the media. Although the emphasis on preventative detention on the grounds of public protection was modified in the Draft Mental Health Bill (DH 2004), this too received a critical reception, with some commentators considering that it lacked the guiding principles set out in relevant policy documents (Thornicroft and Szmukler 2005). Proposals for preventative detention were finally dropped before the final draft of the Mental Health Bill was passed and became the Mental Health Act 2007 (HMSO 2007), which was implemented in October 2008. The aspects of most relevance for personality disordered offenders are a single broad definition of mental disorder as 'any disorder or disability of the mind' and the replacement of the 'treatability' clause with one relating to the availability of 'appropriate treatment'.

Meanwhile, there had been significant changes in criminal justice legislation, all aimed at increasing public protection. Several of these related specifically to sex offenders; the Sex Offenders Act 1997 (HMSO 1997) was updated by the Sex Offences Act (HMSO 2003b), with the addition of four civil orders, including Sexual Offences Prevention Orders (HMSO 2004), designed to protect the public from harm. The Criminal Justice Act (HMSO 2003a), relevant for both violent and sexual offenders, included the provision of sentences of Imprisonment for Public Protection (IPP), usually imposed with a short set period to be served, based on the duration of a fixed sentence for the same offence. The IPP sentences are imposed on offenders considered, on the basis of previous convictions, to be a high risk of further serious offending. These measures, relating to both sexual and violent offenders, are clearly aimed at offenders who are persistently antisocial and criminal and would include those whose offending is driven by Antisocial Personality Disorder (ASPD) as well as other personality disorders. Alongside these legislative changes there have been major developments in the management of offenders in the community with the statutory establishment of Multi-Agency Public Protection Arrangements and Panels (MAPPA and MAPPPs) through the Criminal and Court Services Act (HMSO 2000).

The demise of the original proposals on preventive detention and increased emphasis on the additional criminal justice provisions, together with service developments arising from the DSPD programme, have resulted in some commentators adopting a cautiously positive view of the

DSPD initiative (Mullen 2007; Tyrer 2007). Service developments within the DSPD programme have included a number of different approaches (some of which are described below) to the treatment and management of groups of individuals who were previously excluded from accessing treatment due to the severity of their personality dysfunction. Changes in the legal framework have also had an impact on the prison DSPD units with a growing number of referrals of men serving IPP sentences.

Meeting the criteria for DSPD

The term DSPD is not a psychiatric diagnosis but was proposed to describe those offenders with severe personality disorder who, by virtue of their behaviour that can be linked to their personality disorder, present a high risk to others (Thornton 2001). The operational definition, as used within the DSPD programme, comprises three components as outlined in Text Box 16.1.

With respect to the first criteria, the determination of high risk for DSPD is carried out in the first instance using established static risk measures. In the case of violent offenders, the main tools used initially were the Risk Matrix 2000/V Scale (Thornton et al 2003), the Violence Risk Appraisal Guide (VRAG; Quinsey et al 1998) and the historical items from the Historical/Clinical/Risk Management-20 (HCR-20; Webster et al 1997). Following DSPD Expert Advisory Group recommendations, the Risk Matrix/V Scale and VRAG were replaced with the static items of the Violence Risk Scale (VRS; Wong and Gordon 1999), whereas the use of historical items for HCR-20 was retained. In the case of sexual offenders, the tools used are Risk Matrix2000/S scale and Combined Risk scale (Thornton et al 2003), and Static-99 (Hanson and Thornton 2000) together with historical items from HCR-20.

In practice, much of this risk assessment can be carried out from an offender's records alone. If the offender meets the high-risk criteria and is considered suitable for DSPD assessment (usually after admission to a DSPD unit), the static risk measures are reviewed and dynamic risk assessment is undertaken using the Clinical and Risk Management items of HCR-20 and the dynamic items of VRS. Dynamic risk assessment of sexual offenders is carried out using the

---

Box 16.1 Threshold criteria for DSPD

1. An individual meets the *high risk* criteria of the definition if he or she is *more likely than not* to commit a serious violent or sexual offence such that a victim might suffer physical and/or psychological harm from which it would be difficult or impossible to recover. ('More likely than not' refers to a probability of re-offending of >50% within the next 15 years)

2. The presence of severe personality disorder is determined in one of three ways:

   a. A Psychopathy Checklist List-Revised (PCL-R; Hare 1991) score of 30 or above

or

   b. A PCL-R score of between 25 and 29 and at least one distinct personality disorder (DSM-IV or ICD-10 diagnosis) other than ASPD

or

   c. Two distinct personality disorder diagnoses (DSM-IV or ICD-10), one of which is ASPD

3. Evidence of a *functional link* between the high-risk behaviour and the personality disorder(s)

Structured Assessment of Risk and Need (SARN; Sex Offender Treatment Programme 2004) or the Sex Offender version of the Violence Risk Scale (VRS-SO).

Alongside the development of DSPD units and the debate concerning the use of mental health legislation to manage high-risk offenders, there was another debate about assessing risk in the clinical management of MDOs. Research indicated that using unstructured and unaided clinical judgement was both unreliable and inaccurate. This led to the development of a number of tools commonly referred to as actuarial risk assessment instruments, which did not include elements of clinical judgement. These instruments, for example, the VRAG and Static-99, conceptualize the risk of violence solely in terms of probability of future violence, ignoring other facets of risk. They use fixed and explicit algorithms, developed based on the data from known groups of recidivistic and non-recidivistic violent offenders and patients, to estimate the specific probability or absolute likelihood that a person will engage in violence in the future (Hart et al 2007). Although enthusiasm for their use initially abounded, the limitations of the strictly actuarial tools were soon realized, in so much that many of them used only static factors such as age, gender, history of previous offending that did not change over time and, as such, purely actuarial instruments were insensitive to treatment change and had a limited use in monitoring rehabilitative potential. Among others, the Scottish Executive (2000), who reported on serious violence and sexual offenders, recommended that the most appropriate and useful empirical approach to risk assessment is 'structured clinical judgement'. One such risk assessment instrument, the HCR-20 (Webster et al 1997), has been internationally validated and combines static actuarial information with clinicians' knowledge of the offenders current situation and likely future responses (Maden 2005). However, structured methods should inform clinical judgement but cannot replace it (Monahan 1992).

With respect to the third criteria, Thornton (2001) set out some guidance for clarifying the functional link between high-risk behaviour and personality disorder. One necessary criterion is that the individual's personality characteristics (as identified by either personality diagnosis or the positively scored PCL-R items) played a *major role* in their offending, that is, that the offence(s) would probably not have occurred if those personality characteristics had been absent. The other necessary criterion is that the behaviour associated with the personality disorder(s) was evident in at least two harmful offences perpetrated by the individual.

There is no doubt that establishing the functional link has caused considerably more difficulty for clinicians working in DSPD units than establishing either of the other two criteria (see Text Box 16.2 for clinical examples). It is generally accepted that it is insufficient to base the link only on the characteristics of ASPD, as this diagnosis is mainly based on past antisocial and criminal behaviour. The objective of the DSPD programme is not to treat criminality as such but to reduce the risk of violent and sexual re-offending linked to other types of personality dysfunction.

Severe personality disorder, psychopathy and DSPD

Although there is no agreed definition of 'severe personality disorder', all clinicians working with individuals with these conditions recognize a clinical level of severity. Much of the difficulty in defining severity arises from the categorical approach of both the DSM (American Psychiatric Association 2000) and ICD (WHO 1992) classification systems. While continuing to work with the diagnostic categories, many clinicians use a dimensional approach in formulating treatment readiness and need of those with personality disorder. Stone (2007) described a continuum of personality disorder from low severity, where personality disorder shades into the normal population, through to high severity, where it denotes the concept of psychopathy. Tyrer (Tyrer and

Box 16.2 Vignettes illustrating the functional link

(Phrases in bold are terms used in the formal descriptions of psychopathy and personality disorder)

- Mr X funded his drug use by carrying out robberies. He identified the homes of elderly or vulnerable people, gained entry by posing as a Council official and then threatened the victim with violence before taking money and valuables. His choice of potential victims and his behaviour towards them once inside the homes showed **callousness and lack of empathy together with a glib and superficially charming** approach to **con/manipulate** victims to gain entry, that is, affective and interpersonal aspects of psychopathy

- The majority of Mr Y's offences involved violence towards women and culminated in a homicide. This pattern began with an assault on his first girlfriend after she went out with another boy. The pattern recurred and escalated with other women; his violence always occurred at the point a relationship ended or when Mr Y suspected that the woman was seeing someone else. There was clear evidence of **unstable and intense interpersonal relationships** and his violence as an expression of **frantic efforts to avoid abandonment;** traits of borderline personality disorder

- Mr Z believed that he was very attractive to women and met several through his work as a hairdresser. He had many sexual encounters and brief relationships with women who bought him gifts, for example, designer clothes. At the time of his index offence he was short of money and robbed a female stranger. He became enraged when she pulled his hair and strangled her. There was evidence of a **grandiose sense of self-importance;** he was **preoccupied with fantasies of his attractiveness and sexual prowess** and his relationships were marked by **interpersonal exploitation**. In the context of these narcissistic traits the pulling of his hair was a severe threat to his self-image

Johnson 1996) developed a dimensional system based on diagnosis with five levels of severity: no personality disorder, personality difficulty, simple personality disorder, complex personality disorder and severe personality disorder. He applied the term 'complex personality disorder' to those with one or more personality disorders from more than one DSM cluster and the term 'severe personality disorder' to those whose personality disorder causes severe disruption to the individual and society.

Research studies of populations with known high levels of personality disturbance have shown a high level of co-morbidity of all types, that is, dual diagnosis of Axis I disorder (mental illness and/or substance abuse) with personality disorder or the diagnosis of two or more personality disorders in one individual as diagnosed using the DSM (American Psychiatric Association 1994). Of particular relevance to DSPD are Coid's studies (Coid 1992; Coid et al 1999) of patients detained in high secure hospitals under the category of Psychopathic Disorder, and prisoners in special units in the prison service. The majority of this cohort would have met DSPD criteria and Coid found high levels of co-morbidity, both between Axes I and II and across Axis II. In DSPD terms, evidence of ASPD alone, that is, evidence of conduct disorder before age 15 and of a pervasive pattern of disregard for and violation of the rights of others (American Psychiatric Association 1994), is insufficient to meet DSPD criteria. A high proportion of prisoners serving sentences of 4 years or more in the United Kingdom would meet criteria for ASPD (and many would also meet criteria for an additional diagnosis of substance abuse) but would not necessarily meet DSPD criteria. Borderline personality disorder (BPD) is probably the commonest personality disorder diagnosed in mental health services, with at least some increase in provision of services in recent years, but the vast majority of these individuals do not meet DSPD criteria. In DSPD services, there has been some debate (in terms of Tyrer's dimensional understanding of severity, although this is not an agreed part of DSPD criteria) as to whether the combination of antisocial and borderline personality disorder (both Cluster B disorders) is sufficient to meet DSPD criteria. However, in view of the seriously impaired personal and societal function of many offenders with this combined diagnosis, they are usually considered to reach the DSPD criteria. Among those who meet DSPD criteria, as set out by Thornton (2001), and who begin treatment on one of the DSPD units, some of the most challenging individuals are those who meet criteria in terms of psychopathy alone (see Text Box 16.3 for definitions), as these men tend to experience little subjective distress and have limited insight into their personality disturbance, and those who have co-morbid diagnoses of personality disorder spanning all three DSM clusters (e.g. a combination of paranoid, antisocial, narcissistic and obsessive–compulsive personality disorder diagnoses).

As having a high score as measured by the PCL-R is one of the threshold criteria for admission to a DSPD unit, psychopathy is a key construct in the DSPD programme, yet as Cooke (Cooke et al 2007) eloquently explains, considerable debate surrounds the core features of this construct. Cooke (Cooke et al 2007) argued that a fundamental criticism of the PCL-R as a measure of psychopathy is that it confounds two distinct constructs, personality disorder and

Box 16.3 Personality disorder, definitions and criteria relevant to DSPD

Severe personality disorder: No generally accepted definition of severity but DSPD criteria are met if there is a diagnosis using DSM-IV or ICD-10 criteria of two (or more) personality disorders, of which one is ASPD

Psychopathic disorder: A legal (not clinical) term used in the Mental Health Act 1959 and 1983 (England and Wales) for one of the four categories of mental disorder under which an individual can be detained. It was defined as 'a persistent disorder or disability of mind (whether or not including significant impairment of intelligence) that results in abnormally aggressive or seriously irresponsible conduct on the part of the person concerned'. Under the 1983 Act, there was an additional condition for detention, that is, that 'treatment is necessary to alleviate or prevent deterioration of his/her condition'. In clinical practice, this category was usually applied to individuals with personality disorder, but the definition allowed for wider usage, for example, individuals of average intelligence who were violent in the context of autistic spectrum disorder. This term is no longer relevant since the introduction of the Mental Health Act 2007. This Act uses a single broad definition of mental disorder, and where detention for treatment is proposed there must be evidence that 'appropriate treatment is available'

Psychopathy: In international forensic practice this term is applied to the combination of interpersonal, affective, lifestyle and antisocial traits and is measured by the PCL-R. The checklist, as devised and revised by Hare (Hare 1991, 2003), was derived from the work of Cleckley (1941) and includes 20 items with maximum score of 40. Assessment is based on collateral and interview evidence and individuals scoring 30 or more (25 in the UK) meet the criteria for psychopathy criminal behaviour. Cooke emphasized that in the DSPD programme individuals are detained because of the assumption of a functional link between their personality disorder and the risk they pose. As Mullen (2007) continues, if the measure of psychopathy, that is, the PCL-R, and the construct of psychopathy are not distinct, and the instrument incorporates the behaviour it is supposed to be measuring, there is a confounding circularity. Mullen paraphrases Wootton (Wootton 1959) to concisely illustrate this tautology: 'Why does he keep committing crimes? Because he is a psychopath. How do you know he's a psychopath? Because he keeps committing crimes.'

To examine the key constructs of psychopathy, the PCL-R has been subjected to statistical analysis using factor analysis to tease out the nature of the multivariate relationships among the latent variables (constructs) that together influence the item ratings observed empirically. In the original description of the PCL-R (Hare 1991), the majority of the 20 items were divided into two factors, the first relating to aspects of interpersonal style and the second to impulsivity and antisocial behaviour. Cooke and Michie (2001) found that items that tapped antisocial behaviour were relatively poor indicators of psychopathy and therefore largely excluded them from their 3-factor model, thus diminishing the tautological relationship between the construct and what it is attempting to measure.

In Cooke's model (Cooke et al 2005; Cooke and Michie 2001), a superordinate trait of psychopathy overarches three factors: arrogant and deceitful interpersonal style, specified by items such as glibness/superficial charm, grandiose sense of self-worth, pathological lying, and conning/manipulative; the second factor, referred to as deficient affective experience, is specified by lack of remorse or guilt, shallow affect, callous/lack of empathy and failure to accept responsibility for own actions; the third factor, impulsive and irresponsible behavioural style, is specified by need for stimulation/proneness to boredom, irresponsibility, impulsivity, parasitic lifestyle and lack of realistic, long-term goals. Hare and colleagues (Hare 2003; Hare and Neumann 2005) responded to the 3-factor model by presenting a 4-factor model – essentially the three factors of Cooke and Michie (2001) plus a fourth factor comprising five items relating to criminal behaviour, that is, poor behavioural controls, early behaviour problems, juvenile delinquency, revocation of conditional release and criminal versatility.

Fundamentally, there is disagreement as to whether criminal behaviour is a core construct of psychopathy. Hare (Hare and Neumann 2005) argued that it is and that PCL-R items relating to criminal behaviour are indicators of important psychopathic traits; furthermore that the exclusion of antisocial behaviour in the 3-factor model decreases the usefulness of the PCL-R for predicting violence and aggression. Cooke and colleagues (Cooke et al 2007) rejected the contention that criminal behaviour plays a central role in diagnosing psychopathy; instead, they view such behaviour as a sequela of the disorder (Cooke et al 2004; Skeem and Cooke 2007).

In clinical practice in DSPD services, the total score on PCL-R assessment is the guideline for determining whether the individual meets the severe personality disorder component of DSPD criteria in terms of psychopathy. However, for subsequent psychological treatment, the antisocial behaviour/criminality items are of less importance compared with the interpersonal, affective and lifestyle characteristics. Thus, in treatment settings, the debate about 3-factor or 4-factor models is of limited clinical relevance as the more important characteristics for treatment are reflected by either Cooke's three factors or the first three of Hare's four factors.

It could be argued that as the relationship between psychopathy and criminal behaviour is pivotal in the DSPD service, where people are detained on the basis that there is a functional link between their personality disorder and their high-risk behaviour, it is important to rigorously elucidate the constructs of psychopathy that underpin the measure – a measure that is used as a threshold for both detention and access to intensive treatment services. Furthermore, understanding the constructs underpinning psychopathy can inform thinking about the psychological processes involved in the disorder, inform theories of causation and should aid the development of more effective treatment interventions.

Another concern for those individuals assessed as psychopathic on the PCL-R, for clinicians working with them and for research, is the question as to whether the psychopathy score changes over time or in response to treatment. As the assessment of psychopathy by the PCL-R requires the use of all available collateral information (many practitioners would not undertake a full assessment if documentation is scanty) as well as interview, the score is taken as a lifetime measure. A number of items, for example, early behavioural problems and juvenile delinquency, are clearly static, but there has been little research so far to determine whether measurable change can occur in the interpersonal and affective items.

For those unfamiliar with the PCL-R and for many individuals who undergo PCL-R assessment, the terminology of both the individual items (such as glibness/superficial charm, pathological lying, parasitic lifestyle) and the factor descriptors seem pejorative. A negative and judgemental tone is evident in both popular (Hare 2003) and professional (Meloy and Reavis 2007) accounts of psychopathy. The challenge for those working clinically with individuals with high PCL-R scores is to recognize the full range of personality disturbance these scores reflect and to deal transparently, creatively and compassionately with the individuals concerned. Each of the treatment approaches described below attempt to do this in different ways.

The treatment of severe personality disorder and psychopathy

It has been widely accepted that randomized controlled trials (RCTs) are the 'gold standard' for research in health settings, and this standard has been enshrined in the Cochrane database (Higgins and Green 2006). In the field of personality disorder, there have been two main views concerning research approaches; first, that despite the difficulties of conducting research with individuals with personality disorder, the RCT remains the preferred approach; the second, that due to the heterogeneity of individuals with personality disorder, other more clinically based research methodologies (including qualitative research) will better fit the experience of treatment.

Following the publication of the Review of Health and Social Services for Mentally Disordered Offenders chaired by John Reed (DH and HO 1992), a review of treatment and research issues in relation to psychopathic and antisocial personality disorder was commissioned and carried out by Dolan and Coid (1993). These authors found great difficulty in reaching definite conclusions concerning the effectiveness of treatment for personality disorder owing to the variety of methodologies employed and lack of clear outcome measures used in many of the studies reviewed. Following proposals for the DSPD programme, a systematic review of psychological and pharmacological treatments for severe personality disorder was undertaken (Warren et al 2003). This research group found that the main treatment approaches and associated research fell into three main groups: those that targeted offending behaviour, those that focused on symptoms associated with personality disorder, for example, self-harm or substance abuse, and those addressing core personality structure and function. Conclusions about positive treatment outcomes mainly related to the research on specific symptoms, but some optimism was expressed about therapeutic community treatment approaches. Duggan (Duggan et al 2007) carried out a systematic review of RCTs of treatment of personality disorder published up to 2002 and then repeated the review to include reports of RCTs published between 2002 and 2006. As they included only those studies where participants met DSM or ICD diagnostic criteria for personality disorder, many studies in the criminological literature were excluded. Twenty-seven studies met the inclusion criteria, of which 14 related to BPD, 6 to mixed personality disorder and only 2 to ASPD.

They found useable outcomes for most of the individual studies, but any comparison across studies using meta-analytic techniques to combine data was hampered by the heterogeneity of the data. The authors conclude that their findings are similar to many preceding reviews 'in that good-quality evidence from properly conducted studies of psychological interventions in personality disorder that might aid the practitioner is sparse'.

In relation to the treatment of psychopathy, Hare himself expressed considerable pessimism (Hare 2003). In their review of treatment, Harris and Rice (Harris and Rice 2006: 568) concluded that 'there is no evidence that treatments yet applied to psychopaths have been shown to be effective in reducing violence or crime'. They based this on their belief that psychopaths are 'fundamentally different from other offenders', with 'an evolutionarily viable lifestyle strategy that involves lying, cheating and manipulating others'. However, Hemphill (Hemphill and Hart 2002) argued that although there is a lack of evidence for reliable and effective treatments for psychopathy, there is no evidence that it is untreatable. Broadly speaking, treatment interventions in psychopathy have focused on two approaches; those aimed at reducing PCL-R scores and hence treating underlying personality structure (with associated therapeutic pessimism), and those aimed at reducing re-offending behaviour. In a review of the risk of criminal recidivism and psychopathy, Douglas (Douglas et al 2006) suggested that work to prevent re-offending should continue but that it would be misguided to adopt an attitude of resignation towards the treatment of the personality structures underlying psychopathy.

Psychologists working in the Correctional Service of Canada have a good track record of methodologically sound criminological research. Seto's (Seto and Barbaree 1999) follow-up study of sex offenders treated in a prison Sex Offender Treatment Programme (SOTP) became very influential as they found that good treatment behaviour was associated with increased recidivism, particularly in men scoring 15 or above on PCL-R. This finding led to the exclusion of prisoners with high PCL-R scores from standard offending behaviour programmes in UK prisons. Barbaree's (2005) follow-up on the same cohort, with more-complete recidivism data, found no statistically significant interaction between psychopathy and treatment behaviour. Following publication of this finding, there was some relaxation of admission to treatment programmes for prisoners with high PCL-R scores, but there is still considerable caution about allowing individuals with high scores on the interpersonal and affective factors of psychopathy to access offending behaviour programmes.

A number of other contributions are relevant to how treatment models have developed in DSPD services. Bateman and Tyrer's expert paper (2002), published to accompany the NHS personality disorder initiative 'No longer a diagnosis of exclusion' (National Institute for Mental Health in England 2003), rated available mental health treatments for personality disorder by efficacy and generalizability. Dowsett and Craissati (2008) followed the same approach to appraise the treatments available to offenders in England and Wales. They also addressed issues of denial of offending, especially in sex offenders, and the role of motivational interviewing. The issue of motivation and readiness for treatment has been considered more specifically in relation to high-risk offenders with personality disorder by Howells and Day (2007). They described a Multifactor Offender Readiness Model that recognizes that there are programme, organizational and environmental factors as well as those internal to the offender (cognitive, affective, volitional, behavioural and identity) that may interfere with engagement in and completion of treatment.

The DSPD programme

The government proposals for a DSPD programme were first made public in early 1999 and were soon followed by the Green Paper (HO and DH 1999). Despite the ensuing controversy, practical planning began for the four initial sites for DSPD services, to be located within the high secure prison estate and in high secure NHS provision. The first pilot project opened at HMP Whitemoor in September 2000 and has since developed into the Fens Unit. It occupies an existing prison wing, adapted to provide interview rooms and office space for clinicians in what were previously prisoner cells. The first pilot project in high secure hospitals began on an existing ward at Broadmoor Hospital in 2003. Meanwhile, organizational planning and construction work went ahead for new buildings at three sites: the Westgate Unit at HMP Frankland and the Peaks Unit at Rampton Hospital, both of which opened in spring 2004, followed by the Paddock Centre at Broadmoor Hospital in autumn 2005.

Planning also began for NHS medium secure and community services that opened to patients during 2006/7. The medium secure sites are in South and East London and Newcastle-on-Tyne. Community services have been developed in South-East and South London and in Newcastle. The Millfield Unit in East London uses a modified therapeutic community approach to treatment, but the other medium secure and community services use cognitive behavioural treatment programmes.

All of these services are for men, reflecting the relatively lower rate of offending in women and the much smaller proportion of women who meet DSPD criteria. A small service for women has been developed at the Primrose Unit at HMP Low Newton. The main treatment approach is dialectical behaviour therapy (DBT) with emphasis on reduction of self-harm, an approach with a proven evidence base, although not yet in MDO populations (Linehan et al 2006).

These units, in their infancy, are currently under evaluation and, to date, few individuals have completed their treatment. For those in NHS units, progression will be gradual through relevant levels of security, that is, high to medium then to a dedicated hostel or follow-up by a community forensic mental health team. A high proportion of participants in the prison units are life-sentence prisoners who will progress through the levels of security within the prison service. The progression of the IPP prisoners now being referred to the prison DSPD units is as yet unclear. Prisoners serving a fixed sentence, who have completed part of the treatment programme, must be released on completion of the mandated custodial portion of the sentence. In some cases, a prisoner is released to approved premises (probation hostel) with probation supervision and mental health follow-up, if this can be arranged. In other cases, the individual may be referred to an NHS unit, at the appropriate level of security, with a view to transfer to continue treatment, beyond the end of sentence if this is deemed necessary. Under the terms of the Mental Health Act 2007 (HMSO 2007), it is likely that 'appropriate treatment' will be available only to such individuals in dedicated personality-disorder services in both NHS and independent sector hospitals (the latter accessed through NHS gate-keeping arrangements). The cognitive treatment approaches adopted by three of the high secure units are described below.

Cognitive treatment models in DSPD units

Chromis programme; Westgate Unit, HMP Frankland

Chromis (HM Prison Service 2005) is a complex and intensive programme that aims to reduce violence in high-risk offenders whose level or combination of psychopathic traits disrupts their ability to engage in treatment and change. Chromis is an accredited programme that has been specifically designed to meet the needs of highly psychopathic individuals and provides participants with the skills to reduce and manage their risk. It also focuses on the identification and provision of external risk management in response to the particular circumstances and contexts within which participants live their lives. The programme was developed by forensic psychologists following a detailed review of the literature on psychopathy.

The programme can be completed within 2 to 3 years and consists of five treatment components accompanied by a progression strategy. The first component, Motivation and Engagement, introduces participants to the 'strategy of choices'. This is a way of engaging with participants which reinforces their choice and self-responsibility while providing clear and consistent risk management. This is particularly helpful in setting and maintaining boundaries and dealing with resistance. It is also used as a basis to motivate participants to constructively engage in treatment and sets the overall tone of transparency.

The core modules of the programme focus on developing the skills and self-responsibility of participants. The Creative Thinking Component enables participants to understand, develop and then generalize creative thinking skills. The Problem Solving Component helps participants to develop skills in defining and resolving problems together with critical reasoning. The Handling Conflict Component focuses on the skills needed to understand, avoid and resolve conflict situations in pro-social ways. The Cognitive Self-change Component addresses styles of thinking and types of behaviours associated with past violence to enable participants to reduce the risk of future violence. This component also has a strong emphasis on generalization work and behavioural monitoring. It includes the development of an individual relapse-prevention plan as an essential part of preparing for progression and resettlement.

The programme is delivered by multidisciplinary teams. Participants are always seen by two members of staff, even during assessment. Treatment sessions are delivered in a mixture of individual and small group sessions. This offers flexibility to run the session in a way that maximizes learning. Chromis is delivered as part of a broader treatment framework and participants can engage in other activities in parallel with treatment. There is a strong emphasis on staff competence and safety, and on the whole organization being sufficiently aware of the programme to provide a supportive culture.

Violence Reduction Programme (VRP); Paddock Centre, Broadmoor Hospital and Wadden Ward, part of the Forensic Intensive Psychological Treatment service (FIPTS), Bethlem Royal Hospital, South London

This cognitive behavioural treatment programme was developed at the Regional Psychiatric Centre, Saskatoon, in Canada and has been described by its authors (Wong et al 2007) and Maden (Maden et al 2004).

The programme is based on risk–need–responsivity principles as follows; the highest-risk offenders should have priority for treatment; treatment need focuses on criminogenic factors and responsivity allows for adaptation to individual abilities. The main criminogenic factors identified are the social and peer support of antisocial attitudes and behaviour; dysfunctional behaviours such as aggression, manipulation and impulsivity; dysfunctional attitudes and poor emotional regulation. Both static (historical) and dynamic (ongoing personal and situational) risk factors are assessed using the VRS (Wong and Gordon 1999) and progress is monitored by regular reassessment of those factors identified as the individual's treatment targets. An essential aspect of both initial and ongoing treatment assessments for individuals is the modified Transtheoretical Model of Change as described by Prochaska (Prochaska et al 1992).

The five stages of change are pre-contemplation, contemplation, preparation, action and maintenance. An individual may be at different stages in relation to specific treatment targets at any one time, and guidance is provided for therapists concerning each stage with an expectation that the patient will move through the stages of change, although progression may not be linear. The stages of change model is also integrated into the three phases of the main programme. The first phase, covering the pre-contemplation and contemplation stages, includes initial assessment and identification of treatment targets, motivational work and development of the therapeutic alliance leading to commitment to change. The second phase, covering the preparation and action stages, includes the recognition of behaviour patterns linked to violence, followed by the acquisition of skills for cognitive, emotional and behavioural change. The third phase, based on ongoing action then maintenance stages, focuses on relapse prevention.

The VRP is usually delivered over periods of 6 to 8 months in Canada and a small pilot programme (4 participants, 2 controls) has been delivered over 7 months at the Close Supervision Centre at HMP Woodhill (Wong et al 2007). At the Paddock Centre, the VRP is delivered through an intensive programme of group work reinforced by individual motivational work over approximately 2 years. Programme delivery is led by clinical and forensic psychologists, supported by therapy assistants, with out-of-session support being provided by nursing staff. This programme is also the main treatment approach in the FIPTS medium secure and community services in South London.

Cognitive Interpersonal Model; Fens Unit, HMP Whitemoor

This model (Butler et al 2005) brings together theoretical understanding and treatment approaches described by a number of clinicians and researchers, most notably Young (Young et al 2003) and Livesley (2003). The model is based on a number of assumptions outlined in Text Box 16.4.

The overall aim of the treatment programme is to facilitate change in each prisoner. While treatment needs are identified by individual case formulation, the therapeutic changes expected will include increased flexibility of thinking with reduction of cognitive distortions, access to and management of a range of affects (anger having been the predominant affect for many participants), reduced impulsivity and improved interpersonal relationships with peers and staff. A strong emphasis is placed on the development of a therapeutic alliance with the individual therapist as well as with fellow group members and facilitators.

The model recognizes the importance of emotional experience in facilitating change. All staff, whether or not they are directly involved in therapy, are provided with guidance to facilitate their interactions with prisoners so that these provide opportunities to reinforce new emotional experiences. Treatment is delivered through individual therapy (provided by therapists from a range of clinical backgrounds) and a progressive programme of group work that aims to address affective and interpersonal dysfunction related to personality disorder and psychopathy before the prisoner progresses to groups focusing on offending, addictive behaviours and healthy sexual relationships. Prisoners remain in the same group throughout treatment and sessions are facilitated jointly by clinicians and prison officers.

Box 16.4 Conceptual underpinning of the Fens unit treatment model

- It must be capable of meeting multiple needs of diverse clients with diffuse problems and varying levels of insight and motivation
- Personality has a survival function and treatment must enable an individual to find less dysfunctional ways of meeting his needs
- In order to achieve change, treatment must challenge pre-existing expectations
- A profound emotional experience is necessary for change
- The treatment of offenders who have been traumatized requires attention to their own trauma

There is a strong emphasis on ensuring treatment integrity with recognition that this involves adapted and cooperative ways of working for all members of the multidisciplinary team, both prison officers and clinicians. Although no prisoners have completed the programme to date, a number of men have shown signs of internal change, as evidenced by a reduction in the frequency of their violent behaviour and other disciplinary infractions, as compared with their pre-treatment level.

The experience of treatment for participants and staff

Well before the development of DSPD services the challenges and pitfalls of managing and treating offenders with personality disorder had been widely recognized by clinicians and academics (Coid 1992; Hare 1993) and also by statutory inquiries (Fallon et al 1999). Consequently, each of the new-build DSPD units was designed with small living units (10–12 places) and each DSPD team placed a strong emphasis on the need for training (both induction and ongoing) and supervision for staff. The central DSPD team have arranged multi-site meetings to manage, develop and research the programme and to provide a forum so that all grades of multidisciplinary staff can share their experiences.

With treatment programmes planned to last two or more years, sustaining the engagement and motivation of the participants is crucial. Although all participants meet criteria for 'severe personality disorder', they may present in a variety of ways, for example, charming but inauthentic, overtly hostile, impulsive, repeated self-harming, anxious to please, garrulous, withdrawn. Each of these presentations or behaviours can seriously interfere with treatment unless it is overtly challenged and addressed and the underlying cause explored. Another aspect of individual behaviour that may become apparent is behaviour that parallels the individual's behaviour while he was offending. For example, a man who had offended against girls in their early teens and who liked to talk to young petite female staff; a man who had strangled his victim and who put his hands round the neck of another prisoner during an argument. Overt behaviours such as strangling will be challenged by staff and may have disciplinary consequences in the prison units. Other behaviours, reflecting unconscious offence-paralleling processes, may be unobserved by staff or difficult to recognize as such, for example, a man who had sexually offended against adult women who was polite and charming when face to face with female staff but derogatory about women when he thought he would not be overheard. Such behaviours are most likely to come to the attention of those staff in most contact with the patients/prisoners but may not be recognized or challenged unless there is good communication with the experienced clinicians who are able to provide guidance and training.

In addition to individual behaviours there are the challenges that arise through a group of personality-disordered individuals living in close quarters for long periods. These include power struggles (colloquially referred to as the 'alpha male' issue), overt and subtle intimidation, verbal harassment (e.g. use of the term 'nonce' for sex offenders), trading, gambling and sexualized behaviour. Daily exposure to problematic interpersonal behaviour, including that arising from offence-paralleling processes, over long periods will inevitably be draining for staff. In these environments, the maintenance of good communication is vital and should involve staff, of all levels, who are in regular contact with prisoners/patients. High levels of support and regular supervision (both individual and group) is viewed as a necessity for staff, with the recommendation that such support and supervision be provided by staff external to the unit (National Institute for Health and Clinical Excellence 2008: 68–72). It is also helpful for those guiding treatment to have a strong theoretical framework for understanding the interpersonal dynamics of those in treatment and that those clinical leaders share the essentials of that framework with frontline staff.

The framework adopted will depend of the theoretical and professional background of the clinical leaders.

Although the overall treatment models are essentially types of cognitive therapy, many clinicians with experience of providing long-term cognitive therapy have come to recognize the value of concepts that originated in psychoanalysis, such as splitting, projection, transference and countertransference. Some of the ways these are expressed in interpersonal interactions and therapy with personality disordered individuals are described by McGauley (McGauley et al 2007) and Akhtar (2007). For other clinical leaders, a more behavioural approach to understanding problematic behaviour may be more relevant. One such approach has been proposed by Bowers (2002), who described the 'manipulation hexagon' of bullying, corrupting, conditioning, capitalizing, conning and dividing behaviours that may be used by individuals in secure settings to meet either conscious/instrumental or unconscious/interpersonal needs.

Although the treatment models described are primarily cognitive, in practice, all units have needed to make provision for treating the previous traumatic experiences of these men. Both the affective instability inherent in BPD and the added psychological work of dealing with trauma can result in these men being highly affectively aroused at times. If this results in damage to self, others or property there may well be a need for the short-term use of close observation or seclusion (or segregation in prison units) to ensure the safety of all concerned. Many staff and observers expected that there would be considerable violence on the DSPD units. There have been incidents, and some of these have led to the exclusion of a participant from treatment, but few have led to significant injuries. Overall, the incidence of serious violence has been less that in many secure units for the mentally ill or on the main wings of high secure prisons, and less than would be expected from the previous histories of men on the units (Hawes 2006). On some units there has been a rise in self-harming incidents; postulated reasons for the increase include that these incidents occurred as an alternative to harming others or in response to the recovery of traumatic memories. There have also been two suicides and one (probable) accidental death on one of the prison units.

When reviewing the impact on staff of working on these units, there are relatively few surprises. Most units have experienced a variable staff turnover, with some people, across all disciplines and grades, adapting well and remaining in post, while some others, perhaps initially enthusiastic, have quickly become disenchanted and have left. The units have not been immune to the problem of boundary violations that are a recognized feature of most secure institutions and of working with individuals with severe personality disorder (see Chapter 14). A common form of violation is inappropriate relationships between female staff members and male offenders. Some of these seem to be based on romantic fantasy; others on subtle yet powerful conditioning and coercion. Regular clinical supervision together with strong team relationships and astute line management are the main protection against such breaches. For most clinicians these structures were already part of regular practice, but for other staff, for example, prison officers, clinical supervision constitutes a new and unfamiliar experience.

Conclusion

The conviction of Michael Stone for the killing of Lin and Megan Russell catalysed the DSPD programme. Its introduction was a result of the government's dissatisfaction over what it perceived as psychiatrists' failure to intervene when faced with a personality-disordered offender. The initial proposals for DSPD services drew debate from health, legal, political and social systems and from the voluntary sector concerning the tension between public protection and the civil liberties of society's citizens, combining the role of punishment and health care and the ethical role health care professionals would occupy if such proposals were enacted unmodified. It could be argued that this pluralistic debate resulted in a shift away from preventive detention and focused thinking with respect to the ethics of detention, the nature of treatability, the function of treatment and the development of treatment programmes.

A decade or so later, the DSPD programme is established and in the process of its first independent evaluation, which is inevitably focusing more on process, or at best intermediate, rather than final, outcomes (IDEA 2008). Questions remain as to the criteria that will be used for this and future evaluation; over whether there has been a decrease in violent recidivism among those completing the programmes and if so to what extent over how long a follow-up period; over whether there has been a decrease in the level and or severity of their personality disorders (Mullen 2007) or a decreased score on the PCL-R or other measures of personality functioning. Will the variations in the cognitive treatment models yield differing outcomes and how will the 'value for money' criteria be factored into both evaluating the services and assessing outcome?

Much of this chapter has drawn on the work of psychologists and psychiatrists as well as the author's experiences of working on a DSPD unit. However, given that the main burden of the day-to-day care of the personality-disordered offenders treated on DSPD units falls to nurses (or to prison officers), it is relevant to close with reference to nursing research. Bowers (2002) noticed that, despite prevailing negative attitudes towards people with personality disorder, some mental health professionals managed to sustain a positive approach. His research, with nurses working in the three English high secure hospitals, aimed to identify the cognitive strategies used by professionals who maintained these positive attitudes, with a view to developing support structures and training that would nurture such attitudes. The foundations of the positive attitudes he identified included a belief in the uniqueness of individuals and their problems; a moral commitment to values such as honesty, equality, individual value; cognitive and emotional self-management; technical mastery of interpersonal skills such as the art of confrontation, teamwork skill and organizational support. Although this study focused on nurses, his findings are relevant for all other staff members who work in treatment programmes for offenders with personality disorder.

Key points

- The 1990s saw increasing political concern about public protection in relation to homicides committed by MDOs, especially those with personality disorder
- The initial proposals for the DSPD Programme led to considerable debate within health, legal, political and social systems, mainly about the tension between governmental protection of its citizens and their civil liberties
- DSPD services have been established mainly at the level of high and medium security. Each service has developed its own treatment programme based predominantly on cognitive behavioural models
- The initial evaluation of these programmes is currently taking place

References

Akhtar, S. 2007 Disruptions in the Course of Psychotherapy and Psychoanalysis 93–108 in Severe Personality Disorders (Van Luyn, B., Akhtar, S. and Livesley, J. Editors) Cambridge: Cambridge University Press.

American Psychiatric Association 1994 Diagnostic and Statistical Manual of Mental Disorders, 4th Edition DSM-IV. Washington DC: American Psychiatric Association.

American Psychiatric Association 2000 Diagnostic and Statistical Manual of Mental Disorders, 4th Edition Text Revision. DSM-IV-TR Washington DC: American Psychiatric Association.

Barbaree, H.E. 2005 Psychopathy, Treatment Behavior and Recidivism. Journal of Interpersonal Violence 20: 1115–1131.

Bateman, A. and Tyrer, P. 2002 Effective Management of Personality Disorder. London: Department of Health.

Bowers, L. 2002 Dangerous and Severe Personality Disorder: Response and Role of the Psychiatric Team 31–35, 143–160. London: Routledge.

British Psychological Society 1999 Dangerous People with Severe Personality Disorder. Leicester: British Psychological Society.

Buchanan, A. and Leese, M. 2001 Detention of People with Dangerous Severe Personality Disorders: A Systematic Review. Lancet 358: 1955–1959.

Butler Committee 1975 The Butler Committee on Mentally Abnormal Offenders, Cmnd 6244. London: HMSO.

Butler, M., Fox, S., Hawes, V. et al 2005 The Integrated Multidisciplinary Treatment Model for the DSPD Unit, HMP Whitemoor. Unpublished Work.

Cleckley, H. 1941 The Mask of Sanity 1st Edition. St Louis: Mosby.

Coid, J. 1992 DSM-III Diagnosis in Criminal Psychopaths: A Way Forward. Criminal Behaviour and Mental Health 2: 78–94.

Coid, J., Kahtan, N., Gault, S. and Jarman, B. 1999 Patients with Personality Disorder Admitted to Secure Forensic Psychiatry Services. British Journal of Psychiatry 175: 528–536.

Cooke, D.J. and Michie, C. 2001 Refining the Construct Of Psychopathy: Towards a Hierarchical Model. Psychological Assessment 13: 171–188.

Cooke, D.J., Michie, C., Hart, S.D. and Clark, D.A. 2004 Reconstructing Psychopathy: Clarifying the Significance of Antisocial and Socially Deviant Behavior in the Diagnosis of Psychopathic Personality Disorder. J Personal Disord 18: 337–357.

Cooke, D.J., Michie, C., Hart, S.D. and Clark, D. 2005 Assessing Psychopathy in the UK: Concerns about Cross-cultural Generalisability. British Journal of Psychiatry 186: 335–341.

Cooke, D.J., Michie, C., Hart, S.D. and Clark, D. 2007 Understanding the Structure of the Psychopathy Checklist-Revised. An Exploration of Methodological Confusion. British Journal of Psychiatry 190: s335–s341.

Dell, S. 1984 Murder into Manslaughter – The Diminished Responsibility Defence in Practice, Maudsley Mongraph 27 Edition Oxford: Oxford University Press.

Department of Health 2001, Reforming the Mental Health Act. Part 1: The new legal framework. Part II High risk patients Cm5016. London: The Stationary Office.

Department of Health. 2004 Draft Mental Health Bill. Cm6305 London: Department of Health.

Department of Health and Home Office. 1992 Review of Health and Social Services for Mentally Disordered Offenders and Others Requiring Similar Services The Reed Committee, HMSO, London, Final Summary Report, Command Number 2088.

Department of Health, Home Office and HM Prison Service. 2005 Dangerous and Severe Personality Disorder DSPD High Secure Services for Men: Planning and Delivery Guide. DSPD Programme, DH, HO, London: HMPS.

Dolan, B. and Coid, J. 1993 Psychopathic and Antisocial Personality Disorders: Treatment and Research Issues. London: Gaskell.

Douglas, K.S., Vincent, G.M. and Edens, J.F. 2006 Risk for Criminal Recidivism – The Role of Psychopathy 533–554 in Handbook of Psychopathy (Patrick, C.J. Editor) New York: Guilford Press.

Dowsett, J. and Craissati, J. 2008 Managing Personality Disordered Offenders in the Community: A Psychological Approach. Hove: Routledge.

Duggan, C., Huband, N., Smailagic, N., Ferriter, M. and Adams, C. 2007 The Use of Psychological Treatments for People with Personality Disorder: A Systematic Review of Randomized Controlled Trials. Personality and Mental Health 1: 95–125.

Eastman, N. 1999 Public Health Psychiatry or Crime Prevention? BMJ 318: 549–551.

Fallon, P., Bluglass, R., Edwards, B. and Daniels, G. 1999 Report of the Committee of Inquiry into the Personality Disorder Unit, Ashworth Special Hospital Cm 4194–ii. London: The Stationery Office.

Freedland, J. 23 October 2002 Stop This Madness. The Guardian.

Gunn, J. 2000 Future Directions for Treatment in Forensic Psychiatry. British Journal of Psychiatry 176: 332–338.

Gunn, J. and Felthous, A.R. 2000 Politics and Personality Disorder: The Demise of Psychiatry. Current Opinion in Psychiatry 13: 545–547.

Gunn, J., Robertson, G. and Dell, S. 1978 Psychiatric Aspects of Imprisonment. London: Academic Press.

Hanson, R.K. and Thornton, D. 2000 Improving Risk Assessments for Sex Offenders: A Comparison of Three Actuarial Scales. Law and Human Behavior 24: 119–136.

Hare, R.D. 1991 The Hare Psychopathy Checklist-Revised. Toronto, Ontario: Multi-health Systems.

Hare, R.D. 1993 Without Conscience. New York: Guilford Press.

Hare, R.D. 2003 Manual for the Hare Psychopathy Checklist–Revised 2nd Edition. Toronto, Ontario: Multi-health Systems.

Hare, R.D. and Neumann, C.S. 2005 Structural Models of Psychopathy. Current Psychiatric Reports 7: 57–64.

Harris, G.T. and Rice, M.E. 2006 Treatment of Psychopathy – A Review of Empirical Findings 555–572 in Handbook of Psychopathy (Patrick, C.J. Editor) New York: Guilford Press.

Hart, S.D., Michie, C. and Cooke, D.J. 2007 Precision of Actuarial Risk Assessment Instruments: Evaluating the 'Margins of Error' of Group V. Individual Predictions of Violence. British Journal of Psychiatry 49: s60–s65.

Hawes, V. 2006 Reduction of Violence on a prison DSPD Unit. Poster Presented at Royal College of Psychiatrists Annual Meeting, London.

Hemphill, J.F. and Hart, S.D. 2002 Motivating the Unmotivated: Psychopathy, Treatment and Change 193–219 in Motivating Offenders to Change (McMurran, M. Editor) Chichester: Wiley.

Higgins, J.P.T. and Green, S. 2006 Cochrane Handbook for Systematic Review of Interventions 4.2.6, [updated September 2006] Chichester: Wiley.

HM Prison Service 2005 Chromis Manuals, Offending Behaviour Programme Unit.

HMSO 1957 The Homicide Act. London: HMSO, c11.

HMSO 1959 The Mental Health Act 1959. London: HMSO, c72.

HMSO 1983 The Mental Health Act 1983. London: HMSO, c12.

HMSO 1997 The Sex Offenders Act 1997. London: HMSO, c51.

HMSO 2000 The Criminal and Court Services Act 2000. London: HMSO, c43.

HMSO 2003a The Criminal Justice Act 2003. London: HMSO, c44.

HMSO 2003b The Sex Offences Act 2003. London: HMSO, c42.

HMSO 2004 Sexual Offences Prevention Orders 2004. London: HMSO.

HMSO 2007 The Mental Health Act 2007. London: HMSO, c12.

Hobson, J., Shine, J. and Roberts, R. 2000 How Do Psychopaths Behave in a Prison Therapeutic Community? Psychology, Crime and the Law 6: 139–154.

Home Office and Department of Health 1999 Managing Dangerous People with Severe Personality Disorder: Proposals for Policy Development. London: Department of Health.

Home Office and Department of Health 2002 Managing Dangerous People with Severe Personality Disorder: Proposals for Policy Development. London: HMSO.

Howells, K. and Day, A. 2007 Readiness for Treatment in High Risk Offenders with Personality Disorder. Psychology, Crime and Law 13: 47–56.

IDEA – Inclusion for DSPD: Evaluation Assessment and treatment. www.psychiatry.ox.ac.uk/research/researchunits/socpsych/research/DSPD/IDEA. Accessed 20 October 2008.

Jewesbury, I. and McCulloch, A. 2002 Public Policy and Mentally Disordered Offenders in the UK 46–64 in Care of the Mentally Disordered Offenders in the UK (Buchanan, A. ed) Oxford: Oxford University Press.

Linehan, M.M., Comtois, K.A., Murray, A.M. et al 2006 Two-year Randomized Controlled Trial and Follow-up of Dialectical Behavior Therapy vs Therapy by Experts for Suicidal Behaviors and Borderline Personality Disorder. Archives of General Psychiatry 63: 757–766.

Livesley, W.J. 2003 Practical Management of Personality Disorder. New York: Guilford.

Maden, A. 2005 Violence Risk Assessment: The Question Is not Whether but How. Psychiatric Bulletin 29: 121–122.

Maden, A. 2007 Dangerous and Severe Personality Disorder: Antecedents and Origins. British Journal of Psychiatry 49: s8–s11.

Maden, A., Scott, F., Burnett, R., Lewis, G.H. and Skapinakis, P. 2004 Offending in Psychiatric Patients after Discharge from Medium Secure Units: Prospective National Cohort Study. BMJ 328: 1534.

McGauley, G., Adshead, G. and Sarkar, S.P. 2007 Psychotherapy of Psychopathic Disorders 449–466 in The International Handbook of Psychopathic Disorders and The Law Vol 1 Diagnosis and Treatment (Felthous, A. and Henning, S. Editors) Chichester: Wiley.

Meloy, J.R. and Reavis, J.A. 2007 Dangerous Cases: When Treatment Is not an Option 181–195 in Severe Personality Disorders (Van Luyn, B. Akhtar, S. and Livesley, J. Editors) Cambridge: Cambridge University Press.

Monahan, J. 1992 Mental Disorder and Violent Behavior. Perceptions and Evidence. American Psychologist 47: 511–521.

Mullen, P.E. 1999 Dangerous People with Severe Personality Disorder. British Proposals for Managing Them Are Glaringly Wrong and Unethical. BMJ 319: 1146–1147.

Mullen, P.E. 2007 Dangerous and Severe Personality Disorder and in Need of Treatment. British Journal of Psychiatry 49: s3–s7.

National Institute for Health and Clinical Excellence (NICE). 2008 Antisocial Personality Disorder: Treatment, Management and Prevention 68–72 National Clinical Practice Guideline. National Collaborating Centre for Mental Health, Commissioned by the National Institute for Health and Clinical Excellence. Full Guideline Draft.

National Institute for Mental Health in England (NIMHE). 2003 Personality Disorder: No Longer a Diagnosis of Exclusion: Policy Implementation Guidance for the Development of Services for People with Personality Disorder. London: Department of Health.

NHS South East Coast. 2006 Report of the Independent Inquiry into the Care and Treatment of Michael Stone, South East Coast Strategic Health Authority, Kent County Council, Kent Probation Area. www.southeastcoast.nhs.uk

Prochaska, J.O., DiClemente, C.C. and Norcross, J.C. 1992 In Search of How People Change. Applications to Addictive Behaviors. American Psychologist 47: 1102–1114.

Quinsey, V.L., Harris, G.T., Rice, M.E. and Cormier, C.A. 1998 Violent Offenders: Appraising and Managing Risk. Washington DC: American Psychological Association.

Ritchie, J. 1994 Inquiry into the Care and Treatment of Christopher Clunis. London: Department of Health.

Royal College of Psychiatrists. 1999 Response to Home Office and Department of Health 1999 Managing Dangerous People with Severe Personality Disorder: Proposals for Policy Development. London: RCP.

Scottish Executive. 2000. Report of the Committee on Serious Violent and Sexual Offenders. The MacLean Report. Laid before the Scottish Parliament by the Scottish Ministers in June 2000.

Seto, M.C. and Barbaree, H.E. 1999 Psychopathy, Treatment Behaviour and Sex Offender Recidivism. Journal of Interpersonal Violence 14: 1235–1248.

Sex Offender Treatment Programme (SOTP). 2004 Structured Assessment of Risk and Need Sexual Offenders. London: HM Prison Service.

Skeem, J. and Cooke, D. 2007 Is Antisocial Behaviour Essential to Psychopathy? Conceptual Directions for Resolving the Debate. Psychological Assessment. In press.

Stone, M.H. 2007 Treatability in Severe Personality Disorders: How Far Do the Science and Art of Psychotherapy Carry Us? 1–29 in Severe Personality Disorders (Van Luyn, B. Akhtar, S. and Livesley, J. Editors) Cambridge: Cambridge University Press.

Thornicroft, G. and Szmukler, G. 2005 The Draft Mental Health Bill in England: Without Principles. Psychiatric Bulletin 29: 244–247.

Thornton, D. 2001 Operational Definition of Dangerous and Severe Personality Disorder. Unpublished Work.

Thornton, D., Mann, R., Webster, S. et al 2003 Distinguishing and Combining Risks for Sexual and Violent Recidivisim, in Understanding and Managing Sexually Coercive Behaviour. Annals of Academy of Sciences (Prentky, R., Janus, E. and M. Seto Editors).

Tyrer, P. 2007 An Agitation of Contrary Opinions. British Journal of Psychiatry 190: s1–s2.

Tyrer, P. and Johnson, T. 1996 Establishing the Severity of Personality Disorder. American Journal of Psychiatry 153: 1593–1597.

Warren, F., McGauley, G., Norton, K. et al 2003 Review of Treatments for Severe Personality Disorder. Online report 30/03 report. http://www.homeoffice.gov.uk/rds/pdfs2/rdsolr3003.pdf London: Home Office.

Webster, C.D., Douglas, K.S., Eaves, D. and Hart, S. 1997 HCR-20: Assessing Risk for Violence – Version 2 Vancouver: Simon Fraser University.

Wong, S.C.P. and Gordon, A. 1999 Violence Risk Scale. Department of Psychology, University of Saskatchewan. Available at www.psynergy.ca

Wong, S.C., Gordon, A. and Gu, D. 2007 Assessment and Treatment of Violence-prone Forensic Clients: An Integrated Approach. British Journal of Psychiatry 49: s66–s74.

Wootton, B. 1959 Social Science and Social Pathology. Allen and Unwin.

World Health Organisation 1992 ICD-10; Classification of Mental and Behavioural Disorder. Geneva: Author.

Young, J.E., Klosko, J.S. and Weishaar, M.E. 2003 Schema therapy – A Practitioner's Guide. New York: Guilford.

Section 3

Law

Chapter 17

Introduction

Martin Wrench and Bridget Dolan

In this section we focus on those areas of law we considered most relevant to forensic mental health practitioners and allied professionals working with mentally disordered offenders. In our experience of teaching practitioners lacking specialist knowledge in this area, people can find the law intimidating. Our guiding principle is, therefore, that it is better that practitioners know something about the law that relates to their clients and patients than that they know nothing. The reader of this section should not expect to encounter impenetrable legal detail. For those who become very interested in the ideas, or who are required to acquire specialist knowledge, there are a number of well-known relevant legal textbooks they might peruse.

It is important for practitioners to understand how the legal system operates in relation to Mentally Disordered Offenders. Wrench and Dolan's chapter (Chapter 18), 'Law and the Mentally Disordered Offender: an Overview of Structures and Statutes', explains the principles of clinical and legal approaches, on which stand both the structures to process MDOs and the statute law that governs such processing. Sarkar's chapter (Chapter 20), 'Mental Health Law and the Mentally Disordered Offender', describes in detail current, relevant legislation, particularly the 1983 Mental Health Act. It places this Act, itself soon to be replaced by the 2007 MHA, in historical context and also discusses its ethical basis. It is evident from this chapter that seeking a balance between public protection and the rights of the patient is complex. He argues that it can be affected, sometimes adversely, by societal influences, including the media. Equally, the government's wish to allay continuing public concern about the sometimes exaggerated risk posed to the public by mentally disordered offenders has informed the development of new legislation.

Hartford-Bell and Bartlett's chapter (Chapter 19), on 'Mental Health Defences', takes the reader deeper into criminal law. It elucidates how the criminal courts make a determination about the relationship between someone's mental health and their degree of responsibility for a crime, particularly with regard to serious offences, especially homicide. Citing case law they describe and elaborate key concepts, including fitness to plead and stand trial, diminished responsibility, abnormality of mind and insanity and automatism defences. They also describe the role of the expert witness in the judicial process. The last chapter (Chapter 21) in this section, by Lerner and Morris, 'Mentally Disordered Offenders: Childcare Law and Practice', is included because forensic mental health practitioners, irrespective of the setting in which they work, frequently come into contact with clients or patients who are parents or are in contact with children. It is, therefore, vital that they be familiar with the relevant childcare law and practice issues pertaining to it. Lerner and Skinner's chapter provides a clear, comprehensive introduction to the legislation and the responsibilities and duties of professionals with regard to safeguarding children, as well as offering guidelines on effective interagency collaboration.

Chapter 18

Law and the mentally disordered offender: an overview of structures and statutes

Martin Wrench and Bridget Dolan

Aim

To provide an overview of civil and criminal law to which forensic practitioners relate.

Learning objectives

- ◆ To distinguish the basis of legal and clinical approaches to mentally disordered offenders
- ◆ To describe the legal structures within which mentally disordered offenders are considered in the criminal courts
- ◆ To describe, in outline, the range of legislation relevant to forensic mental health practice

---

Introduction

Legislation relating to mentally disordered offenders (MDOs) has developed in a piecemeal way over several hundred years, frequently in response to the anxieties of the ruling class or the public about real or perceived danger from people who have been variously described as 'criminal lunatics', 'the criminally insane', 'the morally insane' in the case of people with personality disorders, or, in the words of the tabloid press, 'psychos', 'perverts' and 'mad axe murderers'. The Criminal Lunatics Act of 1800 was hastily enacted in response to James Hadfield's attempted assassination of George III and the ensuing public outcry about the lack of any judicial means to detain him.

This chapter provides an overview of the current legislative framework and its evolution. It comments on what mental health practitioners working with MDOs need to know and understand about it, including its inconsistencies and inherent tensions. This is increasingly vital as, with the implementation of the Mental Health Act 2007, a more detailed knowledge of mental health law will now be required by a far wider range of professions than was previously the case. Under the un-amended 1983 Mental Health Act (MHA) only social workers (as approved social workers) and psychiatrists (and in some cases GPs approved under s.12) could exercise powers in relation to the compulsory detention, treatment and discharge of patients subject to the MHA. Since November 2008, psychologists, nurses and occupational therapists find themselves in the role of 'Responsible Clinician' (previously Responsible Medical Officer) overseeing a detained patient's treatment. In addition, a similarly wide range of professionals will be empowered to make applications for admission under the new MHA, as they take on the role of an 'approved mental health professional' which was previously only available to the approved social worker.

Bartlett and Sandland (2003: 2), writing on mental health law, quote Michel Foucault's description of the language of psychiatry as 'a monologue of reason about madness'. They add that mental health law is another language of reason about 'madness' that exists at times in a symbiotic relationship with psychiatry and at other times in 'uneasy juxtaposition'. Add to these languages the different professional languages of the mental health professions allied to psychiatry, each with different levels of knowledge of and professional involvement with the law, and the result could be a Babel of mutual incomprehension. What is also problematic is that some of the legal concepts underpinning mental health law, for example, abnormality of mind, the M'Naghten rules and diminished responsibility (see Chapter 19) are based on archaic forms of reasoning about the relationship between 'madness' and violent offending that are no longer supported by clinicians. The legal arguments can themselves seem anachronistic and anything but reasonable, but have a good claim to be rational, that is, there is a discernible logic to them. Bartlett and Phillips (1998) argued strongly that the legal, rational discourse on madness can be further undermined by the messy reality of operating it in complex social arenas. In such arenas, the culturally informed ideologies of the participants, including both professionals and service users, can easily be at odds. The consequences might include both a lack of consensus about decision making and overt micro-cultural conflict in relation to individual patients.

Eastman (2000) has described the 'uneasy juxtaposition' between the law and the mental sciences as a consequence of individuals inhabiting either 'Legal Land' or 'Mental Land' respectively. The inhabitants of mental land and legal land have different cultures, histories and languages: Mental landers are principally concerned with the welfare of psychiatric patients and legal landers with the administration of justice. Of particular relevance to forensic mental health practitioners are 'the inherent tensions between the principles of welfare and justice in relation to much law pertaining to mental disorder'. Eastman noted the extent to which there has been a shift in emphasis in mental science jurisprudence from the traditional welfare model to a justice model focusing particularly on public protection in recent legislation. As evidence, he cites the Crimes (Sentences) Act 1997, the Sexual Offences (Amendment) Act 1999, sections 2(2b) and 4 of the Criminal Justice Act 1991 and the proposals to preventively detain people with severe personality disorder who are considered to pose a grave danger to the public. (HO 1999).

Forensic psychiatry has always been a branch of psychiatry that, of necessity, has placed considerable emphasis on risk to third parties, but the balance has increasingly shifted to placing potential and actual victims nearer the forefront of concern, a change in emphasis towards a form of 'public health psychiatry' that has implications for all mental health practitioners, but particularly forensic practitioners. Clarkson (2005: 254) comments that 'in any society that values liberty, the criminal law ought only to be invoked as a last resort method of social control when absolutely necessary'. He goes on to note that recent Conservative governments and the current Labour government have tended to resort to criminalizing conduct as a first resort. The current government created 661 criminal offences between 1997 and 2004. It seems that politicians currently view criminalizing antisocial behaviour and taking a tough attitude to crime as electorally popular. This clearly has implications for professionals working with a patient group who already elicit little public sympathy or concern for their civil liberties. If mental health practitioners are to work effectively with MDOs, it is crucial that they develop sufficient understanding of the legal framework. They also need to grasp the impact of a move from a welfare to a justice model on developments in and the implementation of mental health law.

Considerable anxiety was expressed by a wide range of professional bodies and some mental health charities, notably MIND, about the proposals for the Mental Health Bill (now the MHA 2007). The proposals were widely criticized for placing public protection above the needs and

---

Box 18.1 Legal and quasi-legal fora

Criminal courts

♦ Magistrates courts

♦ Crown courts

Civil courts

Mental health review tribunals

MAPPA panels

Inquests

Childcare proceedings

---

rights of the patient by, for example, replacing the treatability test as a criterion for detention under the 1983 Act with an 'availability of treatment' criterion (see s.4 MHA 2007). This, to many opponents of the amended Act, gives 'the authorities the right to lock up people indefinitely, irrespective of whether they are in need of treatment' (Independent 2007). In its response to the report of the Joint Committee on Human Rights, the government largely rejected concerns raised about the new MHA's potential failure to comply with the Human Rights Act by the House of Lords and the House of Commons joint committee on Human Rights Legislation (House of Lords 2007).

Whatever the concerns raised about the 2007 amendments to the MHA, it is important, in any event, for mental health professionals to develop an understanding of the interrelationship between the civil liberties, rights and needs of the patient and the protection of an increasingly risk-averse society. Bearing these real-life tensions in mind, this chapter now clarifies the key elements of current law, principally in relation to MDOs; it outlines how the legal system, criminal justice system and mental health services relate and what legal options are available in a range of different circumstances. It also addresses the role of forensic practitioners in other legal and quasi-legal settings (see Text Box 18.1).

The criminal justice system and the mentally disordered offender

For many forensic mental health professionals their first contact with a client arises because of the client's involvement in the criminal justice system. This can be at one of five stages:

1. *With the police*: At the detention and/or charge stage

2. *Pre-trial*: On determining a defendant's fitness to plead

3. *At trial*: Giving opinions on aspects of the crime, including the evidence, the mental element and motivation, or the confession

4. *Post-trial*: Advising on disposal prior to sentencing and

5. *On disposal*: Whether to a prison or a psychiatric facility

Thus an understanding of the legislation and principles applicable at each of these stages is essential; this is explored in greater detail below.

Throughout the process there is a guiding principle. This is embodied in a surprisingly well-known document, Home Office Circular 66/1990 (HO 1990). This states that 'it is government policy that, wherever possible, mentally disordered offenders should receive care and treatment from the health and social services'. The circular outlines the various legal mechanisms by which MDOs can be 'diverted' into the Mental Health System by use of the Mental Health Act 1983 and allied legislation. Other, mainly criminal justice, legislation is in place to govern the reduced criminal responsibility of those with mental disorder, to protect those who are so unwell at the time of trial that they are not fit to be tried and to ensure that psychiatric disorder, where relevant, is taken into account on sentencing.

However, as Bartlett and Sandland (2003: 255) state, diversion has 'never been a blanket policy'. They commented that Part III of the Mental Health Act 1983 'functions more as a threshold than a simple gateway between the two systems'.

Police: detention and charge

There are two options available at this stage; these are the use of Section 136 and diversion schemes early on in the criminal justice process.

Section 136 of the MHA 1983 empowers police officers to remove to a place of safety a person found in a place to which the public have access and who appears to be mentally disordered and in need of care and control. In many cases, although a person may appear to have committed an offence (and in particular a public order offence), the police recognize the expediency of not dealing with the matter through a criminal justice route and use s.136 powers to divert the person into the care of hospitals or social services. Research suggests that s.136 'informal' diversion is 'unlikely to be used when evidence of a notifiable crime is present' (Robertson et al 1996: 176).

Where a more serious crime has been committed, the police will tend not to make diversion decisions themselves using s.136 but leave the decision to the Crown Prosecution Service (CPS) to determine, where there is sufficient evidence to prosecute, whether it is in the public interest to do so. To this end, diversion schemes operate in many Magistrates' Courts and police stations throughout the country and are staffed principally by community psychiatric nurses working alongside CPS teams, with the aim of identifying those with mental disorders and, where appropriate, diverting them to mental health settings. In 2005, there were 136 schemes in existence. A survey by NACRO (Smith 2004) showed wide variation in the staffing levels for the schemes, ranging from one clinician, generally a CPN, to multidisciplinary teams. The survey found that 25% of schemes had had a reduction in funding since the previous year and that 72% of respondents viewed the lack of beds as a barrier to their scheme operating. NACRO, in its recommendations, called for more ring-fenced money to be made available and for the Department of Health to make more beds available to the schemes rather than leave it to the discretion of individual Trusts to provide them. A survey of nine schemes on behalf of NACRO by the Centre for Public Innovation (2005) found that 79% of those seen were White males between the ages of 25 and 55, arrested predominantly for violent crimes against the person, including sexual assault. Many minor offences are filtered out at an early stage in the criminal justice process, as in 37% of arrests no further action is taken if a mental health problem is identified. (Centre for Public Innovation 2005: 18).

More recently, a specialist multidisciplinary unit has been established to identify and divert to mental health services individuals with mental disorder who might pose a threat to VIPs and prominent people. The Fixated Threat Assessment Centre (FTAC) is a joint initiative between the Metropolitan Police and the Department of Health and is staffed by police officers, a forensic psychiatrist, a forensic psychologist and two forensic community psychiatric nurses. It is claimed that this will be 'the most developed such service in the world'. However, concerns have been expressed that such a unit leads to distinctions being blurred between criminal investigations and clinical decision-making.[1]

---

[1] www.timesonline.co.uk/tol/news/uk/crime/article1847697.ece

Where diversion is not employed there are safeguards for mentally disordered persons under s.66 the Police and Criminal Evidence Act, 1984 (PACE). Code of Guidance C, which covers the detention and questioning of subjects, requires the presence of an appropriate adult when a vulnerable suspect is interviewed by police officers or asked to sign a statement or note of interview under caution in relation to an alleged offence. The purpose of having an appropriate adult present is to advise the person being questioned, aid communication with them and to observe to ensure that the interview is conducted properly and fairly without duress.

Pre-trial: fitness to plead

At any stage before the defence case opens, the issue of fitness to plead may be raised by the prosecution, the defence or by the judge. A defendant will not be unfit to plead merely because he or she has a mental disorder. The issue for the courts will be whether, regardless of any mental disorder, the defendant can understand the proceedings and evidence so as to be able to properly put a defence to the charges made against him or her.

At trial: defences

Sanity and accountability for actions are rebuttable presumptions; they are presumed in law unless proved via evidence to the contrary. The special verdict at trial of 'not guilty by reason of insanity' should not be confused with the issue of fitness to plead. 'Insanity' is concerned with mental state at the time of the offence, whereas fitness to plead relates to mental state at the time of the trial.

A plea of diminished responsibility is a specific defence to a charge of murder introduced in the Homicide Act 1957. In contrast to the complete defence of 'insanity', a finding of 'diminished responsibility' is a partial defence, which if successful has the effect of reducing liability for murder to manslaughter. The importance of the defence is that the only possible sentence for murder is life imprisonment, whereas for manslaughter the punishment can range from a life sentence to an absolute discharge.

These two defences are most relevant to cases where the defendant's mental health is an issue (see also Chapter 19).

Post-trial: disposal

Except for the special case of diminished responsibility for murder, having a mental illness short of 'insanity' cannot affect one's liability for a crime. The law requires those suffering with mental illness to be judged to the same criminal standards as everyone else. However, suffering with a mental disorder may have a very significant effect on the sentencing of an offender once convicted.

Even where there has been no mental health issue raised as part of a defence case, psychiatric reports will often be requested by the courts before sentencing. Based on such reports, treatment orders will be made (whether under the Mental Health Act or as a condition of probation).

Part III of the MHA 1983 is concerned with criminal proceedings and gives judges wide powers when dealing with MDOs.

Before trial, a judge can remand an accused person to hospital for assessment or treatment (s.35 and s.36). After conviction, a judge can order hospital admission of an offender suffering with mental disorder (s.37), and the evidence of two doctors (invariably psychiatrists) is required. If, after having heard oral evidence from a doctor, the judge finds that there is a risk of serious harm to others if the offender were released from hospital, the judge can also set restrictions on the offender's future discharge (s.41). This usually also requires that the patient remain under supervision, following their discharge from hospital, by a psychiatrist and a social supervisor (usually a social worker, but probation officers also take on this role). The medical and social supervisors are required to provide regular reports to the Mental Health Unit at the Ministry of Justice.

The MHA also empowers the Secretary of State to transfer sentenced prisoners to hospital if found to suffer with a mental disorder that requires hospital detention (s.47 and s.49). At least two doctors must provide reports in support of the transfer from prison.

The vast majority of criminal prosecutions commence in a Magistrates' Court and will be resolved there unless the defendant exercises a right to request jury trial. Magistrates have powers to impose fines and make community orders but have limited powers of imprisonment.[2] Therefore, in more serious cases, the Magistrates' Court may convict and refer the case to the Crown Court for sentencing. Serious offences, known as 'indictable offences', can only be heard by the Crown Court. Indictable offences will involve the defendant in being remanded in custody or on bail, often for lengthy periods, while awaiting a Crown Court date. As detailed in Sarkar's chapter (Chapter 20), the Magistrates' and Crown Courts have recourse to part III of the MHA 1983 in remanding for psychiatric reports (s.35). Although Magistrates' Courts may not remand for treatment (s.36), both types of criminal courts can make hospital orders post-conviction.

Patients can be detained in hospital at different levels of security depending on the degree of risk they are deemed to pose to the public or themselves. High security is provided by the special hospitals: Broadmoor, Rampton and Ashworth. The next level comprises medium secure units. Patients will usually be transferred to a medium secure unit from a special hospital as part of the rehabilitation process before eventual discharge to the community. Low secure services include a range of types of accommodation, from psychiatric intensive care units through to the locked and lockable wards found in most general psychiatric hospitals.

The principle that a person should be detained in the least restrictive environment is enunciated in the Code of Practice (Department of Health, 2008) and derives from the Reed Report (1994). This guidance is not contained within the MHA legislation itself. However, a welcome provision brought in with the MHA 2007 was is the requirement that the revised Code of Practice shall contain a statement of principles that should inform all decisions made under the MHA; this includes minimizing restrictions of liberty, avoiding discrimination, respecting the patients' wishes, feelings, religion, culture and sexual orientation.

Under the 2008 Code of Practice (and to be compliant with ECHR rights) patients should be discharged from detention as soon as their application is no longer justified. In practice, discharge can come via four routes:

- The Responsible Clinician (previously the RMO) discharging the section under s.23
- More rarely, a discharge by the patient's nearest relative under s.23 (if not then nullified under s.25)
- For restricted patients by the Secretary of State under s.42
- By decision of a Mental Health Review Tribunal under s.72 or s.73. If the RC's duty to discharge when restrictions are no longer needed is adhered to then it should only be in exceptional circumstances that a compulsory detention order is passively allowed to expire

Aftercare under supervision and community treatment

The Mental Health (Patients in the Community) Act 1995 introduced into the 1983 MHA provision for some mentally disordered patients to receive aftercare under supervision (also known as

---

[2] For not exceeding 6 months.

supervised discharge) after leaving hospital following their compulsory detention for treatment. The provisions could only be used where there would be a substantial risk of serious harm to the health or safety of the patient or others, if the patient did not receive aftercare services on leaving hospital and where being subject to aftercare under supervision was likely to help to secure that the patient received those aftercare services.

However, the powers in s.25D MHA in respect of a supervisee were extremely limited. The 'responsible aftercare bodies' could impose requirements on the patient that she or he (1) reside at a specified place and (2) attend at specific places and times for the purpose of medical treatment, occupation, education or training. Yet these additions to s.25 MHA created no power to enforce a patient to undergo treatment in the community, the only power being that to 'take and convey' the patient to a place where they were required to attend for medical treatment. There is no power to treat. It was, not surprisingly, argued that CPNs forcing unwilling patients into their cars and taking them to a hospital where they are then asked to take treatment that they have (presumably) already refused would be little different in its therapeutic effect, and that such action was 'inconsistent with properly exercised assertive care, which rests on painstaking and careful building of a relationship with the patient'. (Eastman 1995: 1081)

However, the MHA 2007 in the face of great resistance from a number of patient and professional bodies, has now taken a further step and replaced 'Supervised Discharge' with 'Supervised Community Treatment' (SCT) and 'Community Treatment Orders' (CTO; see s.32 MHA 2007, s.17a-MHA 1983), the purpose of which is to ensure that the patient receive treatment, or to prevent risk of harm to the patient or others. Many detained patients are at risk of being discharged into the community upon conditions. Such conditions include compliance with community treatment, with failure to comply meaning a potential recall to hospital. The wider range of mental health professionals now permitted to act as 'Responsible Clinicians' under the revised Act will perhaps also find themselves being held responsible should their patient under a CTO re-offend.

The multi-agency public protection arrangements

These arrangements for managing serious sexual and other violent offenders in the community developed from interagency cooperation between the police and probation in the late 1990s. They were met with some suspicion by those health professionals invited to attend the multi-agency public protection arrangements (MAPPA) panels because of the possible consequences with regard to patient confidentiality. Some clinicians were concerned that the primacy of public protection and social control issues would adversely affect the therapeutic relationship.

Sections 67 and 68 of the Criminal Justice and Court Services Act (2000) placed MAPPA on a statutory footing and the provisions of that act were strengthened by sections 325–327 of the Criminal Justice Act (2003). The legislation requires the police, prison and probation services to act jointly as the 'responsible authority' to establish arrangements for assessing and managing the risks posed by sexual and violent offenders. The Criminal Justice Act (2003) imposes a 'duty to cooperate' with MAPPA on a wide range of agencies, including NHS trusts, local authorities, local housing authorities and other landlords who accommodate MAPPA offenders. In 2002/3, there were 52,809 MAPPA offenders. It is not clear, however, what proportion of those were mentally disordered.

Civil law and the forensic mental health professional

Involvement of forensic mental health professionals with the courts is not limited to the criminal justice system. Indeed, many forensic mental health professionals, particularly psychiatrists and social workers, will perhaps be more often involved within the civil legal system. This includes involvement in decisions regarding detention under the civil sections of the Mental Health Act 1983 and in Children Act proceedings (see Chapter 21).

Under the Mental Capacity Act (MCA) 2005, professionals' opinions will perhaps more frequently be sought in respect of best-interest decisions in the Court of Protection. Furthermore, all mental health professionals can find themselves as both factual and expert witnesses in inquests in the Coroners' Courts and within civil negligence litigation.

The MCA came into force in October 2007. Although decisions about the welfare of incapable patients were made earlier under the common law, the MCA now sets out a statutory framework for making decisions on behalf of incapable people. To a large extent, the MCA simply puts the current common law on a statutory footing, formalizing the existing test of capacity[3] and providing a framework for how 'best interests' is to be assessed. The Court of Protection now adjudicates upon controversial capacity and welfare decisions under the MCA, and psychiatrists and social workers in particular will find themselves called upon to give expert opinions in such cases.

Coroners have a very limited jurisdiction to hold inquisitorial proceedings to establish only four matters: 'who' the deceased person was and 'how', 'when' and 'where' they came by their death.[4] With the advent of the Human Rights Act 1998, the impact of Article 2 ECHR (the right to life) is such that the interpretation of the term 'how' has now been expanded in some cases to require a very wide-ranging inquiry into the broad circumstances of a death. Where there has been any violent death or unnatural death (including through self-harm), or where a death occurs in prison, police or psychiatric custody, an inquest will always be held, invariably with a jury.

Forensic mental health professionals can therefore find themselves involved as both witnesses of fact and as expert witnesses commenting on actions of others in such inquiries.

In civil damages claims, psychiatrists and psychologists will often be asked to give expert evidence about any psychiatric injury suffered by the claimant. Expert opinion is always required for a claimant to prove the degree of their psychiatric injury, its causation and its prognosis. Although previously it was the norm to have a psychiatric expert report from both the claimant and the defendant since the advent of the Civil Procedure Rules in 2000, it is now more common for there to be a single 'joint' expert appointed by the court in personal injury cases.

Although negligence claims against psychologists and mental health social workers are very rare in the authors' experience, it is fairly common for 'psychiatric clinical negligence' claims to be brought against Hospitals and Trusts where the standard of the psychiatric and nursing care is called into question. Such claims often arise from alleged failures to prevent suicide, or from alleged diagnostic and treatment errors. In such cases, expert evidence to establish what is a reasonable professional standard of care will be required from an appropriate mental health professional.

Whenever asked to write an expert report for a civil claim, an inquest or an MHRT, the forensic mental health professional has certain duties which should always be observed. The Civil Procedure Rules 1998 (the rules which govern all civil court actions) include at rule 35 a 'Code of Guidance on Expert Evidence' with which all those writing court reports should be familiar. Impartiality is the key for good expert evidence, whether presented in the civil or criminal courts.

---

[3] As set out in the Court of Appeal case of Re MB (Medical Treatment) 2 FLR 426.
[4] Coroners Act 1988 s.11.

Conclusion

The emphasis in this chapter has been on the criminal justice system and the MDOs. This reflects the key areas of activity for the majority of forensic practitioners. However, it has also sought to make clear that the legal landscape affecting MDOs, and for that matter many other psychiatric patients, has altered over the recent past and will do so again. The advent of an amended Mental Health Act would always be significant (Dyer 2006; Eastman 2006). Given the paradigm shifts built into the 2007 MHA, it is likely to have a huge impact on practice, more than any individual Act since 1959. Key changes include the creation of a single category of Mental Disorder, with the concomitant loss of the existing four categories, the removal of the so-called treatability test and the introduction of Supervised Community Treatment. Its contents also show how a changing political climate can alter the practicalities of both detention in hospital and of care delivery (Dyer 2005). As citizens, forensic mental health practitioners must operate within the law, but it seems likely that at least some will find that the 'uneasy juxtaposition' of law and mental health sciences is more difficult to live with than at any other point in their careers to date.

References

Bartlett, A. and Phillips, L. 1998 Decision Making and Mental Health Law 173–188 in Law without Enforcement: Integrating Mental Health and Justice (Eastman, N. and Peay, J. Editors) Oxford: Hart.

Bartlett, P. and Sandland, R. 2003 Mental Health Law: Policy and Practice. Oxford: Oxford University Press.

Clarkson, C.M.V. 2005 Understanding the Criminal Law. London: Sweet and Maxwell.

Department of Health 2008 Code of Practice to the Mental Health Act 1983 (Revised 1999) London: HMSO.

Department of Health 2007 Mental Health Act 2007 – Overview. Accessed on 26 September 2008. www.dh.gov.uk/en/Policyandguidance/Healthandsocialcaretopics/Mentalhealth

Dyer, C. 2005 Draft Mental Health Bill Needs Major Overhaul, Says Committee. British Medical Journal 330: 747.

Dyer, C. 2006 UK Government Scraps Mental Health Bill. British Medical Journal 332: 748.

Eastman, N. 1995 Anti-therapeutic Community Mental Health Law. British Medical Journal 310: 1081–1082.

Eastman, N.L.G 2000 Psycho-legal Studies as an Interface Discipline 83–110 in Behaviour, Crime and Legal Processes: A Guide for Forensic Practitioners (McGuire, J., Mason, T. and O'Kane, A. Editors) Chichester: Wiley.

Eastman, N. 2006 Reforming Mental Health Law in England and Wales. British Medical Journal 332: 737–738.

Home Office. 1990 Provision for Mentally Disordered Offenders, Circular 66/1990, London: HMSO.

House of Lords Paper 2007: 40HL288/04/02/07.

Independent 22 April 2007 Owen, J and Goodchild, S. "Lord Bragg Attacks Mental Health Bill as 'Inhuman, Inefficient and Unfair.' Labour Rebels and Health Experts Fear 'Lock Them-up' Legislation Will Leave Patients Detained Indefinitely".

Nacro 2004 Findings of the 2004 Survey of Court Diversion/Criminal Justice Mental Health Liaison Schemes for Mentally Disordered Offenders in England and Wales: Nacro: London.

Reed, J 1994 Report of the Department of Health and Home Office Working Group on Psychopathic Disorder. London: Department of Health and Home Office.

Robertson, G., Pearson, R. and Gibb, R. 1996, Police Interviewing and the Use of Appropriate Adults'. Journal of Forensic Psychiatry 7: p 297

The Centre for Public Innovation. 2005 Review of the Current Practice of Court Liaison and Diversion Schemes. www.publicinnovation.org.uk

Chapter 19

Mental health defences: the relevance of mental health issues to a legal understanding of crime

Nerida Harford-Bell and Annie Bartlett

Aim

To describe how the criminal courts consider the issue of legal responsibility for criminal behaviour and how they conceptualize and incorporate mental health information.

Learning objectives

- To understand the process of criminal trials and what issues need to be considered by the courts for that process to be just
- To understand the concept of fitness to plead and the consequences of being found unfit to plead
- To appreciate the various defences that a defendant can put forward in a criminal trial and the possible relevance of mental health issues to their defence
- To understand the specific defences that might apply in murder cases

Introduction

Defendants who come before the criminal courts in England and Wales often require courts to consider a variety of mental health issues. This was not always the case. It is only relatively recently that the criminal courts became concerned (to think) about the relevance of someone's mental health to their responsibility for a crime. Famously, Daniel M'Naghten in 1843 killed Sir Robert Peel's secretary, when intending to kill Peel himself, and was acquitted of murder on the grounds of insanity. This case led to public and parliamentary debate at the time.

The public continue to be interested in and perturbed by the small number of cases where a person with a mental health history and previous contact with mental health care providers goes on to kill. Most cases with a mental health component, that are before the criminal courts, relate to much less serious offences and generate much less legal argument.

This chapter is concerned for the most part with issues of legal responsibility for those who are charged with serious criminal offences, particularly murder. However, it also addresses how the courts can think about legal responsibility for a range of cases, including minor crimes, if they think it necessary and in the interests of justice.

To think clearly about this it is necessary to understand how criminal courts work. These issues are covered in Chapter 18. It is also necessary to know who takes part in the process and something about the principles of legal responsibility. It is important to bear in mind that mental

Box 19.1 Criminal justice process and mental health issues

Pre-trial issues

- ◆ Vulnerability of witnesses
- ◆ Fitness to plead
- ◆ Fitness to stand trial

Trial issues

- ◆ Insanity
- ◆ Automatism (sane and insane)
- ◆ Diminished Responsibility
- ◆ Provocation

Post-trial issues

- ◆ Possible mental health disposals
- ◆ Risk Assessments

health issues can be raised at any point in criminal cases but that the way in which they will be raised will depend on the legal stage of the process. Criminal cases can be divided into pre-trial, trial and post-trial issues (see Text Box 19.1).

The most important pre-trial issue is first, the possible vulnerability of witnesses. This means whether, when they gave evidence, they might have needed someone in addition to their lawyers who would be able to help them give a reasonable account of themselves. This would include making sure they have understood the questions and are able to answer free of suggestion or harassment. This is relatively rarely addressed by the court and is not considered further in this chapter. The second important pre-trial issue is whether someone is fit to plead/stand trial[1], and that is dealt with below. However, this chapter is mainly concerned with trial issues, specifically, the different ways in which the law indicates that someone may not be fully responsible for what they have done. This is, of course, quite a different question from whether they actually did the unlawful act. Post-trial issues that can involve psychiatric or psychological issues include provision of recommendations to assist the court in making a mental health disposal or giving expert evidence prior to sentence that will enable the court to consider possible mitigating factors. This chapter discusses the options the courts have in concluding cases, although not (specifically) the issue of mitigation as it does not involve any specific legislation.

Key players in courts where mental health issues are relevant are most often psychiatrists; usually, but not always, forensic psychiatrists. Psychiatrists will offer expert evidence in relation to mental disorders in general but most often into mental illness, often depression, schizophrenia and personality disorder. Expert witnesses can also include psychologists, who will often address levels of intelligence and personality issues. Regardless of the discipline of the expert witness, their job is the same in the end; they need to present clinical information clearly and link it to the legal issues the court is considering. It is rarely the case that it is enough simply to say that someone has a mental health problem. What is important to the court is not only that such a mental health

---

[1] Fitness to stand trial often addresses the physical rather than the mental health of a defendant. This is outside the scope of this chapter.

problem is robustly identified but also that it had a consequence in terms of the case before the court. Given the pace with which the criminal law has changed in the last decade, this can be daunting for the occasional expert witness.

The starting position of all courts in relation to all defendants is that, unless the contrary is proved, a person is responsible for his actions. As will be clear from the following sections, all the parties to the criminal proceedings can bring up mental health issues. The evidence of expert witnesses about these matters is always subject to the decision of the courts, and it will often be contested. This is in the nature of the adversarial system of justice and therefore unlike that which applies in other jurisdictions, where single experts are appointed and their evidence not contested in the same way. It is also true that evidence is contested because, to some extent, the acceptance of the relevance of mental health issues to offending leads to what may be viewed by some as leniency.

Defendant unfit to plead and/or stand trial

The courts recognize that some people do not have the capacity to enter a plea or participate in a trial. In these circumstances, evidence will have to be called, normally from psychiatrists, to establish the requisite lack of understanding. This issue is usually raised by the defence. In this case, the standard of proof demanded is that on 'the balance of probabilities' the defendant lacks the capacity to enter a plea or stand trial. If the issue is raised by the Crown, i.e. the prosecution, it is the usual criminal standard that is 'beyond reasonable doubt'. Expert witnesses need to decide on the following related issues:

- Whether the person understands the nature of the criminal charge and the difference between pleading guilty or not guilty
- Whether they can give instructions to their legal representatives
- Whether they can challenge a jury in the sense that they could exercise their right to object to certain members of the jury as they are selected
- Whether they are able to follow the proceedings of court as their case unfolds

Though this sounds like a straightforward list, in practice it can be hard to establish a robust clinical view. There are cases where the matter is straightforward and all parties would agree, for example, where someone's thinking was profoundly disturbed in a schizophrenic illness such that they were completely 'thought disordered', or where psychosis had rendered them mute, or where they are so learning-disabled that they could never meet the intellectual demands of the court. However, many cases are more debatable, not least because the expert is required to consider to what extent any member of the public would really understand often complex court proceedings.

The issue as to fitness to plead/stand trial is now determined by a judge alone, on the written or oral evidence of two medically qualified practitioners (one of whom has to be approved for the purposes of section 12 of the 1983 Mental Health Act) (see s.4(6) Criminal Procedure (Insanity) Act 1964). After that, and separately, a jury is sworn to determine whether the accused did the act. The fact that a defendant is found not fit to plead or stand trial does not prevent them returning to court at a later date, when their mental health is improved, and being found fit to plead/stand trial at that time. The court can take a view when the person is unfit to plead/stand trial, but if there is evidence of a recovery, the issue of fitness, and thus ultimately of guilt or innocence, can be reopened with another hearing. Where a jury is considering whether the defendant did the act, they do not have to consider what in lay terms might be called motivation. This relates to criminal offences that require particular levels of intent to commit them, for example, knowledge on the part of a defendant that a complainant is not consenting in a sexual assault.

The consequences that flow from a finding of unfitness are various. The options for the court are to impose the following:

- A hospital order with or without a restriction order
- A supervision order
- An absolute discharge (s.5 Criminal Procedure (Insanity) Act 1964)

In effect, the court is allowed to weigh up the gravity of the crime and the needs of the defendant so that the level of public protection is appropriate. This may mean a period, long or short, in a mental hospital, or it may mean being in the community but subject to some constraint. Although these seem like a wide range of possible disposals, in practice they may not fit well with the needs of the defendant. Specifically, where the unfitness arises owing to a lack of intellectual capacity, it is very likely that the sanctions of the court will be otiose. Consider, for instance, the case where a defendant with an assessed mental age of 5 or 6 is living in supported accommodation with a high level of supervision and support and is found to have committed a minor sexual assault. If there are no mental health issues requiring a hospital order, it is questionable that any order should be imposed. The procedures and consequences that the criminal courts bring to bear are, in these circumstances, wholly inadequate and clumsy. In particular, the onerous requirements to register as a sexual offender are absurd in these circumstances where there is lack of intellectual capacity. It is only if there is an absolute discharge that the requirement is avoided. If there is a hospital order or supervision order imposed then the requirement to register arises. In reality, this will mean the person with care of the defendant will have to comply on the defendant's behalf.

Trial issues 1: Insanity and the M'Naghten rules

Insanity at the time of the commission of a crime is merely a situation where the necessary mental element, that is, the capacity to form the intent to commit the specific crime, is lacking, and thus the intent to commit the crime, the *mens rea*, is also lacking. The mental condition recognized by the law as insanity for this purpose is not the same as the range of mental disorders recognized by contemporary psychiatry (APA 1994; WHO 1992). The defence have the burden of establishing legal insanity on the balance of probabilities. If established, it leads to a special verdict of not guilty by reason of insanity. Section 2 of the Trial of Lunatics Act 1883 provides for this verdict. The Act is concerned with responsibility rather than providing any definition of insanity. The verdict is returned by a jury after hearing evidence. The evidence must comprise evidence from two registered medical practitioners, at least one of whom must be approved for the purpose of section 12 of the 1983 Mental Health Act.[2]

Before the jury can return the special verdict of insanity, the prosecution must first prove to the criminal standard, that is, beyond reasonable doubt, that the defendant did the act or made the omission charged. If they fail to do this, the defendant is entitled to an acquittal whether or not he was insane at the time of the alleged act. The test for insanity for this special defence is still that laid down in the series of questions and answers first posited in the case of M'Naghten (1843) 10 CL. & F.200. That is, to establish a defence on the grounds of insanity, it must be clearly proved that, at the time of the committing of the act, the defendant 'was labouring under such a defect of reason, from disease of the mind, as not to know the nature and quality of the act he was doing, or, if he did know it, that he did not know he was doing what was wrong'.

---

[2] That is, they must be duly approved by the Secretary of State as having special experience in the diagnosis or treatment of mental illness.

The status of the insanity defence is interesting. It appears to be used infrequently, with fewer than 10 a year being run successfully recently (HO 2003). This may be for several different reasons. The introduction of the Homicide Act (see below) allowed for a different defence to murder. The old insanity legislation was more limited in its sentencing options, in that it directed individuals requiring treatment in hospital solely to special (now high secure) hospitals; this was inappropriate if the offence was minor. Finally, it is arguable that the understanding of the insanity defence's key element, 'defect of reason', has changed over time. In the past, unreason was synonymous with madness, as in the phrase 'lost their reason'. More contemporary usage of the term reason is confined to cognitive ability, as in 'to reason'; this was a small part of the old meaning. This leaves the expert with an interesting challenge of interpretation. Individuals with significant cognitive problems, for example, dementia or learning disability, are likely to be weeded out of the criminal courts pre-trial, as they will be unfit to plead. Individuals with major mental illness, for example, schizophrenia, may well, perhaps paradoxically, not be construed as insane.

In any case, and confusingly, sanctions follow such a Mad Hatter's verdict; insanity is an acquittal but the court must then make one of three possible orders.[3] These are the same as where there was a finding of unfitness to plead/stand trial (see above). This, therefore, includes an order that the person be admitted to a hospital as specified by the Secretary of State; this may be with or without a restriction as to time. However, where the offence alleged was murder, then the court must make an admission without limit of time. The alternatives are a Supervision Order or an order for the person's Absolute Discharge.

Trial issues 2: Automatism

Automatism is sensibly considered next because of its proximity to insanity. When automatism is raised as a defence to a crime, it is often questioned by judges as to whether in fact one is raising the defence of insanity due to the interpretation of that phrase 'disease of the mind'. This is reflected in the revised judgements on particular cases where the arguments for both automatism and insanity are rehearsed, but the decision at different levels of the court system vary. Automatism has been raised in many sex cases when the defendant asserts the acts complained of must have occurred when he was sleepwalking, although it is open to lawyers to raise it in relation to any criminal charge.

The term 'automatism' means no more than the involuntary movement of the limbs or body. Whether there is evidence of a state of automatism is a matter of law. The jury will decide, but only after a proper foundation for the defence has been laid out. This evidence is likely to be medical or scientific. Once such evidence exists, it is for the prosecution to negate it by proving that the defendant's criminal acts were voluntary, in the sense that they were done when he was fully conscious.

The difficulties in the interpretation of insanity and automatism, which rely on a proper understanding of the phrase 'disease of the mind', are illustrated by the following two cases. In Bratty (1963), the defendant took off a girl's stocking and strangled her with it. The defence called medical evidence to support the contention that Mr Bratty suffered at the time he was alleged to have committed the murder from psychomotor epilepsy. This might have prevented him from knowing the nature and quality of his act. It was said he therefore lacked the requisite *mens rea*. The judge ruled there was no evidence of automatism, that the psychomotor epilepsy amounted to a disease of the mind, and it was therefore a defence of insanity. The case illustrates that whether a particular condition amounts to a 'disease of the mind' within the M'Naghten Rules is not

---

[3]   This is in accordance with the Criminal Procedure (Insanity and Unfitness to Plead) Act 1991.

a medical but a legal question. What is clear is that the actions complained of in Bratty were purposive and not the convulsive, involuntary movement which one associates with an epileptic. The House of Lords upheld this ruling. The precedent has been followed in other cases in the Court of Appeal. In Quick (1973), the Court of Appeal held that the alternative defences of insanity and automatism should have been left to the jury. The trial judge had ruled, following Bratty, that the evidence put forward by the defence of acts done while hypoglycaemic due to an imbalance of insulin amounted to a defence of insanity. Following on this ruling the defendant had promptly pleaded guilty. The Court of Appeal reviewed the authorities on disease of the mind and drew a distinction between a disease of the mind caused by inherent physical disorder and some malfunctioning caused by external factors. This distinction has been applied in later cases.

In Burgess (1991), the defence to a charge of causing grievous bodily harm with intent was that the violence had been inflicted when the defendant was sleepwalking. Expert medical evidence was called on both sides. The trial judge ruled that the medical evidence amounted to evidence of insanity within the M'Naghten Rules. On appeal, it was held that, on a defence of automatism, the judge had to proceed through a two-stage process, deciding first whether there was evidence of automatism, and then whether the evidence showed the case to be one of insane automatism within the M'Naghten Rules, or one of non-insane automatism. It was further held that the judge had correctly concluded that the appellant's state was an abnormality that, although transitory and unlikely to result again in extreme violence, was due to an internal organic condition, which had manifested itself in violence and might recur, and, therefore, amounted to 'a disease of the mind'. The fact that there was a danger of recurrence resulting in violence were factors rendering it more appropriate to categorize the condition as a disease of the mind, but the absence of such factors does not preclude it being a disease of the mind. Although non-insane automatism and insanity appear to have similarities, the consequences that flow from the two defences are very different. The defence of non-insane automatism imposes no burden on the defence. If successful, such a defence results in a complete acquittal. Insanity, on the other hand, must be proved by the defence to the much less onerous civil standard on the balance of probabilities; it results in a special verdict of not guilty by reason of insanity. It is a special verdict, in so far as it is not a complete acquittal but requires one of the three disposals outlined above.

Trial issues 3: Diminished responsibility

The concept of someone's responsibility for criminal acts being reduced or diminished is peculiar to murder. It is a purely statutory defence, introduced for the first time to English Law by the Homicide Act 1957, s.2. The section states:

> Where a person kills or is party to the killing of another, he shall not be convicted of murder if he was suffering from such abnormality of mind (whether arising from a condition of arrested or retarded development of mind or any inherent causes or induced by disease or injury) as substantially impaired his mental responsibility for his acts or omissions in doing or being a party to the killing.

The burden of proof is on the defence, albeit to the civil standard of 'on the balance of probabilities'. Abnormality of mind is a much wider concept than 'defect of reason' within the M'Naghten Rules. Very helpful legal guidance was developed in the case of Byrne, a sexual psychopath who had difficulty in controlling his perverted sexual desires. He strangled a woman and then mutilated her body. On appeal it was held that there was evidence of diminished responsibility to bring him within s.2, and his appeal was allowed. Lord Justice Parker defined abnormality of mind as:

> [A] state of mind so different from that of ordinary human beings that the reasonable man would term it abnormal. It appears to us to be wide enough to cover the mind's activities in all its aspects, not only

the perception of physical acts and matters, and the ability to form a rational judgement as to whether an act is right or wrong, but also the ability to exercise willpower to control physical acts in accordance with that rational judgement.

(Byrne 1960)

The defence of diminished responsibility is much more common than insanity. There is no statutory requirement for medical evidence, although invariably there will be such evidence. In practice, in many cases, the issue of diminished responsibility will be an obvious one on the facts, such as when a mother of hitherto good character inexplicably kills her child while suffering from depression. The defence will obtain a report from a suitably qualified psychiatrist; this will then be submitted to the Crown, who will obtain a report from a second psychiatrist, and if there is agreement about both the clinical issues and their relevance, a plea to manslaughter by reason of diminished responsibility is likely to be tendered and accepted. In such a case there is then no trial.

However, where there is not this measure of agreement the matter will have to be determined by a jury. Even where the evidence appears clear, there will be cases where public interest demands a trial. The case of Peter Sutcliffe, the 'Yorkshire Ripper', was such a case. The prosecution were prepared to accept pleas to manslaughter; the medical evidence was unanimous that Sutcliffe had paranoid schizophrenia and his responsibility was diminished. However, the judge insisted that there should be a trial before a jury, perhaps reflecting the gravity of the charges and the savagery of the killings. A jury was duly put in charge and, having heard all the evidence, including the medical evidence, they convicted of murder. Sutcliffe went to prison, although he was subsequently transferred to mental hospital. The jury have to be directed by the judge on the wider meaning of 'abnormality of mind'; thereafter, the matter is one for them. The jury must consider the medical evidence, but they can, of course, reject the opinions of the expert witnesses, as they clearly did in the case of Sutcliffe. If there is no evidence or facts that could serve to undermine unchallenged, medical evidence supporting a finding of 'diminished responsibility', then a jury should be directed to accept that medical evidence.

Intoxication through drink or drugs can give rise to questions of 'diminished responsibility'. It is important to recognize that, for the most part, intoxication is viewed as a voluntary act and is therefore of no use as a defence against a criminal charge. In Tandy (1989), the defendant was an alcoholic who strangled her 11-year-old daughter after drinking a bottle of vodka. She was clearly suffering from an 'abnormality of the mind' at the time of the killing. The amount of alcohol in her bloodstream would have been lethal for most people. The Court of Appeal upheld her conviction for murder on the basis that her act in taking the first drink of the day was a voluntary one. This is important because it addresses the second arm of the defence, that is, the issue of responsibility. In fact, the medical evidence was divided, as is often the case. The defence contended that her ability to resist drinking had been extinguished by the disease of alcoholism. The prosecution expert's view was that she had control over whether she had the first drink of the day, but once she had the first drink she was no longer under control. Tandy establishes that where alcoholism alone is relied upon for a defence of diminished responsibility the defendant must establish three things. First, that he was suffering from an 'abnormality of mind' at the time of the killing. Second, that the 'abnormality of mind' was induced by the disease of alcoholism; and third, that the abnormality substantially impaired his mental responsibility for the act that caused death. This linkage of the various parts of the defence is useful not just for cases where alcohol is relevant, although most homicides do involve the consumption of some alcohol. The linkage helps us to think about how to present the expert's argument without infringing on the proper territory of the court.

A finding of 'diminished responsibility' leads on to sentencing. The judge is then free to consider further medical evidence. The finding of 'diminished responsibility' does not lead automatically to a mental health disposal, for two reasons. First, the medical evidence may make no such recommendation. Where the 'abnormality of mind' is some version of psychopathy, for example, antisocial personality disorder, it may well be that no mental health disposal is forthcoming. This would be because the assessing clinicians saw no scope for treatment. Where the 'abnormality of mind' is a mental illness it is likely that some treatment would be indicated. Second, the judge need not follow medical advice with regard to the need for care. Owing to the gravity of the offence, judges are most likely to consider the imposition of a Hospital Order (s.37), which can be made with or without restriction under s.41 of the 1983 Mental Health Act. Before a restriction order is made, evidence from two s.12-approved psychiatrists must be before the court. At least one must give oral evidence. The judge is not obliged to follow the recommendations of the psychiatrists with regard to imposing a restriction order. A restriction order is generally made for more serious offences where concerns for public safety override the general principle that the patient's needs are paramount. Responsibility for discharge is accordingly transferred from the RMO (Responsible Clinician in the MHA 2007) and the hospital to the Secretary of State (Ministry of Justice) and the Mental Health Review Tribunal.

Trial issues 4: Provocation

Provocation has long been recognized as a defence to murder but was made statutory by s.3 of the Homicide Act 1957. If successful, it reduces murder to manslaughter. It does not require any medical evidence and the test as to whether provocation is made out is objective. We include it for discussion because it involves a defendant losing self-control, and it has been raised in innumerable 'battered woman' cases where women who have been subjected to violence by their male partners over varying degrees of time have gone on to kill the perpetrator of the earlier violence. It is common in these cases for psychiatric evidence to be called, which can be put de facto towards two defences simultaneously, that is, provocation and diminished responsibility. This is done even though there is a question as to the extent to which any aspect of the provocation defence falls within the province of the psychiatric expert. Provocation differs from the defence of 'diminished responsibility' in that it does not have to be proved by the defence. Once there is evidence that could amount to provocation it is for the prosecution to make the jury sure of the absence of provocation. The courts are sometimes thought to stretch circumstances to found such a defence, as it enables the judge to pass a sentence commensurate with the facts of the case, that is, it takes into account the woman's previous suffering.

The Law Commission (2004) reviewed the law on homicide and sentencing options in multiple jurisdictions and found variation in definition, the significance of the intent to kill and the sentencing options (Law Commission 2004: 22–25). This Commission was tasked with considering the issue of partial defences to murder, that is, both 'provocation' and 'diminished responsibility'; this was also with specific reference to the issue of domestic violence, which had featured in recent case law (Ahluwahlia 1993; Thornton 1996).[4] It made a series of recommendations; these have been partially accepted. These included reforming, but not abolishing, the defence of 'provocation', as well as maintaining the separate defences of 'diminished responsibility' and 'provocation'.

----

[4] The Ahluwahlia Case, which was concluded on appeal in 1992, was led by Southall Black Sisters – www.southhallblacksisters.org.uk – a campaigning group who supported Kiranjit Ahluwahlia through her case and publicized the background issue of domestic violence.

Current sentencing issues

The Homicide Act allows for only one sentence following a conviction for murder and that is life imprisonment. This is different from either a successful defence to murder of 'diminished responsibility or 'provocation', where the judge has a wider range of sentencing options for the lesser conviction of manslaughter. It is in considering the flexibility afforded by manslaughter verdicts that one sees the arguments for the abolition of the mandatory life sentence for murder. However, this flexibility has been eroded by recent legislation and has substantially changed the situation for those with mental health problems convicted of serious offences.

Manslaughter is a serious offence as defined by the Powers of Criminal Courts (Sentencing) Act 2000. People with mental health problems convicted of a second serious offence committed between October 1997 and April 2005 would not be able to be sentenced to a hospital order but would be subject to an automatic life sentence.[5] This sentence might, of course, be served at least in part in a hospital setting if it was deemed appropriate to transfer that person to hospital from prison.

A further change is that anyone convicted of manslaughter after April 2005 would be subject to the Criminal Justice Act 2003. Within this Act are mandatory provisions for assessing danger-ousness and significant risk of serious harm being occasioned. Therefore, even if the defendant is suffering from a mental illness, he or she could still be sentenced to a discretionary life sentence or sentenced for public protection if the criteria are met. Once again, a hospital order is less likely to be imposed than hitherto.

Questions of dangerousness and assessment of risk of serious harm to the public have been brought to the forefront of sentencing by the Criminal Justice Act 2003 for the majority of offences, not all of them obviously very serious offences. The emphasis on protection of the public has also been evident in the passage of the controversial 2007 Mental Health Act and the failed Mental Health Bills preceding it. Provisions for treatment and containment of those persons who present a danger to others have been a focus of public debate (Hansard 1999). It seems likely that future legal changes will be in the direction of more forceful risk management of offenders.

Although to date there has been no erosion of the specific protections and defences available to individuals with mental health problems charged with criminal offences (of any gravity), in practice the changing sentencing climate runs the risk of jeopardizing their care.

References

APA (American Psychiatric Association) 1994 Diagnostic and Statistical Manual 4th Edition. Washington DC: Author.

Hansard 1999: Col 601-3, 5 February.

Law Commission 2004 Partial Defences to Murder Final Report www.lawcom.gov.uk

WHO (World Health Organisation). 1992 International Classification of Diseases 10th Edition Classification of Behavioural and Mental Disorder: Clinical Descriptions and Diagnostic Guidelines. Geneva: WHO.

Cases

Ahluwahlia [1993], 96 Cr.App.R.133.

Bratty v. Att.-Gen. for Northern Ireland [1963] A.C.386, HL.

---

5 Section 109 with a tariff to be served.

Byrne [1960] 2 QB396 (Lord Parker CJ at p. 403).

R v. Burgess [1991] 93 Cr.App.R. 41, CA.

R. v. Quick [1973] Q.B.910, 57 Cr. App.R. 722, CA.

R v. Thornton(No 2) 1996 Cr.App.R 108.

Section 4(6) Criminal Procedure (Insanity) Act 1964.

Section 5 Criminal Procedure (Insanity) Act 1964.

Tandy [1989]1 WLR 350.

Chapter 20

Mental health law and the mentally disordered offender

Sameer P. Sarkar

Aim

To describe how laws are developed to manage mentally disordered offenders (MDOs).

Learning objectives

- To consider the purpose and history of mental health legislation
- To explain how mental health law works in practice
- To appreciate the ways in which mental health law is changing and still developing

---

Introduction

'The law, in its majestic equality, forbids the rich as well as the poor to sleep under bridges, to beg in the streets, and to steal bread.' This famous quote is from French author Anatole France, (pen name of Jacques Anatole Francois Thibault 1844–1924), winner of the 1921 Nobel Prize for literature. One can say that allowing the stealing of bread is hardly fair on the baker, and it would not be much of a society if everyone were sleeping under bridges, begging and stealing. However, faced with the limited options available to the poor, the hungry and the unemployed, breaking existing law may be the only way to survive. Most scholars on jurisprudence (philosophy of law) agree that there is a distinction between the law as it is and the law as it ought to be. Mental health legislation affects those who are vulnerable and stigmatized, and this chapter argues that often there is a gap between how such law is and how it ought to be. This chapter discusses the current, commonly used, mental health legislation. It focuses on the 1983 Mental Health Act (MHA; HMSO 1983) and outlines some of the issues this law failed to resolve. The chapter also describes the legislative changes in and the thinking that underpinned the 2007 Mental Health Act (HMSO 2007). All the references to the legislation will, of necessity, be to that of the law of England and Wales. Scottish law will be referenced separately when relevant.

Origins of the current framework and legislative principles

Legislation governing the involuntary hospitalization of mentally disordered patients has evolved since the first law of this kind was enacted in the eighteenth century. At that time, it was directed at vagrants by means of various Vagrancy Acts. These Acts gave way to the Criminal Lunatics Act in 1800. The County Asylums Act of 1808 paved the way for the proliferation of large local asylums that provided the bulk of psychiatric care until recently (Jones 1993: 36–37). Bluglass and Bowden (1991) noted that between 1808 and 1891 more than 20 Acts of Parliament were passed that were concerned with the care of the mentally ill in institutions. In the 65 years following the Lunacy Act 1890 there were a further seven Acts (eight including the Mental Health Act 1983), as well as numerous amendments.

It is obvious, from the very titles of these Acts, that originally mental health legislation was designed to care for (and perhaps protect) the unfortunate, the poor and the misfits. The earliest mental hospitals, following the stipulations of the 1808 Act, were built close to the edge of large towns. Asylums were often self-sufficient, not least because the standards of care laid down by the parliamentary reformers required that patients be offered work and other occupations if they were able. Despite oversight by regulatory authorities, public asylums were isolated institutions, and throughout the nineteenth century there was concern about possible abuse of patients, particularly the possibility of illegal detention (Jones 1993: 93–111). Although these concerns existed, fear of the mad was also prevalent, and Jones links this fear as one which may have resulted in the increasing numbers of the insane (see Bartlett this volume Chapter 1).

Both the police power of the state (the power to stop untoward behaviour) and the *parens patriae* power (the power of state to care for citizens, as if it were the parent) have been the jurisprudential basis for mental health legislation, especially in relation to the MDO. Not surprisingly, there have been stark polarities in the political interpretation of these powers, and the pendulum has swung from care to custody, and back to care again.

The Mental Health Act 1983 as amended 2007: background

This statute set out in detail the various provisions whereby compulsory powers of detention and treatment could be applied. For a detailed discussion on the 1983 Act the reader is referred to Jones (2003). The Mental Health Act (2007) was passed and given the Queen's assent in 2007, which makes further, substantial amendments to the 1983 Act. Known as the Mental Health Act 2007 (MHA 2007), this Act was implemented in 2008 with a revised Code of Practice relating to the new Act (DH 2008).

The twentieth century saw the passing of three major pieces of mental health legislation: the Mental Treatment Act 1930 and the Mental Health Acts of 1959 and 1983. Other smaller statute provisions were passed but were less important. The Mental Treatment Act 1930 was the first Act to allow for voluntary treatment. By 1957, 75% of all admissions to mental hospitals were voluntary (Bluglass and Bowden 1991). The 1959 Mental Health Act removed compulsory admissions from the Justices of the Peace and also introduced Mental Health Review Tribunals (MHRTs) for MDOs. The 1983 Act focused on safeguards and procedures relating to disorder and its treatment. For this reason, Eastman and Peay (1999: 1) called the Mental Health Act 1983 a 'misnomer' because it did not promote mental health but emphasized the framework for compulsory treatment. However, one could argue that providing the framework and safeguards with which mental health care is delivered is a legitimate societal, and hence legislative, goal, irrespective of whether it is called a Mental Health Act or Mental Health (compulsory treatment) Act. The government announced its intention to reform the Mental Health Act 1983 in September 1998. Reform was a long process and included the publication of a Green Paper, a White Paper and a Draft Bill, and a revised Draft Bill in 2004 (DH 2001, 2004). Parliament then established a Scrutiny Committee of Peers and MPs to report on the proposals. In March 2006, the government abandoned its plans to pursue a new Act and instead decided to amend the 1983 Act.

A fundamental assumption in mental health ethics is that overriding an individual's personal autonomy is justified if they lack capacity to exercise that autonomy. Mental health law worldwide (save in Scotland) assumes that the patient is by default capacitous or 'competent' but that their mental disorder has caused them to lose the capacity to make treatment decisions for themselves. Most jurisdictions require some assessment of capacity before legislation is invoked. This is not the case in English law. Detention under the 2007 MHA is possible even if the patient is able to make decisions for themselves and even if they are accepting treatment. The main justification for detention offered by the Act is risk, that is, risk to self or others. If the patient has a mental disorder and poses a risk, they can be detained in hospital. 'Risk' is not defined in the Act, and there are no procedural standards or safeguards about the assessment of risk.

Application of the 1983 Act as amended 2007: general practice

To apply the 2007 MHA the patient must be suffering from a 'mental disorder'. According to the Act, mental disorder means any disorder or disability of mind. In the preceding 1983 MHA, mental disorder was broken down into four categories: mental illness, psychopathic disorder, mental impairment and severe mental impairment. In the 2007 Act there is a single definition of mental disorder, and the four categories of mental disorder have been abolished (MHA 2007 s.1). For completeness, a discussion of the limitations of these categories follows, as these limitations contributed to their removal.

Curiously, although the other three categories were clearly defined, the term mental illness was not defined in the 1983 Act. The deliberations of various authorities with respect to the absent definition are summarized by Jones (2003: 12–13), who noted that the Butler Committee (1975 para.1.13) defined mental illness as 'a disorder which has not always existed in the patient, but has developed as a condition overlaying the sufferer's personality'. In 1974, Lord Justice Lawton said that 'mental' and 'illness' are ordinary words of the English language, with no particular medical or legal significance, which should be construed in the way that ordinary, sensible people would construe them. 'In this case the lay person would have said, "Well, the fellow is obviously mentally ill."' Lawton's 'man-must-be-mad' test clearly has the advantage of brevity (Hoggett 1984), and it echoes US Supreme Court Justice Kennedy's phrase that 'the term mental illness is devoid of any talismanic significance' (Kansas v. Hendricks 2002). However, it could be argued that adopting the Lawton view would mean that only a fraction of the population the Act was intended to apply to would be included; quiet madness would perhaps go unremarked by ordinary sensible people. In practice, psychiatrists often included schizophrenia, mood disorders and organic disorders within the legal category of mental illness.

Mental Impairment, severe mental impairment and psychopathic disorder were separately defined in s.1 of the 1983 MHA. These definitions suffered from the same criticism of being non-discriminating and tautological. It is important to remember that the 1983 MHA categories were not psychiatric diagnoses and were not synonymous with either the DSM-IV-TR (American Psychiatric Association 2000) or ICD-10 (WHO 1992) diagnoses of schizophrenia, mood disorders, organic disorders and other syndromes. Although it was true that most people with psychotic disorders were detained under the category of mental illness, and most people with personality disorders were detained under the category of psychopathic disorder, there was considerable research evidence (Blackburn et al 1990, 2003) to suggest that these old legal categories of detention bore little relationship to the patients' actual psychopathology. The categories were legal measures, designed by parliamentary draftsmen to ensure that the right people were detained for the right legal purposes.

In general adult psychiatric practice, despite increasing use of the compulsory admission sections of the 2007 MHA, many patients will be informal and receive treatment voluntarily. The 2007 MHA gives certain approved professionals and doctors powers to detain, assess and treat patients for their mental disorder without their consent and in the face of a flat refusal. It sets out in detail how long patients may be detained for assessment and treatment without consent, how they can appeal, and measures for their release from legal detention. For most patients, detention will end naturally when their mental state has improved; for others, they will seek a review of their detention by a Mental Health Review Tribunal. For details of the workings of Tribunals the reader is referred to Eldergill (1997).

In addition to the single definition of mental disorder, the 2007 MHA introduced key changes with respect to the criteria for detention and the role of professional groups (see Text Box 20.1 for key changes). For a full description of the Act the reader is referred to Bowen (2007).

The repeal of the four categories of mental disorder potentially extends the group of people who are liable to detention for treatment under the 2007 Act, as disorders not previously covered can now be included, such as head injuries in adulthood. With respect to being detained for the purposes of treatment (rather than assessment), the 2007 Act abolishes the 'treatability test', replacing it with an 'appropriate medical treatment' test. 'Appropriate' is defined as being appropriate to the patient's case, 'taking into account the nature and degree of the mental disorder and all other circumstances of his case'. The definition of treatment has also been widened in the 2007 Act to include psychological interventions, nursing and specialist mental health habilitation, rehabilitation and care. The Act widens the pool of professionals eligible to perform specific roles. The Approved Mental Health Professional (AMHP) replaces the role of the approved social

---

Box 20.1 Mental Health Act 2007; key changes from the 1983 Act

- ◆ Single broad definition of mental disorder
- ◆ Criteria for detention
  - • Must have a mental disorder
  - • Nature or degree of the mental disorder warrants detention in hospital for assessment or for treatment
  - • The person ought to be detained in the interests of their own health and safety or for the protection of others
  - • Appropriate medical treatment is available
  - • Treatment cannot be provided unless the person is detained under that particular section of the Act
  - • An application for either admission for assessment or for treatment is made on the written recommendation of two registered medical practitioners
- ◆ Professional roles; broadening of the group of practitioners who can take on the functions previously performed by approved social workers and responsible medical officers.
- ◆ Amends the criteria for being a nearest relative or for being displaced as a nearest relative
- ◆ Independent mental health advocates will be available to patients
- ◆ Adults with capacity can refuse to accept electroconvulsive therapy (ECT) treatment even if they are detained under the Act. ECT treatment can still be given in an emergency
- ◆ The introduction of Supervised Community Treatment
- ◆ Changes in the referral procedure to Mental Health Review Tribunals
- ◆ The introduction of age-appropriate services for inpatients under the age of 18

Box 20.2 Mental Health Act sections affecting mentally disordered offenders

- Section 35/36: Transfer of accused but unconvicted defendants to hospital from courts
- Section 37: Allows for the detention of convicted offenders in hospital for treatment, as an alternative to a custodial sentence. Similar to a section 3
- Section 38: Transfer of offenders convicted but not yet sentenced for a trial of treatment (usually used to assess treatability of personality disorder)
- Section 41: A Restriction order, attached to section 37 in cases where there is a concern that the patient presents a risk of serious harm to others if released. It gives the Ministry of Justice some control over the patient's detention
- Section 45A: Allows for a convicted offender to be committed to treatment in hospital before a prison term is imposed
- Section 45B: Allows for section 45A offenders to be subject to the restrictions as in Section 41
- Section 47: Allows for the transfer of sentenced prisoners to hospital for treatment
- Section 48: Allows for transfer of unsentenced prisoners to hospital for treatment
- Section 49: Allows for sections 48 and 49 offenders to be subject to the restrictions as in Section 41

worker, and nurses, occupational therapists and psychologists can apply to train as an AMHP. Likewise, the pool of professionals who can take on the role of approved clinicians (AC) and responsible clinicians (RC) is no longer restricted to doctors but includes chartered psychologists, first level nurses, occupational therapists and social workers. The purpose is that patients will be able to have the most appropriately skilled AC appointed as their RC, although some decisions in the management of the patient must still involve a registered medical practitioner.

Mental health legislation for MDOs

Since Roman times, it has been recognized that a minority of psychiatric patients may commit offences under the influence of mental illness. The 1860 Criminal Lunatics Act allowed for the detention of such patients as an alternative to prison custody. Broadmoor Hospital was built in 1863 to house such offenders, who had been previously detained in a variety of settings, none designed explicitly for that purpose. Although MDOs can be subject to the ordinary MHA measures, there are particular legal measures set out in part III of the Act that deal with offenders who need psychiatric treatment and supervision (see Text Box 20.2).

Early diversion from court or custody

Court Diversion Schemes were designed to provide appropriate intervention for people with mental disorder charged with a criminal offence (HO 1990; James and Hamilton 1992).[1]

---

[1] This is different from situations requiring the use of Section 136 where a person's behaviour might normally result in a criminal charge but where the police are required to focus initially on the possibility of a mental disorder causing someone in a public place to behave in a sufficiently unusual way to warrant being taken to a place of safety for further consideration.

The primary function of court diversion is the transfer of people with a mental disorder from the criminal justice system to hospital, if their condition warrants this. Alternative outcomes, for example, outpatient follow-up, are not uncommon (Purchase et al 1996). Contrary to popular belief, prosecution is not necessarily discontinued.

The accused may be admitted to hospital under a section of the MHA 2007, or recommendations made for his treatment and care once the case is settled. Magistrates' Courts provide a convenient and timely opportunity to assess the accused; defendants appear promptly after brief periods spent in police custody. Defendants are then remanded either on bail or in custody. Offenders may also be seen in the community, on bail, or in prison on remand.

MDOs can be brought to hospital for assessment through at least two other routes. Section 35 (s.35) allows an accused person (except for those convicted of murder), on the order of a Magistrates' Court or the Crown Court, to be remanded to a specified hospital for a report on his mental condition. As with other sections of the 2007 Act, the accused must be suspected of suffering from a mental disorder. This has to be confirmed by oral or written evidence of a registered medical practitioner. In addition, there must be written or oral evidence from the approved clinician who would be responsible for the patient (or another designated person representing the managers of the hospital) that arrangements have been made for his admission to that hospital within seven days of making the order. For busy services with beds blocked, this can be a disincentive to using these provisions of the Act. An 'accused person' includes any person awaiting trial or those who have been tried and convicted and are awaiting sentence (except persons convicted of murder because the punishment of life imprisonment is fixed in law). The duration of the order is 28 days and renewable for up to 12 weeks on oral or written evidence of the approved clinician. Although a registered medical practitioner needs to provide evidence for the initial detention, the s.35 can be renewed on the evidence of the approved clinician, who may or may not be a doctor. The accused person is not required to be present in court when an application for further remand is made.

Patients detained under s.35 can be treated against their will under limited circumstances but only using the powers under part II s.2 or s.3. The courts have stated that this is appropriate (i.e. that parts II and III of the Act can co-exist and operate independently of each other). It has been shown that psychiatrists do not mind using the 'dual section' approach when they are faced with the prospect of treating someone against their will. However, there is a separate provision for treatment while on remand under s.36 of the 2007 Act. This is essentially the same as s.35 in scope but with the exceptions that it can only be passed by the Crown Court and that it requires the written or oral evidence of two registered medical practitioners. Orders are made initially for a period of 28 days, renewable for up to 12 weeks in total, in blocks of 28 days. Although two registered medical practitioners need to provide evidence for the initial detention, the s.36 can be renewed on the evidence of the responsible clinician, who may or may not be a doctor. Under both these sections, the accused may obtain an independent report on his mental condition from either a registered medical practitioner or approved clinician of his choosing and apply to the Court on the basis of it for the remand to be terminated.

Assessment and treatment of convicted offenders

Provisions exist for ordering admission to hospital for MDOs who are already convicted, depending on whether they have been sentenced (s.37) or are awaiting sentencing (s.38). Provision also exists for placing an MDO on a Guardianship Order under the care of the local social services authority (s.7).

For those offenders who have been convicted of an offence where it is thought more appropriate that they be treated in hospital rather than serve a prison sentence, s.37 of the 2007 MHA may be used. This order, often known as a 'Hospital Order', can be imposed by either a Magistrates' Court or the Crown Court. It is available for all offences except those whose penalty is fixed in law, that is, murder. Curiously, there is also provision that in extreme cases, where a Magistrates' Court is satisfied that the accused did the act, or made the omission charged, the court may, if it thinks fit, make a hospital order without conviction.

For the order to be made three conditions that have to be fulfilled:

◆ The offence is not one whose penalty is fixed by law

◆ The court is satisfied on the written or oral evidence of two registered medical practitioners (at least one of them being approved under s.12 of the Act) that the offender is suffering from a mental disorder as defined in s.1 of the MHA 1983 as amended 2007

◆ The court is of the opinion having regard to all the circumstances including the nature of the offence and the character and antecedents of the offender and other means of disposal available to the court that this is the most suitable mode of disposal available to the court

For a hospital order to be made, the court must also be satisfied on the written or oral evidence of the approved clinician who would have overall responsibility for the patient's case (or some other person representing the hospital managers) that arrangements for admission will be made within 28 days of the order being made. In cases where, despite earlier assurances, the bed is not made available (by no means a rare situation), the Secretary of State can make a direction for the accused to be admitted into another suitable hospital. Under the 2007 Act, the court must be satisfied that 'appropriate medical treatment' will be available to the offender in hospital and that the purpose of this treatment is to alleviate or prevent the worsening of the disorder or one or more of its symptoms or manifestations. The hospital order operates like the civil section 3 in that appropriate medical treatment may be given involuntarily and patients may in time appeal against detention to a Tribunal.

A similar order is available to the courts on conviction but before final sentencing, and is called an 'Interim Hospital Order' (s.38). This section of the Act gives the court powers to assess whether treatment is going to be beneficial and hence whether hospital is a suitable disposal option. If not, the case should be dealt with by a criminal justice route. This order is available to the courts for a period of up to 12 months. Prior to the 2007 Act, this section was most often used for an individual with a personality disorder where there was uncertainty about the patient's 'treatability'. Now that the treatability test has been repealed it remains to be seen how this section will be used.

Restriction orders

Section 37 of the 2007 MHA can be employed in conjunction with s. 41, which is called a 'restriction order'. This allows for restriction of the patient's movement and liberty at the discretion of the Ministry of Justice. When combined it is called a hospital order with restrictions (s.37/41). Section 41 is only applied to those MDOs who are thought to be particularly dangerous in terms of the risk of future violence. A restriction order can only be passed in conjunction with a hospital order and on a strict criterion that 'it appears to the court, having regard to the nature of the offence, the antecedents of the offender and the risk of his committing further offences if set at large, that it is necessary for the protection of the public from serious harm'.

A restriction order is always passed with a hospital order but a hospital order is not necessarily accompanied by a restriction order. In the majority of cases, orders are passed without limit of time; however, prior to the 2007 Act they could also be passed for a limited time (5% of all restriction orders). In the case of R v. Nwohia (1996), the Court of Appeal said that unless there is some foundation in the medical evidence for saying that the patient can be cured within a particular time period, it would be indeed unwise to put a limit on a restriction order. The Butler Committee (1975) recommended that limited restriction orders be removed from the statute books. However, they remained because, in certain cases, it was thought possible to predict consequent to recovery from an illness that led to the offence (e.g. endogenous depression) when the patient would cease to be dangerous. The 2007 Act has now removed this provision (s.40). Restriction orders are serious measures and can be passed only by the Crown Court, and can be made only if at least one of the two registered medical practitioners whose evidence was taken into account in making the s.37 gives oral evidence at the sentencing court.

Two points need to be made. First, the term 'antecedents' is construed by judges to include not only previous convictions but also accounts of previous unprosecuted dangerous behaviour made in psychiatric reports (subject to defence objections); some judges may also take account of previous unsuccessful treatment. A history of violence is of particular concern, especially if it appears that the violence is escalating. Second, the term 'serious harm' is not the same as serious risk of harm. The Butler Committee wanted to ensure that a restriction order is not passed for the petty recidivist because there is virtual certainty that he will persist in committing similar offences in the future. Serious harm also refers to the possibility of future serious harm as opposed to proven past serious harm. Hence a restriction order can be passed on an offender who has had no history of previous violence but has a potential for causing serious harm in the future. It is not necessary that the harm should be purely physical; a risk of serious psychological harm may also attract a restriction order.

Patients detained under a restriction order require ministerial consent before discharge, transfer and leave of absence. The Ministry of Justice also requires that the responsible clinician send regular reports on the mental state of the patient. There is guidance on the areas these reports need to cover but at the very minimum they should address the patient's current understanding of their offence, their level of insight into their mental disorder and their risk of re-offending. The restrictions remain in force even when the patient is conditionally discharged but cease to have effect once an absolute discharge from the section is made. A restriction order can be lifted only by the Secretary of State or by a Mental Health Review Tribunal if it orders an absolute discharge.

Section 41 is a legal measure. It is viewed by some as a very useful adjunct to treatment and by others as a further restriction of liberty. Irrespective of the view taken, there is no doubt that recidivism in post-discharge mentally disordered offenders is less than would be anticipated from the Offenders Index, which takes into account the demographics of an individual and their offending history (Ly and Howard 2004). It seems likely that the combination of both psychiatric and social supervision contributes to this, if only by ensuring that offenders are not completely socially isolated.

Mental Health Review Tribunals

The MHRT has the responsibility of hearing applications or referrals concerning people detained under the 2007 MHA. The point at which an individual can make an application depends on the nature of their detention. The Tribunal members are appointed by the Lord Chancellor and Secretary of State of the Ministry of Justice and are independent of the detaining authority.

The MHRT's substantive powers are limited to determining whether the conditions for continued detention are made at the time of their review. However, they have no powers to review the validity of the initial detention, and they cannot make any orders in respect of future treatment or placement of the patient. The Tribunal can order the discharge of a detained patient if it is not satisfied that the criteria for detention are met. The Tribunal can discharge both unrestricted and restricted patients (s.41) but can only recommend the discharge of transferred prisoners or patients on hospital and limitations directions (s.45A, a hybrid order, see below) as the final decision is taken by the Secretary of State.

Applications can be made to the MHRT by the patient and their nearest relative (s.66, s.69, s.70, s.75) and referral can be made by the Secretary of State (s.67 or s.71). There is also a duty for hospital managers to make a referral in some limited circumstances (s.68). Patients detained on s.37 can make their first application to the MHRT after 6 months and before 12 months of detention, and then in any subsequent period of 12 months.

Assessment and treatment of prisoners

Prisoners are subject to the same safeguards against enforced medical treatment as an ordinary citizen; the Mental Health Act does not apply in prison. A prisoner who develops a mental disorder while serving a sentence may be offered psychiatric treatment by NHS in-reach teams or doctors providing basic medical cover in prisons (Sainsbury Centre for Mental Health [SCMH] 2007). However, the 2007 MHA allows for the transfer of both remand and sentenced prisoners to hospital if required. If a prisoner refuses treatment and their mental disorder means they are a risk to themselves or others they can be assessed for transfer. The 2007 Act may be used in the same way as for a non-prison population. In other words, to be removed from prison to hospital the Secretary of State must be satisfied, by reports from at least two registered medical practitioners, that the person is suffering from a mental disorder, the nature and degree of which makes it appropriate for him to be detained in hospital for medical treatment, and that appropriate medical treatment is available for him. Furthermore, patients transferred to hospital from prison under the 2007 MHA who are still within the timeframe of their original prison sentence are, in the main, discharged back to prison. Although possible, it is rare for such a patient to be discharged directly into the community.

Sentenced prisoners may be transferred under the provisions of s.47 of the Act, which acts in the same way as the hospital order (s.37). For prisoners who are not yet sentenced, persons remanded in custody, civil prisoners and those detained under either the Immigration Act 1971 or under s.62 of the Nationality, Immigration and Asylum Act 2002, there is provision under s.48 of the 2007 Act for their transfer to a hospital on the direction of the Secretary of State. The same criteria must be met as for s.47 but in addition, the person must be 'in urgent need' of treatment. The definition of 'urgent' is not clear and has often been interpreted narrowly. Hotopf (Hotopf et al 2000) remarked that between 1984 and 1996 the use of this section increased sixfold. The Reed Report (1992), the last major governmental review of the management of MDOs, suggested that this section should be applied where a doctor would recommend inpatient treatment if the same person was seen as an outpatient or in the community.

Sections 47 and 48 almost always have a restriction on discharge attached to them. This restriction direction is set out in s.49 of the 2007 Act and, although it theoretically only applies to cases when the 'Secretary of State thinks fit', it is an almost universal accompaniment to a hospital direction (s.48 or s.47). There are no statutory criteria regarding what constitutes 'fit', and it is entirely at the Secretary of State's discretion. The Secretary of State is not allowed to make a time-limited restriction direction. Section 49 has the same effect as a restriction order (s.41). The responsible clinician under the 2007 Act must send a report to the Secretary of State on s.49 patients, as for s.41 patients. When the offender is sentenced to a fixed term of imprisonment the restrictions will automatically cease on expiry of that sentence. The transfer direction (s.47) in this case is regarded as a 'notional' s. 37, but the restrictions cease. There is no way of reimposing them save for a new sentence for a new offence. The 2007 Act has left these provisions unchanged except that the responsible clinician replaces the responsible medical officer.

The numbers of people transferred from prison to hospital vary year on year but in the 1990s were between 700 and 800. Fewer than half of these were transferred as sentenced prisoners. In 2003, 67% of restricted patients admitted to hospital were prison transfers, the rest being on court orders, that is, s.37/41 (Ly and Howard 2004). Court and prison admissions account for less than 10% of all formal admissions to mental hospitals (Hotopf et al 2000).

In 1997, the Crime (Sentencing) Act gave rise to a piece of inventive legislation; the hybrid order (s.45A and s.45B). This legislation was developed because of concerns that offenders detained under the 1983 MHA under the category of psychopathic disorder, who did not respond to treatment, could not be sent to prison. This order allows the sentencing judge to commit the offender to both a prison term and hospital treatment. Limited to England and Wales, s.45A of the Act empowers the Crown Court, at the time of sentencing, to give direction for a prisoner's immediate admission and detention in a hospital, together with a direction (s.45B) that they are subject to special restrictions as in s.41. Although under the 1983 Act hybrid orders were available only to patients detained under the category of Psychopathic Disorder, the abolition of categories in the 2007 Act means that these sections can now be applied to anyone who has a mental disorder, within the meaning of the Act, and has been convicted before a Crown Court of an offence the sentence for which is not fixed by law. Under the 1983 Act, these orders were rarely used but kept on the statute books because it gave judges additional options; it remains to be seen whether they will be used more frequently in the future now that they can be applied to a wider group.

The jurisprudence of offender treatment

The existing legal framework clearly attempts to address both the need of offender patients for protection and treatment and the need to protect the public from any risk these individuals might still pose. However, there are a number of ways in which the current legislation is still ethically unjust; it may also conflict with other legal frameworks (see Text Box 20.3).

Ethical conflict

The first way in which the legislation may be seen to be ethically unjust is in its failure to ensure access to resources. Although the standard of the services offered inside prisons has seen a marked improvement in recent years, owing to the care being tendered through an NHS-contracted

---

Box 20.3 Problems with the existing legal framework

Ethical problems
- Unequal access to resources
- Public protection at the expense of service provision
- Assumptions of guilt
- Inadequate consideration of the link between mental health problems and offending

Legal problems
- Incompatibility with the 1998 Human Rights Act
- Absence of due process

service, prison staff still express concern that there are far too many mentally ill prisoners who are not covered by existing services or indeed existing legislation (Wilson 2004). The rate of suicide for both men and women is higher in prison than in the general population; remand prisoners are especially at risk (Shaw et al 2004). Outside prison, men are more likely to commit suicide than women, but the position is reversed inside prison; although suicides may now be diminishing in women (HO 2007; The Corston Report).

The second way in which the legislation may be unjust is in the balance of legal powers, which emphasize public protection over service provision. All the legal developments over the last 20 years that affect MDOs, such as the hybrid order, The Criminal Justice Sentencing Act 2002 and the 2007 MHA have emphasized risk reduction rather than access to treatment.

Every citizen is entitled to have their case heard by their peers (as represented by a jury) and have their guilt established in open court. Finite sentences may be considered fair, and even in the case of murder the penalty is fixed by law such that prisoners know when they will be eligible for release. The provision of the hospital order (with or without restrictions) potentially flouts these principles. A hospital order can be passed even when an offender has not been tried by a jury, or even without conviction being recorded if the court is satisfied on available evidence that he or she did the act or committed the omission (see above). In cases of unfitness to plead, the offender can be sentenced based on the 'trial of facts' which, by definition, does not need the offender's participation. More seriously, an offender can be diverted from the criminal justice/penal system without any determination of his culpability. The danger is that it will be assumed that they committed the act. This is, of course, different in cases of murder (manslaughter due to diminished responsibility) and the cases of insanity, but the majority of hospital orders are made on offenders who do not fit into either category. The law simply requires that the person is 'then suffering from mental disorder', which means at the time of trial, not at the time of the offence.

This situation raises an issue as to whether mental health legislation is being used inappropriately. Jurisprudentially, for mental health legislation to apply there should be some connection between the mental disorder and the offending. It is sometimes assumed that there is a connection, where there is none: for example, when offenders on remand become mentally ill and are transferred to hospital. They may then receive a hospital order, despite or perhaps because they have made a good recovery with treatment. However, if there was no relationship between the offending and their subsequent illness on remand, and they are no longer ill, the continuation of a hospital placement can seem peculiar. The addition of any type of restriction order means that such offenders are likely to be detained longer in secure treatment than they would have spent in custody for the same offence (Dell and Robertson 1988).

Legal conflicts

There have been legal challenges to English Mental Health legislation on the grounds of incompatibility with the Human Rights Act (HRA). In one recent case (R(H) v. Mental Health Review Tribunal [2002] EWHC 1522 (Admin); [2002] QB 1), the court found that it was incompatible with the HRA for the burden of proof detainee. Patients argue that they are detained without any involvement in the decision, and then have to prove either that they are no longer ill or that they are no longer a risk. This carries a heavy burden of proof. This burden is particularly problematic when the patient's own doctor gives evidence as both a professional and expert witness at MHRTs. Other bases for an HRA challenge include the length of time it takes for patients to have Tribunals and the failure to provide supervision for conditionally discharged patients.

Another major concern that has arisen out of the current mental health legislation is that the existing law provides little due process protection. Any detention, however justified, is a definite restriction on liberty. Apart from the incompatibility noted with regard to the burden of proof, there appears to be a similar but less discussed difficulty of evidentiary problems. In determining legality of detention, the Tribunals (which act as courts) apply a civil standard, that is, 'on the balance of probabilities'. However, some would argue that, in relation to liberty, procedural due process demands at least a stricter standard, such as 'preponderance of evidence' (about 75%–80%), if not the criminal standard of 'beyond reasonable doubt'. Not only is the standard of proof lighter for a serious matter such as liberty but the quality of evidence that is admitted in MHRTs would ordinarily be considered non-permissible, even in civil courts. Medical evidence is often uncontested, so that the Tribunal remains an essentially inquisitorial process (establishing truth) rather than adversarial, even though the matters examined are of a very serious nature. These include not only restriction of liberty, but in many cases, enforced medication too (Sarkar and Adshead 2005).

The role of the state: the Ministry of Justice and MDOs

The Ministry of Justice (previously the Home Office) has a role in MDO jurisprudence and law, primarily in relation to public safety. This frequently conflicts with the duty of mental health staff to promote patients' welfare (Eastman 2006a). To its credit, the Ministry of Justice's outlook on how to best manage the risks from MDOs has been transformed in recent years, notably as a result of litigation but also due to internal reform and more direct liaison with clinicians (Ministry of Justice 2007). The fact that the Ministry of Justice has the power to discharge or authorize leave for restricted patients says something about public confidence in clinicians' ability to predict risk. This power, despite repeated challenges in various courts, has remained unchanged for over two decades and remains unchanged in the 2007 Act.

For the purposes of the following section the Ministry of Justice is to be read as the Mental Health Unit (formerly C3 division of The Home Office). Besides case working with MDOs, (mainly patients on restriction orders), the Ministry of Justice has a policy unit whose remit includes education and research. Major policy initiatives, such as the Dangerous and Severe Personality Disorder programme (HO and DH 1999; see Chapter 16) and the reform of the Mental Health Act were Home Office projects, devised jointly with the Department of Health. The Ministry of Justice is also responsible for liaising with government agencies for input into other legislation connected to the public safety agenda. The Ministry of Justice does not purport to be welfare-oriented; neither does it purport to be a penal agency, although all of Her Majesty's Prisons and detention centres are administered by departments within it. As a public body, its decisions are open to judicial reviews and human rights challenges.

In addition to approving leave and transfer of those subject to part III of the 2007 MHA, the Ministry of Justice also is an interested party in all MHRTs involving a restricted patient. The Secretary of State has to file and comment on all reports submitted to MHRTs, both those of the applicant and the health authority. In straightforward cases, this takes the form of attaching a list of convictions and the antecedents of the index offence, and a comment on the suitability of the plan proposed by the responsible clinician in the name of the clinical team. The Secretary of State's submissions have the same probative value as any report presented, and although the Secretary of State is rarely represented in hearings, a hearing is not deemed to have been proper if the MHRT has not had the Secretary of State's comments. In more contentious cases, usually relating to patients detained in high security, the Secretary of State can instruct psychiatrists to prepare an additional report and have his or her position represented by barristers and lawyers.

The Secretary of State has a vital role in discharging restricted patients. Any restricted patient can be discharged, either conditionally or absolutely, if the Secretary of State deems fit, without the intervention or determination by an independent tribunal. If the Secretary of State is convinced, on representation from the responsible clinician or other professionals, that a discharge is appropriate (because it does not increase risk to the public), he or she can agree to any course of action, including a discharge. Conditional discharge on these grounds, initiated by the health authority, although rare, does occur, and depends on the merits of the individual case and the quality of the submissions. Absolute discharge through this route is understandably rarer.

Recent legislative developments

Prompted by the Michael Stone case (Hansard 1999), the Blair government focused some attention on people who were dangerous and had personality disorder (Mullen 1999). Joint thinking between the Department of Health and then Home Office led to proposals to change the law relating to mental health detention (see Chapter 16). The government established a scoping committee, chaired by Professor Genevra Richardson, to review the then 1983 Act and make recommendations for its future. The Richardson Report (1999) was widely welcomed by psychiatrists and patient groups. Notably, this report elucidated and made explicit the principle of reciprocity; that deprivation of liberty on the grounds of mental illness needed to be matched by the delivery of treatment and care for that illness. Further, the Richardson Committee suggested linking mental health detention with a determination of incapacity. The committee suggested that only in very serious cases, where serious harm was an issue, could there be a case for compulsion in a capacitous patient.

The government rejected almost all of the Richardson Committee's recommendations and proposed the first of its own Mental Health Bills, with their overt agenda of public protection (Montcrieff 2003). The professional disquiet that followed resulted in the proposals for pre-emptive detention on grounds of risk being dropped, although some psychiatrists argued that psychiatry could be involved in public protection in the context of the criminal justice system with psychiatry in a 'secondary, supporting role' (Coid and Maden 2003: 406). The government tabled two new Mental Health Bills in succession without giving the reason for the withdrawal of the first (DH 2001, 2004). The second draft bill was viewed as an improved version of the earlier one, although it did not address the issue of compulsion in relation to capacitous patients. The definition of mental disorder was expanded, the 'treatability' requirement for Psychopathic Disorder dropped, and proposals were made to make the tribunal system that reviews detention more efficient.

Whether or not those reforms were timely and wise, the publication of the second draft bill in 2004 achieved something rarely seen in the history of psychiatry. Opposition to the Bill was so universal that, for the first time, mental health charities and other pressure groups united with the Royal College of Psychiatrists (with whom they are often at loggerheads). At scrutiny stage, The Joint Parliamentary Committee also raised a number of objections, mostly on procedural issues (Eastman 2006b). The government announced that it would incorporate its proposed changes to 'amend' rather than replace the existing 1983 MHA, and this has resulted in the MHA 2007. This vindicated the many observers who claimed that the 1983 Act was workable and that its minimal working difficulties could be solved by amendments. Capacity issues have not been addressed in what is now the 2007 MHA; perhaps because the Mental Capacity Act 2005 came into force in 2007. In Scotland, however, a capacity-based Mental Health Act has been enacted (the first in an English-speaking Western democracy) and appears to be working well (see Chapter 35). When the 2007 Mental Health Act received the Queen's assent, approximately 10 years of legislative attempts to reform mental health legislation was at last put to rest. However, some of the concerns and criticisms that accompanied the 1983 Act and subsequent mental health bills still remain.

Conclusion

MDOs may receive treatment under ordinary mental health legislation, like other patients. More often they receive assessment and treatment under specific legislation that emphasizes the need for the public to be protected from such patients. One consequence is that forensic patients' wishes and needs, and a reasonable assessment of their risk, can be overridden by the fears of others. Repeated and widely publicized homicide inquiries can reinforce the public perception that psychiatric services exist only to protect the public from dangerous madmen. This may make clinicians more defensive. With the 2007 MHA now in place, it may be argued that not only is there a gap between how mental health legislation is and how it ought to be, but that the gap has widened.

References

American Psychiatric Association. 2000 Diagnostic and Statistical Manual of Mental Disorders 4th Edition Text Revision (DSM-IV-TR). Washington DC: American Psychiatric Association.

Blackburn R., Crellin C.M., Morgan E.M. and Tulloch R.M.B. 1990 Prevalence of Personality Disorders in a Special Hospital Population. Journal of Forensic Psychiatry 1: 43–52.

Blackburn R., Logan C., Donnelly J. and Renwick S. 2003 Personality Disorders, Psychopathy and Other Mental Disorders: Co-morbidity among Patients at English and Scottish High-security Hospitals. The Journal of Forensic Psychiatry and Psychology 14: 111–137.

Bluglass, R. and Bowden P. 1991 Principles and Practice of Forensic Psychiatry. Edinburgh: Churchill Livingstone.

Bowen P. 2007 Blackstone's Guide to The Mental Health Act 2007. Oxford: Oxford University Press.

Butler Committee. 1975 The Butler Committee on Mentally Abnormal Offenders, Cmnd 6244. London: HMSO.

Coid, J. and Maden, T. 2003 Should Psychiatrists Protect the Public? British Medical Journal 326: 406–407.

Dell, S. and Robertson, G. 1988 Sentenced to Hospital: Offenders in Broadmoor. Oxford: Oxford University Press.

Department of Health 2001, Reforming the Mental Health Act. Part 1: The New Legal Framework. Part II High Risk Patients, Cm5016. London: The Stationary Office.

Department of Health. 2004 Draft Mental Health Bill, Cm6305. London: Department of Health.

Department of Health, Mental Health Act 1983: Code of Practice 2008 Edition: Code of Practice 2008 Revised.

Eastman N.L.G. 2006a Can there be True Partnership between Clinicians and the Home Office? Invited commentary on . . . The Home Office Mental Health Unit. Advances in Psychiatric Treatment 12: 459–461

Eastman, N. 2006b Reforming Mental Health Law in England and Wales. British Medical Journal 332: 737–738.

Eastman N.L.G. and Peay J. 1999 Law without Enforcement: Integrating Mental Health and Justice. Oxford: Hart Publishers.

Eldergill, A. 1997 Mental Health Review Tribunals: Law and Practice. London: Sweet and Maxwell.

Hansard, 1999, 5 Feb, column 601–603.

HMSO. 1983 The Mental Health Act 1983, c12. London: HMSO.

HMSO. 2007 The Mental Health Act 2007, c12. London: HMSO.

Hoggett, B. 1984 Mental Health Law. London: Sweet and Maxwell.

Home Office. 1990 Provision for Mentally Disordered Offenders. Circular 66/90. London: Home Office

Home Office. 2007 The Corston Report, Executive Summary: A Report by Baroness Jean Corston of a Review of Women with Particular Vulnerabilities in the Criminal Justice System. London: Home Office.

Home Office and Department of Health. 1999 Management of Dangerous and Severe Personality Disorder. www.homeoffice.gov.uk/rds/pdfs2/occ79outcome.pdf

Hotopf, M., Wall, S., Buchanan, A., Wessely, S. and Churchill, R. 2000 Changing Patterns in the Use of the Mental Health Act 1983 in England, 1984–1996. British Journal of Psychiatry 176: 479–484.

James, D.V. and Hamilton, L.W. 1992. Setting Up Psychiatric Liaison Schemes to Magistrates' Courts: Problems and Practicalities. Medicine, Science and the Law 322: 167–176.

Jones, K. 1993 Asylums and After. A Revised History of the Mental Health Services: From the Early 18th Century to the 1990s. London: Athlone.

Jones, R.M. 2003 Mental Health Act 1983 Manual. London: Sweet and Maxwell.

Ly, L. and Howard, D. 2004 Statistics of Mentally Disordered Offenders 2003. National Statistics. London: Department of Health.

Ministry of Justice. 2007 Mental Health Unit Bulletin. No 1. Available to download at www.mentalhealthunit.com/guidance.html; accessed on 5 May 2008.

Montcrieff, J. 2003 The Politics of a New Mental Health Act. British Journal of Psychiatry 183: 8–9.

Mullen, P.E. 2003 Should Psychiatrists Protect the Public? A New Risk Reduction Strategy, Supporting Criminal Justice, Could Be Effective. British Medical Journal 326: 406–407.

Purchase, N.D., McCallum, A.K. and Kennedy, H.G. 1996 Evaluation of a Psychiatric Court Liaison Scheme in North London. British Medical Journal 313: 531–532.

Reed, J. 1992 Review of Mental Health and Social Services for Mentally Disordered Offenders and Others Requiring Similar Services: Vol. 4: The Academic and Research Base. Final Summary Report. Cm. 2088 London: HMSO.

Richardson, G. Chair Expert Committee 1999 Review of the Mental Health Act 1983. London: HMSO.

Sarkar S.P. and Adshead G. 2005 Black Robes and White Coats: Who Will Win the New Mental Health Tribunals? British Journal of Psychiatry 186: 96–98.

Sainsbury Centre for Mental Health (SCMH). 2007 Mental Health Care in Prisons Briefings 32 www.scmh.org.uk

Shaw, J., Baker, D., Hunt, I.M., Moloney, A. and Appleby, L. 2004 Suicide by Prisoners. National Clinical Survey. British Journal of Psychiatry 184: 263–267.

Wilson, S. 2004. The Principle of Equivalence and the Future of Mental Health Care in Prisons. The British Journal of Psychiatry 184: 5–7.

World Health Organisation 1992. ICD-10; Classification of Mental and Behavioural Disorder. Geneva: World Health Organisation.

Cases

Kansas v. Hendricks 1997, 521 U.S. 346.

R v Nwohia 1996 1 Cr. App. R. (S) 170, CA.

R(H) v. Mental Health Review Tribunal 2002 EWHC 1522 (Admin); [2002] QB 1.

Chapter 21

Childcare law and practice for forensic mental health practitioners

Sarah Lerner and Lib Skinner

Aim

To provide an overview of childcare legislation and practice as it relates to forensic mental health.

Learning objectives

♦ To outline the relevant childcare legislation and guidance relating to parents with severe mental health problems

♦ To describe the policies, decision-making procedures and agencies that enable effective interagency collaboration in protecting children

♦ To discuss and suggest solutions to practice dilemmas that may arise in working with mentally disordered offenders who are parents or otherwise closely involved with children

---

Introduction

Research in a range of countries shows high rates of psychiatric morbidity in adult populations (Andrews et al 2001; Jenkins et al 1997), and it is not surprising to observe that mental health difficulties in parents are common. Jenkins et al (1997) in the United Kingdom found 1 in 5 have alcohol or drug dependence and 16% have an anxiety or depressive disorder. Research has also demonstrated the impact mental health difficulties in a parent can have on his or her children (Cleaver 2001; Mowbray et al 2000; Seeman and Gopfert 2004). These can often result in disorganized parenting or neglect, and sometimes serious or even fatal abuse. Nevertheless, with the right support many mentally ill parents can look after their children. This is likely to be less true in the field of forensic mental health, where the nature of parents' offences, combined with their diagnosis, may suggest that they are too dangerous to care for, or even have contact with, their children.

Parents' rights and responsibilities

The Children Act 1989 defines who has 'parental responsibility' for any child under 18. A parent, or other person with parental responsibility for a child, is defined as having 'all the rights, duties, powers, responsibilities and authority which by law a parent of a child has in relation to the child and his property'.[1]

---

[1] s.3(2) Children Act 1989.

In English law there is no comprehensive statutory definition of these rights and responsibilities.[2] The law says that parents must maintain their children, provide them with food, clothing, medical care and accommodation until they reach 16,[3] and make sure their school-age children receive full-time education.[4] Parents caring for children under 16 commit a criminal offence if they ill-treat or wilfully assault, abandon or neglect them.[5] Those who do so because of mental illness may have a defence in criminal proceedings. Other childcare matters are mainly dealt with by the family courts.

Most parents are left to make their own decisions about how to bring up their children. Parents are presumed to be best placed to understand and meet their children's physical, emotional, educational and developmental needs, and children are expected to thrive best if they remain in their parents' care. There have to be cogent reasons for authorities to come between parents and their children. When parents' mental states affect their ability to care for their children or have contact with them, the state, or a relative, is more likely to intervene.

In cases where, for example, the illness is short term, it may not be necessary for any formal arrangements to be made. A person with parental responsibility can ask someone else to exercise it on his or her behalf under s.2(9) Children Act 1989, although it would be prudent for that person to have written authority in case of queries from any authorities. Under s.3(5) of that Act, a person caring for a child without parental responsibility is entitled to do anything reasonable to safeguard or promote the child's welfare.

Where a more formal approach is needed, proper decision making in this area requires understanding and communication between mental health and childcare professionals, although this is not always easy to achieve. Government guidance emphasizes the importance of professionals and agencies working together, especially where children are at risk.

Children at risk

When a local authority suspects that a child is suffering or likely to suffer 'significant harm', the local authority has a duty to investigate under s.47 of the Children Act 1989.

'Harm' means ill-treatment or the impairment of health or development. 'Ill-treatment' can include abuse of a non-physical nature, including exposure to domestic violence. 'Health' means physical or mental health. 'Development' means physical, intellectual, emotional, social or behavioural development.

Local authorities should ensure that children are seen, where this is reasonably practicable, to decide whether action is needed to safeguard children or promote their welfare. If access is refused they should consider taking legal action. Local authorities cannot avoid taking action because parents deny them access. Other local authorities, such as education authorities, housing authorities, health authorities, NHS trusts and so on, are required to provide relevant information to a local authority carrying out an investigation. In such cases, they are permitted to disclose confidential information without a parent's consent. Usually a child protection conference will be convened when a child is believed to be at risk. Professionals from different agencies will pool information about the family, and the parents will be consulted. A decision will then be made as to whether the child's name should be placed on the child protection register and on the plan to be put in place to ensure the child's protection.

---

[2] See chapter 9, 'Children's Rights and the Developing Law' by Jane Fortin, 2nd Edition 2003.
[3] s.1 Child Support Act 1991 and s.1(2)(a) Children and Young Persons Act 1933.
[4] s.8 Education Act 1996.
[5] s.1 Children and Young Persons Act 1933.

A parent who is unable to provide adequate care because of mental illness may agree that a child should be taken into care temporarily. He or she can make an agreement for the child to be accommodated under s.20 of the Children Act 1989 without court proceedings. In this case, the local authority does not acquire parental responsibility, and the child can be removed by the parent at any time. It is also difficult for the local authority to make long-term plans for the child.

Some parents may decide that they will not be able to care for their children in the longer term and neither will other family members. They can agree to them being placed for adoption, or actually adopted, without getting involved in court proceedings. If a mother gives consent before her child reaches 6 weeks of age, her consent will allow placement of the child only until that date.[6] Parents can also withdraw their consent to placement or adoption provided an application for adoption has not actually been made, but this may well result in court proceedings and the court dispensing with their consent if the child's welfare requires it.

This chapter looks at some common practice issues for mental health professionals, in the context of this legislation and related guidance, as it affects parents with mental health problems and their families.[7]

Practice issues for mental health professionals

Working together

Lord Laming presided over the inquiry into the death of Victoria Climbie, who was physically and mentally abused, and then murdered, by her great aunt and partner, after various agencies failed to identify or assess Victoria's needs. In his report (Laming 2003), Lord Laming emphasized the importance of support for families in protecting children and the fact that a child's needs and those of his or her family are often inseparable. Lord Laming also stressed that effective support for children and their families requires multidisciplinary input from a number of agencies.

In 2003, Pavitt carried out an overview of serious case reviews (previously called Part 8 reports) (Pavitt 2003). She explained that, according to 'Working Together to Safeguard Children'(DH 1999), the main purpose of a serious case review is to look at the factors concerned in the death or significant harm of a child. This includes consideration of abuse. There is a need to learn lessons to prevent further, similar tragedies. The reviews also seek to improve interagency working and ensure that children are safeguarded. Pavitt considers cases going back to the 1970s and comments with reference to Victoria Climbie (Pavitt 2003):

> The common denominators of poor information sharing, inadequate documentation and recording, lack of inter-agency communication, poor supervision of practitioners and above all lack of co-ordinated strategic planning to enable the tracking of vulnerable children from area to area, which have been highlighted in the other cases reviewed, are all too familiar and have once again been found wanting in Victoria's case.

Falkov (1996) reviewed a hundred cases of fatal child abuse and found that one-third of the parents had psychiatric disorders. The importance of the mental health professionals in this field is evident.

The Children Act 2004 s.11 places a duty on Strategic Health Authorities, designated Special Hospitals, Primary Care Trusts, NHS Trusts and NHS Foundation Trusts to make arrangements to ensure that, in discharging their functions, they have regard to the need to safeguard and

---

[6] s.52 Adoption and Children Act 2002.

[7] The Appendix (pp–pp) gives the interested reader more information on the detail of statute law in this area.

promote the welfare of children. Under the Act, Children's Trusts are being set up as a response to Lord Laming's report and aim to bring together all services for children and young people in an area. These include social services, education and health. There is a common assessment framework for all services and a children and young people's plan. Health bodies will be included through children's and maternity services, and mental health trusts will be pooled in through Child and Adolescent Mental Health Services (CAMHS). These agencies, as well as the police, probation and youth-offending teams, will have shared aims, not only to protect children from harm or neglect but also to improve their physical and mental health, emotional well-being, education, training and recreation, social and economic well-being, and their contribution to society. The agencies are required to work together in furtherance of these aims, to share information and resources and carry out joint assessments where appropriate.

The revised guidance 'Working Together to Safeguard Children'(DH 2006) is a lengthy document containing material on how to safeguard children in different situations. The document deals with the duties of health services in detail, and states (DH 2006: 48):

All health professionals who work with children and families should be able to

- ◆ Understand the risk factors and recognise children in need of support and/or safeguarding
- ◆ Recognise the needs of parents who may need extra help in bringing up their children, and know where to refer for help
- ◆ Recognise the risks of abuse to an unborn child
- ◆ Contribute to enquiries from other professionals about children and their family or carers
- ◆ Liaise closely with other agencies, including other health professionals
- ◆ Assess the needs of children and the capacity of parents/carers to meet their children's needs, including the needs of children who display sexually harmful behaviour
- ◆ Plan and respond to the needs of children and families, particularly those who are vulnerable
- ◆ Contribute to child protection conferences, family group conferences and strategy discussions
- ◆ Contribute to planning support for children at risk of significant harm, e.g. children living in households with domestic violence or parental substance abuse
- ◆ Help ensure that children who have been abused and parents under stress (e.g. those who have mental health problems) have access to services to support them
- ◆ Play an active part, through the child protection plan, in safeguarding children from significant harm;
- ◆ As part of generally safeguarding children and young people, provide ongoing promotional and preventative support, through proactive work with children, families and expectant parents
- ◆ Contribute to serious case reviews and their implementation.

Working Together to Safeguard Children also provides guidance as to steps to be taken in individual cases. The importance of health professionals having access to advice and support from named and designated child safeguarding professionals and undertaking regular training is emphasized. So too is the role of adult mental health services, including those providing general adult and community, forensic, psychotherapy, alcohol and substance misuse and learning disability services. They have a responsibility in safeguarding children when they become aware of, or identify a child at risk of harm. This may be as a result of a service's direct work with those who may be mentally ill, a parent, a parent-to-be, or a non-related abuser, or in response to a request for an assessment of an adult perceived to represent a potential or actual risk to a child or young person. These staff need to be especially aware of the risk of neglect, emotional abuse and domestic abuse. They should follow the child protection procedures laid down for their services within their area.

In addition, adult mental health staff should 'routinely record details of patients' responsibilities in relation to children, and consider the support needs of patients who are parents and of their children . . . using the Care Programme Approach'(DH 2006: 61).

Assessments of children in need are carried out in accordance with the 'Framework for the Assessment of Children in Need and Their Families'(DH 2000). This is to be used to gain an understanding of the child's developmental needs, the capacity of parents or caregivers to respond appropriately to those needs, including their capacity to keep the child safe from harm and the impact of wider family and environmental factors on the parent and child. The provision of appropriate services need not and should not wait until the end of the assessment process.

What the above-quoted 'Working Together to Safeguard Children' document does not address in detail are the difficulties experienced on the ground within social services and health authorities when mental health professionals, particularly adult services, and children's services need to work together. The new legislation and guidance contemplates unified assessments for children but does not explain how integrated services for all family members are to be achieved where adults with children have specific health needs.

The issue of integrating children's services and adult mental health services is at the core of the training manual 'Crossing Bridges' (Falkov 1998). This proposes an approach for clarifying how practitioners in specialist adult and children's services can prioritize arrangements for jointly supporting families in which mentally ill adults and dependent children live together. It suggests that opportunities for joint working exist at every stage from initial referral to assessment and treatment (Falkov 1998: 141):

> Staff in each service must respond according to the degree of urgency. Whilst there must be a priority on safety and the needs of the 'core' client/patient, ascertaining the needs of other family members at the same time will facilitate comprehensive assessment and planning of joint working opportunities.

If the situation is urgent,

> Workers in adult services must address the needs of an acutely disturbed adult, but will also be aware of the presence of children and will consult with colleagues in children's services as appropriate. This may require an urgent joint assessment or there may be options to make arrangements for joint assessment at a later stage. An adult worker faced with a child emergency should undertake a joint assessment with a member of the children and families team. Similarly a childcare practitioner faced with an adult mental health emergency should have the support of a colleague from mental health services.

(Falkov 1998:143)

Various suggestions are made for joint working, including the following:

- Formal and informal meetings and discussions
- Attending each other's meetings (case discussions, ward rounds, CPA (care programme approach) reviews, CP (child protection) conferences)
- Establishing a regular forum for reviewing cases and developing or modifying local protocols
- Joint visits can be vital for example to facilitate communication between parents and children about mental illness and to provide explanations about mental illness for parents and children (Falkov 1998: 143)

The Parental Mental Health and Child Welfare Network has been set up to promote joint working between social care and health staff working with parents with mental health problems and their children in adult mental health and children's services. The network has been set up by the Social Perspectives Network (SPN) on behalf of SCIE. It has a website (www.pmhcwn.org.uk) that contains a wealth of useful information for those working in this area.

Dilemmas for the adult mental health worker

Crossing Bridges (Falkov 1998) describes a range of parent–child interactions for parents or carers with a severe mental illness, from child fatalities and serious abuse and neglect at one end of the spectrum to a high level of care at the other.

This range may be at the root of the conflict often felt by adult mental health workers who are concerned about the children of their adult patients or clients. The adult workers will be understandably concerned for the welfare of their adult clients, and may fear that referral to children's services will provoke a draconian response, through the instigation of child protection procedures, whereas it is support that the family requires.

The Children Act 1989 s.17 places a duty on local authorities to provide a range of services to promote the upbringing of children by their families. The adult will also be entitled to an assessment of their need for community care services under the National Health Service and Community Care Act 1990. The child, if he or she is providing care for the adult, may be entitled to a carer's assessment. The adult may receive services under a variety of pieces of community care legislation, including the Mental Health Act 1983 s.117, and may also be subject to the CPA. The result of all of the above might be the provision of services such as help in the home, attendance of a CPN (community psychiatric nurse) to assist with medication, and attendance for children at nursery or after-school clubs, all of which could take pressure off young children who feel the need to escape their home situation. Thus, a referral to social services may well help children to remain at home, rather than lead to their removal.

The adult worker may also be concerned about their duty of confidentiality. Guidance exists on this in various publications (www.everychildmatters.gov.uk). Working Together (DH 1999: 36) states as follows:

> Where there is a need to share information, professionals need to consider their legal obligations, including whether they have a duty of confidentiality to the child. Where there is such a duty, the professional may lawfully share information if the child consents or if there is a public interest of sufficient force. Where there is a clear risk of significant harm to a child, or serious harm to adults, the public interest test will almost certainly be satisfied. However there will be other cases where practitioners will be justified in sharing some confidential information in order to make decisions on sharing further information or taking action – the information shared should be proportionate.

Decisions in this area need to be made by, or with the advice of, people with suitable competence in child protection work, such as named or designated professionals or senior managers.

Parents admitted to hospital

If parents are admitted to hospital, it may be possible to make alternative arrangements for their children's care with family members on an informal basis, or the children could be accommodated under s.20 Children Act 1989.

Adult workers, especially nurses and hospital doctors, have a crucial role to play in ensuring that appropriate contact with children is maintained. Children's services may have to assess whether it is in the best interests of a child to visit a patient. All inpatient mental health services must have policies and procedures relating to children visiting inpatients as set out in the Guidance on the Visiting of Psychiatric Patients by Children in Home Office and Local Authority Circulars (HSC 1999:222; LAC (99) 32) to NHS trusts. There is specific guidance referring to visits to Ashworth, Broadmoor and Rampton (HSC 1990: 160), which sets out the assessment procedure to be followed. There is also guidance in the Code of Practice to the Mental Health Act 1983

(DH 1999). A visit by a child should only take place following a decision that such a visit would be in the child's best interests. The guidance emphasizes the importance of facilitating a child's contact with its parents or other key family members, wherever possible. Staff should think creatively about how to make the visit a positive experience. Clearly, joint working with children's services is vital to ensure that parents are supported in making arrangements to see their children. It will be necessary to consider where in the hospital the visit should take place and to ensure there is a child-friendly space available.

When it comes to discharge planning, consideration should of course be given to childcare issues, and to inviting children's social workers to CPA or s.117 aftercare planning meetings.

Mental health workers should be aware of the role of their Primary Care Trust's (PCT) designated doctor and nurse, whose duty it is to take a strategic lead on child protection across the PCT area. They should also be aware of their Trust's named nurse for child protection, who is accountable for child protection matters to the appropriate designated professional and to whom designated professionals provide advice and support.

Court proceedings

When there are court proceedings, the adult mental health professional may become involved in a variety of ways, as detailed in Text Box 21.1.

Capacity issues

If a person with a mental illness involved in court proceedings appears to be mentally incapable of instructing a solicitor, a psychiatrist may be asked to certify whether he or she is competent to do so. In other words, what is at stake is whether they can understand the nature of the proceedings and give coherent instructions on the issues in dispute. If certified as incapable they will require a litigation friend, and the official solicitor will normally take on this responsibility, instructing a solicitor to act in the person's 'best interests'. This may conflict with their wishes, as, for example, where the official solicitor believes that contact with her child may be detrimental to the mother's mental health. It is therefore important for the psychiatrist to understand that a person's competence or otherwise to instruct a solicitor will not be taken to imply competence or incompetence in other areas, such as her ability to care for her child, care for herself, manage her financial affairs, or live in the community. If the psychiatrist becomes aware that a person he or she certified as incapable is now capable of instructing a solicitor, he or she can provide a certificate of capacity, and the official solicitor's involvement will cease.

Box 21.1 Role of mental health professionals

+ Relevant and appropriate sharing of information with child agencies
+ Assessment of capacity to instruct solicitors
+ The nature of mental health problems clarified for the court
+ Risk assessment of parents
+ Facilitation of contact where a parent is detained
+ Assisting patients to understand their situation and ensuring adequate legal representation

Expert evidence

A report from an adult psychiatrist may be directed by the court in private law proceedings (e.g. where one parent has a mental illness and there is a dispute between the parents over the child's residence) or in public law care proceedings (e.g. care proceedings). An example in either case might be that the child's mother has chronic depression and is finding it difficult to care for the child. An adult psychiatrist may be asked for a report on the mother's mental state, symptoms, day-to-day functioning, any substance abuse, how long she is likely to remain ill, what treatment she will be getting and the likelihood of compliance with treatment and relapse. Questions may also be asked about her physical and emotional availability and responsiveness to the child and the risk of her becoming violent to the child or harming herself. The report may be requested from the treating psychiatrist or from an independent expert. In either case, the report must be objective. The expert's duty is to the court. A treating psychiatrist must be aware that if he or she writes a report in a case in which there is a potential risk of harm or prejudice to the child's welfare, it may be necessary to disclose the risk, thus breaching his or her patient's confidentiality, or to make a recommendation that is contrary to her interests and well-being. A person's medical records, including hospital records and nursing notes, are sometimes disclosed within family proceedings if this is considered necessary by the court.

A report from a forensic psychiatrist (dealing with risk assessment) may be required, commonly when there is a risk of sexual abuse or where drug or drink abuse is an issue.

The psychiatric evidence will be considered alongside other expert evidence. This may include the evidence of a child psychiatrist on any emotional harm suffered by the child, the evidence of a paediatrician on the nature and likely cause of any physical injury to the child or the evidence of the child's social worker or an independent expert on the mother's general parenting ability.

It is important that experts stick to their own areas of professional expertise. They must express opinions only in these areas and not seek to resolve disputed issues of fact (such as whether a person has used illegal drugs or committed violence). These issues should be decided by the court and often will be, in advance, to assist the experts.

The end of the case

If the child is to remain with the parent, it is important that there are agreed arrangements for liaison between mental health professionals and children's social services. These may include crisis plans in case of relapse or the need for further intervention. Clearly mental health professionals will have to be involved in contributing to the plan.

Whatever the outcome, the mental health professional has an important role in helping patients to understand the situation, and to ensure that he or she has legal advice before, during and after the court process.

Considerations for professionals in medium and high secure units and other forensic settings

Issues for nurses and other professionals dealing with patients in these settings are of necessity different to those of professionals working in the community or ordinary psychiatric hospitals. Their patients will often have committed a serious offence and may be ill and potentially dangerous over a number of years, resulting in a long period of detention in hospital. It is fair to say that where a person is convicted of a serious violent or sexual offence, their chances of being able to care for a child are remote, unless there is convincing evidence of likelihood of change within the child's timescale. Where a person is likely to be in hospital for a long time, for example, under a restriction order, other arrangements will have to be made for the child. It is likely that the only realistic issue for the patient will be some form of contact with the child, rather than the possibility of resuming care.

The mental health nurse can, in accordance with the hospital policy, facilitate a patient's request for contact with the child and ensure that the appropriate procedures are followed in consultation with the hospital social worker, named nurse, or designated professional. If face-to-face contact cannot be arranged, consideration could be given to indirect contact by letter or even telephone, but this must be done in consultation with those responsible for caring for the child, for example, family members or social services.

Where a child is placed with a relative, there may be intense family opposition to the patient seeing the child. This can be particularly difficult where the patient has harmed a family member and the individual child may be opposed to contact. If a child has been placed with foster carers under a care order, the care plan may deal with the issue of contact. If a child has been placed with a special guardian, or with adopters, the court should consider the issue of contact when making the necessary orders (see above). In many cases, to provide security for carers and children alike, contact with parents will cease if the child is placed outside the family. However, there will be cases where the child would benefit from some contact with the birth parent.

Conflict between the child's welfare and that of the parent

In many cases, parents with mental health difficulties will be more concerned than anyone to ensure their children's welfare. If possible, they will want to receive treatment and support to be able to care for their children at home. To achieve this it is important that professionals work together and ensure the needs of both adults and children are identified and appropriate services are provided. Both children's services and adult mental health services should aim to keep children at home with their families if possible and cooperate to provide the necessary support.

Removal of children from their parents should always be the last resort. Mental health professionals can help parents obtain legal advice when necessary to ensure that they are properly assessed. If assessments show they are unable to care for their children, a placement within the extended family should be found if possible. This is often more acceptable to the parent than placement away from the family. Where this cannot be achieved, mental health professionals have an important role to play in ensuring contact, if appropriate, and can also help patients understand and cope with their situation.

If the patient is properly advised and supported, it is likely that conflicts will be minimized.

Conclusion

Mental health problems are common. Having a child is common. The problems that this chapter has considered are, therefore, common. Forensic practitioners are used to dealing with adults who pose significant risks to others. To conceptualize them as people with children and rather ordinary parental experiences and feelings can require considerable imagination. It is also true that some forensic patients will pose risks to their own and other children, and may themselves be painfully aware of that.

The law described in this chapter supports workers who find themselves in these delicate clinical encounters. Such workers are not expected to be lawyers. Nonetheless, forensic practitioners must pay heed to the law and need to know when it might be invoked. The law and its detailed guidance are intended to support forensic practitioners in often complex interagency work, where the final decisions may rely on their clinical work and the evidence they provide to the courts.

References

Andrews, G., Henderson, S. and Hall, W. 2001 Prevalence, Co-morbidity, Disability and Service Utilisation: Overview of the Australian National Mental Health Survey. British Journal of Psychiatry 178: 145–153.

Cleaver, H. 2001 When Parents Issues Influence Their Ability to Respond to Children's Needs 273–286 in The Child's World: Assessing Children in Need (Horwath, J. Editor) London: Department of Health.

Department of Health (DH) 1999 Code of Practice to the Mental Health Act 1983. London: The Stationery Office.

DH 2000 Framework for the Assessment of Children in Need and Their Families. London: The Stationery Office.

DH 2006 Working Together to Safeguard Children: A Guide to Interagency Working to Safeguard and Promote the Welfare of Children. London: The Stationery Office.

Department of Health, Home Office 1999 Working Together to Safeguard Children: A Guide to Interagency Working to Safeguard Children. London: Department for Education and Employment, The Stationery Office.

Falkov, A. 1996 A Study of Working Together Part 8 Reports: Fatal Child Abuse and Psychiatric Disorder. London: Department of Health.

Falkov, A. 1998 Crossing Bridges. Lambeth Healthcare NHS Trust, Lewisham Social Services, Southwark Social Services and the Department of Health.

Home Office Circular HSC 1990/60.

Home Office Circular HSC 1999/222.

Jenkins, R., Bebbington, P., Brugha,T. et al 1997 The National Morbidity Surveys of Great Britain – Initial Findings from a Household Survey. Psychological Medicine 27: 775–789.

Local Authority Circular LAC 99 32.

Lord Laming 2003 The Victoria Climbie Inquiry: Report of an Inquiry. London: The Stationery Office.

Mowbray, C.T., Oyseman, D. and Bybee, D. 2000 Mothers with Serious Mental Illness. New Directions for Mental Health Services 88: 73–91.

Pavitt, J. 2003 The Role and Effectiveness of the Named Nurse in an Acute Hospital' Unpublished Doctoral Dissertation quoted with permission of the King's College, University of London.

Seeman, M.V. and Gopfert, M. 2004 Parenthood and Adult Mental Health 8–21 in Parental Psychiatric Disorder: Distressed Parents and Their Families (Gopfert, M. Webster, J. and Seeman, M.V. Editors) Cambridge: Cambridge University Press.

Childcare law and practice

Lib Skinner and Sarah Lerner

Parents' rights and responsibilities

The status of 'parental responsibility' is now automatically given to mothers, and to fathers who were married to them at or after the child's birth,[1] and to unmarried fathers of children registered after 1 December 2003 who are named on the birth certificate. Otherwise, unmarried fathers, stepparents and registered civil partners can acquire parental responsibility for their child or their partner's child by registering a parental responsibility agreement, or applying to a family court for a parental responsibility order.[2] An unmarried father involved in his child's life who applies to the court is increasingly likely to be granted parental responsibility, unless he is unable to play a positive role, for example, because of mental illness. The court can, however, cancel a parental responsibility order or agreement if it considers this appropriate.[3]

It is important, when advising parents, partners or other relatives, to find out whether they do have parental responsibility, as it can affect their rights to make decisions about a child, or to automatically be a party to any proceedings involving the child. If a person acquires parental responsibility by means of an agreement or a parental responsibility order, it does not mean that another person, for example, the mother, will lose it.[4] She will still be able to make decisions about the day-to-day care of a child who is living with her, unless the court orders otherwise.

Childcare disputes between family members

Many disputes about childcare between those with or without parental responsibility can be resolved by negotiation and agreement or mediation with the help of a trained mediator. Advocates may help to support the parent through this process. In some cases, family group conferences may be convened by social services, involving parents and other relatives or friends of the family, in the hope that the family can reach agreement themselves. For example, it might be agreed that a mother will look after her child unless she becomes unwell, when a selected family member will provide support or respite care for the child, and ensure that the mother seeks medical help. Otherwise, a grandmother may step in to look after the child while the parent is in hospital and agree contact arrangements with the parent. If an agreement is reached, it may not be necessary to apply to the court, unless an order is considered necessary to make the agreement legally binding.

If necessary, a parent or other interested person can apply to the family court for orders on any issues relating to a child's upbringing, the most common issues being contact and residence.

---

[1] s.2 Children Act 1989
[2] s.4 and 4A Children Act 1989
[3] s.3 (2A) Children Act 1989
[4] s.2 (6) Children Act 1989

A non-parent without parental responsibility may need permission from the court to apply.[5] In urgent cases, an application may be made without notice to the other party, for example, where a father is attempting to remove his child from the mother's care without her agreement; but in general, anyone with parental responsibility ought to be notified of the application. Individuals interested in the dispute may apply to be made parties to the proceedings. A family court can encourage the parties to reach agreement, perhaps involving an officer from the Children and Family Court Advisory and Support Service (CAFCASS).

If agreement cannot be reached or an order is necessary, orders the court can make under s.8 of the Children Act 1989 include the following:

- Contact orders, saying who is to be allowed contact with the child
- Residence orders, to decide with whom the child should live
- Specific issue orders, to decide particular issues affecting the child's upbringing (e.g. their health or education)
- Prohibited steps orders, for example, to prevent the child's removal by another person

An order may have conditions attached, for example, that contact should be supervised, or take place at a certain time or place. Once served, an order will be legally binding. In certain circumstances, a party breaching the order may be fined or committed to prison.

A person making an application to the court or responding to an application should be encouraged to seek legal advice from a solicitor specializing in family law, who may be able to represent them in the court proceedings. The solicitor may be able to obtain public funding from the Legal Services Commission, depending on the person's means. Their opponent's income will not be taken into account when assessing their means.

Individuals without parental responsibility for the child, for example, other relatives, may apply for orders under s.8, in some cases subject to the court giving them permission. In December 2005, special guardianship orders[6] were introduced for long-term carers (e.g. grandparents) who assume responsibility for a child because the parents are unable or unwilling to care for him. Non-parents who are granted either residence or special guardianship orders acquire parental responsibility for the child for as long as the order lasts.[7] A special guardianship order, unlike the other orders mentioned, also suspends the exercise of parental responsibility by others who have it. A parent may apply for the order to be discharged but will first have to show that the circumstances have changed since the order was made. However, unlike adoption, special guardianship is not irreversible, and does not give the child a new parent. It may therefore be appropriate if, for example, a parent is unable to care for a child owing to severe and persistent mental illness but will remain in contact with the child.

Certain actions usually require the consent of every person with parental responsibility for the child: taking the child abroad or changing the child's name (unless the court's permission is obtained), or agreeing to the child being placed for adoption or actually adopted. If a parent does not have parental responsibility, he or she will not automatically be a party to care or adoption proceedings, although he or she ought to be notified of the application and advised to seek legal advice about getting involved in the proceedings.

---

[5] s.10 Children Act 1989
[6] s.14A Children Act 1989
[7] s.14C Children Act 1989

When the court decides disputes about childcare it has to apply the principles of the Children Act 1989. Its paramount consideration must be the child's welfare. There is a welfare checklist that has to be considered in each case. The checklist includes the following:

1. The ascertainable wishes and feelings of the child, considered in the light of his age and understanding
2. The child's physical, emotional and educational needs
3. The likely effect on the child of any change of circumstances
4. The child's age, sex, background, or other relevant characteristics
5. Any harm the child has suffered or is at risk of suffering
6. How capable each of his parents, and any other relevant person, is of meeting his needs
7. The range of powers available to the court

There is a presumption that no order will be made unless it will be beneficial to the child and that delay in deciding the case will be prejudicial to the child's welfare.[8]

The court will consider evidence, including that of the parents and others involved with the care of the child. Often, expert evidence will also be obtained, and this may include adult psychiatric evidence.

Expert reports may be ordered under s.7 of the Children Act 1989, to provide the court with information, or under s.37, if the court considers care proceedings may be appropriate, for example, because none of the parties to the proceedings appears able to care for the child.

Local authorities and children in need

If a child is living with parents or other close relatives and is not thought to be at risk, local authorities are often reluctant to intervene unless the parents ask for help. However, under s.17 of the Children Act 1989, they are under a duty to safeguard and promote the welfare of children within their area who are 'in need' by providing a range and level of services appropriate to their needs. Children in need are those whose health and development are likely to be adversely affected without the provision of services, or who are disabled. The local authority should follow up any referral from another agency and assess the child's particular needs in the context of their family circumstances. They are also under a duty to promote the upbringing of children within their families, where this is consistent with the previous duty.

In theory, this should mean support being offered to the family before the child is put at risk, not simply when considering the child's removal into care.

Local authorities, in practice, rely heavily on the parents' cooperation when assessing the need for services to improve a child's well-being rather than to protect him from harm or neglect. The United Kingdom has signed up to the UN Convention on the Rights of the Child, which focuses on the child's right to develop to his or her full potential, but this is not directly enforceable in individual cases. Local authorities do have to comply with Article 8 of the European Convention for the Protection of Human Rights and Fundamental Freedoms, incorporated into domestic law by the Human Rights Act 1998. This prohibits them from interfering with both the parent's and the child's right to respect for their private and family life, unless the interference is in accordance with the law and necessary, for example, to protect the child's health, rights and freedoms, and is proportionate to achieving that aim.

---

[8] s.1 Children Act 1989

Where there is a conflict between a parent's right to bring up a child without state interference and the child's right to protection from harm, it is well established that the child's right has precedence. The situation may not be so clear when the child is apparently not at immediate risk of harm.

There is no formal registration procedure for children in need who are also not considered to be at risk. This can make it difficult for agencies to share or access information about particular children. If the government's plans for a national online directory of children[9] are successful, then, subject to strict controls, authorized practitioners will be able to find out who else is working with a particular child. This should streamline sharing of information and referrals to support services.

Child protection and the courts

When an initial investigation shows that legal action is needed to protect a child, the local authority normally holds a strategy meeting to decide what action is needed.

To remove a child from home urgently or, if appropriate, to prevent a child's removal – for example, from hospital by a mother after the birth – the police may take the child into police protection for up to 72 hours,[10] and will then hand the child over to the local authority for accommodation to be arranged.

Where a local authority is refused access to a child, or it or another person believes a child would otherwise be at risk of significant harm, an application may be made for an emergency protection order[11] to remove the child to other accommodation, or alternatively, to prevent the child's removal. This is only a temporary measure. The order will last up to 8 days, and can be extended, only on an application by a local authority or the NSPCC, for a further 7 days. The court may also require assessments, disclosure of a child's whereabouts by any individual, and, where appropriate, may exclude an alleged abuser from the home where the child is living, if the child's carer agrees.[12]

If a child needs to be assessed and the parent does not consent, the court can make a child assessment order[13] with or without the child being removed from the parent's care, for up to 7 days, where there is reasonable cause to suspect the child is suffering or likely to suffer significant harm.

None of the above measures gives the local authority parental responsibility for the child. Instead of or in addition to these measures, a local authority or the NSPCC may start care proceedings on the grounds that a child is suffering or likely to suffer significant harm attributable to the care he is receiving – or expected to receive – not being what it would be reasonable to expect a parent to give him, or the child being beyond parental control (the threshold criteria).[14] If the court is satisfied that there are reasonable grounds for believing that these criteria are met, it may – pending the final outcome – make interim care orders or interim supervision orders[15] that can be renewed up to the final hearing. At the final hearing, if the court is satisfied that the child was suffering or likely to suffer such harm, it may make a final care order or supervision order, but only if the order is necessary to protect the child.

---

9 www.everychildmatters.gov.uk/deliveringservices/contactpoint
10 s.46 Children Act 1989
11 s.44 Children Act 1989
12 s.44A Children Act 1989
13 s.43 Children Act 1989
14 s.31 Children Act 1989
15 s.38 Children Act 1989

Under an interim or final care order, the local authority will share parental responsibility for the child with anyone who has this already.[16] The child may be removed from home and placed with a foster carer or relative, for example, or may remain at home under a plan agreed with the local authority and approved by the court. If an interim care order is in force and the carer agrees, an alleged abuser can be ordered to stay away from the home where the child is living.[17]

Parents involved in care proceedings can obtain public funding for legal representation from the Legal Services Commission without a means test.

The child will, in most cases, be a party to the proceedings, represented by a solicitor, usually instructed by a Children's Guardian arranged through CAFCASS. In some cases, however, an older child may be able to instruct his or her solicitor directly.[18] The court will be presented with allegations and evidence relating to the threshold criteria and a care plan setting out the arrangements proposed for the child's care. Usually, care proceedings last between 9 months and a year, but they can last a lot longer.

Early on in the proceedings a timetable will be fixed for assessments by experts, for example, psychiatric reports in the case of parents with possible mental illness or personality disorders or a history of substance abuse, paediatricians' reports and/or child psychiatrists' reports where the child may have suffered physical or emotional harm, and assessments of parenting ability in respect of parents and other potential carers. Sometimes the parent and child may undergo an assessment in a residential unit, for a period of, say, 3 months, so the interactions between the parent and child can be observed. Sometimes the child will be placed in foster care and contact between the child and the parent observed at a contact centre. The children's guardian will also make enquiries and provide a report.

Experts may differ as to whether the parents can care for the child safely, whether there is a risk of relapse, or a prospect of improvement with treatment. Further reports may be needed if the situation changes.

Other family members who wish to be assessed as potential carers may wish to apply to be joined as parties to the care proceedings. Non-parents applying for public funding for legal representation will have to undergo a means test.

Once all the evidence has been obtained, the court will decide what order, if any, should be made.

If a final supervision order[19] is made, it will last for up to 12 months, but can be renewed to a maximum of 3 years if necessary. Under a supervision order, the local authority does not share parental responsibility, but a supervisor is appointed to advise, assist and befriend the child, and should visit the child at least every 6 weeks. The child may remain with the parent or be cared for by someone else. The supervision order will enable the local authority to identify any need for further support or intervention. The local authority can apply for a care order if at any time a supervision order is no longer thought adequate to protect the child from harm.

If a final care order is made, it will last until the child is 18,[20] unless a residence order, special guardianship order, placement order or adoption order is later made, or a successful application is made for its discharge. While the care order is in force, the parents should be consulted on all decisions relating to the child,[21] and be involved in regular reviews of the care plans. There will be

[16] s.33 Children Act 1989
[17] s.38A Children Act 1989
[18] s.41 Children Act 1989
[19] s.35 Children Act 1989
[20] s.91 Children Act 1989
[21] s.22 Children Act 1989

a complaints procedure if disputes arise.[22] Unless the court decides otherwise, local authorities have a duty to promote contact between children in care and their parents, and if contact is refused, the parent can apply to the court for a contact order.[23]

Where the child is to be placed with a relative, foster carer, or prospective adopter, the care plan should state whether the parent will be allowed direct contact with the child, and if so, how often. Alternatively, there may be indirect contact by letters or exchange of photographs or school reports.

If the plan is for adoption, the court may make a placement order,[24] authorizing the child's placement for adoption, either with the parents' consent, or if it is satisfied that this should be dispensed with. Once adopters are found and the child has been placed with them, they will acquire parental responsibility for the child. After 10 weeks, they can apply for an adoption order,[25] which will make them the child's legal parents, and extinguish the parental responsibility of the birth parents, the local authority, and any others who may have shared it with them.[26]

Unless the parents have requested otherwise, they should be told about the adoption application. However, they will not be able to oppose it if a placement order has been made or they have consented to adoption, unless there has been a change of circumstances since then, and the court gives them permission.[27] Consent of the parents to the adoption can be dispensed with if the child's welfare requires it, but before making a placement order or an adoption order, the court must consider whether any members of the birth family could care for the child or have contact with him, and whether any contact orders are appropriate. Very similar principles apply under adoption law as under the Children Act 1989. The child's welfare will be the paramount consideration.[28]

The needs of the child, the birth parents and the adopters for support services should be assessed; for example, for counselling services. Arrangements have been made to assist adopted persons over 18 to trace their birth parents, and, if they wish it, to assist their birth parents to trace them, subject to certain safeguards.[29]

---

[22] s.26 Children Act 1989
[23] s.34 and Schedule 2 para 15 Children Act 1989
[24] s.21 Adoption and Children Act 2002
[25] s.42 Adoption and Children Act 2002
[26] s.46 Adoption and Children Act 2002
[27] s.47 Adoption and Children Act 2002
[28] s.1 Adoption and Children Act 2002
[29] s.80 Adoption and Children Act 2002

Section 4

Ethical aspects

Chapter 22

Introduction to ethics

Gwen Adshead

Ethics is the discourse of 'ought' and 'should'; that is to say, it is the type of discussion we get into when we wonder what the right thing is to do. The study of what makes an action or position 'good' or 'right' is the study of 'morality'; ethics in health care is putting morality into action.

When we talk about ethics in forensic mental health care, we are talking about how forensic professionals decide what to do when faced with an ethical dilemma. Most ethical dilemmas have a number of features in common, even if they seem different on the surface. They usually involve a clash of moral principles, or a tension between observing a moral principle (e.g. always tell the truth) and the possible consequences of doing so. Ethical dilemmas, especially in psychiatry, often involve spending time considering different people's perspectives. This is often at a time when people feel anxious and therefore want to resolve things quickly. In forensic mental health, many ethical dilemmas involve a tension between the professional duty to care for the patient and to put their interests first (as most professional codes demand) and real anxiety that respect for the patient's interests may result in others being put at risk of harm.

There are at least two ways to approach the subject of ethics: ethical principles can be understood and ethical reasoning about real-life ethical dilemmas can be rehearsed. This section of the book attempts to do some of both. In Chapter 23, 'Principles of Ethical Reasoning in Forensic Psychiatry', core ideas are laid out with reference to the world of the mentally disordered offender. In Chapter 24, 'Ethical Issues in Secure Care', these principles are seen in action as they are applied to clinical settings. The final chapter (Chapter 25), 'Ethical Roles, Relationships and Duties of Forensic Mental Health Clinicians', takes this further. It explores some of the ideas in greater detail. It addresses how professional roles in health and social care as well as in the course of multi-agency work can generate ethical tensions and how these can be resolved.

The overall intention of this section is to leave the reader with increased skills in ethical reasoning and argument. This should build on the existing skills many readers will already have as practitioners in the forensic field. Unlike philosophy, practitioners deal with real cases where painful decisions do have to be made. Forensic professionals have a duty to make sure that they make the best-quality decisions that they can make: decisions that are honest, informed, humane and thoughtful.

Chapter 23

Principles of ethical reasoning in forensic psychiatry

Gwen Adshead

Aim

This chapter sets out ways of thinking about ethical reasoning in forensic psychiatry.

Learning objectives

- To understand the nature of ethical reasoning
- To appreciate the different approaches to making ethical arguments
- To understand how ethical dilemmas arise in forensic practice
- To understand why ethical reasoning is an important skill for forensic practitioners

Introduction

This chapter will draw on the established bioethics literature. At the same time, it shows how forensic practice challenges that literature and its principles in important ways. The terms 'psychiatry' and 'psychiatrists' are used throughout, reflecting the author's personal training and familiarity. Everything that is written here can apply to all forensic health care practitioners.

Theories of ethical reasoning

'Mores' and 'ethics' have Latin and Greek roots, respectively. Both once meant the 'customs' or 'habits' of groups of people; over time, both words have acquired slightly different meanings. 'Moral' has come to mean 'good', such that something that is immoral is bad, and 'morality' is the study and definition of that which is 'good'. Although some people also use 'ethics' as shorthand for 'good', for example, 'this is ethical', this should be considered a misunderstanding. 'Ethos' came to mean 'character', and ethics is thus about how to be a good character. Having established (by the study of morality) what a good person is, ethical reasoning is the process of deciding how people should act, so as to be a good person. For forensic professionals, ethical reasoning will relate to the ideal of the 'good' practitioner.

Ethics, therefore, is always about people reasoning and thinking, about applying a process of reflection. Rather than something being 'ethical', it makes more sense to say, 'This is ethically justifiable, because . . .'. Ethical reasoning is also about values, personal and professional, individual and social. Values are those beliefs, attitudes and feelings that inform and frame our personal judgements. Such values are, as it were, the 'spine' of our moral identity. Values are based on our experiences and our relationships. As they can change over time, ethical reasoning can come to different decisions at different times. Above all, ethics is the discourse of 'ought'

Box 23.1 Examples of approaches to ethical reasoning

- ◆ Consequentialist e.g. Utilitarian: Do that action which will maximize the best consequences
- ◆ Principlist e.g. Deontological: Do that action which reflects an over-riding moral intention
- ◆ Four principles of medical ethics
  - Respect autonomy of each patient
  - Do good for your patient (beneficence)
  - Avoid harm for patients (non-maleficence)
  - Respect for justice

and 'should'. Whenever we find ourselves using the words 'ought' and 'should' we know that we have moved from a factual discussion to an evaluative one; we are doing ethical reasoning.

The bioethics literature has expanded over the past 20 years. There has been an increase in different approaches to bioethical reasoning. The main approaches have between a *principles* (or deontological) approach and a *consequentialist* approach (Text Box 23.1)

A *principles* approach to ethical reasoning advises decision makers to apply ethical principles, such as 'do no harm', or 'always tell the truth'. An obvious problem is that there is no guidance as to what to do when principles clash. A *consequentialist* approach advises taking that course of action that brings about the best consequences: the problem here is that it is not always clear:

1. Who gets to decide
2. Which consequences will count
3. Over what time period

Consequentialist approaches emphasize the moral implications of the consequences of any chosen action. In contrast, deontological approaches emphasize the intentions of the actor, and the moral principles that inform his thinking and reflections on the ethical dilemma at hand. Deontology emphasizes the moral duties that arise between people, and how a reasonable understanding of these duties will help us to answer the question, 'What *should* I do in this situation?' as opposed to, 'What *can* I do?'.

Ethical reasoning and psychiatry

Two key assumptions are made here. First, decisions of enormous ethical import are taken on an almost daily basis in medicine, especially psychiatry. This implies that ethical dilemmas are not separate from the clinical realm, but are part of the bread-and-butter of clinical practice. It will not be possible for clinicians to avoid ethical issues by saying 'that would never happen in real life', or 'that's just a value judgment; you can't make value judgements'. Clinicians have to make ethical decisions and the challenge is to ensure that these are high-quality decisions.

The second assumption is that medical ethics is dominated by consequentialist approaches. This is problematic for psychiatry. It is not surprising that consequentialist ethics are important in medicine. All medical practice is teleological in nature; medical students are taught to act in ways that will bring about the best consequences for their patients. Utilitarianism and beneficence are built into the clinical framework of medicine; this is why clinicians so often confuse 'I can do this treatment' with 'I should do this treatment'. It is possible for those practising medicine (as described in the subsequent chapter) to conflate facts and values (Fulford 1989).

Although consequentialist reasoning in medical ethics seems obviously the most valid, there are problems when this type of thinking dominates in psychiatry, especially forensic psychiatry (Adshead and Sarkar 2004). First, consequentialist reasoning relies heavily on facts but psychiatry as a body of knowledge is low on facts and high on values. Although there is an evaluative component to all medical diagnosis and practice, the ratio of fact to value is much lower in mental health work than it is in say, orthopaedics or dermatology. Many 'facts' in psychiatry depend on the perspective of the assessor and may change with further information; much evidence is conflicting in nature. Psychiatrists are constantly evaluating whether behaviour or thoughts are 'normal' compared to the standards of the individual, that is, 'He's not normally like this', and the standards of a group, that is, 'We don't do this in our culture'. Thus when a psychiatrist says that he or she is just making a decision on the facts, we can bet that he or she is also making an ethical decision about values as well. The other problem is that consequentialist reasoning relies heavily on good-quality facts. If it is a fact that a good consequence will follow if a course of action is taken, then this will be used to justify that action, even if it also breaches an ethical duty, such as honesty. If the facts are uncertain, then the justification is much less reasonable.

A good example of this problem is in the area of risk assessment. Risk assessment and management are seen as necessary, clinical activities for all mental health practitioners. Risk assessment is part of hospital policy and drives other aspects of practice such as documentation, information sharing and use of mental health legislation; all of these have ethical implications in their own right. However, risk assessment itself is a type of consequentialist analysis. It is not just an account of what the facts are likely to be in the future, it is an evaluative analysis of the likely harm that might befall individuals. It also considers the costs to individuals and to large social groups. The very term 'risk' is shorthand for 'risk of harm', where the ethical imperative is assumed to be 'Prevent or avoid all possible harms'. Risk assessment is also subject to the usual criticisms of consequentialist reasoning. First, there is uncertainty as to which consequences are considered most important. Second, there may be a conflict of ethical principles and in the pursuit of one ethical ideal another may be violated.

There is another reason why consequentialist reasoning is not sufficient in psychiatry and needs to be backed up by deontological reasoning. Many people with psychiatric disorders break social rules, especially criminal laws. Psychiatrists, especially forensic psychiatrists, spend time evaluating whether an individual chose to break the rules or was internally compelled to by an abnormal mental state. This means that psychiatrists need to be thoughtful about how people form intentions and what the capacity to keep the rules means for any individual. Depending on what the psychiatrist says, blame or excuse will be attributed to someone who breaks the rules. Even if the consequences are the same, for example, lengthy detention in some sort of locked environment, it is significant whether people are held responsible for their actions. Psychiatrists fulfil an important social role in this process.

Decisions, decisions: ethics in mental health practice

Traditional accounts of bioethics and medical law assume a reasonably competent patient who can take decisions based on available information and their own view of the world. Doctors have a duty to respect their patients' autonomous choices, help patients make good-quality choices by providing them with information that is well and warmly communicated, and act in ways that are just to the patient and others. Doctors must generally tell the truth, not gossip and not behave illegally. Arguably a higher standard of behaviour is expected of them because they have to be trusted not to exploit other people's vulnerability.

Mental health practice makes this all more complicated (Bloch and Chodoff 2004; Radden 2002). First, mental disorders impair an individual's autonomy to make good-quality decisions in many situations, including treatment. Most mental health legislation assumes that mental disorders make people likely to refuse treatment that may actually help them because their disorder impairs their capacity to make a good-quality decision. Compulsory treatment is justified on the basis that the treatment refusal does not represent the 'real' choice of the patient; that he or she is not 'himself or herself'. Just as unconscious patients in intensive care may later say 'thank you' to their doctors for making it possible for them to recover, so when the mentally ill patient is his or her 'real self' again, he or she will be grateful for the treatment that has helped him or her to recover.

Psychiatrists often find that they are dealing with patients who lack capacity to make decisions for themselves, and they may be pushed into making decisions for their patients. This would be difficult enough, although this type of weak paternalism is common in medicine. However, psychiatrists may also find that although they are the clinical experts in the assessment of mental capacity, the patient does not accept their findings. It is important to remember that lack of individual capacity justifies others as well as doctors making decisions on one's behalf. In mental health work lack of capacity can justify compulsory detention, compulsory treatment and the removal of social privileges, such as voting. Assessments of mental capacity have enormous ramifications for the people with mental disorders.

Second, psychiatry tends to take a much broader view of beneficence and non-maleficence than other branches of medicine. Non-maleficence, in the form of risk assessment, has arguably moved from 'Do no harm' to 'Prevent all future harm'; this is a greatly expanded and probably impossible duty. A duty of beneficence to individuals has also become confused with a duty of beneficence to the public; only in mental health can a patient be detained for treatment for a condition that may cause danger to others alone. Most jurisdictions have legislation that makes it possible to detain people with infectious diseases for treatment of their condition, which will at least benefit *them* as well as others, that is, they will get better. In England and Wales, mental health legislation takes this one step further in making it lawful to detain people for treatment which should prevent deterioration, that is, not necessarily generate improvement in their condition. The consequence of this process is, de facto, to reduce someone's re-offending. This could be seen as a 'health gain', as health legislation is used to justify detention. Imprisonment can achieve the same health gain, but is seldom conceptualized in this way.

If mental health care practitioners do include a duty to protect the public among their ethical and professional duties, then this will inevitably mean that at some point the wishes of the patient and the wishes of society will clash. However, unlike other health care professionals, who can say hand-on-heart that their duty is to their patient, mental health professionals usually find that they have to negotiate this clash with the patient, in a way that is disturbing for all concerned. Unlike child protection cases, where it is assumed that the child's interests are paramount (and reporting of concerns is mandatory for some professionals), mental health workers can find that the guidance available to them is incomplete with regard to whose interests should prevail.

In these circumstances, it can happen that psychiatric patients' interests are seen as less morally compelling. This brings up the issue of respect for justice as part of morally justifiable practice in medicine. Justice in general medicine, as in psychiatry, involves fair access to resources. In psychiatry, professionals frequently encounter the vulnerable or the mentally ill and find themselves in positions of power and authority, backed by legislation. They have perhaps more opportunity than other health workers to exploit their positions, something that is inherently unjust.

Radden (2002) has argued that psychiatric practice is so different from general medical practice that it needs an ethical approach of its own. To some extent, this has been made explicit by the fact that internationally, psychiatrists have developed Codes of Ethics specifically for psychiatry (Sarkar and Adshead 2003). If we accept that psychiatry confronts specific ethical questions, we may also wish to examine the extent to which this is additionally true for forensic psychiatry, owing to its proportionately greater use of detention and its contact with an offending population.

Forensic psychiatry: locked in (and locking in) syndrome

There are two competing ethical principles running through forensic psychiatric practice: benefi-cence and justice (Adshead and Sarkar 2005). Whether it is the justice of the courtroom, or the social justice needed in secure treatment centres, forensic practitioners do not have an option on justice. They equally have the same obligations to treat all patients with respect, deal honestly with patients, and not share clinical information with others without the patient's consent.

Locking in

Forensic psychiatrists operate in two particular domains; in lockable facilities for offenders with mental health problems (prisons or forensic psychiatric hospitals), or in courts, where the ques-tion of how, why or whether an offender is to be locked up is determined. As we have seen, the psychiatrist may have a significant influence on whether an offender gets locked up in prison or hospital, or whether he gets locked up at all. Psychiatric testimony can be used in the criminal courts to determine the issues of guilt, mitigation and length of sentence, and disposal, that is, where the offender should go to serve their time. Appelbaum (1997) has suggested that in these circumstances the relationship between the forensic psychiatrist and the alleged offender is differ-ent, and gives rise to different duties. It is not that the evaluee's welfare is of no importance. Rather, the psychiatrist has a duty to the justice process, which is as great, if not greater, than the duty to the evaluee.

This argument seems compelling for the following reasons. First, our duties to each other arise out of our relationships. It seems obvious therefore that different relationships give rise to different duties; for example, we may be curious about the man who, when he sees both his son and a stranger in peril, saves the stranger in preference to his son. Arguably we have greater, more complex and more wide-ranging duties to people the longer we know them, the closer we are to them, and the more intimate the context. In a medical context, for example, patients may have different relationships with their GPs than with the surgeon who operates on them only once for a minor complaint. This is usually reflected in the ways that patients and their different doctors talk to each other. The purpose of the relationship is different; one is time limited, dis-crete and comparatively superficial; the other is ongoing, takes in different domains of the patient's life and can go very deep. It therefore makes sense that the psychiatrist who is only see-ing an offender for the court process has a different relationship with him than if they were in therapy together.

Second, as citizens, we all have an interest in ensuring that the justice process is as informed, diverse and complex as possible. This requires having access to good-quality expert testimony on issues before the court. The process of justice means that in an adversarial system, both sides need access to good-quality expert testimony. Justice is valuable because it concerns our freedom: both our freedom from interference and our freedom to be ourselves (Berlin 1969). For justice to flourish, the courts will need access to psychiatric testimony. This need not deprive any offender/ evaluee of treatment; it means only that the functions of treatment and expert evaluation will be distinct because the relationships are distinct.

This distinction is the nub of the counter-argument against psychiatrists as experts in the criminal court (and other legal fora, but the criminal court is most potent in this regard). It is argued that an evaluee will not make this distinction and will not appreciate that the doctor's testimony will not necessarily be in his or her interests. This may be particularly so if the evaluee is mentally ill or otherwise lacking in capacity. The only possible response to this is to acknowledge that there is a chance that this will happen and to take steps to try and ensure it does not. This means advising the evaluee repeatedly and clearly that the psychiatrist is not there as 'his or her' doctor.

Locked in

There are also unusual ethical dilemmas associated with forensic psychiatric care in locked settings (such as prisons or forensic psychiatric facilities). Some of these ethical dilemmas are the dilemmas that arise in the context of long-stay residential care for people with disabilities and disorders. When patients enter secure hospitals and prisons, they join a community: a community of the rejected, unwanted and unattractive. They also join a community of people who need help – who are dependent on the staff of the hospital not only for their welfare but also for control of their environment. Forensic practitioners know that they have a duty not only to care for their patients but also a duty to control them.

Forensic practitioners in locked settings find themselves with daily, not to say hourly, dilemmas, and have to decide whose interests come first. A primary dilemma is to balance the safety of the institution against the needs of any individual patient. A secondary dilemma is to balance the potentially competing needs of individual patients. Patients who attract staff attention may do so at the expense of the apparently undemanding, withdrawn individual. It might be said that these are better construed as clinical issues, but this neglects the fact that ethical and clinical domains overlap. Deciding to attend to one patient's needs over another's involves thinking about the following:

1. Ethical duties to both patients
2. The consequences of our actions, and failures to act
3. Our duties to the other patients on the ward
4. Our duties to the institution
5. Our duties to preserve resources

All these issues are ethical ones: about what we should do if we want to be 'good' practitioners. We know what we can do, clinically. We also know what we can do legally as well as the legal justification for our actions. However, neither clinical textbooks nor the law can help us to decide what we should do, morally.

Ethical tensions commonly arise in relation to information sharing and the duty to preserve confidential material. In general medicine and outpatient psychiatry, patients have rights over their own clinical information, which cannot be disclosed without their consent. As we shall see in later discussions, most clinicians want to disclose information about patients when they think that the patient presents a danger to others. Most professional guidance and legal advice supports breaching confidence to avoid serious harm.

In locked-in settings, patients (and prisoners) find out things about each other (and staff) that fall outside the normal domains of confidentiality. It is not uncommon for staff in secure psychiatric units to say, 'The patients know more than I do', including about fellow patients' health. This is not necessarily due to incompetent boundary keeping. It is more to do with the fact that the patients are living together in a loosely networked community, where news travels. This is not to say that staff should abandon attempts to keep personal information private and to treat clinical material with respect. However, there may be a need to think about autonomy and confidentiality in a different way.

Ethical reasoning in practice

Ethical dilemmas arise because of 'collisions' and differences between the interests and values of different groups or individuals; these may be irreversible and irreconcilable (Berlin 1969). Such situations cause anxiety, and decisions made when people are anxious are often not good decisions. Text Box 23.2 sets out the key points of ethical reasoning.

Best-quality ethical decision-making takes time: time to reflect on the nature of the issues and where the main tensions lie. There may be an ethical tension between the needs of an individual and the group. There may be an ethical tension between two members of the same family. Such tensions may relate to two conflicting ethical duties. It can feel like a decision must be made in a hurry, but this feeling is usually an index of the anxiety of one or more of the parties involved. It is rare in mental health that there will not be time to sit down and reflect for an hour with one or two colleagues. In fact, the more serious the issue, the more time it takes to do it justice. It might be argued that not making time to address the ethics of a decision indicates a lack of respect for all concerned. Again, actuarially speaking, decisions made in a hurry may miss certain vital pieces of information, which would otherwise be highly relevant (Surowiecki 2004).

The next step is elucidate the 'should' question or questions, so that the ethical dilemma is clearly set out, for example, 'Jim is smoking cannabis in his room; should I tell the police?' Note that this example sets out the facts from the evaluation. It paves the way for the following question: this is what is happening, what should I do about it, if I want to be a good practitioner? There may be facts that are relevant. This may include factual evidence that this has happened, the effect it has had on Jim and the evidence base about cannabis and mental health. These facts are relevant, but they do not determine the appropriate course of action. They will be part of the process of ethical reasoning.

The different perspectives of the different participants also need consideration. It may be helpful to set out how each party might see the issue in terms of the consequences and the principles involved. One way of considering this is to use the terms 'insult' and 'injury': What *insults* to human respect and dignity will arise from different courses of action? What *injuries* might arise from different courses of action? Even if the consequences are good, will the insult to feelings or dignity be so great as to diminish their benefit? It is important for all to express their view, and to be heard, partly not to miss out on any dissenting view that might contain important information

Box 23.2 Ethical reasoning in forensic practice

- ◆ Take the time necessary
- ◆ What is the 'should' question?
- ◆ Explore perspectives of all parties
- ◆ Insults and injuries
- ◆ Explore feelings aroused by the dilemma
- ◆ Keep a record of discussions

but also because it is likely that someone's view will be overridden in the end. Their sense of injury may be reduced if they feel they have had their say.

It may sometimes be helpful to discuss relevant legal cases. It cannot be emphasized adequately that the law is *not* the whole or complete answer to ethical dilemmas: ethics guides law, not the other way around. If one needs convincing that law and ethics are not the same, one need only look at the twentieth century race laws of Germany and South Africa, which were legal but not ethical. However, legal approaches to previous or similar ethical dilemmas will provide examples of how others have gone about the reasoning process.

It is also worth noting what negative feelings are associated with the ethical dilemma and asking the main protagonists about the feelings that are aroused. The reasoning process is likely to be clarified and enriched if people can speak honestly about their feelings. For example, if a staff member can say, 'If we do this, I feel it is being deceitful', this helps. This kind of transparency reduces the emotional temperature and elucidates another ethical principle for discussion. It may be, in this particular situation, that the patient really is to be deceived, and the sooner that this is accepted as a reality, the sooner the discussion can move on to the ethical issue, which is whether the deception can be justified.

Finally, all hospital professional and legal protocols would advise writing notes of the discussion and the decision. Although this is not an ethical point as such, it is evidence of the process of thinking. There are often many right answers to an ethical dilemma but only one can be chosen. To make it clear that the solution was arrived at by way of a good-quality discussion and not a knee-jerk response is to demonstrate respect for the patient. In forensic psychiatry many ethical dilemmas have significant consequences for patients. If we were in their situation, we would want to know that time and effort had been made to understand our views.

References

Adshead, G. and Sarkar S.P. 2004 Ethics in Forensic Psychiatry. Psychiatry 3: 15–17.

Adshead G. and Sarkar S.P. 2005 Justice and Welfare: Two Ethical Paradigms in Forensic Psychiatry. Australian and New Zealand Journal of Psychiatry 39: 1011–1017.

Appelbaum, P. 1997 A Theory of Ethics for Forensic Psychiatry. Journal of the American Academy of Psychiatry and Law 25: 233–247.

Berlin, I. 1969 Two Concepts of Liberty 118–172 in Four Essays on Liberty. Oxford: Oxford University Press.

Bloch, S. and Chodoff, P. 2004 Psychiatric Ethics. Oxford: Oxford University Press.

Fulford, K.W.F 1989 Moral Theory and Medical Practice. Cambridge: Cambridge University Press.

Radden J. 2002 Notes towards a Professional Ethics for Psychiatry. Australian and New Zealand Journal of Psychiatry 36: 52–59.

Sarkar S.P. and Adshead, G. 2003 Protecting Altruism: A Call for A Code of Ethics in British Psychiatry. British Journal of Psychiatry 183: 95–97.

Surowiecki, J. 2004 The Wisdom of Crowds. New York: Anchor Books.

Chapter 24

Ethical issues in secure care

Gwen Adshead

Aim

This chapter describes ethical issues that arise when working with mentally disordered offenders (MDOs) with severe psychopathology in secure environments.

Learning objectives

- ◆ To be able to discuss how an ethical understanding can contribute to the care of mentally disordered offenders
- ◆ To articulate the tension created by the ethical duty of care and control
- ◆ To understand the impact on autonomy of impaired capacity
- ◆ To outline the reasons why boundary violations within the therapeutic relationship are unacceptable

Introduction

Forensic psychiatric treatment often involves long-stay residential psychiatric care, where patients are detained for years. This type of care (which used to be the norm) is now increasingly unusual in psychiatric services, so that health care professionals may find themselves facing clinical problems that they did not meet in training, which places emphasis on community care and service user autonomy. Working in long-stay residential secure care with patients who have severe psychopathology of various kinds raises ethical dilemmas for health care professionals. What follows complements the discussion of ethical principles in the previous chapter by describing the ethical dilemmas in their clinical context and some practical approaches for dealing with them.

Background

The people who are detained in secure care have, by definition, been the cause of fear and serious harm to others in the wider community to which they belonged. They are also individuals with serious mental illness and severe personality disorders, often in combination; they frequently have histories of substance misuse and rule-breaking behaviours going back into early childhood. Although they are usually detained under only one Mental Health Act category (such as mental illness or psychopathic disorder), it is important to remember that these categories are legal constructs that bear little relationship to actual psychiatric diagnosis. Co-morbidity is the norm, so that most patients are struggling with multiple types of psychiatric problems simultaneously, which explains why they are often slow to respond to treatment and frequently relapse.

Furthermore, patients in secure care suffer from two other handicaps. First and foremost, they are people who have often experienced significant abuse and neglect during their early childhood (Coid 1992; Heads et al 1997; Mueser et al 2002). It is rare to find a forensic patient who has *not* suffered from physical, sexual and emotional abuse by caretakers; more commonly they have experienced all three. Some patients may have been placed in social security care from an early age and then had multiple changes of carer within the social care system; this can result in further abuse by state-appointed carers. These childhood experiences apply equally to men and women; men tend to have suffered more physical abuse and women more sexual abuse, but overall the prevalence of childhood abuse is the same in both sexes for people with serious mental disorders (McFarlane et al 2001).

What this means in practice is that these patients do not easily make therapeutic alliances with health care professionals. Rather, they tend to see them as potentially persecutory figures, who have to be kept at bay by a variety of means, including aggression, deception and seduction. Often forensic patients set up relationships with staff that are a repetition of early abusive relationships with previous attachment figures (Adshead 1998). Working with such disturbed people is emotionally draining for staff, who need ample time for reflection and concentration if they are to establish a 'secure base' for therapy, and not get caught up in toxic re-enactments (Aiyegbusi 2003). Even with support and supervision, staff may still find themselves in painful dilemmas about how best to manage a patient who seems unable to engage therapeutically (Adshead 1996).

The second disadvantage faced by forensic patients is that they are survivors of a disaster, where they were the disaster. They have to come to terms with what they have done, the impact of their offences on their own lives and that of their community. This is especially true for those who have killed, where there is no possibility of reparation. It is also true for those who have acted in non-fatal, but frightening or cruel ways. These patients have to be able to accept the reality of their capacity for cruelty, which involves the experience of painful feelings of shame, hopelessness, regret and guilt. These would be horrible feelings for anyone to experience, but they are even more of a challenge for people whose childhood experiences have left them with poor affect control and poor regulation of arousal.

Helping patients to take appropriate responsibility for their actions and the emotional states that either engendered or flow from them is the challenge faced by mental health professionals. It is possible to discuss this challenge in terms of the delivery of clinical care (see Adshead & McGauley, Chapter 14, p 179). At times it is also necessary to stand back from the immediate clinical action and consider the issues facing patients and staff from an ethical perspective. This ethical understanding is much more than a theoretical approach because it can then be very properly used to inform the clinical intervention.

The advantage that secure settings provide is time. They can also offer a type of physical environment that will help patients eventually to feel safe enough to engage in this painful psychological process. Forensic settings can also provide a multidisciplinary approach to treatment, essential for people with multiple types of problem. Staff also need time to build up therapeutic relationships, especially to make and maintain the boundaries that are necessary to manage relationships that will inevitably endure over months and years, rather than weeks. These therapeutic relationships will be governed by the tension between care and control, concepts of capacity, consent and confidentiality and professional ethical codes that are sometimes violated.

Staff have to relate to patients in different ways at different times. At one moment, a member of staff may be offering a therapeutic space to talk about a traumatic memory from early childhood; the next, they may have to physically restrain the patient, who may be threatening them or other people. Unwanted behaviours of patients may arise in individuals lacking capacity to take responsibility for their behaviour. This in turn may pose complex dilemmas related to the issue of consent. Disclosure of information about violence and past trauma, in particular, will force staff to address the need for confidentiality and safe therapeutic space balanced against the safety of third parties. Equally, staff have to manage different types of intense feelings aroused in them by patients, sometimes sympathy, sometimes hatred. Extreme feelings about patients that are neither acknowledged nor understood can lead to a range of boundary violations, including sexual contact and physical abuse. From the point of view of professional ethics, forensic health care professionals have a complex duty of care that explicitly includes a truthful relationship with the patient.

The 'two hats' problem: care and control

It has long been recognized that forensic professionals have dual ethical obligations: to their patients and to third parties who may be at risk from those patients. This notion of dual obligations is complex, and practitioners can be uncertain as to the correct course of action. The General Medical Council (2006) states (for doctors) that it is their ethical duty to make 'the care of your patient your first concern' but also says that there is a duty to manage resources fairly, which would indicate some sense that the patient's care may not be the only concern for the doctor. Similarly, what concerns the patient may not be the same as the doctor's concern; the case of a man who sought to ensure that he be tube fed even if unconscious or dying, suggests that although doctors have to respect their patients' wishes, they do not have to do whatever the patient requests them to do (Burke 2005).

Most health care professional codes are similar. Social workers (including mental health social workers), however, have an overriding duty of care to protect children; they are mandated to report to the local authority any concerns they have about a child at risk. In mental health teams, this may mean breaching patient confidentiality and that the patient suffers the 'harm' of being distressed and bereft. The key issue here is that there are times and occasions where the duty to the patient and their concerns will be 'trumped' by a duty to someone else.

Mental health services have always had to face the issue of responsibility for the protection of others. In Roman times, for example, there was an assumption that those family members who had the care of the mentally ill were responsible for their behaviour. As mental health services have developed, so they have been seen to be responsible for the behaviour of their patients. Department of Health guidance (DH 1994) suggests that if a criminal defendant has been in psychiatric care in the six months prior to his offence, there should be a health authority inquiry into the circumstances of his offence and the care he received. There seems to be an expectation that mental health services have a duty to manage the risk posed by their patients, which includes the protection of others who may be at risk.

There are a number of ethical issues that arise from this. The first is the scope of the duty of care to third parties:

1. How far should a professional go in protecting others?
2. How certain do they have to be of their facts?
3. Do they have to get the patient's consent to discuss their concerns?

There have been some legal cases on this issue, both here and in the United States. In the United States, the Californian Supreme Court ruled that therapists had a duty to 'warn and protect' any identifiable victim (Tarasoff 1976). 'Protection' could be effected by using relevant mental health legislation. In a similar case, the English courts found that health care professionals might have a duty of care to named individuals, who could be potential victims (Palmer 1998). The proposed

Mental Health Bill for England and Wales lays a duty on mental health care professionals to detain people who pose a risk to themselves or others and to share information with others to manage risk.

The second ethical issue is to decide what advice needs to be given to patients about professionals sharing information. Patients may understand that forensic staff cannot offer complete privacy and confidentiality of personal information. If there is an apparent risk to the patient's health, or to the welfare and safety of others, then forensic health care professionals do have a duty at least to discuss it with other professionals and to assess the risk. Therapeutically, patients can understand the need for staff to have this discretion to be able to keep their environment safe and secure in every sense. Ethically, it makes sense to advise patients on admission that there is limited confidentiality in relation to security issues. It should however still be possible to offer a stricter duty of confidentiality in relation to personal details, which are not so relevant to security. Giving advice like this is not only respectful of patients' dignity but also models a process of honesty and transparency, which is itself containing and trust-enhancing.

The most important impact of the dual obligations is the therapeutic one. Forensic mental health professionals will always have to operate on the boundary between their patients' concerns and society's concerns; sitting on a boundary is not always comfortable. Clinically, professionals may have to face their patients' rage and disappointment that they cannot always put their concerns first. Professional carers may find it difficult to disappoint patients and resent being made to feel like a jailer or policeman. Alternatively, mental health professionals may sometimes get caught up with the public safety role to such an extent that that they lose sight of the patients' vulnerability. In worst case scenarios, as happened in Ashworth Hospital in the early 1990s (DH 1992), staff can be physically abusive to patients in the name of 'control', or, as happened later in the same hospital (Fallon et al 1999), collude with patients in the name of 'care'. The take-home message is that being both a carer and a controller requires increased clinical competencies; forensic professionals have to have enhanced therapeutic skills if they are to manage the boundary well.

Capacity, consent and confidentiality

A key ethical principle in health care is that patients' autonomy should be respected, and patients should be free to consent or refuse treatment. The legal duty to get consent from patients before starting treatment reflects this ethical principle of respect for autonomy. The law assumes that patients making decisions have the psychological competence to do so; if they do not, someone else may, in certain circumstances, offer advice or recommendations about their treatment.

These key ethical and legal principles have to be rethought for psychiatric service users. For a start, many patients' capacities to make choices of any kind are compromised by their mental illness (there are also many physical disorders that also compromise autonomy, but that is a separate matter; see Sarkar and Adshead 2002). Second, the choices that many psychiatric patients do make may seem to be a product of psychopathological mental processes, such as delusions or hallucinations. For example, the choice to obey a command hallucination is scarcely an autonomous choice, or one that staff should automatically encourage or respect. Finally, most countries have some sort of mental health legislation because it is accepted that there are circumstances where people with mental illnesses may refuse to have treatment because they have no insight, and it is painfully necessary to force treatment on the patient involuntarily, without their consent, even in the face of their refusal.

Forensic health care professionals will be working with people with a compromised capacity to make different types of choice. It will not always be possible to respect their autonomy and support their chosen plan of action. For instance, an informal patient may wish to leave the hospital grounds to go to the local shop. Although he has a legal right to go, if the staff thought he was very unwell at that point, they might conclude that his wish to go should not be respected. The staff have legal powers to stop him from going, a reflection of the state's concern to protect people who cannot make choices for themselves. Forensic mental health care professionals are under the same duty of care as other mental health professionals, that is, to help the patient achieve a level of autonomy and self-care.

In secure settings, staff will have to deal with patients who are detained under mental health legislation and are unhappy about it. Their feelings of being coerced and exploited have an impact on the therapeutic relationship. Clinically, patients need to be allowed to express these feelings and have them understood. Ethically, patients may need help to understand how the wider community, from which they have come, manages its fear of people like them and the purpose of the mental health law to which they are subjected. Staff will also have to think about how they manage the increased power that they have over detained patients; bodies like the Mental Health Act Commission and the Prison Inspectorate exist because it is widely accepted that detained patients are at risk of exploitation and abuse by both staff and fellow patients. Sad, but true.

Finally, as described above, there are limits on confidentiality. This is a particular issue for forensic professionals who have to liaise with Multi-agency Public Protection Panels, charged with monitoring patients who are thought to be risky to others. At a practical level, staff need regular training in confidentiality. Wards or units need easy-to-read information sheets for patients. Given that staff will have to breach confidentiality from time to time, there is an ethical imperative to inform patients of this fact. In terms of justice, it is important to keep reminding patients of our dual obligations as forensic practitioners, and to acknowledge the tension that this causes in the therapeutic relationship. Staff need access to reflective practice time in their work to think about these tensions.

Boundary violations

Boundary violations are those activities by staff which reflect their personal responses to the patient that take them out of their professional role. The psychological origins of boundary violations and some suggestions for management are described in Adshead (Adshead & McGauley Chapter 14, p 179). This chapter discusses the *ethical* aspects of boundary violations.

Although most practitioners know that boundary violations are wrong, there is often very little discussion during training about why they are wrong. For instance, probably all mental health professionals know that it is professionally unethical to have sexual relationships with patients. They may not realize that this is a prohibition going back to antiquity. There are two ethical frameworks for understanding why it is wrong; one is in terms of consequences, the other is in terms of ethical principles or duties. There is ample evidence that sexual relationships with patients can cause harmful consequences, especially for psychiatric patients who are already struggling with psychological distress (Jehu and Davis 1994). In terms of duties, health care professionals who have sexual relationships with patients are exploiting the vulnerability of those in their care. Even if there were no harmful consequences, and even if the patient seemed to be agreeing to the relationship, it would still be an abuse of power. For many psychiatric patients, such an abuse of power by an authority figure will be a replication of particular events in their childhood, which explains why such violations are more likely to involve patients with histories of sexual abuse or borderline personality disorder (Kluft 1989).

Staff have a professional duty not to exploit the inherent vulnerabilities of the staff–patient relationship, especially in psychiatric services, where patients are particularly vulnerable. Staff also have a duty to protect themselves, by getting supervision for their work with especially difficult patients. An emphasis on the duties of the profession, and not the consequences, reinforces the ethical identity of the professional.

An emphasis on non-exploitation also helps us to see how boundary violations include many more activities than sexual ones. For example, consider the possibility that a member of staff borrows a significant sum of money from a patient. Even though no harm might result and no matter how apparently friendly the relationship between the patient and the staff member, it might be argued that the staff member would be exploiting their position of authority for their personal benefit. They would have stepped out of a professional and into a personal role.

As discussed in Chapter 14, there are many reasons why boundary violations are common in mental health practice, and not all of them are harmful. There are undoubtedly occasions where a member of staff will bring something of their personal experience into the professional inter-change, in a way that is less exploitative and intended to be helpful to the patient. For instance, if a patient is bereaved, their key worker may talk about their own experiences of loss and how they coped. Although such a conversation may involve self-disclosure, it is non-exploitative, intends benefit to the patient and does not satisfy the key worker's own psychological needs. However, if the key worker were to become tearful, such that the patient comforted them, this would be moving into the realm of the exploitative.

Both clinicians and managers will appreciate that this is a complex area, where it may be difficult to set hard and fast rules. It is, however, possible to set two rules: first, that staff have a duty not to exploit the vulnerabilities of patients; second, that sexual/emotionally mutual rela-tionships with patients *always* constitute exploitation. Ethically, staff have a duty to seek advice from trusted colleagues if and when they become aware of slippage in their professional role with a patient. Clinical managers, supervisors and institutions have a duty to take these concerns seri-ously and not act too hastily before there has been ample time for reflection and understanding of what has taken place. It is easy for both patient and staff concerns to be either ignored or acted on so swiftly and rigidly that important information, or opportunities for learning, may be missed.

Authenticity and truth-telling

Health care professionals are under an ethical obligation to tell the truth to their patients. At one level, this is no surprise. There is nothing about being a health care professional that gives one an option on honesty. There is legal authority that states that doctors must tell the truth when asked direct questions by patients about their condition and treatment, regardless of the consequences.

The ethical emphasis in health care has changed over the last 50 years, from beneficence to autonomy. It used to be accepted that doctors and nurses would sometimes not tell the truth to patients about their conditions, in case it might distress them. The message here seemed to be that health care professionals should not do anything that might cause a patient distress. Now the ethical imperative favours respect for autonomy, the patient is the one who is 'expert by experience'; they are the ones who generally should take the lead in managing their illness. The health care professional provides advice and information, which the patient is free to refuse. The patient controls all the information about himself or herself that he or she gives to the doctor. Thus the relationship is more one of partnership than dependency.

The obvious objection to this is that many patients are highly dependent on health services and need help in taking decisions. As stated above, the basis of most mental health law rests on the assumption that professional carers provide help and protection to their psychiatric patients. There is an added concern, which is that many psychiatric patients come to services because they are distressed, or cope with distress badly. Mental health care professionals may therefore feel an extra pressure not to distress patients further, by giving them potentially upsetting information, even when this is very relevant information.

This argument could be applied to forensic psychiatric patients, who are both vulnerable by virtue of their illness and the legal restraints imposed. Clinicians may be tempted not to tell the patient all the details of their case or their professional opinion because of the risk of distress. There is also the question of risk of harm as a possible consequence. Clinicians may fail to give patients information, or speak frankly to them, because of the risk that the patient will be angered and may act violently or threateningly.

As we have seen before, in terms of consequences, this may make good sense. However, there are two counterarguments that need consideration. First, it is not particularly respectful to withhold the truth from patients, or to deceive them, even for a good reason. In terms of harmful consequences, we may also need to consider the effect on the patient of finding out subsequently that one has lied to them, or been in some other way inauthentic.

Second, there is an issue of modelling authenticity. Most forensic patients have grown up in environments where people cannot be trusted to speak truly. They themselves have often acted in ways that are dishonest, and their dishonesty is often thought to be an aspect of their psychopathology. There is an extra duty on forensic mental health care professionals to pay special attention to authentic and honest communication. Not only does it pay attention to a principle of virtue, it also may have the effect of fostering trust. Patients value professionals who are 'straight' with them, even if they have uncomfortable things to say. There is also an important therapeutic need to model talking about uncomfortable issues because most patients will have to talk about very uncomfortable issues indeed during their therapeutic journey.

Honesty and authenticity seem essential components of an ethical approach to communication, even if in the short term it may cause the patient some distress.

Respect for justice

This chapter ends with a brief discussion of the importance of attending to one of the major principles of medical ethics, respect for justice. This ethical principle is one that often gets overlooked in favour of doing good, or not doing harm. In forensic psychiatric secure care there is an urgent need for professionals to pay attention to justice.

First, as forensic professionals, we are part of the criminal justice system that expresses condemnation of antisocial behaviour on society's behalf. We have no brief to be punitive (this is the prerogative of the court), but we are allied to a social system of judgement of personal behaviour. We are therefore at least partly bound by the same code of justice as the rest of the system.

Second, we have the care and control of individuals who have been deprived of liberty by a court. The possibilities for exploitation are great, not least because the patients can be so provocative. Respect for justice may help us to keep our negative feelings in check, therapeutically.

Finally, forensic mental health care professionals have dual ethical obligations. They cannot escape having concerns about risk to third parties as a result of knowledge that they acquire during their work. They may be required to act in ways that the patient feels is harmful to them, such as detaining them for lengthy periods, telling the Ministry of Justice about their behaviour on the ward or warning a possible identifiable victim. Given that we have the means, the opportunity and occasionally the obligation to act in ways that are unwelcome to patients, we need to pay the highest attention to justice and the process of justice. We need to be able to say, hand on heart, that we acted fairly and honestly towards patients, especially when we take steps that they vehemently oppose. In the end, it is a matter of respecting other human beings and recognizing how we would like to be treated.

Conclusion

This chapter has demonstrated that, without the capacity to formulate ethical argument within clinical discussion, even the most experienced practitioner risks uncertainty and sub-optimal clinical practice. This is a consequence of the gravity of the problems of individuals incarcerated in secure care. Their sensitivities and rights warrant respect, but their extreme behaviours and experiences must also be incorporated into multidisciplinary discussion. Part of this discussion needs to include a rigorous rehearsal of the ethical conflicts and wide-ranging and sensitive debate in coming to conclusions.

Key points

- Care of Mentally Disordered Offenders requires consideration of obligations to both the patient and to third parties
- Mentally disordered offenders often lack capacity which will affect the ethical duty to respect the autonomy of the patient
- Boundary violations are unacceptable because they constitute exploitation of the patient, whether or not harm results
- Patients' early experiences of dishonesty and abuse make it particularly important for staff to establish transparent and truthful relationships

References

Adshead, G. 1996 Written on the Body 110–115 in. A Practical Guide to Forensic Psychotherapy (Welldon, E. and Van Velsen, C. Editors). London: Kingsley.

Adshead, G. 1998 Psychiatric Staff as Attachment Figures. Understanding Management Problems in Psychiatric Services in the Light of Attachment Theory. British Journal of Psychiatry 172: 64–69.

Aiyegbusi, A. 2003 Forensic Mental Health Nursing: Care with Security in Mind 167–192 in A Matter of Security: The Application of Attachment Theory to Forensic Psychiatry and Psychotherapy (Pffafflin, F. and Adshead, G. Editors). London: Kingsley.

Coid, J. 1992 DSM-III Diagnosis in Criminal Psychopaths: A Way Forward. Criminal Behaviour and Mental Health 2: 78–95.

Department of Health. 1992 Report of the Committee of Inquiry into Complaints about Ashworth Hospital Vol I and II. London: HMSO.

Department of Health. 1994 Guidance on the Discharge of Mentally Disordered People and Their Continuing Care in the Community. LASSL 944. London: Department of Health.

Fallon, P., Bluglass, R., Edwards, B. and Daniels, G. 1999 Report of the Committee of Inquiry into the Personality Disorder Unit, Ashworth Special Hospital. Vol II. London: The Stationary Office.

General Medical Council. 2006. Good Medical Practice.

Heads, T., Taylor, P. and Lees, M. 1997 Childhood Experiences of Patients with Schizophrenia and a History of Violence: A Special Hospital Sample. Criminal Behaviour and Mental Health 7: 117–130.

Jehu, D. and Davis, J. 1994 Patients as Victims: Sexual Abuse in Psychotherapy and Counselling. Chichester: Wiley.

Kluft, R. 1989 Treating the Patient Who Has Been Sexually Abused by a Previous Therapist. Psychiatric Clinics of North America 12: 483–500.

MacFarlane, A.C., Bookless, C. and Air, T. 2001 PTSD in a General Psychiatric Inpatient Population. Journal of Traumatic Stress 14: 633–645.

Mueser, K., Rosenberg, S.D., Goodman, C.A. and Trumpetta, S.L. 2002 Trauma, PTSD and the Course of Severe Mental Illness: An Interactive Model. Schizophrenia Research 53: 123–143.

Sarkar, S.P. and Adshead, G. 2002 Treatment over Objection: Mind, Bodies and Beneficence. Journal of Mental Health Law 7: 105–118.

Cases

Burke c GMC and others 2005 EWCA.Civ10003. 3 WLR.1132.

Palmer v Tees HA and Another. June 1 1998 Court of Appeal, Times law Report.

Tarasoff v Regents of the University of California et al (cal 1976)131 Cal Rpt 14, 551 P2d34.

Chapter 25

Ethical roles, relationships and duties of forensic mental health clinicians

Nigel Eastman, Daniel Riordan and Gwen Adshead

Aim

This chapter describes special ethical problems inherent to forensic mental health practice and how different roles and relationships within forensic teams can lead to different understandings of ethical duties.

Learning objectives

- To understand more about the special ethical problems inherent within forensic mental health care and appropriate methods of ethical reasoning about those problems

- To appreciate the differences in ethical duties between the different professional roles

- To understand more about roles and relationships in forensic practice and their ethical implications

Introduction

Professional governing bodies recognize the importance of ethical decision making and publish guidelines (BASW 2003; BPS 2006; GMC 2006; NMC 2006) that are mostly based upon two theoretical approaches: consequentialist and principles-based ethics (see Chapter 23). However, as Radden (2002) argues, there are particular aspects of psychiatric practice (such as loss of mental capacity, involuntary treatment and the management of risk of harm to self or others) that suggest that traditional ethical reasoning can fall short in helping practitioners to negotiate complex ethical issues within mental health care.

If this is true for general mental health care, the problem is further emphasized in forensic mental health care, where other people, apart from the patient and (for example) doctor, have both clinical and legal interests in the patient's care, and a right to claim that their interests should also be reflected within the health care professional's duty of care. Each forensic patient will therefore usually find himself or herself at the centre of a network of professional relationships, where different professionals have different roles. Within this, professionals must not only relate to the patient, they must also relate to each other, while still keeping their ethical duty to the patient in mind.

Forensic mental health care professionals therefore need different ways of thinking about their ethical duties in the context of their different roles and relationships from those adopted within general mental health care. In this chapter, we use the different theoretical models of ethical reasoning to look at some of the practical dilemmas faced by multidisciplinary teams.

Relationships and ethical duties

A criticism of traditional approaches to medical ethical dilemmas has been the failure to think about the nature of the relationships involved; yet these are often at the heart of problems in decision making being difficult (Gilligan 1993). This is particularly true in psychiatry, where problems in relationships are often both at the heart of mental distress and also relevant to the therapeutic alliance and treatment outcome (Adshead 2002).

Forensic psychiatric patients usually have many different relationships with different professionals; from the moment they are first assessed until the, often much later, moment when they are discharged from forensic care. And the ethical nature of any one relationship may itself change over time, or between circumstances. For example, nurses may find themselves acting as therapists but then physically restraining the same patient, when they become disturbed.

Forensic mental health care is awash with complex ethical dilemmas, and practitioners can become frustrated by the apparent lack of a coherent framework with which to address them. Our natural wish for a quick, 'right or wrong' answer can increase frustration when facing what seem 'insoluble' dilemmas. However, ethics is essentially not about 'answers' but 'process'. That is, understanding the 'ethical nuts and bolts' of a particular situation, what consequences, rights and duties are 'in play' and what is implied ethically by making one choice rather than another. What is required is 'ethical insight', that is, knowing what you are doing ethically when you do it. Put another way, there is always the need ultimately to 'bite the ethical bullet', but this should be done with clear insight into the ethical implications of the *way* in which an ethical dilemma is resolved.

We discuss in greater detail common examples of ethical dilemmas from forensic practice in the next sections: assessment, treatment and treatment roles, risk management and detention.

Assessment

Within forensic mental health care there is particular emphasis laid upon assessment; whether, this is assessment for admission, assessment of risk, assessment for treatment, or assessment directed towards consideration of a legal question. It is crucial that the assessor think carefully about the nature of the relationship between himself or herself and the subject of assessment, given the purpose of the assessment. Yet commonly the subject may also be, or have been, a patient of the assessor, within a previous clinical context. Alternatively, the clinician conducting the assessment may have had no prior clinical relationship with the subject. For example, they may be carrying out the assessment at the request of the court, having had no previous knowledge of the person or with no intention of any future relationship. Thus there is commonly a 'dual role' to be negotiated by the clinician, who may retain a duty of clinical care to a patient and yet also have a duty to the court, either (or both) in terms of its pursuit of justice or the protection of others.

This latter problem is emphasized in criminal proceedings, where (usually) psychiatrists or psychologists may be asked to assess whether a defendant has a mental disorder, its relevance for guilt or innocence of a given crime, what sort of sort of treatment is indicated (if any) and what risk the person represents to others. Here the legal question asked by the court may bear no relevance to mental health 'care', but solely relate to whether the person should be convicted or to the length of imprisonment. It follows that, for example, the psychiatrist who is instructed by the prosecution will not necessarily have the defendant's welfare at heart. Hence for example, a defendant is unlikely to want a life sentence but the prosecution may be seeking this outcome and may want to use psychiatric evidence to justify this. Even a psychiatrist instructed by the defence may be addressing questions entirely unrelated to treatment. The problem of relationships is even more complicated if the defendant has previously been a patient of the assessor, so that the psychiatrist will have information about them that would normally be known only to someone with in a therapeutic role. The 'defendant' may not have wished to tell 'his' or 'her' doctor about certain things if he or she had known that it 'might get to a court'. Hence, there can be complexities concerning roles, both for the 'patient' (or 'defendant') and the clinician. Furthermore, there may often be the simultaneous wearing of two hats, both by the clinician and by the defendant/patient.

Crucial to approaching the problem of 'dual roles' is to be very clear about which roles are 'in play', and in relation to what, both for the clinician and the patient/subject. Such clarity should extend to the clinician being explicit and open with the patient/subject about the situation between them, be it 'sole role' or 'dual roles'. For example, one might say, 'Although I am a doctor, and although I am asked to see you by your lawyers, I am not here to consider whether you need treatment, or what treatment. I am here to assist the court in answering the question of . . .' Where the doctor is instructed by the Crown, the same clearly applies. In either case, it is also crucial to make it plain that the doctor is not there either to support or attack any defence that the defendant may put forward. The doctor is there solely to provide medical evidence that is potentially relevant to the defendant's legal situation. Similarly when undertaking risk assessments, one might say, 'Although I normally work with you as your nurse, today I am concentrating on assessing what sort of risk you pose to others, which may be used in your Mental Health Review Tribunal.'

Some people have argued that if one is transparent in this way about the different roles that one is taking, the patient can decide whether or not to participate in the interview, and therefore, there is no remaining ethical problem. Against this position, however, is the argument that it may be hard, perhaps impossible, for a prisoner not to see the assessing doctor or nurse as a healer and helper in the usual way; they may then unconsciously relax into the traditional way of relating to a health care professional and ignore the fact of dual roles. Indeed, the very reason that the clinician is there conducting the assessment is that they have clinical skills that will elicit information, which would be unlikely to be elicited by non-health professionals. Empathy, for example, therefore becomes a tool directed not towards patient benefit but towards the administration of justice. This problem is especially likely if there has been a therapeutic relationship between assessor and assessee, and is why assessments directed towards solely legal purposes should generally not be conducted by clinicians with either a past, or ongoing, clinical relationship with the assessee.

When the clinician necessarily maintains two roles simultaneously, or cannot avoid coincidence of different past and present roles, there is a question about which one should take ethical precedence, or how the balance between the two should be struck. Indeed, it can be argued that this 'balancing of distinct roles' is inherent to all forensic, perhaps even all, health practice, because every clinician always remains a 'citizen', with duties to the state. Alternatively, the clinician might ask, 'To what extent should I maintain the strict role which usually accords with my profession, for example, "doctor", or to what extent should I "take on" roles usually accorded to other professions or agencies in society, for example, as an agent of public protection?' In an increasingly 'multi-agency' world of mental health care, the latter can become emphasized, because clinicians increasingly 'rub up against' non-welfare, justice-related agencies. Certainly there will be 'cooperation' between health and welfare agencies and justice agencies. However, there is a risk that mutual cooperation may lead to contamination of one another's usually accepted social roles.

The latter is a particular issue in relation to risk and its assessment. Forensic mental health care professionals have skills and expertise in the assessment of risks posed by their patients. Normally, this is pursued within the context of the overall care of the patient. However, risk assessments may now be communicated into Multi-agency Public Protection Arrangement (MAPPA) Panels, established by statute and with which health Trusts are required to cooperate. Deciding what clinically derived information, for example, to give to MAPPA Panels is difficult, and there is a danger of simply 'describing all there is to describe', if only because sieving out what information is disclosable on the accepted 'breach of confidence' legal principles is time-consuming.

Assessments for legal purposes are not only conducted for courts, they are also carried out for the Ministry of Justice. Restricted inpatients are the subject of annual reports to the Ministry of Justice, which have to be supplied by their treating Responsible Clinician (RC). In this context, the extent to which psychiatrists see themselves 'in partnership' with the Ministry of Justice in managing 'restricted patients' is debatable (Srinivas et al 2006). Partnership would suggest common goals for the patient being agreed and operated for the patient. Yet frequently, the Ministry of Justice will oppose not only what the patient wants in terms of treatment, leave or transfer, but also what is recommended by the RC and the clinical team. This suggests that 'partnership' is a misnomer for the relationship between the two agencies (Eastman 2006).

Treatment and treatment roles

The very definition of what are the boundaries of proper forensic mental health practice is the subject of debate and dispute. One model, the 'traditional' therapeutically based ethical position, argues that the essence of such practice requires there to be *some* benefit arising to the patient, beyond merely the reduction of his/her risk of offending. An alternative model posits that forensic mental health care is centrally concerned with reducing risk, both to others and to the individual who is mentally disordered.

Another way of putting this dispute is to consider the extent to which forensic mental health care is about making patients 'feel better' or making them 'behave better'. The hope is, of course, that our treatments will do both. However, there may be ways of making the mentally disordered behave better which do not make them feel better. This may be to convert 'care' into 'management'. That is, if we just concentrate on making patients behave better, there is essentially little difference between secure forensic mental health care and other forms of public protection, including prison. The picture is further complicated by introducing (non-clinical) forensic psychologists into forensic mental health care settings, mainly in relation to treating personality disorder, to run 'offender management programmes'. This suggests that some NHS units are 'hybrids' of hospital and prison, with all/some the staff being similarly hybrid in their functions and roles.

How different forensic practitioners approach this question will have a significant impact upon their clinical practice *and* on the extent to which they are prepared to apply their skills to entirely *non-therapeutic goals*, that is, interventions that do not benefit the patient (other than by reducing their offending) but do benefit society by reducing risk. These interventions include not only treatment in secure institutions but also assisting courts, through providing risk assessments that can lead to longer, or indeterminate, sentences. Other contexts include providing reports to Tribunals which are solely directed at risk (either on behalf of the Ministry of Justice or the patient himself or herself) in relation to a patient's potential transfer or discharge.

Some might argue that if a patient is admitted to a secure psychiatric service, then all interventions are 'therapeutic' since, even though they may also reduce risk, there will be benefit to the patient; indeed, they will have a 'care plan'. This is an argument that is more sustainable in relation to patients with psychotic symptoms, such as delusions or command hallucinations, assuming that such symptoms can be linked causally to their offending. In these circumstances, it is clear that any therapeutic intervention for the psychosis will also be 'therapeutic for the risk'. However, this is not always the case, for example, with regard to people with personality disorders, or deviant sexual behaviour. Such patients may not really want treatment for the cognitive and affective distortions that give rise to their offending; they do not want to 'feel better', or may not 'feel better'.

They may understand that they have to behave better but they may not accept that their beliefs and attitudes about their offending are wrong.

Different members of the clinical team may take up different positions concerning the role of treatment. Nursing and social work professionals may feel that their duty is to bring benefit to the patient. Some forensic psychiatrists and psychologists may be more inclined to see reduction of risk as a 'therapeutic' goal, even if the patient does not agree. And, mental health legislation exists to ensure that people with mental disorders receive treatment, even if they do not think they need it and are resistant to receiving it. The counter-argument is that mental health legislation is directed at mental health care, not solely public protection. Indeed, in England and Wales we have a Mental Health Act, not a Mental *Disorder* Act.

A common argument put forward by forensic practitioners who veer more towards the 'risk reduction' philosophy is that it is in a patient's interests not to let him re-offend. This can most obviously be seen as a valid argument for mentally disordered individuals who lack the capacity to form the intention to commit given offences, for example, some of those who are grossly thought-disordered. However, such individuals will not sometimes, in any event, be found guilty of offending, and/or will receive a Mental Health Act disposal. By contrast, where a person has the capacity to be held responsible, it can be seen as 'their decision' whether to offend or not.

Risk reduction and confidentiality

The increasing reluctance of society and government to accept 'risk' implies that forensic clinicians may sometimes be drawn into activities that are entirely non-therapeutic. They can then be instrumental in assisting in 'preventive detention' by way of detention in hospital in the absence of real therapeutic benefit, or extended imprisonment. This may include being drawn into risk assessment where there is no prospect or intention to offer treatment, or 'real treatment'.

The Criminal Justice Act (2003) makes provision for fairly inflexible application of 'imprisonment for public protection' (IPP) based on 'detention until safe for release'. Such sentences can include the setting of very low 'tariffs' ('the punishment fitting the crime'), so that the bulk of any period of detention occurs through the continuance of risk. Against government expectations, as argued, the numbers of such sentences is already large, some 3,000 at the time of writing. It is increasingly common for an IPP to be imposed based on a risk assessment carried out by a psychiatrist or psychologist, with no prospect or intention of treatment. In addition to the problem of the forensic expert stepping out of any therapeutic role (which *may* be justified on the grounds of the clinician owing a duty to justice as a citizen) there is also a concern that the risk assessment tools or techniques used to justify such detention are neither adequately reliable nor sufficiently valid to justify their use in the taking of such grave decisions (Logan 2003).

Risk assessment may be of limited benefit to the patient or prisoner, albeit that discussion of risk behaviours is routine in both probation and therapeutic practice. Indeed, they may see it as potentially harmful to them, in that if someone's risk appears to others to have increased, their liberty may then be restricted, or further restricted, irrespective of their wishes. Even if this does not happen, details of their situation and condition may be communicated to others, including without their consent. Such a breach of confidentiality can be justified on the grounds of risk reduction.

The requirement of keeping confidence within medical practice rests primarily upon the principle of respect for autonomy, and has long been considered sacrosanct in medicine. It dates back to the fifth century BC and is enshrined within the Hippocratic Oath (Miles 2003).

> Whatever I see or hear in the lives of my patients, whether in connection with my professional practice or not, which ought not to be spoken of outside, I will keep secret, as considering all such things to be private.

Breaching confidence is legally and ethically acceptable when the patient has given their consent, where the law requires disclosure (either under Statute, including by way of a Court Order) or where there is a public interest in disclosure (Dolan 2004). In a forensic mental heatlh context, the latter is usually referred to as the Egdell principle; that is, non-consensual breach of confidence is permissible where there is a significant risk of serious harm to others in the absence of such a breach.

The Criminal Justice Act 2003 made provisions enforcing a 'duty to cooperate with the MAPPA process' for a range of criminal justice and health and social care agencies, within 'multi-agency working'. However, this does not include a duty to disclose information per se, which is still governed by case law (Royal College of Psychiatrists Guidance document, see www.rcpsych.org.uk).

At times, the 'perceived right' to disclose on the part of a doctor (or presumably other mental health professional) will be used. However, it is not yet clear whether the real effect of the Criminal Justice Act 2003, in which much disclosure will sit, will result effectively in a lowered threshold for disclosure where it occurs within MAPPA Panels. Certainly, whether lawful or not, the nature of MAPPA Panels is such that there will likely be pressure in that direction. The different duties of employers and practitioners that follow from this Act are also relevant to the extent and volume of disclosure. The need for public bodies, for example NHS Trusts, to support government initiatives aimed at public protection may be relevant in this regard. It is possible that there could be conflict for the clinician between their perception of their duty to their profession, or professional body, and their duty to their employer. Ultimately, of course, voluntary disclosure of information is the most desirable means of communication with justice agencies, and the doctor will wish to seek consent from his/her patient before offering disclosure. However, the very nature of the information potentially to be disclosed will often discourage the patient from consenting.

If the clinician adopts the assumption that ultimately their primary aim is one of risk management and public protection, then this will set a potential for conflict between forensic psychiatry and core medical ethics. In the latter context it can be argued that the *primary* role of forensic psychiatry should be the treatment of patients with mental disorder, for their benefit, with coincidental (albeit intended and important) benefit to the public. Within traditional medical ethics, therefore, 'prevention of re-offending' cannot amount to adequate justification for *non-consensual* detention aimed solely at risk reduction. Certainly, that is a stance which is capable of protecting the social role of mental health services from simply being that of jailer. That is, there must be 'some scintilla of benefit' to the patient arising from treatment other than mere risk reduction (Eastman 2006).

One further ethical tension relating to risk assessment solely for criminal justice purposes lies in the forensic practitioner applying skills and approaches that are essentially derived from being a mental *health* professional directed towards an entirely non-clinical purpose. Empathy is used by practitioners to foster trust and to encourage disclosure of sensitive information for the 'patient's' benefit. It is used for a different purpose in criminal-justice-related risk assessment, where defendants may incriminate themselves within the process.

Health care ethics and the law

Health care ethics privilege patient autonomy, beneficence to the individual and non-maleficence. In contrast, law privileges justice. Legal process can result in the loss of person's liberty. It is only by a legal process that an individual's rights can be overruled for the benefit of others. This means that there can be a challenge to professional ethical principles when forensic practitioners move from a clinical context into a legal one. In addition, the law, in being an instrument of the state, reflects the political forces (albeit Statute law made by Parliament can be interpreted, and even ruled, 'unlawful' by the courts under the Human Rights Act). There is therefore certainly no guarantee that law and legal practice will always be consistent with professional ethics, be they medical or other.

Forensic practitioners find themselves involved in a variety of legal settings, including criminal and civil courts, as well as a variety of Tribunals whose decisions are subject to judicial review (including Mental Health Review Tribunals). In the criminal courts, the fact, nature or extent of the person's guilt is explored and sentence imposed; in the civil courts, a wide variety of questions are addressed, covering every aspect of the human condition.

A central theme in forensic mental health practice is the potential for conflict that is ever-present between the duty to the individual 'patient' versus the duty to assist in the pursuit of justice. As we have already observed, such 'dual role' dilemmas can be responded to in the following ways:

1. Forensic psychiatrists (for example) are first and foremost doctors, and their primary concern should be therapeutic benefit to the patient. Their role should be such as to be directed always towards the benefit of the individual patient and never solely towards public protection.

2. Forensic practitioners are not only doctors but are also citizens and have a duty to participate in the legal system of the state.

3. Forensic practitioners are similar to public health practitioners; violence is a public health issue and they help to protect the public from harm specifically by providing not only treatment to mentally disordered offenders but also expert opinion to the state. This is an overall 'good' and so trumps any necessary individual loss of liberty.

4. When a doctor assesses a subject for the courts who has never been his patient the assessment is to assist the court in the pursuit of justice. The doctor is not carrying out treatment, and the subject is not a patient. The doctor may be properly described therefore as a 'forensicist' (a term that has been used in the United States, although not much in the United Kingdom).

5. Whatever the stated reason for the assessment, there is always a potential therapeutic alibi, given that a forensic practitioner may well uncover disorder which requires treatment, and can be treated. Hence, according to this argument, forensic practitioners are never compromised in their social role of pursuing mental health by taking part in the court process, since they may discover disorder which can and should be treated.

6. Doctors operating in the court arena do so under the general ethical framework of *justice ethics*; hence it would be unethical to deny the court process expert psychiatric testimony, which is needed in order for justice to be done, including to the defendant (Adshead and Sarkar 2005).

Consequently, one solution to the dilemma faced by the professional who is both clinician and citizen, owing a duty to both individual patients and the state, is to be prepared to 'assist the state' (as a citizen) so long as there is 'the rule of law', and/or so long as the state is (democratically) 'good enough'. Hence, a clinician might refuse to assist the 'not good enough' state, or the state where the rule of law is absent; but, where that is not the situation, he or she may accept that he or she has dual responsibilities and that these must somehow be balanced at least so as, in some measure, to satisfy the clinician's duty to both the individual and the state.

Another way to think about the relationship between health care and the law is to see them represented in two sets of agencies whose purposes are inevitably in some degree of ethical conflict or tension, in terms of their individual primary purposes. Such tension is not necessarily destructive; however, since it can be a productive tension born of the need to represent both 'public protection' and 'offender patient rights (including to health care per se)' (Eastman 2006). That is, the tension produces a proper balance between pursuit of the interests of society and that of the individual.

Detention and civil law: Mental Health Review Tribunals

Mental Health Review Tribunals (MHRTs) examine the legality of the detention of a patient in hospital under the Mental Health Act 1983, amended by the Mental Health Act 2007, and have a duty to discharge a patient from hospital who is not found to satisfy the statutory requirements for detention; alternatively, they have the power to conditionally discharge patient who is the subject of a 'restriction order' if they deem that the patient can lawfully continue to be subject to recall. Each Tribunal is made up of a legal chair (the president), a lay member and a psychiatrist (the medical member); the president is a judge if the patient is under a 'restriction order'.

The ethical situation for forensic psychiatrists with regard to MHRTs is somewhat similar to the relationship with criminal courts. There is similarity, in that Tribunals are legal, not clinical bodies, and so many of the 'problems of relationship' for the clinician which apply to courts also do so in relation to Tribunals. However, there are differences, in that Tribunals administer law specifically related to (non-consensual) mental health care. As a direct result, the role of the professional giving evidence to a tribunal is 'directly and necessarily dual'. For example, the RMO has no choice about whether to give evidence about his patient, and their treatment, since the whole basis for the Tribunal sitting is 'about' that treatment.

The position of the medical member of an MHRT is particularly ethically and legally problematic. As a member of a legal Tribunal, but also a psychiatrist, his or her role in terms of the patient's welfare is somewhat blurred. The members are required clinically to interview the patient, and material from this interview is 'evidence' to the rest of the Tribunal. At the same time, they are charged with reviewing the evidence that will justify detention, so that they are, in effect, acting as both witness and judge.

This dual role can pull the clinician into ethical difficulty, particularly because the medical member gives 'evidence' without it being challenged by the lawyer for the patient. The medical member is therefore some sort of 'medico-legal hybrid' who somehow applies both a clinical ethical framework and, very different, legal duties. Yet the medical and legal discourses operate very differently (see above). So the doctor on the Tribunal perhaps attempts to translate between the two discourses. However, it is debatable whether such translation is achievable, especially where it is embodied within one individual.

There is also a problem concerning the nature of the evidence given by the different participants. The RMO is giving evidence as to the clinical care and treatment of his particular patient and is therefore a witness as to fact. However, the RMO is also invited to give an opinion as to whether the grounds for detention are made out, and so is also acting as an expert witness, including potentially on behalf of the Trust that employs him or her and detains the patient. This can also create problems within the therapeutic relationship between doctor and patient.

Conclusion: the role of values

This chapter has suggested that specific approaches might be needed to address ethical dilemmas in mental health care, and especially so within forensic mental health care. We have suggested some approaches to practical ethical reasoning aimed at better addressing these issues, albeit leaving practitioners with having often to choose between different approaches. In so doing we have paid attention in particular to the fact that forensic mental health practitioners inevitably deal, almost constantly, with social values and law, as well as with legal agencies and process. We have also tried to make plain that, even within clinical practice per se, clinicians inevitably apply their own corporate professional, personal, or even societal or state-originating values, not only to how they deal with the justice system but also to the very stuff of clinical practice. Hence, for example, determination of diagnosis, or what is 'treatment', or whether someone is 'treatable' represents a mixed science and value judgement.

More obviously, a solely values-based decision is deciding whether to carry out a risk assessment for a court that has in mind the possibility of imposing an IPP. Similarly, setting a threshold of risk in terms of recommending discharge, or not, to an MHRT very clearly involves normative judgement, for example, deciding what is an 'acceptable' level of risk for discharge. The context of recent reform of the Mental Health Act towards greater control over patients, including those in the community, and with removal of a 'treatability', or 'therapeutic benefit' test, has inevitably given rise to reconsideration of, and even dispute about, what constitute proper professional values within psychiatric practice, including consideration of whether libertarian and not just therapeutic/safety interests should be given weighty consideration (Sarkar and Adshead 2005).

Making value judgements is inherent to all clinical practice in any health care context. However, the operation of values is both 'obvious' and somewhat 'special' within forensic mental health practice, by virtue of the inherently hybrid nature of such practice and by virtue of its unusual degree of association with the justice system. What is crucial, however, is awareness of the role of making value judgements within everyday practice on the part of the practitioner, that is, 'values insight'. There may not be a 'right' answer to each ethical dilemma faced by any forensic clinician; there may not even be general agreement about what should be the answer. Whatever answer is arrived at by any clinician with respect to any dilemma must be 'ethically thought out' and 'justified'. Practice that is *un*ethical is practice that is pursued without reasoned ethical thinking. That is, practice that is ethically 'blind'.

References

Adshead, G. 2002 A Different Voice in Psychiatric Ethics 56–62 in Health Care Ethics and Human Values (Fulford, K.W., Dickenson, D. and Murray, T. Editors). Oxford: Blackwell.

Adshead G. and Sarkar S.P. 2005 Justice and Welfare: Two Ethical Paradigms in Forensic Psychiatry. Australian and New Zealand Journal of Psychiatry 39: 1011–1017.

BASW (British Association of Social Work). 2003 Code of Ethics. London: BASW.

BPS (British Psychological Society). 2006 Code of Ethics and Conduct. London: BPS.

Dolan, B. 2004 Medical Records: Disclosing Confidential Clinical Information. Psychiatric Bulletin 28: 53–56.

Eastman N. 2006 Evidence to the Joint House of Lords, House of Commons Parliamentary Scrutiny Committee for the Draft Mental Health Bill, published in Joint Committee on the Draft Mental Health Bill (2005), HL Paper 70-II, HC 95-II, pages 339–348, London, The Stationary Office.

Eastman, N. 2006 Can there be True Partnership between Clinicians and the Home Office? Advances in Psychiatric Treatment 12: 459–461.

Gilligan, C. 1993 A Different Voice 2nd Edition. Cambridge MA: Harvard University Press.

GMC (General Medical Council). 2006 Good Medical Practice. London: GMC

Logan, C. 2003 Ethical Issues in Risk Assessment Practice and Research 72–86 in Ethical Issues in Forensic Mental Health Research (Adshead, G. and Brown, C. Editors). London: Kingsley.

Miles, S. 2003 xiv The Hippocratic Oath and the Ethics of Medicine. Oxford University Press, US.

NMC (Nursing and Midwifery Council). 2006 Code of Conduct. London: NMC.

Radden J. 2002 Notes towards A Professional Ethics for Psychiatry. Australian and New Zealand Journal of Psychiatry 36: 52–59.

Sarkar, S.P. and Adshead, G. 2005 Black Robes And White Coats: Who Will Win the New Mental Health Tribunals? British Journal of Psychiatry 186: 96–98.

Srinivas, J., Denvir, S. and Humphreys, M. 2006 The Home Office Mental Health Unit. Advances in Psychiatric Treatment 12: 450–458.

Section 5

Social policy

Chapter 26

Introduction to social policy and the mentally disordered offender

Annie Bartlett

This section considers the evolution of 'political' concepts applied to those who have a combination of mental health problems and offending behaviour. It describes the emergence and current use of the term mentally disordered offender (MDO). The term MDO and other concepts historical, for example, criminal lunacy, as well as contemporary, for example, DSPD, are useful starting points for a discussion of social policy in this area.

Put simply, it is significant whether someone is framed within the language of health or of criminal justice and whether they are seen as suitable for treatment or punishment. Equally, the bald dichotomies of health and criminal justice and of treatment and punishment are unfair to all the agencies involved. The intentions, formal roles and practice of agencies involved with MDOs are more nuanced; they often combine elements of both treatment and punishment. It is to some extent unfashionable to suggest that locking up people is a punishment but if it is, then clearly both health and criminal justice agencies do this. Similarly, treatment, in some form, happens in both criminal justice and health settings.

The section demonstrates how social policy and its implementation in relation to MDOs, however they are defined, derives from the views and often competing interests of government departments, statutory agencies in health and social care, the voluntary sector and the criminal justice system. MDO policy and practice, regardless of its origin, has always grappled with the dichotomy of treatment and punishment, as well as with its institutional manifestations; this formidable dichotomy acts simultaneously to inform and constrain discourse in this domain of thinking, and remains very powerful.

In two of the chapters in this section, 'Organizational and Conceptual Frameworks and the Mentally Disordered Offender' (Chapter 27) and 'Prison Mental Health Care' (Chapter 28), the history of relevant services is outlined along with developments of policy and practice. In Chapter 29, 'Current Service Provision for Mentally Disordered Offenders', the current state of services is considered. This describes the complex system that attempts to deliver holistic care and risk management within a multi-agency system.

Two key issues for this section are: first, the legitimacy of recent changes in policy; and second, the adequacy of the strategic development and implementation of policy that has followed. Policy is clearly influenced by the overall philosophy of mental health care, not least because MDOs constitute a small subset of all mental health service users. Policy will also shift according to the current understanding of the origins of criminality in those with mental health problems. The wishes of three distinct arms of government (the Home Office, the Ministry of Justice and the Department of Health) come into play, sometimes cooperatively and sometimes with the potentially conflicting agendas of public safety and patient care. Legislative initiatives are an important component of the final governmental view but not the only clue to government thinking.

Consultations and guidance from government also signal the direction of travel. The MDO's own voice, as such, is relatively absent from this debate although there are lobby groups (e.g. MIND, Women in Secure Hospitals, Revolving Doors Agency, NACRO) and other agencies (e.g. Mental Health Act Commission) that, in part, advocate and represent their perspectives. Forensic practitioners have developed an evidence base that also informs best practice in the field. Finally, media coverage in this field is important; tabloid and other journalistic interests have exerted considerable leverage in the name of public opinion, on coercive practice, in particular, in the old Special Hospitals and the so-called psychiatric homicides.

As practitioners, we have a therapeutic armoury of pharmacological and psychological treatments unthinkable a hundred years ago. Yet much of what we do, particularly when working with MDOs, does not relate to therapeutic efficacy but to the current, and no doubt temporary, resolution of more profound questions of stigma, the acceptability of coercive intervention, societal understanding of risk and moral responsibility.

It would be cheering if this section were to convince the reader that the care of the MDO is evolving in a simple, positive fashion. However, the jury is out on the wisdom of recent policy; it is for readers to weigh up the arguments themselves. As fashions in care change it is salutary to reflect on the extent to which these changes are evidence-based. It also remains to be seen how the fundamental shifts in policy witnessed since 1992 have resulted in real or useful changes in clinical practice, that go beyond compliance with the latest mandate.

Chapter 27

Organizational and conceptual frameworks and the mentally disordered offender

Annie Bartlett and Sue Kesteven

Aim

To outline the origins of the systems used in England and Wales to help and manage mentally disordered offenders (MDOs).

Learning objectives

- To understand the chronological development of forensic services in England and Wales
- To explain the current concept of the MDO
- To relate the concept of the MDO to social policy and provision

---

Introduction

Each historical period has its own ways of describing difference, that is, of categorising those who are in some way out of the mainstream, not like everyone else. The last two hundred years in England and Wales has seen society do this in various ways. The development of a powerful discourse on madness, inextricably linked with both a medically driven illness model and the institution of psychiatry (see Bartlett this vol. pp 5–20), is one way. One facet of this discourse, but an important one, is the attention given to individuals who break the law and are also mad. The language used to describe this, rather modest, number of people has changed over time. So too have the services set up specifically to deal with the problems they cause themselves and the problems they cause the rest of society. Who these people are, how we, in the broadest sense, think about them, and what we have provided to assist and monitor them is the subject of this chapter. A more detailed understanding of current service provision is covered in the next chapter.

The main term in use at present is mentally disordered offender (MDO). Like its ancestor, 'criminal lunatic', it is both immediately clear and not clear what is being described. It is not so much that its meaning is actively debated, rather that, to understand it, we should consider what is included in its meaning when used. This is a practical question for practitioners and also an important social policy issue. Within the social policy arena the shifting and ambiguous meanings of terms are licence for social change; nowhere has this been seen more clearly than in the altered understanding of Mental Disorder in the 2007 Revised Mental Health Act.

This chapter will look first at the historical background to current service provision, from which the term MDO emerges, and second, at the different usages of this now ubiquitous term, and third, the implications for treatment.

Historical service provision

The linkage of 'lunacy' and risk has a long history. As far back as 1482, English common law allowed for the lawful containment of dangerous lunatics (Allderidge 1979). There was no statute law until the Vagrancy Act of 1714, which conceived of the 'furiously mad and dangerous' and made explicit provision for their care, perhaps because the authority of common law was insufficient. The passage of the 1800 Criminal Lunatics Act enshrined the term in statute and can be viewed as reactive policy-making; it followed the high-profile attempt on the life of the then King, George III. Throughout the nineteenth century there was concern about the plight of pauper lunatics, often construed as inappropriately placed, and a newfound optimism about the likely success of humane treatment (Jones 1993: 60–77). The Criminal Lunatics Act of 1860 was the first to provide specific assistance for them, and followed what would now be called a needs assessment indicating they were in a range of unsatisfactory placements, that is, prison, private madhouses, county asylums and the Bethlem hospital (Walker and McCabe 1973: 5). Broadmoor Criminal Lunatic Asylum opened in 1863 and was soon full.

Parker (1985) documented in detail the piecemeal planning of further specific provision, involving turning part of Parkhurst prison into a temporary 'criminal lunatic asylum'. At the end of the nineteenth century, it was recognized that additional provision was needed and Rampton, another asylum, not a prison, opened in 1912. Legislation dealing with mental deficiency came into force in 1913, but there was little clarity in capacity plans for individuals deemed to be dangerous mental defectives. Various placements were developed. Systems of management for what came to be the three main institutions for criminal lunatics and dangerous mental defectives exemplify the conceptual fluctuation to which they were subject. We see in the first half of the twentieth century the creation of both an 'Institution' and of 'Hospitals' with varied input from the Ministry of Health and the Home Office.

In 1959, after the long deliberations of the Percy Commission, legislation about learning difficulty (as mental deficiency has come to be known), mental illness and personality disorder were combined in a single Mental Health Act. These categories are salient, as their relationship to clinical categories had to be established, and was over subsequent years. The most controversial category was psychopathic disorder, as professional support for its inclusion was lukewarm (Ramon 1986). The categories were of enduring significance, lasting well into the next century unchanged.

Special hospitals

At the same time, the 1959 Mental Health Act (MHA) created the term 'special hospital' to describe Broadmoor, Rampton and Moss Side. The tensions between ideas of care and custody were played out both in the significant role of the Prison Officers' Association, as the main union in the special hospitals, and in the continuing role of the Home Office in relation to discharge of restricted patients. Although many patients were sent to special hospitals from the criminal justice system, admissions did not invariably go through the courts or prison. It was also the case that after the 1959 Act women were more likely than men to be admitted to the special hospitals without being successfully prosecuted (see Bartlett 1993 for fuller discussion of patient cohorts).

By 1960, patients in the three special hospitals were legally and clinically diverse, with Broadmoor taking more of the mentally ill and psychopathically disordered. Length of stay over subsequent decades waxed and waned (see Bartlett 1993) but was never less than 5 years. There were no other designated forensic services in England and Wales. Most psychiatric practice elsewhere was preoccupied with the deinstitutionalization of less-dangerous mental health patients (Raftery 1992). Special hospital patients had difficulty moving out either to the community or to less-secure hospital settings. Eastman (1993) considered the Percy Commission to have neglected planning of secure services and to be responsible for the de-skilling of staff in relation to violent patients.

In 1961, a government working party (Ministry of Health 1961) mooted the possibility of regional secure units and recommended expansion of maximum secure hospital placements for psychopathically disordered individuals. In 1974, Park Lane was opened for this population. In 1989, Moss Side and Park Lane merged into Ashworth and all three special hospitals then came under the newly created special hospital service authority (SHSA). By 1991, the population of the three special hospitals was 1,740, of whom 20% were women. Most patients were detained under mental illness but a quarter were held under psychopathic disorder (SHSA 1991).

The hospitals were thought to be stigmatizing by ex-patients and by other commentators (Bowden 1981). Media interest led to inquiries into standards of care, specifically the balance of security and therapy. These were considered as on a continuum where the consequence of a preoccupation with security meant the absence of therapy and vice versa (see Text Box 27.1).

In the early 1990s, there were calls to close the special hospitals (Bluglass 1992; Dillner 1992). The newly created SHSA had to respond with speed and vigour. It recruited more clinical staff, introduced more general management of a kind found in the rest of the NHS (Anderson 1988) and grappled with the dominance of the Prison Officers' Association. By the end of the 1990s, the tide had turned. The Fallon Report (Fallon et al 1999) resonated with previous calls to close the special hospitals, but now it was in the context of anxiety about legitimate control and supervision of dangerous patients. The Tilt Report (2000) led to enhanced security in all three hospitals. In future they would cater for those who really required that level of security, fewer than in the past. The developing discourse of risk and risk management in other areas of mental health in the late 1990s could be argued to have contributed to their survival.

Medium secure services

In the mid-1970s both the Butler (HO 1975) and Glancy Committees (DHSS 1974) had made recommendations as to forensic need at a more local level than the three national high secure units. Such regional units were intended to assist the rate of discharge from the special hospitals, which was recognized as too slow (Dell 1980), and which continued to be unsatisfactory in subsequent decades (Bartlett et al 1996; Murphy 1990) and created a significant population of people who were over-detained (Dell and Robertson 1988; Maden et al 1995). The Butler and Glancy recommendations coincided with concern that substantial numbers of prisoners needed transfer

---

Box 27.1 Special hospitals' inquiries

- 1975 Broadmoor: too great an emphasis on security (Gostin 1977)
- 1981 Broadmoor: 'modern and humane system of care' post escape (Hamilton 1985)
- 1988 Broadmoor: security stifles therapeutic initiative (HAS 1988)
- 1980 Rampton: outdated institutional practices with inadequate emphasis on rehabilitation and individuality
- 1990 Rampton: improved but still rigid (DH 1989)
- 1992 Ashworth: too like a prison, control and discipline replace therapy. Inappropriate admissions. Racist staff (DH 1992)
- 1999 Ashworth: loss of control of the Personality Disorder Unit (Fallon et al 1999)

from prison to hospital. The Glancy recommendation of 20 beds per million of the population was adopted, but Regional Health Authorities were slow to respond.

The number of regional secure beds crept up to 555 in 1991 (Murray 1996). Money allocated to the regions for their creation had been diverted elsewhere (Parker 1985). The Reed Committee, whose remit was to review the whole system of care for MDOs, recommended a total of 30 beds per million – 1,500 – which was half way between the original Butler and Glancy target (DH/HO 1992).

Subsequent expansion in medium secure provision has been startling, especially when set against the slow pace of the late 1970s and 1980s. Laing and Buisson (2006) report 2,886 medium secure beds by 2006 with a further 1,800 beds in the private sector. Early secure provision was idiosyncratic, with varied design and function, often in adapted buildings. By 2007, the DH was sufficiently concerned about security in the now large number of units to create core standards. Although they do not deal exclusively with physical security, this is undoubtedly their focus (DH 2007b). In the London area, expansion of NHS medium and low secure beds has been by a factor of 366%, from 207 in 1996 to 758 in 2006 (Bartlett et al 2007).

There is a complex background to this sea change in practice. Key has been the developing climate of risk aversion. A range of measures designed to improve risk management came in the wake of detailed examination of 'psychiatric homicides' (DH 1998; Munro and Rumgay 2000). Measures included Supervision Registers (Bindman et al 2000), Section 25A Supervised Discharge, the Criminal Justice Act 2003 and the promotion of MAPPA, rigorous implementation of CPA/117 (DH 2000) and a range of formal risk assessment tools introduced and promoted in clinical practice (Gray et al 2004, 2008, DH 2007a; McKenzie and Curr 2005). Despite this, the National Confidential Inquiry into Suicide and Homicide (NCISH 2006) reviewed 249 homicides by individuals in current or recent contact with mental health services and found no increase or decrease in the number of homicides committed by the mentally ill between 1999 and 2003, echoing Gunn and Taylor's pessimism (1999) that changes in treatment regime would effect a reduction in such cases of violence.

Concepts and meaning

Definitions

The focus of this chapter is the 'political' concepts used to address offending behaviours and mental health problems as they occur together in single individuals. Their relationship to other categories within the professional mental health literature, or within criminology, will always require elucidation. A chronological perspective of service development shows how concepts are seldom static; the terms used change over time and new terms are introduced into the discourse of policy. In the twentieth century, criminal lunacy has fallen away to be replaced with MDO. Asylums became hospitals. Perhaps in this century we will see hospitals being replaced by 'unit' or 'service'; both terms are in use in forensic settings and are essentially devoid of the medical overtones of 'hospital'. Importantly, existing terms can also be (re)defined by deliberate intent or through regular use. The concept of 'mental illness' in the 1959 and 1983 MHAs was never defined but acquired meaning through use. The concept of mental disorder, also in both MHAs, has been altered in the 2007 MHA.

Mentally disordered offenders

The concept of the MDO is fluid. This can be seen in light of the historical expansion of the range of services provided to those with a combination of offending behaviour and mental health problems.

No single definition of the term has received general acceptance. As Peay (1994) put it, 'The term "mentally disordered offender" means many things to many people.'

There have been a number of attempts to describe those who fall into this category. In its original guidance in relation to MDOs, the Home Office (1990) described the group concerned as 'mentally disordered persons who commit, or are suspected of committing, criminal offences'. A similar definition is used by the Reed Review (DH/HO 1992: 115): 'A mentally disordered person who has broken the law . . . this term is sometimes loosely used to include mentally disordered people who are alleged to have broken the law.'

Breaking the law could cover anything from speeding in a car to murder, so, in fact, these definitions barely constitute a definition.

This is not to say that offenders with mental disorder are never dangerous, but simply to give a sense of proportion. To reflect the broad spectrum of individuals who might be described as MDOs, NACRO (2009) adopted a broad definition that encompasses those who repeatedly commit relatively minor offences as well as those whose level of disorder and dangerousness makes them a risk to the public:

> Those who come into contact with the Criminal Justice System because they have committed or are suspected of committing a criminal offence and: who may be acutely or chronically mentally ill; those with neuroses, behavioural and/or personality disorders; those with learning difficulties; some who, as a function of alcohol and/or substance misuse, have a mental health problem; and any who are suspected of falling into one or other of these groups. It also includes those offenders in whom a degree of mental disturbance is recognized, even though that may not be severe enough to bring it within the criteria laid down by the *Mental Health Act 1983* and those offenders who, even though they do not fall easily within this definition – for example, some sex offenders and some abnormally aggressive offenders – may benefit from psychological treatments.

'Mental disorder' is the overarching term that has been used in section 1 of the 1983 Mental Health Act. It comprised one or more of four types of disorder, that is, mental illness, psychopathic disorder, mental impairment and severe mental impairment and the exclusion clauses. Three of the categories in section 1 were defined, but mental illness was not. The implication of the term mental disorder is that anyone satisfying one or more of these categories is potentially subject to the compulsory powers of the Act, for example, compulsory hospitalization for assessment and treatment.

It has never been entirely clear whether 'mentally disordered offender' was supposed to refer only to those individuals who might fall within the relevant sections of the Act and who were arrested and/or before the courts or whether some other and/or broader concept was intended. The Code of Practice (DH 2008: 298) refers to mentally disordered people, obviously in the legal sense, who come into contact with the criminal justice system.

NACRO have taken at one level a helpfully broad view, with the intention clearly expressed of going beyond this. This use might allow individuals access to MDO services to assist them and might also reflect the complexity of many people's problems. It also represents a creeping medicalization of issues traditionally seen as more the remit of the Criminal Justice System, that is, sexual offending. Sexual offending per se is, first of all, offending, that is, a behaviour, often indicating a lifelong sexual preference amounting to sexual deviance. Sexual deviance, often phrased as an identity, that is, 'He is a sexual deviant', was excluded from the 1983 Act. Also, dependence on alcohol or drugs was never in itself grounds for inclusion under the 1983 Mental Health Act. NACRO's approach, scooping up those who would otherwise fall outside the compulsory powers of the Act, might be criticized if it transpired that MDOs were to be subject, at some point in the future, to measures imposed rather than services accepted.

The revisions to the concept of mental disorder which form part of the 2007 Mental Health Act seem to move precisely in this direction. They remove the sexual deviation exclusion clause and pave the way not for voluntary treatment but for compulsory intervention in this area. They abolish the legal concepts of mental illness, psychopathic disorder or mental impairment or severe mental impairment and use a broader definition of mental disorder, that is, 'any disorder or disability of mind'. This definition makes no explicit reference to current diagnostic systems such as ICD-10 (WHO 1992) or DSM-IV (APA 1994). Even if it did, the implications for the forensic world in the field of personality disorder are potentially profound. Personality pathology is very common in offender populations and the MHA 2007 also reduces the emphasis on compulsory treatment having any actual benefit.

The changing climate of risk: DSPD

It is also arguable that, whatever might be intended by government or related professionals, the publicity associated with what has come to be known as 'psychiatric homicide' skewed public perceptions of MDOs. Although cases like those of Michael Stone (Francis et al 2006) and Christopher Clunis (NE Thames and SE Thames Regional Health Authorities 1994) are exceptional, they received substantial and disproportionate media coverage when compared with other homicides. Such journalism is often sensational. It is not newsworthy that someone with schizophrenia got a job last week; it is if they killed someone. The combination of criminal trial and the review of events within the NHS can also lead to prolonged coverage (Blom-Cooper et al 1995; South West London SHA 2006). Most media attention has been given to cases where horrific crimes had been committed by individuals with schizophrenia. The DH had recognized the link (DH 1998); the Michael Stone case is the exception to this.

The opportunity to rehearse important policy issues within a public arena is part of the consultation and reform process. However, decisive action may undermine a more deliberate, and deliberated, change in policy. Jack Straw, then Home Secretary, personally intervened in the case of Michael Stone. His statement in Parliament (Hansard 1999) led directly to both an attempt at a new Mental Health Act involving preventive detention (DH and HO 2000) and to the creation of units designed to deal with a new category of person, that is, DSPD units (Eastman 1999; Mullen 1999). Although the intention was to generate rapid action, in fact, the debates around the most controversial elements of these proposals spanned several years and in part are unresolved. It is hard to argue against the idea that that the MDO of the early 1990s has become the dangerous madman of the 2000s.

DSPD is an important new addition to the social policy canon on mental health issues. In effect, it is a sub-category of MDO. In 1999, the Home Office and Department of Health (DH/HO 1999) put forward proposals for managing dangerous people with severe personality disorder. The phrase 'dangerous and severe personality disorder' (DSPD) was coined to describe 'people who have an identifiable disorder to a severe degree, who pose a high risk to other people because of the serious antisocial behaviour resulting from their disorder' (DH/HO 1999: 12).

These are people whose offending behaviour is at the serious end of the scale; they commit crimes such as murder, manslaughter, arson, serious sex offences, or grievous bodily harm. According to the consultation paper, by far the majority of these individuals are either in prison or are detained in hospital under the 1983 MHA. The numbers are small; the government estimated around 2,000 adult men fell into this category, together with tiny numbers of young men between the ages of 18 and 20 and also of women (DH/HO 1999).

The introduction of this term is significant. The term, a government invention, has acquired a life of its own. There are now DSPD services, treatment programmes and evaluations

Box 27.2 Mentally disordered offender: issues in definition

- May or may not refer to section 1 of the 2007 Mental Health Act
- May include mental health problems historically excluded by section 1 of the 1983 Mental Health Act
- Covers a range of offending behaviours from minor to grave
- Can refer to those involved in criminal justice proceedings or those actually convicted

(HO, HMP Prison Service and DH 2006; MoJ/DH 2008a, 2008b), mainly for men but with a small number of prison beds for women. This is remarkable as the term neither has obvious clinical meaning nor does it appear in statute law, unlike the term 'mental disorder'. It also, importantly, brings together the idea of dangerousness and a particular clinical entity, that is, personality disorder. This was never true of 'criminal lunatic' or of 'MDO'; it encapsulates a change in the mindset away from the liberalism of the early 1990s that was most visible in the principles of the Reed Review of Services for MDOs (DH/HO 1992).

Principles of treatment for MDOs: a social policy perspective

Given the uncertainty surrounding the term MDO, it is unsurprising that there is equal uncertainty about the implications for treatment. MDOs would constitute a part of three distinct populations: first, those in prison, second, those in hospital, and third, those living in a community setting.

The comprehensive ONS prison survey (Singleton et al 1998) found that, before entering prison, 40% of women prisoners and 20% of male prisoners had been receiving help or treatment for a mental health problem. There were high levels of psychiatric morbidity in the prisoner population, ranging from neurotic disorder (66% of female prisoners, 59% of male remand and 40% of male sentenced prisoners), to functional psychosis (14% of women prisoners, 10% of male remand and 7% of male sentenced prisoners) and personality disorder (50% of women prisoners, 78% of male remand and 64% of male sentenced prisoners). However, the level of psychiatric morbidity is not an indication of a comparable level of dangerousness. Only a small proportion (21.4% in 2007) of offenders sentenced in the Crown Courts had committed offences of violence against the person (MoJ, 2008a).

The epidemiology of prison populations suggests that very high numbers of incarcerated individuals have mental health problems that could, and should, be treated. Estimates of offender populations in the community are harder to establish, and they have not been subject to the same epidemiological scrutiny. Most prisoners are on fixed-term sentences or remanded prior to a community disposal; it is not credible that their mental health problems dissolve on release. There is an additional small population of individuals held in secure hospitals, recent estimates suggest 800 high secure beds and 3,500 medium secure beds in July 2007 in England and Wales (Rutherford and Duggan 2007).

The case for treatment of the MDO population will depend on the nature of the condition, the efficacy of any treatment intervention and the availability of such an intervention. From a social policy perspective in relation to MDOs, critical elements are also likely to include the possibility of treatment affecting future offending and the overall cost-benefit equation, that is, the amount it would cost to treat a given number of patients with what level of anticipated improvement.

The case of mental illness

For many mental health problems it is taken for granted that treatment gets people better, e.g. schizophrenia, anxiety and depression. The government, like clinicians, has a straightforward attitude to mental illness. It has been consistent for more than 15 years in placing the responsibility for MDOs with major mental illness with the NHS (DH/HO 1992; HO 1995, 1990). It has funded both prison in-reach services (SCMH 2007) and more local secure hospital beds (DH 1998; DH/HO 1992) in an attempt to provide adequate services. It is held that if the small number of people whose mental illness makes them violent is clinically well managed, this will reduce the risk to the public. This policy also has a humanitarian aim: it differentiates places of punishment from places of treatment. This is, of course, to gloss over the fact that prisons can treat and hospitals incarcerate. Successive Mental Health Acts have endorsed the view that the mentally ill need correct placement; many of its provisions, and the whole of Part III, are intended to move people out of the criminal justice system into the NHS. People worry about adequate bed numbers, slow speed of transfers and a possible lack of aftercare but the broad social policy issue is uncontroversial. The ill need NHS care, whether or not they are criminal and/or violent.

The case of personality disorder

This is all much less obvious in the case of personality disorder. This is relevant as so many of the MDO population suffer from personality disorders. There is continuing debate about the effectiveness of treatment for personality disorders, that is, whether interventions alter any measurable aspect of personality functioning (NICE 2008a, 2008b). There is further debate about whether any treatment interventions reduce the risk of re-offending. Both these issues are crucial in designing services that incarcerate individuals for long periods of time. This needs to be set against what appears to be an imperative to treat or manage MDOs in the name of public safety (Mullen 1999).

Forensic hospital services in the United Kingdom and elsewhere have always assessed and treated individuals with personality disorder, when it is linked with serious offending or the likelihood of serious offending. Much of this treatment, though not all, for example, Henderson Hospital and Portman Clinic, has been on a compulsory basis. In the last two decades this compulsory treatment has been in the context of the 1983 Mental Health Act. This explicitly indicated that treatment must be either 'likely to alleviate or prevent a deterioration' in someone's condition. For a small number of relatively serious offenders, the clinical judgements made are that hospital treatment will help. The total number of patients detained, with restriction orders, under the 1983 MHA category of psychopathic disorder in hospital was 465 (Rutherford and Duggan 2007). For an even smaller number of people with personality disorder and some offending, who seek help voluntarily, some community treatment might be available.

This leaves a very large number of individuals in the prison system whose personality problems coincide with and perhaps are causally linked to offending, of different levels of gravity. The prison population in England and Wales is approximately 80,000 (MoJ 2008a). Singleton et al (1998) suggested that half of all women prisoners and more than half of all male prisoners have at least one personality disorder, more than 40,000 individuals at any one time. Currently, specific treatment is thin on the ground, and very few people are offered treatment. Crisis management is a necessity in prison (see Chapter 28), but therapeutic communities in prison are small in number when compared with the potential size of the clinical task. The correctional regimes in other jurisdictions as well as the prison service in England and Wales do however deliver programmes designed to reduce re-offending, that is, not designated as therapeutic, to significant numbers of the personality-disordered in prison (NICE 2008a: 165–194).

This paradoxical situation exemplifies the indecision mental health services display about treating personality disorder. Estimates of morbidity are not usually matched by robust assessments of prisoners' capacity to engage in or benefit from treatment. If they were, even allowing for large numbers of prisoners who might reject help, it seems likely that the sheer size of the demand would crush the health service.

The financial cost of NHS involvement with so much of the prisoner population could also be a constraint. Such a major ideological shift in the role of the prison system still provides no guarantee that it would reduce crime. Currently, the prisons, which cost less per inmate than the NHS costs per psychiatric inpatient, bear the costs at a rate of £37,500 per inmate per year (MoJ 2007). A medium secure hospital bed in the NHS in London costs, on average, £146,000 per patient per year (Bartlett et al 2007). Pragmatism, and government concern about very violent and serious sexual offenders, even though they may be the hardest to help, has determined that considerable resources have gone into, as yet, untested and resource-intensive DSPD programmes located partly in high secure hospitals and partly in prison (see Chapter 16).

Conclusion

The shape, size and location of MDO services for personality-disordered offenders are determined not only by consideration of financial costs and treatment effectiveness (the criteria by which many health interventions are judged) but also by the complex societal and governmental view of people they consider, rightly or wrongly, to be very dangerous.

The distinction made above between the treatment options for the mentally ill and the personality-disordered is, however, misleading. It misses out what is apparent to many clinicians, that is, the clinical and social complexity of many individuals who might fall within the term MDO. Their clinical problems are frequently far from straightforward. Dual and triple diagnoses are common (Bartlett 2007; Dolan and Davies 2006), with mental illness often compounded by addiction and personality disorder. Such problems emerge alongside other factors contributing to social exclusion: poor literacy, unemployment and housing problems (SEU 2002). This is one of the reasons why the organization of services designed both to monitor and assist them is in turn very complex.

Forensic services are predominantly institutionally based, either in secure hospitals or in prisons. They are therefore out of step with other components of mental health care that have been increasingly community-based since the 1960s. They have been caught up in a wave of adverse publicity about serious crimes committed by a small number of individuals with major mental health problems. Since 1992, the changes have gone in a single direction, that is, towards a culture of surveillance, inside and outside institutions, possibly tempered by therapeutic initiatives and the real move out of high secure care. The expansion of institutional care has been at the level of low and medium secure beds whose security has undergone recent scrutiny and enhancement. It remains true, however, that secure hospital populations are dwarfed by the highly morbid prison populations whose often short length of stay and dispersal procedures can defeat even the most determined health professional. The measures led by government in the last 15 years to focus on risk discourage health professionals from tolerating risk and, in turn, this may jeopardize the establishment of long-term, nurturing therapeutic relationships in which risk management can be embedded.

Financial power has been allocated to local NHS Commissioners; this weakens the independence of even large NHS Trusts and certainly of individual clinicians to effect change or maintain the status quo. A crucial historical dichotomy has been clinical risk and individual autonomy. In the future, with high cost/low volume services of uncertain efficacy, it may be more important to balance clinical risk and financial cost.

References

Allderidge, P. 1979 Hospitals, Madhouses and Asylums: Cycles in the Care of the Insane. British Journal of Psychiatry 134: 321–334.

American Psychiatric Association. 1994 Diagnostic and Statistical Manual 4th Edition. Washington DC: Author.

Anderson, F. 1988 Special Hospitals Set to Get General Management. The Health Service Journal 12th May: 521.

Bartlett, A. 1993 Rhetoric and Reality: What Do We Know about the English Special Hospitals? International Journal of Law and Psychiatry 16: 27–51.

Bartlett A. 2007 Women in Prison: Concepts, Clinical Issues and Care Delivery. Psychiatry 6, 11: 44–48.

Bartlett, A., Cohen, A., Backhouse, A., Highet, N. and Eastman, N. 1996 Security Needs of South West Thames Special Hospital Patients 1992 and 1993. No Way Out? Journal of Forensic Psychiatry 7: 256–270.

Bartlett, A., Johns, A., Fiander, M. and Jhawar, H. 2007 London Secure Forensic Units Benchmarking Study. London: NHS London.

Bindman, J., Beck, A., Thornicroft, G., Knapp, M. and Szmukler, G. 2000 Psychiatric Patients at Greater Risk and in Greatest Need: Impact of the Supervision Register Policy. London: Department of Health.

Blom-Cooper, L., Hally, H. and Murphy, E. 1995 The Falling Shadow: One Patient's Mental Health Care 1978–1993. London: Duckworth.

Bluglass, R. 1992 The Special Hospitals Should be Closed. British Medical Journal 305: 323–324.

Bowden, P. 1981 What Happens to Patients Released from Special Hospitals? British Journal of Psychiatry 138: 340–354.

Dell, S. 1980 Transfer of Special Hospital Patients to the NHS. British Journal of Psychiatry 136: 222–234.

Dell, S. and Robertson, G. 1988 Sentenced to Hospital: Offenders in Broadmoor. Oxford: Oxford University Press.

DH (Department of Health) 1989 Prejudice and Pride. A Report about Rampton Hospital Ten Years After the Boynton Report.

DH (Department of Health). 1992 Report of the Committee of Inquiry into Complaints about Ashworth Hospital Vol. I and II. London: HMSO.

DH. 1998 Modernising Mental Health Services: Safe, Sound and Supportive. London: Author.

DH. 2000 Effective Care Co-ordination in Mental Health Services: Modernising the Care Programme Approach. London: Author.

DH. 2007a Best Practice in Managing Risk. London: Author.

DH. 2007b Executive Summary, Best Practice Guidance: Specification for Adult Medium-Secure Services. www.DH.gov.uk/publications

DH. 2008 Code of Practice Mental Health Act 1983. London: TSO.

Department of Health and Home Office. 1992 Review of Health and Social Services for Mentally Disordered Offenders and Others Requiring Similar Services. Final Summary Report. London: HMSO.

Department of Health and Home Office. 1999 Managing Dangerous People with Severe Personality Disorder: Proposals for Policy Development. London, July.

Department of Health and Home Office. 2000 Reforming the Mental Health Act Part II: High Risk Patients. London: HMSO.

DHSS (Department of Health and Social Security). 1974 Revised Report of the Working Party on Security in NHS Hospitals Glancy Report.

Dillner, L. 1992 Special Hospitals under Review. British Medical Journal 305: 334.

Dolan, M. and Davies, G. 2006 Psychopathy and Institutional Outcome in Patients with Schizophrenia in Forensic Settings in the UK. Schizophrenia Research 81: 277–281.

Eastman, N. 1993 Forensic Psychiatric Services in Britain: A Current Review. International Journal of Law and Psychiatry 16: 1–26.

Eastman, N. 1999 Public Health Psychiatry or Crime Prevention? Government's Proposals Emphasise Doctor's Role as Public Protectors. British Medical Journal 318: 549–551.

Fallon, P., Bluglass, R., Edwards, B. and Daniels, G. 1999 Report of the Committee of Inquiry into the Personality Disorder Unit, Ashworth Special Hospital Vol. 1. London: The Stationery Office.

Francis, R., Higgins, J. and Cassam, E. 2006 Report of the Independent Inquiry into the Care and Treatment of Michael Stone. South East Coast Strategic Health Authority, Kent County Council and Kent Probation.

Gostin, L.O. 1977 A Human Condition. The Law Relating to Mentally Abnormal Offenders. Observations, Analysis and Proposals for Reform. London: MIND.

Gray, N.S., Snowden, R.J., MacCulloch, S.I., Phillips, H.K., Taylor, J., MacCulloch, M.J. 2004 Relative Efficacy of Criminological, Clinical, and Personality Measures of Future Risk of Offending in Mentally Disordered Offenders: A Comparative Study of HCR-20, PCL:SV and OGRS. Journal of Clinical and Consulting Psychology 72: 523–530.

Gray, N.S., Taylor, J. and Snowden, R.J. 2008 Predicting Violent Recidivism Using the HCR 20. British Journal of Psychiatry 192: 384–387.

Gunn, J. and Taylor, P.J. 1999 Homicides by People with Mental Illness: Myth and Reality. British Journal of Psychiatry 174: 9–14.

Hamilton, J. 1985 Special Hospitals 84–125 in Secure Provisions: A Review of Special Services for the Mentally Ill and Mentally Handicapped in England and Wales (Gostin, L. Editor) London, Tavistock.

Hansard. 1999 15 Feb col 601–603.

Health Advisory Service (HAS). 1988 DHSS Social Services Inspectorate Report on Services Provided by Broadmoor. HAS–SSI–88. SHI, July.

HO (Home Office). 1975 Report of the Committee on Mentally Abnormal Offenders (The Butler Report). London: HMSO.

HO. 1990 Provision for Mentally Disordered Offenders: Circular 66/90 London: Author.

HO. 1995 Mentally Disordered Offenders: Interagency Working: Circular 12/95 London: Author.

Home Office, HM Prison Service and Department of Health 2006 Dangerous and Severe/Complex Personality Disorder High Secure Services: Planning and Delivery Guide for Women's DSPD Services (Primrose Programme). www.dspdprogramme.gov.uk

Jones, K. 1993 Asylums and After: A Revised History of the Mental Health Services: From the Early Eighteenth Century to the 1990s. London: Athlone.

Laing and Buisson. 2006 Mental Health and Specialist Care Services UK Market Report (cited in Rutherford and Duggan 2007).

Maden, T., Curle, C., Meux, C., Burrow, S. and Gunn, J. 1995 Treatment and Security Needs of Special Hospital Patients. London: Whurr.

McKenzie, B. and Curr, H. 2005 Predicting Violence in a Medium Secure Setting: A Study Using the Historical and Clinical Scales of the HCR-20. British Journal of Forensic Practice 7(3): 22–28.

Ministry of Health. 1961 Special Hospitals. Report of a Working Party. London: HMSO.

MoJ (Ministry of Justice). 2007 Securing the Future: Proposals for the Efficient and Sustainable Use of Custody in England and Wales (Carter Review). www.justice.gov.uk/docs

MoJ. 2008a Sentencing Statistics 2007 England and Wales Ministry of Justice Statistical Bulletin. www.justice.gov.uk/sentencing-statistics-2007.pdf

MoJ 2008b Titan Prisons. www.justice.gov.uk.

Ministry of Justice and Department of Health (MoJ/DH). 2008a Dangerous and Severe Personality Disorder (DSPD) High Secure Services for Men: Planning and Delivery Guide. www.dspdprogramme.gov.uk

Ministry of Justice and Department of Health 2008b Forensic Personality Disorder Medium Secure and Community Pilot Services: Planning and Delivery Guide (Part of the DSPD Programme). www.dspdprogramme.gov.uk

Mullen, P.E. 1999 Dangerous People with Severe Personality Disorder. British Proposals for Managing Them are Glaringly Wrong – and Unethical. British Medical Journal 319: 1146–1147.

Murphy, E. 1990 September. Letter to the Guardian.

Munro, E. and Rumgay, J. 2000 Role of Risk Assessment in Reducing Homicides by People with Mental Illness. British Journal of Psychiatry 176: 116–120.

Murray, K. 1996 The Use of Beds in the NHS Medium Secure Units in England. The Journal of Forensic Psychiatry 7: 504–524.

NACRO. 2009 www.nacro.org.uk/mhu/about/faqs.htm#q1

NCISH (National Confidential Inquiry into Suicide and Homicide). 2006 Avoidable Deaths: Summary of Findings and Recommendations. www.medicine.manchester.ac.uk/suicideprevention/nci/Useful/avoidable_deaths.pdf

NICE. 2008a ASPD Treatment, Management and Prevention www.nice.org.uk/nicemedia/pdf/APSDFullVersionConsultation.pdf

NICE. 2008b Borderline Personality Disorder Treatment and Management www.nicemedia/pdf/BorderlinePersonalityDisorderNiceGuidelineforConsultation.pdf

NE Thames and SE Thames Regional Health Authorities. 1994 The Report of the Inquiry into the Care and Treatment of Christopher Clunis (Ritchie, J.H. Editor). London: Stationery Office Books.

Parker, E. 1985 The Development of Secure Provision, 15–69 in Secure Provision: A Review of Special Services for the Mentally Ill and Mentally Handicapped in England and Wales (Gostin, L. Editor). London: Tavistock Publications.

Peay, J. 1994 Mentally Disordered Offenders 1119–1160 in The Oxford Handbook of Criminology (Maguire, M., Morgan, R. and Reiner, R. Editors) Oxford: Oxford University Press

Raftery, J. 1992 Mental Health Services in Transition: The United States and the United Kingdom. British Journal of Psychiatry 161: 589–593.

Ramon, S. 1986 The Category of Psychopathy: It's Professional and Social Context in Britain 214–240 in the Power of Psychiatry (Miller, P. and Rose, N. Editors) Cambridge: Polity Press

Rutherford, M. and Duggan, S. 2007 Forensic Mental Health Services: Facts and Figures on Current Provision. London: The Sainsbury Centre for Mental Health.

SCMH (Sainsbury Centre for Mental Health). 2007 Briefing 32 Mental Health Care in Prisons. London: Author.

SEU (Social Exclusion Unit). 2002 Reducing Re-offending by Ex-prisoners. London: Author.

South West London SHA. 2006 The Independent Inquiry into the Care and Treatment of John Barrett London: NHS London.

Special Hospitals Service Authority. 1991 SHSA Review 1991.

Singleton, N., Meltzer, H. and Gatward, R. 1998 Psychiatric Morbidity among Prisoners in England and Wales. London: ONS.

Tilt, R., Perry, B., Martin, C. et al. 2000 Report of the Review of Security at the High Security Hospitals. London: Department of Health.

Walker, N. and McCabe, S. 1973 Crime and Insanity in England Vol. 2: New Solutions and New Problems. Edinburgh: University Press.

World Health Organisation 1992 International Classification of Diseases 10th Edition. Classification of Behavioural and Mental Disorders: Clinical Descriptions and Diagnostic Guidelines. Geneva: WHO.

Chapter 28

Prison mental health care

Crystal Romilly and Annie Bartlett

Aim

To describe the development of mental health care in prison.

Learning objectives

- To understand the prison policy context in which mental health services are situated
- To be aware of the nature and prevalence of mental health problems suffered by prisoners
- To know the current models of mental health service delivery in prison
- To understand the issues generated by the policy of equivalence in health care

Introduction

Health care in prisons is something of a paradox. One type of institution, a prison, designed as part of a criminal justice system, has to accommodate health care, the activity of another large institution, the National Health Service (NHS). The values of these two institutions are different but in part overlapping. This chapter situates health care in the context of the prison; it shows how policy initiatives over time have led to the transformation of the nature and quality of health care, specifically mental health care.

The role of health care professionals and their capacity to be effective was, and is, inextricably linked with the purpose and nature of the prisons in which they work.

What is prison for?

It is helpful in the United Kingdom context to realize that in the eighteenth century, prisons were predominantly places where people waited for other punishments such as transportation, hanging or paying fines. Imprisonment was not the punishment per se. It was only as transportation came to an end in 1840, and with the reduction in the use of the death penalty, that imprisonment itself became the punishment.

Liberal commentators were decrying prison conditions as far back as the eighteenth century. A landmark publication was 'The State of the Prisons' by John Howard (1777), in which he described the 'filthy, corrupt-ridden and unhealthy' conditions. Subsequent reforms were designed to deal with the unruly and unhealthy nature of existing prisons. The emphasis in the early nineteenth century was on making imprisonment unpleasant. It was designed to have a regime of unremitting work, minimal comforts, a barely adequate diet and minimal contact with friends and family. A major problem with the reforms, which were born of good intentions, was the capacity of governors to inflict additional punishments above and beyond the original sentence.

These were imposed for breaches of prison rules. Punishments such as solitary confinement, the treadmill, flogging, and bread and water diet could follow minor infringements (McGowen 1998).

It is only fairly recently that in the United Kingdom we have become used to the mantra that imprisonment or the deprivation of liberty *is* the punishment and should not extend to excessively harsh living conditions and, in particular, should not sentence the prisoner to substandard health care. In practice, the prison serves multiple purposes. These currently include not only deprivation of liberty but also deterrence, retraining and education, and preparation for deportation. In some other jurisdictions, it remains the case that prisons are places where individuals are tortured (with or without the approval of the state) and prepared for judicial execution (Amnesty International 2008).

An outline history of prison health care

Prison health care was considered in Parliament in 1774 and the Health of Prisoners Act became statute (Awofeso 2005). The prison medical service began in 1877 (Smith 1999).

Mental health care has always been an important component of prison medical care. Even in the fifteenth century there was some provision for dangerous lunatics to be confined in prison, Bridewells and at home. Legislation came into force in the nineteenth century to enable the transfer of mentally ill prisoners to asylum care (Parker 1985: 25–26). A major difficulty in transferring mentally ill prisoners to hospital, then as now, was the lack of secure psychiatric facilities. Broadmoor, the first asylum designed for the criminally insane, opened in 1863 (Walker and McCabe 1973).

Under the Prisons Act of 1877, prisons came under the control of the Home Office, and the first full-time medical inspector of prisons was appointed. The Gladstone Committee (1895) was responsible for introducing prison rules. Some of these are still relevant to health care in prison now. The Committee also introduced association and a structured working day (with wages) into the prison regime and recommended specific mental training for prison doctors.

Sir Alexander Paterson became prison commissioner in 1922 and was a force behind further reforms. The Howard League for Penal Reform was also started in that year by Margery Fry. Experimental psychological treatment was underway from the 1930s, and Grendon Underwood, a therapeutic prison, was opened in 1962 (Bowden and Bluglass 1990; Genders and Player 1995). This followed interest in therapeutic communities within psychiatry more generally.

After World War II there was a rapid expansion of prison health care. This was modelled on military sickbays and 'sick parades'. Health care officers were recruited from discipline staff. There was concern about variable standards among prison doctors, both in terms of clinical competence and professional integrity in relation to their prisoner patients. There has been increasing recognition about the ethical position and pressures operating on isolated doctors who are employed by a custodial institution. The birth of the NHS in 1948 was an opportunity lost; the Prison Medical Service (PMS) was not included. In 1964, the Royal College of Physicians and, in 1979, the Royal College of Psychiatrists, argued for the PMS' inclusion but they were ignored (Smith 1999).

Recent policy developments in prison health care

Continuing concern about medical recruitment and training in prison was voiced by the Home Office and Department of Health in 1989 (HO/DH 1989) and by three Royal Colleges in 1992 (Royal College of Physicians et al 1992). Organizational reform began to be seriously considered in 1990. The Efficiency Scrutiny (HO 1990) recommended the introduction of the purchaser/provider model into prison health care. HMCIP (1996) went on to introduce the idea of equality of care between prisons and the NHS as well as supporting the involvement of the NHS in service delivery. It also highlighted the problem of discontinuous care consequent on the constantly shifting prison population.

A degree of momentum for reform built up in the late 1990s. In 1999, the Future Organization of Prison Health Care (DH/HMPS 1999) was published. It introduced the concept of 'equiva-- lence', whereby it was argued that prisoners should have access to the same range and quality of health care as the outside community. This continues to inform commissioning of services and their delivery, and has proved to be conceptually and practically powerful. It reiterated the concerns about quality of medical care provided in prison. It recommended needs assessments in view of the evidently poor health of prisoners. More important, it held back from calling for full integration of prison health care into the NHS. The NHS was known to be reluctant and the Prison Officers' Association was recognized as a powerful and potentially obstructive trade union. However, it did argue for a 'formal partnership' between the Prison Service and the NHS and effectively paved the way for what followed. In 2001, 'Changing the Outlook' (DH 2001) supported the development of a quality workforce, including enhanced links with the NHS, but also thought that full integration of the PMS into the NHS was vital.

In the last three years, this process of integration has begun to materialize. The piecemeal introduction of NHS services into prisons has acquired organizational formality with the transfer of commissioning responsibility for prison health care to Primary Care Trusts (PCTs). In 2006, Partnership Boards comprising representatives from the prison and the PCT were set up. They are intended to provide strategic rather than operational management, and represent a new way of working both for the PCTs and the prisons, as they are required to agree in order to proceed. This recognizes that the PCTs and prisons are culturally distinct and that both have steep learning curves to follow if they are to make the Boards work.

Several challenges threaten the advances of recent years. The prison population continues to expand, rising to approximately 80,000 in England and Wales in 2006 (HO Home Office 2007 Population in Custody 2006). The introduction of indefinite life sentences in the 2003 Criminal Justice Act has stressed the prison system and threatens to create a cohort of elderly prisoners, with no hope of release and with all the health problems that accompany old age. Service delivery is variable in different prisons, with the balance of primary and secondary services not always ideal (SCMH 2007a). There has been no published work on the quality or efficacy of the Partnership Boards. Commissioning models vary even in discrete geographical areas such as London. PCTs not actively involved in commissioning services may have no real interest in prison services despite large numbers of their populations being incarcerated in them and released from them. The status and quality of needs assessments is unclear, although a national template now exists. As services within prison have developed, driven by the concept of equivalence, it has been recognized that the nature and morbidity of the prison population, who are not a community in the ordinary sense, may pose insuperable challenges to equality of care with the external community.

Prisoners suffer poor mental and physical health by comparison with the general community (Potts 2000; SCMH 2007a; Watson 2001). This multiple pathology is compounded by aspects of social exclusion (poor or non-existent housing, not part of the regular labour market) and chaotic lives (Bartlett 2006; PRT 2005; SEU 2002; Williamson 2006). Low rates of registration and engagement with general practice compromise their ability to access appropriate health care (Howerton 2007; Mezey 2007; SEU 2002). Against this background, prisons do seem able to provide compensatory care to some extent (Plugge 2006).

Mental health in prison

Poor mental health in prisoners has been the focus of much research over the years. Service delivery models, increasingly cognizant of this, have changed a great deal in the last 10 years. However, partly because of the nature of the prison environment, several problems continue to cause great concern, notably suicide and self-harm, transfers to hospital and compulsory treatment in prisons.

Morbidity

An interest in psychiatric morbidity in the prison population is not new but methodological variations have confounded comparisons over time and across jurisdictions. In the years up to 1978, only five studies used internationally standardized measures (Coid 1984). It is striking that, however measured, early studies found high rates of 'sub normality'.

More recently, Shaw (2001) reviewed the major epidemiological studies, of which the following have proved to be the most influential. Gunn's team (Gunn et al 1991; Maden 1996; Maden et al 1994) took a 5% sample of male sentenced prisoners and a 25% sample of female sentenced prisoners in England and Wales to assess levels of psychiatric morbidity (see Text Box 28.1). This was the first study not to simply count cases but to examine treatment needs too.

Most of those recommended for transfer to hospital – 52 (3%) men and 12 (5%) women – had psychotic illnesses, but smaller numbers had organic disorders, neurosis, personality or sexual disorders. Another 90 (5%) men and 25 (9%) women required more assessment in prison, 96 (5%) men and 20 (8%) women were judged suitable for therapeutic community, and 179 (10%) men and 56 (22%) women required outpatient treatment that could be given within the prison.

Issues raised in this survey include the following:

♦ Not all individuals requiring transfer to hospital had been ill at the time of the offence

♦ Psychiatric evidence might not have been considered at trial

♦ Some individuals had been judged unsuitable for hospital because of difficult or violent behaviour

♦ Some individuals had become ill after imprisonment

♦ Not all individuals with psychosis warranting hospital transfer had been identified by the prison doctors.

By extrapolation, the authors calculated that about 1,450 sentenced prisoners in England and Wales required hospital treatment.

Box 28.1 Sentenced prisoners

	Women (n = 258)		Men (n = 1,751)	
Psychosis	4	1.6%	34	1.9%
Neurosis	40	16%	104	6%
Personality Disorder	46	18%	177	10%
Alcohol abuse/dependence	24	9%	203	12%
Drug abuse/dependence	67	26%	203	12%
Mental handicap	6	2.3%	11	0.6%

Adapted from Maden 1996: 74.

The prevalence of psychiatric disorder among male remand prisoners revealed higher rates of disorder (Brooke et al 1996). Overall, 5.5% of the sample had some form of psychosis. This would imply far higher proportions requiring transfer to hospital than from the sentenced prisoners group.

The ONS survey (Singleton et al 1998) produced far higher figures for rates of mental disorder in prisoners and the gravity of the findings was reinforced by the differences between prison and community figures (Meltzer et al 1995). A frequently quoted finding from the ONS results is that fewer than 10% of prisoners have no mental disorder, 20% have one diagnosis, and the remaining 70% have two or more diagnoses; so, for example, they may suffer from mental illness, personality disorder, and substance abuse problems. A proportion of these individuals may be very difficult to manage safely within the prison but can be rejected by outside NHS services, especially if clear treatable mental illness is hard to demonstrate.

Fazel and Danesh (2002) undertook a systematic review of serious mental disorders among prisoners across several Western countries, amalgamating sentenced and remand prisoners, and men and women. It is striking that despite drawing on surveys from several countries and over a broad timespan, rates for psychotic illnesses and major depression are fairly consistent across countries, perhaps because of greater diagnostic consensus for these disorders. Their overall conclusion was that about one-seventh – or 14% – of all prisoners across relevant countries suffer from psychosis or major depression. This result is considerably higher than the Gunn studies but similar to the ONS results for male and female remand prisoners.

Rates of mental disorder can be useful for service planning and constitute part of the needs assessment now required by PCTs commissioning services. However, the relationship of prison statistics to community prevalence will depend on jurisdiction-specific approaches to crime (definitions of crime, rates of crime, detection, prosecution and the use of prison for remand and sentencing) (see Chapter 3). The UK rate of imprisonment (139/100,000) is the highest among the old EU countries (Walmsley 2003). Similarly, the responsiveness of the health service will determine the ease with which prisoners are moved from the penal system to health care and alter prison prevalence figures.

Service delivery

The delivery of mental health care in prisons has undergone major changes with the introduction of 'prison in-reach teams'. Reed and Lynne (2000) documented the state of mental health care prior to this. They found so-called inpatient units ranged between 3 and 75 beds in the 13 prisons reviewed. No doctor had specialist mental health training, but one-quarter of nurses did. Periods of seclusion lasted 50 hours on average. There was little therapeutic activity and the quality of care fell way below that of the NHS.

The introduction of in-reach was intended to ensure multidisciplinary approaches to care using the model of the Community Mental Health Team (CMHT) (DH/HMPS 1999). This was to be aimed at prisoners with severe and enduring mental illness (SMI). As these teams have become established, several issues are evident. First, the teams are small, and they operate with limited guidance (Steel et al 2007). Second, there is a need for forensic expertise, if not forensic practitioners, because of the need to work with the criminal justice system. Third, to restrict the service to SMI is to ignore the often complex personality pathology of prisoners.[1]

---

[1] The prison service has for many years provided therapeutic community options to small numbers of prisoners, for example, Grendon Underwood and previously the Scrubs Annexe and Barlinnie. Recent expansion has been in the area of DSPD services (see Chapter 16).

HMCIP (2007), reviewing the function of the in-reach services, found that only 19% of such teams thought they could meet prisoners' needs. Most were nurse-led services with variable access to other mental health professionals. Referrals ran at high levels and caseloads were 33 per worker. Two in 3 clients had some kind of care plan but only half of them knew about it. Seventy-five percent of the clients had previous contact with mental health services, but only 59% of the previous providers had been contacted. Pyszora and Telfer (2003) had previously estimated that 2.5% to 7% of new prisoners a year would be eligible for enhanced CPA.

Despite what are widely accepted as improvements in service delivery, mental health care in prisons still faces huge challenges. Some of these are a product of prison regime. The governor and their deputies will ultimately determine movement of prisoners around the prison, including in and out of health care units as well as between prisons. Prisoners are subject to a uniform timetable for activities during the day. The mix of discipline and health staff in health care settings as well as on the wings creates challenges for successful joint working, given that the aims may be different and issues of confidentiality differently managed (the Inmate Medical Record is essentially the governor's property).

Equivalence and transfers to hospital

There are several dimensions of the concept of equivalence worthy of further discussion. Equivalence could mean that mental disorder among prisoners should be treated in an equivalent way to physical disorder. This is not the case at present. If a prisoner develops an acute physical problem, he or she is sent to the local Accident and Emergency department for assessment and possible treatment. He or she will be admitted to hospital there if the assessing doctors think it appropriate. They may not be popular patients and can be returned to prison with some haste, but they are at least seen and treated. The same cannot be said for acute mental health problems. A prisoner will be sent to hospital only if the physical effects of self-harm or attempted suicide require assessment and treatment in hospital. If a prisoner needs hospitalization for an acute mental disorder, and even if assessed in prison by the prison consultant psychiatrist, he or she cannot be admitted straight to the relevant external unit as he or she would if seen 'on call' by the relevant senior clinician. The patients wait in prison for an additional assessment and then are subject to the procedures of the Ministry of Justice or the courts for suitable transfer. This may take several months and may be to do with one or more of the following reasons:

◆ Difficulty identifying appropriate external team

◆ Reluctance of team to accept responsibility for patient who is an NFA (no fixed abode) or does not have a GP

◆ Delay in attending prison for assessment

◆ External team unfamiliar with courts and other aspects of forensic practice

◆ Disagreement between external and prison teams about diagnosis and management

◆ Restricted scope of the section 48 urgent treatment order

◆ Lack of availability of low secure and medium secure hospital beds

Transfer delays have a long history and have been well researched. Dell et al (1993) found transfer requests for women resulted in placement difficulties, especially when personality disorder or mental handicap was involved. Robertson et al (1994) found severely mentally ill men charged with minor offences could be remanded for long periods due to transfer delays. Isherwood and Parrott (2002) still found delays in the transfer of the severely mentally ill, and Reed (2003) argued this was predominantly the fault of the external NHS. The Department of Health has focused on this issue in recent years (DH 2005), but there is continuing debate about realistic time scales for transfers given the lack of availability of beds in the external NHS. McKenzie and Sales (2008) found a reduction in the transfer times from 11 weeks to 7 weeks following the introduction of the guidance. Medium secure beds were particularly hard to access.

Equivalence and compulsory treatment in prison

One of the reasons transfers to psychiatric hospital are important is that the Mental Health Act 1983 does not apply in prisons. A prison health care centre is not classed as a hospital under the National Health Service Act 1977; consequently, psychiatric patients cannot be compulsorily treated in prison under statutory powers. The ethos of 'equivalence' suggests that 'hospital wings' with their 'inpatients' should be just that. In fact, they do not have the same facilities as the external NHS. Their capacity to operate therapeutically is inevitably compromised by their additional need to operate within the prison regime. Finally, such wings are also required to mix up prisoners with physical and mental health needs (Wilson 2004), which would be unthinkable in the external NHS.

The absence of Mental Health Act powers has traditionally meant that psychotropic medication in prison was given without consent only in emergencies, on a common law basis. This is permitted when it was judged necessary to prevent serious harm to the patient or others if not administered. Restrictive prison procedures require two doctors to sign and approve the treatment, one of whom should be a consultant psychiatrist and one of whom should be present when the treatment is given. In practice, this limits the frequency. Many individuals in need of regular medication refuse it (McKenzie and Sales 2008).

Some psychiatrists have been arguing that we should be more willing to give medication to severely psychiatrically unwell prisoners who lack the capacity to give or withhold informed consent, if it is judged in the best interests of the patient (Wilson and Forrester 2002). These authors cite the case of Re F, where it was stated that it was acceptable to do this 'to save life, prevent deterioration or ensure improvement in the patient's physical or mental health'. It is also true that compulsory medication alone, although useful, does not equate to the package of care available in hospital.

Linked to this debate is the view that prison hospital wings, suitably improved and staffed, should be brought under the aegis of the Mental Health Act. This would mean that prisoner-patients can be treated compulsorily if unable or unwilling to consent, as happens in some other jurisdictions (see Chapter 31). Wilson and Forrester argued that now the Department of Health is taking over prison health care, there is an opportunity to reconsider the function of prison hospital wings (Wilson and Forrester 2002). They advocate that wings should become hospitals to which the Mental Health Act is applicable so that psychiatrists working in prison can begin to treat their patients in an equivalent way to those outside. Wilson recognized that more than a change in legislation is required: 'A properly multidisciplinary team of trained staff will be needed with proper facilities and a varied and productive range of therapeutic activities for patient-prisoners' (Wilson 2002: 6).

Legislation would bring with it the statutory protections of the Act, including regular inspections by the Mental Health Act Commission, rather than just the Chief Inspector of Prisons or the Independent Monitoring Boards. The shift towards this position is perhaps driven by the sense that the NHS will never have enough secure psychiatric beds to accommodate the numbers of prisoners needing transfer. Currently, there is an ethical difficulty in leaving such patients languishing in prison for many weeks or months, waiting for a hospital bed.

Suicide and deliberate self-harm

Both suicide and deliberate self-harm have been important issues in prison health in recent years. Completed suicide in prison has consequences for the person's family and friends and for the institution concerned. The pressure group Inquest has played an important role in highlighting deaths in custody (Hill 2008). As with community-based psychiatric homicides, suicides in prison can have significant repercussions for staff. There is a stark contrast between the status of prison suicide and suicide in the community or in psychiatric hospital.

Between 1972 and 1987, the rise in completed suicide in prison was proportionally in excess of the rise in the prison population (Dooley 1990). Hanging was the most common method and a third of successful suicides had a psychiatric history. It became clear that the remand period was a high-risk period and that nearly half of these people had committed previous acts of self-harm. The study found that almost half were seen by a doctor in the week before death, but in only one in six was suicidality noted. These figures from the Dooley paper indicate that it is a minority, albeit a significant and important minority, whose suicide occurs in the context of mental disorder. Leibling (1994) argued from strong empirical material that the prison environment was also relevant to suicide, something echoed in the HMCIP's report (1999). This report emphasized the idea of the healthy prison in which cultural and relational factors contributed to suicide prevention and not simply mental health measures. The suicide rate continued to rise but dropped between 2003 and 2006, rising again in 2007 (HMCIP 2008; Shaw et al 2004). The Chief Inspector of Prisons' report (HMCIP 2008) noted the recent rise, and observes that this is disproportionate to the rise in the prison population. Twenty percent of self-inflicted deaths take place in the first 7 days of incarceration. Self-inflicted deaths are more common in local and female prisons. There seems to be a complex relationship of rates within particular prisons to levels of overcrowding, mediated by the vulnerability of types of prisoners and prison specific regimes (Personal Communication SCG 2008).

Suicidal thoughts and history of deliberate self-harm are common among prisoners. Singleton et al (1998) reported that 15% of male remand prisoners and 27% of female remand prisoners had made a suicide attempt in the previous year. Among sentenced prisoners, 5% of men and 9% of women had self-harmed (as opposed to making a suicide attempt) in the current prison term. The authors estimated that a prisoner has a sevenfold risk of suicide compared with someone in the community, especially, but not exclusively, if they suffer from mental illness or disorder. Many of those at risk will fall in the personality disorder/substance abuse spectrum and are extremely unlikely to be accepted for transfer to an outside hospital.

Another perspective on this is that if you take a young person with all the markers of social exclusion and, very probably, at least one mental disorder, arrest and charge him, strip him of all autonomy, reduce his contact with significant people in his life, take away his drugs and alcohol and place him in a prison cell for up to 19 hours per day, it is perhaps surprising that there are not more acts of deliberate self-harm and self-inflicted deaths. Prisons are high-risk environments with a small number of mental health workers. ACCT training, designed to assess and manage prisoners at risk of self-harm, is now widespread among prison staff; there is support for shared responsibility between health workers and discipline staff. The Safer Custody Group figures suggest that the rates of self-harm are just beginning to fall, but there were more than 22,000 incidents in 2007. HMCIP (2008: 22) reported variable compliance with ACCT guidance, with examples of both 'in-depth understanding and multidisciplinary care planning and reviews' and also of poor practice and inadequate managerial checks.

The approach to preventing suicide in prison should be to offer more humane care to everyone (the whole healthy institution), scrupulous health screening, including obtaining prior medical records when appropriate, and improved mental health care – primary, secondary and tertiary – for those with mental health problems.

It is ethically unacceptable to remove only the means of committing suicide, without taking steps to alleviate the distress that makes the individual want to kill himself or herself.

Simply removing ligature points in cells, fixing beds to the floor, placing someone in a strip cell or maintaining one-to-one observation, is a very limited and inadequate response to distress. Prevention is important but is only the beginning. Institutional pressures or personal circumstances can create distress, but that can sometimes respond to simple measures. A little sympathy, flexibility or professionalism, and sitting down and talking with the prisoner, can alleviate problems and/or pave the way for a better understanding of them.

Furthermore, many suicides occur within a short period of release from prison (Pratt et al 2006). This emphasizes both the vulnerable nature of the prison population and the importance of discharge arrangements for all prisoners, including those with mental health problems in the broadest sense as well as for those with serious mental illness.

Primary care, public health and substance misuse

Effective mental health services are secondary services and are dependent on effective primary care in prisons.

There is a mixed economy of primary care at present (SCMH 2007b), with variable models of primary care. There are no norms for staffing levels that take into account the high morbidity and complex needs of prisoners. No national data exist on the range or type of primary care clinicians in prisons. There is no training structure for prison GPs, and only one-third have experience of psychiatry as senior house officers. Having said that, there appear to have been sustained improvements in primary care across the prison estate (HMCIP 2008), and there is evidence that serious chronic conditions such as diabetes and renal failure can be well managed in a prison setting (Williamson 2006).

The boundaries between primary care and mental health or other secondary-tier services can be unclear. Consequently, cases that could be dealt with by primary care or substance misuse can be referred to mental health in-reach teams. In-reach teams can be at risk of being overwhelmed, burnt out, feeling they are fighting obstructions both within and without the prison, as well as trying to negotiate the custodial issues, and distracted from their core task of managing people with serious mental illness (SCMH 2007a). This is made worse where there is an absence of permanent staff in primary care. Primary mental health care remains an aspiration, rather than a reality (SCMH 2007b). Access to psychological therapies is limited, and there is unmet need in relation to minor but potentially debilitating mental disorders (Durcan and Knowles 2006).

There is also concern about the adequacy of the basic prison screening tool to pick up mental health issues. The realities of detection are illustrated in the personal account by one of the authors (CR) in Text Box 28.2.

Substance misuse, particularly crack cocaine and opiates, is a major problem among prisoners. Thirty-eight percent of prisoners are drug users on reception into prison. Fifty-thousand prisoners a year access detoxification services. Rates of Hepatitis B and C are high among intravenous drug users. Twice as many prisoners smoke as in the general population (see Williamson 2006). Many of these prisoners will be co-morbid for mental health problems.

Aftercare and resettlement

Most prisoners are in custody for less than 6 months and then return to their community, so prisoner-patients should be viewed as part of the mainstream. The importance of continuity in medical care between prison and the outside world is stressed in prison guidance (PSO 3050). Equivalence should mean that no one with mental health problems should leave prison without discharge arrangements being made. The complexity of prisoners' health problems, as well as their social needs, may mean that they do not fit neatly with external services (Durcan and

Box 28.2 Personal view: screening at reception

Anyone who has witnessed the reception process in action at a busy local prison will have some idea why screening is so imperfect in terms of identifying health problems. From my own observations, prisoners begin to arrive at the prison in the late afternoon in Securicor vans, which have been doing the rounds of courts picking up their passengers. These vans continue to arrive well into the evening. The pressure is on in the reception area to get everyone processed, fed, and 'banged up' in a cell, in time for the day shift to hand over to night staff at about 8pm. There is heavy throughput and limited time and privacy. There are procedures for reception health care staff to screen for mental disorder, substance misuse history and vulnerability to self-harm, in which case they refer the prisoner to the duty doctor (who sometimes cannot be found); the system is flawed. Many prisoners will have had a difficult day, having left prison early in the morning (very possibly a different prison from the one to which they are returned in the evening) and having been locked within a cubicle or 'sweatbox' in the prison van while all the collections and drops are made. They will have spent several hours in the cells at court, other than when appearing in court themselves. They then have a similar return journey to prison – it could be a 12-hour day. Most people would be staggered to see the 'toilet cubicle' they are locked into within the van. The rules state that they should have a break to stretch legs, to relieve themselves or have a cigarette no less than every 2 hours. They may well be frightened and distressed because of their circumstances. These are not conditions that encourage candid rapport between prisoner and health professional or promote disclosure of sensitive issues. Primary care staff in reception should begin the process of liaising with the GP and getting background information. This may not happen – it is too busy, too late to contact anyone in most surgeries and the prisoner is not registered with a GP or withholds or cannot recall details.

Knowles 2006), each of which may have a limited remit and be a long way from the kind of 'one-stop shop' envisaged by the Corston Report (HO 2007). Forty-nine percent of prisoners have no permanent accommodation on release (RDA 2002). Continuity of care is dependent on such an address, which permits GP registration. The particular needs of prisoners with mental health problems should also be seen against the background of very variable compliance nationally with resettlement guidance for all prisons and prisoners (HMCIP 2008).

Conclusion

Even now, despite the extra resources and staff devoted to prison mental health care, provision is still far from adequate, given the level of need. Moreover, if this is true now, when the prison population is approximately 80,000, how much truer will it be when the prison population rises to the expected 100,000 forecast by 2010?

References

Amnesty International. 2008 Broken Prisoners Report. thereport.amnesty.org/document/47

Awofeso, N. 2005 Making Prison Health Care More Efficient. British Medical Journal 331: 248–249.

Bartlett, A. 2006 Female Offenders. Women's Health Medicine 3: 91–95.

Bowden, P. and Bluglass, R. 1990 Principles and Practice of Forensic Psychiatry. London: Churchill Livingstone.

Brooke, D. Taylor, C., Gunn, J. and Maden, A. 1996 Point Prevalence of Mental Disorder in Unconvicted Male Prisoners in England and Wales. British Medical Journal 313: 1524–1527.

Coid, J. 1984 How Many Psychiatric Patients in Prison? British Journal of Psychiatry 145: 78–86.

Dell, S., Robertson, G., James, K. and Grounds, A. 1993 Remands and Psychiatric Assessments in Holloway Prison. British Journal of Psychiatry 163: 640–644.

DH Department of Health 2001 Changing the Outlook. A Strategy for Developing and Modernising Mental Health Services in Prisons. London: Department of Health.

DH 2005 Procedure for the Transfer of Prisoners to and from Hospital under Section 47 and 48 of the Mental Health Act 1983: Version 3 London: Department of Health.

DH/HMPS (Department of Health and HM Prison Service) 1999 The Future Organisation of Prison Health Care. Report by the Joint Prison Service and National Health Service Executive Working Group. London: Department of Health.

Dooley, E. 1990 Prison Suicide in England and Wales, 1972–87. British Journal of Psychiatry 156: 40–45.

Durcan, D. and Knowles, K. 2006 Policy Paper 5 London's Prison Mental Health Services: A Review. London: The Sainsbury Centre for Mental Health.

Fazel, S. and Danesh, J. 2002 Serious Mental Disorder in 23,000 Prisoners: A Systematic Review of 62 Surveys. Lancet 359: 545–550.

Genders, E. and Player, E. 1995 Grendon: A Study of a Therapeutic Prison. Oxford: Clarendon Press.

Gladstone Committee Report 1895 Edwards and Hurley 1997.

Gunn, J., Maden, A. and Swinton, M. 1991 Treatment Needs of Prisoners with Psychiatric Disorders. British Medical Journal 303: 338–341.

HMCIP HM Inspectorate for Prisons 1996 Patient or Prisoner? London: Home Office.

HMCIP 1999 Suicide is Everyone's Concern London: Home Office.

HMCIP 2007 The Mental Health of Prisoners. London: HM Inspectorate of Prisons.

HMCIP 2008 HM Chief Inspector of Prisons for England and Wales Annual Report 2006/07. London: The Stationary Office.

HO Home Office 1990 Report of an Efficiency Scrutiny of the Prison Medical Service. London: Author.

HO Home Office 2007 Population in Custody October 2006. www.homeoffice.gov.uk/rds/omcs/html

HO Home Office 2007a The Corston Report: a Report by Baroness Jean Corston of a Review of women with Particular Vulnerabilities in the Criminal Justice System. London: Author.

HO/DH Home Office and Department of Health 1989 The Prison Medical Service in England and Wales in the Recruitment and Training of Doctors. London: Home Office and Department of Health.

Howard, J. 1777 The State of the Prisons in England and Wales. Warrington.

Howerton, A., Byng, Campbell, J., Hess, D., Owens, C. and Aitken, P. 2007 Understanding Help Seeking Behaviour among Male Offenders: Qualitative Interview Study. British Medical Journal 334: 303–306.

Isherwood, S. and Parrott, J. 2002 Audit of Transfers under the Mental Health Act from Prison – The Impact of Organisational Change. Psychiatric Bulletin 26: 368–370.

Liebling, A. 1994 Suicide amongst Women Prisoners. Howard Journal 30: 1–4.

Maden, T. 1996 Women, Prisons and Psychiatry: Mental Disorder Behind Bars. Oxford: Butterworth Heineman.

Maden, T., Swinton, M. and Gunn, J. 1994 Psychiatric Disorder in Women Serving a Prison Sentence. British Journal of Psychiatry 164: 44–54.

McGowan, R. 1998 The Well Ordered Prison England 1780–1865 71–99 in The Oxford History of the Prison: The Practice of Punishment in Western Society. (Morris, N. and Rothman, D.J. Editors). Oxford: Oxford University Press.

McKenzie, N. and Sales, B. 2008 Procedures to Cut Delays in the Transfer of Mentally ill Prisoners to Hospital. Psychological Bulletin 32: 20–22.

Meltzer, D., Gill, B., Pettigrew, M. and Hinds, K. 1995 OPCS Surveys of Psychiatric Morbidity in Great Britain, Report 1: the Prevalence of Psychiatric Morbidity among Adults Living in Private Households. London: HMSO.

Mezey, G. 2007 Improving the Mental Health of Offenders in Primary Care. British Medical Journal: 334: 267–268.

Parker, E. 1985 The Development of Secure Provision 15–65 in Secure Provision (Gostin, L. Editor) London: Tavistock.

Plugge, E. 2006 The Health of Women in Prison. Personal Communication.

Potts, 2000 HIV/AIDS in Federal Prisons: Canada's National Response. HIV Prevalence Plus 2, 2: 1–3.

Pratt, D. Piper, M., Appleby, L., Webb, R. and Shaw, J. 2006 Suicide in Recently Released Prisoners: A Population-based Cohort Study. Lancet 368: 119–123.

Prison Reform Trust (PRT) 2005 Bromley Briefings Prison Factfile. London: Prison Reform Trust. www.prisonreformtrust.org.uk

PSO (Prison Service Order) 3050 Continuity of Health Care for Prisoners. Issue No: 254 10/2/2006.

Pyszora, N. and Telfer, J. 2003 Implementation of the Care Programme Approach in Prison. Psychiatric Bulletin 27: 173–176.

RDA (Revolving Doors Agency) 2002 Where Do They Go? Mental Health, Housing and Leaving Prison. London: RDA.

Reed, J. 2003 Mental Health Care in Prisons. The British Journal of Psychiatry 182: 287–288.

Reed, J. and Lyne, M. 2000 Inpatient Care of Mentally Ill People in Prison: Results of a Year's Programme of Semi-structured Inspections. British Medical Journal 320: 1031–1034.

Robertson, G., Dell, S., James, K. and Grounds, A. 1994 Psychotic Men Remanded in Custody to Brixton Prison. British Journal of Psychiatry 164: 55–61.

Royal College of Physicians, Royal College of General Practitioners, Royal College of Psychiatrists 1992 Report of the Working Party of Three Medical Royal Colleges on the Education and Training of Doctors in the Health Care Service for Prisoners. London: Home Office.

SCMH (The Sainsbury Centre for Mental Health) 2007a Briefing 32 Mental Health Care in Prisons. London: SCMH.

SCMH 2007b Getting the Basics Right: Developing a Primary Care Mental Health Service in Prisons Policy Paper 7. London: SCMH.

SEU (Social Exclusion Unit) 2002 Reducing Re-offending by Ex-prisoners. London: SEU.

Shaw, J. 2001 Prison Health Care Forensic Mental Health R and D Expert Paper www.nfmhp.org.uk/expert paper.htm

Shaw, J., Baker, D., Hunt, I.M., Moloney, A. and Appleby, L. 2004 Suicide by Prisoners: National Clinical Survey. British Journal of Psychiatry 184: 263–267.

Singleton, N., Meltzer, H. and Gatward, R. 1998 Psychiatric Morbidity among Prisoners in England and Wales. London: ONS.

Smith, R. 1999 Prisoners: An End to Second Class Health Care? British Medical Journal 318: 954–955.

Steel, J., Thornicroft, G., Birmingham, L. et al 2007 Prison Mental Health Inreach Services. British Journal of Psychiatry 190: 373–374.

Walker, N. and Mc Cabe, S. 1973 Crime and Insanity in England. Vol 2: New Solutions and New Problems. Edinburgh: Edinburgh University Press.

Walmsley, R. 2003 World Prison Population List 4th Edition. Findings 188 www.rds.homeoffice.gov.uk/rds/pdfs2/r188.pdf

Watson, R. 2001 Drug Users Receive Worse Care in Prison than in the Community. British Medical Journal 323: 654.

Williamson, M. 2006 Improving the Health and Social Outcomes of People Recently Released from Prisons in the UK: A Perspective from Primary Care. www.scmh.org.uk/criminaljustice

Wilson, S. 2004 The Principle of Equivalence and the Future of Mental Health Care in Prisons. The British Journal of Psychiatry 184: 5–7.

Wilson, S. and Forrester, A. 2002 Too Little, too Late? The Treatment of Mentally Incapacitated Prisoners. Journal of Forensic Psychiatry 13: 1–8.

Chapter 29

Current service provision for mentally disordered offenders

Annie Bartlett and Sue Kesteven

Aim

To evaluate current service provision for mentally disordered offenders (MDOs).

Learning objectives

- To describe the roles of agencies involved in the assessment, treatment and management of mentally disordered offenders (MDOs)
- To examine the strengths and weaknesses of current service provision for MDOs

---

Introduction

The mentally disordered offender (MDO) is a little like a spider in a web of organizations, but the web is not of their own making. Attracting the label of MDO, like many labels linked with either crime or madness, is stigmatizing. It comes into play as a consequence of a combination of mental health problems and offending behaviour. Figure 29.1 illustrates the potential relationships of the different agencies with some involvement in the lives of MDOs; it highlights their complex interconnectedness. Not all agencies will be involved at any one time with a given individual. For some, dealing with MDOs is only a minor part of their workload. For others, it is their sole task. The career of an MDO can be long and their involvement with agencies will change over time. One factor remains constant, that is, that for the most part their involvement with these agencies is seldom voluntary, even if they do ultimately derive some benefit. There is no empirical study to indicate what proportion of MDOs, however defined, finally truly exit from the web; nor is there a proper understanding of pathways of care.

The range of agencies include criminal justice (Magistrates' and Crown Courts), prisons (including prison mental health), legal representation (solicitors and barristers) and the Crown prosecution service, NHS and private sector units (secure, non-secure and community services), voluntary sector organizations, hostels, supported living schemes, work placements, Social Services (part of inpatient and aftercare, child welfare issues), police and probation.

Bartlett and Kesteven (Chapter 27) documented the historical development both of the concept of the MDO and of the services designed to assist them. It is too much to say that there has been a flurry of policy-making activity recently, but policy continues to change. The consequence of policy innovation and change is that there are significant shifts in the scope and range of agencies involved in the care of MDOs. This is because although such organizations are capable

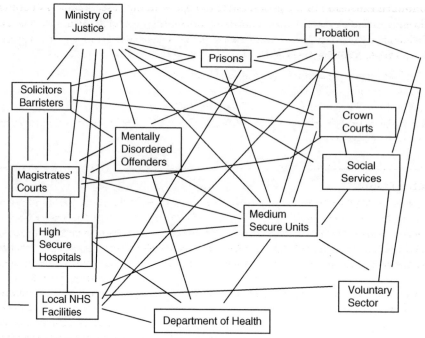

Fig. 29.1 The complex web of interconnections between MDOs and organizations.

of independent development and evolution, one of the main drivers for this is the policy and financing that comes from the state. Specifically, we have seen the following:

◆ Continuing reduction in the size of the high secure hospital estate, from 1,700 beds in 1991(SHSA 1991) to 800 in 2007 (Rutherford and Duggan 2007)

◆ Creation of Enhanced Medium Secure Hospital Services for women

◆ Creation of the DSPD programme in prison and in the NHS (high and medium secure beds and aftercare provision) (MoJ/DH 2008a, 2008b)

◆ Guidance on diversion from custody of MDOs (HO 1990, 1995) and the creation of a range of diversion schemes (Blumenthal and Wessely 1992; James and Hamilton 1991; Joseph and Potter 1993): approximately 150 in 1999 and possibly fewer today (NACRO 2005, 2008). Lord Bradley has undertaken a review of these schemes as there continues to be uncertainty about adequacy and efficacy

◆ Multiple Criminal Justice Acts were passed under the Blair governments. The 2003 CJA created the obligation for agencies involved in the interagency management of MDOs and other offenders, including the NHS, to cooperate to enhance risk management

◆ Multiple changes in guidance and legislation to enhance supervision of MDOs (Supervision Register, Section 25A) culminated in the 2007 MHA. This MHA has broadened the definition of mental disorder and altered the threshold for compulsory hospitalization and community treatment (2007 MHA)

◆ Creation of the Offender Management System to promote continuity of supervision for all convicted offenders (NOMS 2006)

◆ Continued expansion of the prison estate to cope with increased numbers of sentenced prisoners, including the increased number on indefinite sentences (4,619 in July 2008), many of whom have complex mental health needs that are challenging for prison in-reach services (SCMH 2006, 2007; Steel et al 2007)

The following vignettes[1] are designed to illustrate different levels and kinds of contact with this complex system and how individual offenders can experience different pathways of care. They underline the essential ambiguity of the term MDO, as rehearsed in the previous chapter, and emphasize how different the clinical and offending issues may be, from person to person, as well as how they evolve over time.

Vignette 1: Ann

Ann is a 45-year-old White British woman who has been in prison on eight occasions. Her offending is minor with only two convictions for assault occasioning actual bodily harm (AOABH). She is never sentenced to long periods but inevitably, as the number of convictions rises, her sentences are longer. She uses alcohol and cannabis when in the community. When she came into prison on this occasion she required alcohol detoxification. She has had several male partners and one or two female partners over the years. These relationships have been characterized by volatility on her part, sometimes by violence from her partners. She has three children and has struggled hard to look after them. Two have been adopted and now, during her most recent period of imprisonment, the third is up for adoption. *Social services* are interested in her criminal record and her mental health problems as they consider the future of her child. *Local mental health services* are slow to come to *the prison* to assess her. They have previously suggested that because the working diagnosis is one of Borderline Personality Disorder they have little to offer. Ann, in prison, is overwhelmed with a sense of failure as a mother and repeatedly self-harms, on one occasion dangerously. She is in touch with the addiction team in prison, and they recommend she seek help voluntarily and use *a voluntary sector organization*, AA, when she leaves, as she does not want to return to her violent partner. She knows no one where she moves and is unknown to local services. She will see her *Probation* Officer once every two weeks.

Vignette 2: Ralph

Ralph is a 25-year-old Black British man who suffers from paranoid schizophrenia. He had behavioural problems in childhood. He did poorly at school and his mother, his sole carer, could not have him at home. In his mid-teens he went into care. Feeling rejected by his family, his law breaking and his drug use escalated. During his first period of imprisonment, he was the victim of racist bullying. After this he became increasingly paranoid and was admitted to hospital with what initially appeared to be a drug-induced psychosis and was subsequently recognized as paranoid schizophrenia. His family and particularly his sister tried to support him but in the context of relapsing illness he stabbed his mother. The *Crown Court* imposed a s.37 hospital order with a s.41 restriction order. He was admitted to a *medium secure hospital* service. He did well and was discharged under supervision (conditional discharge and MAPPA reviews) to a hostel run by a *voluntary sector agency*. He remains in close contact with services but feels pessimistic about many aspects of his life. He is tentatively resuming his formal education. His family ties have been disrupted, and his mother no longer feels able to see him.

Vignette 3: Colin

Colin is a 30-year-old White British man with bipolar illness. He managed his illness well until his wife left him two years ago. Since then he has had three brief periods of time in hospital, and his employers feel they can no longer keep him on. He is angry at what is happening to him and this engenders a sense of despair

---

[1] These vignettes are not based on real people but are designed to illustrate real care pathways.

independent of his illness. He is erratically compliant with his mood-stabilizing medication and accosts a woman of his wife's age on the street one night and threatens her. Passers-by intervene, he hits one of them and he is arrested. He is assessed by the Court Diversion Scheme in the *Magistrates Court* as in need of a PICU bed, and it is suggested he might be diverted to hospital and the charges dropped. There is no PICU bed and he is remanded into custody. Four weeks later a *private sector* bed is approved. By now he is very ill, having refused medication in prison. At one point, he is forcibly medicated in prison and for the most part is confined to his cell on 3-man unlock. He has assaulted officers and has further charges pending. The CMHT from his *local NHS Trust* appear less keen to look after him and ask the local forensic service to review him in the private placement with a view to an NHS *medium secure bed*.

Vignette 4: Malcolm

Malcolm is a 49-year-old White British man with a primary sexual interest in children. He was a teacher and was first convicted of child sex offences in his early thirties. He has offended since then and is on the Sex Offenders Register. During his last period of imprisonment he was attacked in a prison workshop. On release he has become depressed. He seeks the help of his GP who refers him to *local NHS mental health services*. They notify MAPPA and refer him for the first time to the *local forensic service* for risk assessment in their Sex Offender Service. Review of his housing situation in the MAPPA panel meeting suggests it is very close to a local school and *the police* decide to step up the level of his monitoring as information from the forensic Sex Offender Service suggest that his depression may increase his risk of offending.

The point of the vignettes is not so much what the characters they portray have in common but what they do not have in common. Yet all may, but will not necessarily, be considered mentally disordered offenders. The nature of the agencies involved is different in each case, and over time has altered for them as individuals. They move between the criminal justice system and the welfare systems in ways that can seem appropriate but also inappropriate and arbitrary. Two things emerge from the vignettes. Having diagnosable mental health problems does not necessarily lead to getting help at the right time. Equally, a lifetime of offending punished by the criminal justice system does not preclude referral to the NHS.

It is easy to polarize the agencies involved. In practice, many will have both social welfare and public safety functions, but they will differ in terms of what they actually do and the balance of these two functions.

Strengths and weaknesses of systems to manage MDOs

From within a single agency the rest of the system or potential system to manage a single MDO may not be clear or the role of the other agencies well understood or accepted. To some extent, the agencies have complementary roles, but equally they can be construed as being at odds with each other. This is most apparent in relation to the issue of public protection and is exemplified in the difficult task of MAPPA panels that coordinate thinking about dangerous MDOs as dictated by the Criminal Justice Act 2003. The MAPPA process encourages interagency sharing of risk information while also acknowledging the different working practices of criminal justice and health professionals.

Interagency working has been recognized as difficult to achieve well for more than 15 years and was one of the rationales for the Reed Report (DH/HO 1992). Barriers to effective work include conceptual discordance, ignorance of other professionals' roles, resource constraints, practice imperatives and logistical difficulties. Interagency work relates to a single point in time.

Continuity of care within and between agencies adds a further layer of complexity. There are established mechanisms in both health and the criminal justice systems to encourage this (DH 2005; PSO 3050), but there is evidence that much of this good practice guidance remains aspirational (HMIP 2007; NACRO 2007). Within mental health services the Care Programme approach (DH 1999) attempts simultaneously to plan for the future and to keep all staff involved in someone's care aware of key concerns. The recent emphasis in the revised guidance (DH 2008) is on individuals with complex health and social care needs in contact with multiple agencies, who pose a risk, including, specifically, those in prison or other residential criminal justice settings. The Offender Management System is designed to achieve much the same for the criminal justice system, where sentence planning is formalized. The Offender Management System and CPA do not apply in the same timeframe. The OMS requires assessment of an offender pre-sentence, followed by 'end-to-end' management led by a philosophy of 'continuity, consistency, commitment and consolidation' (NOMS 2006), and the CPA is used not only for MDOs but also for many non-offender patients.

An intended consequence of both systems is that care pathways be established and relevant agencies made aware of their involvement with an individual MDO at the right time. However, mapping of MDO care pathways in health is poor. There is limited information on the origins and sequelae of different care episodes; research is usually confined to the next step of the care pathway but seldom does justice to the complexity of any moment in it or to the life course of the individuals concerned (Coid et al 2007; Edwards et al 2002; Grounds et al 2004; Jamieson et 2002; Maden et al 1999; MoJ 2007). Criminal justice processing is inherently unpredictable, especially if it involves a jury. In addition to the 'in-principle' processing issues, there are in practice other aspects of institutional work that affect the overall efficacy of assessment, placement and sometimes treatment of MDOs. These are outlined in Table 29.1.

Table 29.1

Agency	Function	Strengths	Weaknesses
Ministry of Justice	Oversight of prison transfers and other restricted patients (s.37/41). Policy development, most recently on mental health legislation and the DSPD programme	National awareness of the size and constitution of the MDO population. Liaison with DH about key policy areas, for example, Mental Health legislation	Main role is protection of the public. Health concerns or the welfare of the MDO secondary
Prison service	Custodial care of MDOs	Recent enhanced health care provision with the advent of NHS/Prison Partnerships and PCT commissioned health services. Prison can be thought of as a mental health polyclinic, as primary, secondary and tertiary mental health practice can be delivered under one roof	In-reach teams stretched. Lack of clarity as to the proper focus for their work. Delays in the transfer of the severely mentally disordered to hospital settings are well recognized. Historical concerns regarding quality of staff in prison health settings
Probation	Reduction of re-offending in offender population inside and outside prisons. Assess and supervise individual offenders and implement a range of interventions	Interventions offered address behavioural problems associated with some mental disorders. Robust risk assessment undertaken with OASys (Offender Assessment System)	Lack of clinical expertise

(continued)

Table 29.1 (continued)

Agency	Function	Strengths	Weaknesses
Solicitors and barristers	Representation within court and Tribunal Systems of their clients' interests	Commitment to individual clients. Capacity to instruct and cross-examine mental health experts	Small number of mental health legal specialists. Possible lack of awareness of catchment area basis of mental health services
Crown Courts	Responsible for adjudication of serious crime	Smaller number of cases allow for detailed consideration of pre-trial, per-trial and post-trial mental health issues	Concern about the value of an adversarial system when calling for mental health experts
Magistrates' Courts	Responsible for the adjudication of less-serious criminal offences. There are lay and stipendiary magistrates	Cases resolved faster than Crown Courts. Courts often host diversion schemes for more rapid identification of the MDO population	Most cases do not have a mental health component
Local NHS facilities	Mainly concerned with the assessment and management of individuals with severe and enduring mental illness. Specialist services dedicated to MDOs with serious offences	Links with non-statutory local support with regard to housing and employment. Less stigmatizing than forensic services	Staff not orientated to concepts of the CJS or used to considering the practice issues arising from court appearances or remands in custody
Medium secure units	Specialist units embedded in large NHS Trusts designed to meet the needs of MDOs convicted of serious offences	Specialist detailed assessment and comprehensive management of MDOs on an inpatient and usually community basis. High staff-to-patient ratios. Recent introduction of national standards for all medium secure services	Delayed discharges due to absence of proper care pathways. Current standards of care more robust in relation to security and less so in relation to patient care. Length of stay now considerably greater than that anticipated by original service specifications. Lack of clarity about therapeutic programmes
High secure hospitals	Three hospitals to serve England and Wales. Take MDOs considered to pose a high risk to public safety. Host two of the four DSPD units	Specialist service to patients who have committed serious offences. Slow throughput allows for careful consideration of the patient and holistic care. Well funded. High staff–patient ratios	Distant from patients' homes. Previous concern about an inappropriate balance between custody and therapy in staff approaches to patients
Department of Health	Responsible for strategic direction of service development for forensic and non-forensic mental health services. Local strategy devolved in part to Strategic Health Authorities and to be implemented by NHS Commissioners	Capacity to assemble and review evidence base for policy development. Political will can triumph over the entrenched views of other vested interests, for example, mental health professionals, Trade unions	Political will can ignore evidence. Bureaucratic delay can derail policy initiatives

Table 29.1 (continued)

Agency	Function	Strengths	Weaknesses
Voluntary Sector	Provision of aftercare accommodation and related services to discharged or released populations. Working closely with the Statutory sector on individual cases	Provide more normalizing environments to stigmatized groups. Enhance risk management through monitored step-down facilities	A patchwork quilt of services with gaps in certain geographical areas and can have unpredictable skill mixes
Social Services	Both integrated into forensic services in the NHS and play a major role in care of at-risk children. In forensic services under-take in-depth assessments within MDTs. Historically exclusive role in implementation of MHA and supervision of RO. Crucial role regarding income/work/housing	Provide a more holistic view of patients than other disciplines. ASW training provided in-depth understanding of medico-legal framework of care	Concern nationally about capacity/quality of work of Social Services with regard to at-risk children

Conclusion

MDOs are enveloped and sometimes engulfed by a wealth of professionals. The position of MDOs is unenviable. They and their actions are the subject of multiple, and sometimes competing, discourses on violence and crime. Their own wishes and the discourse of rehabilitation can be drowned out by a set of intrusive, stigmatizing practices. Such practices currently emphasize risk and can lose sight of common humanity. However, for those who reach the threshold for ener-getic intervention, there may be benefits in terms of dedicated, committed staff and the provision of services to minimize future risk.

MDOs are on the horns of a dilemma; none of the options usually available to them are straight forwardly desirable. In fact, their situation is made easier in one way in that they have little choice about who they encounter. For the most part, both health and criminal justice agen-cies speak for them, and in turn decide for them. Their identity as an MDO is likely to bring them into contact with multiple agencies from health and criminal justice whose interest in public safety or individual need will vary considerably, and whose ability to deliver joined-up care will be com-promised in part by the inherent difficulty of coordinating such services.

References

Blumenthal, S. and Wessely, S. 1992 The Extent of Local Arrangements for the Diversion of the Mentally Abnormal Offender from Custody. Birmingham, L. et al. (2007) Prison Mental Health In-reach Services. The British Journal of Psychiatry 190: 373–374.

Coid, J., Hickey, N., Kahtan, N., Zhang, T. and Yang, M. 2007 Patients Discharged Form Medium Secure Psychiatric Services: Reconvictions and Risk Factors 190: 223–229.

DH (Department of Health). 1999 Effective Care Co-ordination in Mental Health Services: Modernising the Care Programme Approach: A Policy Booklet. London: Department of Health.

DH. 2005 Offender Mental Healthcare Pathway. London: Department of Health.

DH. (Department of Health) 2008 Refocusing the Care Programme Approach: Policy and Positive Practice Guidance. London: Department of Health.

Department of Health and Home Office. 1992 Review of Health and Social Services for Mentally Disordered Offenders and Others Requiring Similar Services. Final Summary Report. London: HMSO.

Edwards, J., Steed, P. and Murray, K. 2002 Clinical and Forensic Outcome 2 Years and 5 Years after Admission to a Medium Secure Unit. Journal of Forensic Psychiatry 13: 1, 68–87.

Grounds, A., Melzer, D., Fryers, T. and Brugha, T. 2004 What Determines Access to Medium Secure Psychiatric Provision? Journal of Forensic Psychiatry and Psychology 15: 1–6.

HM Inspectorate of Prisons. 2007 The Mental Health of Prisoners.

Home Office. 1990 Circular No. 66/90 Provision for Mentally Disordered Offenders. London: Home Office.

Home Office. 1995 Circular No. 12/95 Mentally Disordered Offenders: Inter-agency Working. London: Home Office.

James, D.V. and Hamilton, L.W. 1991 The Clerkenwell Scheme: Assessing Efficacy and Cost of a Psychiatric Liaison Service to a Magistrates' Court. British Medical Journal 303: 282–285.

Jamieson, L. and Taylor, P.J. 2002 Mental Disorder and Perceived Threat to the Public: People Who Do Not Return to Community Living. British Journal of Psychiatry 181: 399–405.

Jamieson, E., Butwell, M., Taylor, P. and Leese, M. 2000 Trends in Special (High Secure) Hospitals I: Referrals and Admissions. British Journal of Psychiatry 176: 253–259.

Joseph P. and Potter, M. 1993 Diversion from Custody II: Effect of Hospital and Prison Resources. British Journal of Psychiatry 162: 330–334.

Maden, A., Rutter, S., McClintock, T., Friendship, C. and Gunn, J. 1999 Outcome of Admission to a Medium Secure Psychiatric Unit. Short and Long Term Outcome. British Journal of Psychiatry 175: 313–316.

MoJ (Ministry of Justice) 2007 Statistics of Mentally Disordered Offenders 2006 England and Wales ONS. www.justice.gov.uk/publications

MoJ/DH (Ministry of Justice and Department of Health). 2008a Dangerous and Severe Personality Disorder (DSPD) High Secure Services for Men: Planning and Delivery Guide. www.justice.gov.uk

MoJ/DH. 2008b Forensic Personality Disorder Medium Secure and Community Pilot Services: Planning and Delivery Guide (Part of the DSPD Programme). www.justice.gov.uk

NACRO. 2005 Findings of the 2004 Survey of Court Diversion/Criminal Justice Mental Health Liaison Schemes for Mentally Disordered Offenders in England and Wales. www.nacro.org.uk

NACRO. 2007 Effective Mental Health Care for offenders @: the Need for a Fresh Approach. London: NACRO.

NACRO. 2008 Criminal Justice Liaison and Diversion Schemes: A Focus on Women Offenders. London: NACRO.

NOMS. 2006 Offender Management Model. www.noms.justice.gov.uk/managing-offenders

PSO (Prison Service Order) 3050 Continuity of Health Care for Prisoners. Issue No: 254 10/2/2006.

Rutherford, M. and Duggan, S. 2007 Forensic Mental Health Services: Facts and Figures on Current Provision. London: SCMH.

SCMH (Sainsbury Centre for Mental Health). 2006 London's Prison Mental health Services: A Review. London: SCMH.

SCMH. 2007 Briefing 32 Mental Health Care in Prisons. London: SCMH.

SHSA (Special Hospitals Service Authority Review). 1991 SHSA Review 1991.

Steel, J., Thornicroft, G., Birmingham, L. et al 2007 Prison Mental Health In-reach Services. The British Journal of Psychiatry 190: 373–374.

Section 6

International

Chapter 30

Introduction

Annie Bartlett

Much of the rest of this book relates to practice in England and Wales. In forensic mental health, it can be hard for busy practitioners to look beyond their own immediate work horizons. If and when they do, it is often to the US literature. This is curious, given the absence of an equivalent welfare state and huge differences in health care and penal policy and practice.

This section is designed to whet readers' appetites for a more truly international perspective on policy and practice. The section is not comprehensive; there are parts of the world it was hard to reach. Without apology, the contributions that follow are serendipitous. The authors were left to their own devices to write about countries they knew, addressing forensic topics they found intrinsically interesting and/or important. Authors were chosen because of their personal experience of working outside of England and Wales.

The result is a series of reflections on the mental health and legal systems elsewhere. The authors in this section address mental health policy and practice and the dilemmas that result; this includes discussion of culturally specific social and ethical values. These are, of course, themes that feature in the rest of the book.

This section highlights the often reactive nature of public policy and legal imperatives. Specifically, it becomes clear that it is not only in England and Wales that the direction of practice can be affected by serious crime involving the mentally disordered. The contributions of John Crighton (Scotland), Ceri Evans (New Zealand) and Madleina Manetsch (Switzerland) show how the precise impact on practice varies by jurisdiction. The complexity of the State informs the structure of forensic and other health services. In pieces by Sameer Sarkar (USA), Rob Ferris (Australia) and Madleina Manetsch (Switzerland), countries with different federal styles, this is explored to emphasize the delicate balance of power and influence between local and national legislation. The continued relevance of old colonial systems of thought is seen in the concepts underpinning mental health legislation in Australia, India and New Zealand as well as in the United States. These countries have gone down their own post-independence development routes; these routes are multidimensional. Revised legislation is only one of these dimensions. Their choices, as nation states, are culturally attuned to the needs of their own multi-cultural populations. Different approaches to health care and penal policy are particularly evident in Jaydip Sarkar's contribution on India and Trudie Rossouw's contribution on South Africa. The dilemmas of custodial care and concern about prison conditions are highlighted by both authors in helpful comparison to the European context. Contributions by Emma van Hoecke (Netherlands) and Madleina Manetsch (Switzerland), writing on countries always independent of historical Anglo Saxon jurisprudence, delineate alternative understandings of responsibility for violent actions by those suffering from mental health problems.

Within any jurisdiction, clinical and legal practice will differ from place to place. This selection of international chapters shows up different issues of difference. A key question is the extent to which such international comparison is valuable. If it is, how could it best be undertaken? The nature of any more rigorous comparison, going beyond forensic tourism, is up for debate. There are crucial variations in resource, styles of inquiry and juridical systems. These issues are challenges for current and future practitioners; this section is a jumping-off point.

Chapter 31

Forensic psychiatry in Australia

Rob Ferris

Aim

To describe an overview of service developments for mentally disordered offenders and to outline the legal framework in which they are assessed and managed.

Learning objectives

◆ Familiarity with heterogeneity of legislation and forensic mental health services in Australia

◆ Appreciation of particular issues: the forensic mental health of the indigenous population and the relative disadvantaging of rural population

---

Introduction

Australia has a present-day population of about nineteen million people. They live on a land mass roughly the same size as the Continental United States. The first human settlement, by people today known as Aborigines and Torres Strait Islanders, began tens of thousands of years ago. It was not until 1788 that it was followed by settlement from elsewhere, Great Britain. The principal reason for this more recent settlement was the establishment of a penal colony to relieve over-crowding in British prisons. This element of the country's history has some relevance for today's forensic psychiatry; a subspecialty of medicine that has taken a long time to become established in Australia.

Since 1901, Australia has been a federation of six states and two territories, each with its own legislature, mental health legislation, criminal codes, correctional service and public health system. Although the federal government exerts some homogenizing influence on state functions, there are effectively eight forensic mental health systems. Both the public and private sector make a substantial contribution to services for mentally disordered offenders (MDOs).

Public funding of health comes mainly from the Commonwealth Government, through its universal health insurance scheme (Medicare) and grants to each state and territory. States are responsible for delivering and funding public health services. Australia has a high proportion of prison inmates in private prisons – 17% of the total prison population. Civil forensic psychiatric services are privately funded.

As recently as the 1980s, forensic psychology and psychiatric practitioners were few and far between and worked mainly in private practice. They were mainly concerned with assessing, reporting and, less often, providing expert evidence to courts. Very few either worked in prisons or were based in secure hospitals. The past two decades have seen major changes. Today, the range and number of forensic mental health professionals has expanded and services routinely employ nurses, social workers and occupational therapists as well as psychologists and psychiatrists. The majority are now engaged in providing treatment services.

There has been a corresponding expansion in academic posts. The first Chair in forensic psychiatry was established at the University of New South Wales in 1991, and a number of other major Australian universities have since followed suit. There are now professorial posts in both forensic psychology and, more recently, forensic nursing. University-based training programmes have been developed for all relevant professional groups. The Australian and New Zealand Association of Psychiatry, Psychology and Law (ANZAPPL) was founded by a single private practitioner in 1978. It has since helped foster interdisciplinary dialogue and academic interest in forensic mental health. The Royal Australian and New Zealand College of Psychiatrists established its section of forensic psychiatry in 1988. A two-year advanced training programme in forensic psychiatry is now well established in Australia and New Zealand, together with an accreditation and credential process.

Given the complex structure of the Australian federal system, this chapter constitutes an overview of recent developments in the services for the assessment and treatment of mentally abnormal offenders in Australia and the legal context in which they operate. It is not possible in this volume to describe local services and their variation in the different states and territories. Nor will further reference be made to work in the civil field, despite the latter's importance in the history of forensic mental health, and, particularly, forensic psychiatry (Mullen 2000).

The legal context

Australian law derives from the common law of England. With the passage of time, it has increasingly deviated from the original colonial model. In addition, individual states differ significantly from each other. Queensland, Western Australia and Tasmania have codified their criminal law and are therefore known as 'code' states or jurisdictions. New South Wales, Victoria and South Australia remain common law jurisdictions. This has implications both for the possible mental health defences to criminal charges and, post-conviction, for the courts in the sentencing practices.

In 1995, the Standing Committee of Attorneys General of the States and the Commonwealth of Australia promulgated a Model Criminal Code, intended for adoption by all Australian jurisdictions (Criminal Code Act 1995). This new Criminal Code included a new mental health defence to criminal charges of mental impairment. This was essentially a codification of the original English M'Naghten Rules, which relate to the concept of disease of the mind (see Chapter 19). According to the original M'Naghten Rules, the presence of a 'disease of the mind' in an individual might be judged to affect someone's responsibility for a criminal action. In the new Australian Code, disease of the mind was extended to include, explicitly, severe personality disorder. This inclusion resonates with the historical and ongoing debates in the United Kingdom about the place of psychopathic disorder and personality disorder in criminal and mental health case law and legislation (Eastman 1999; Hansard 1999). The new Australian Code also added inability to control conduct to the original limbs of the legislation, which concerned knowledge of the nature and quality of the criminal act and of its wrongness.

Although Australian states may apparently have given some support to this attempt at harmonization of the law, in practice the Model Code has been modified and applied in disparate ways. For example, South Australia has not included severe personality disorder as a condition capable of producing mental impairment (Criminal Law Consolidation Amendment Act 1995). Victoria has not included the volitional element concerning control of conduct in its mental impairment legislation (Crimes Act 1997). New South Wales has ignored the Model Code altogether in reforming its diminished-responsibility provisions, and it retains its existing insanity defence legislation (Mental Health [Criminal Procedure] Act 1990).

Regarding the defence of diminished responsibility to a charge of murder, only Queensland, Western Australia and New South Wales (also the Northern Territory and the Australian Capital Territory) have adopted it.

Australia went its own way in relation to intoxication as a defence to criminal acts. The result was something very different from English law. The Australian High Court, in the case of O'Connor (1980), decided, by a 4:3 majority, that intoxication could be considered by a jury when deciding whether a defendant had acted voluntarily and intentionally. This decision was contrary to the British House of Lords decision in Majewski (1977). The Majewski judgement held that intoxication could not be relevant in crimes involving basic (general) intent, only in crimes of specific intent. The O'Connor decision (1980) was followed by widespread predictions of a flood of unjust acquittals of defendants taking advantage of this 'drunk's defence'. Although research by the relevant state's Law Reform Commission in 1986 (Law Reform Commission of Victoria 1986) found little evidence of this having happened, the common law states affected by this decision have recently introduced legislation tending to follow Majewski. This followed the 1997 acquittal of a well-known rugby league footballer charged with serious assault (Victorian Law Reform Committee 1999).

A variety of treatment options for MDOs are available to the Australian criminal courts: findings of unfitness to plead or mental impairment lead, in practice, to detention in hospital. In some jurisdictions, including the Commonwealth, courts may release people into the community, either unconditionally or with conditions that may be without limit of time. Final release from such orders may be the responsibility of the Executive (as in Western Australia and New South Wales) or the court (as in Victoria, South Australia and Tasmania).

If a mentally ill offender is convicted in an ordinary way of a criminal offence, that is, without a particular mental health defence being invoked, courts in all Australian jurisdictions have a range of mental health disposals available, including orders requiring treatment in hospital or the community. Some jurisdictions (as in Victoria) have so-called hybrid orders. These enable courts to impose a sentence that may be served in either prison or a forensic mental health service, depending on the offender's mental condition and treatment needs (Fox 1999). These hybrid orders have been criticized for placing clinicians in the ethically invidious position of having to declare their patients fit for punishment (Mullen 2000).

Legislation allowing indeterminate sentences to be imposed following conviction for offenders variously deemed to be habitual criminals, or violent, dangerous or sexual offenders, has been available in most Australian jurisdictions for a long time. The criteria for application of the legislation have varied. The model used, together with those found in Canada and New Zealand, has been described as a community protection model. This differs both from that found in the United States (with its emphasis on Civil Commitment on completion of a determinate sentence) and some European countries, where there has been a clinical model with an emphasis on treatment rather than public protection (Connelly and Williamson 2000), although this may be changing.

In Victoria, the passage of the Community Protection Act 1990 was driven by public concern about the release of one man, a violent repeat offender named Garry David. This bespoke legislation allowed a state Supreme Court Judge to authorize his indefinite detention. This was subject to the need for regular review that ended only with his death in 1993. It was, at the time, the only piece of Australian legislation allowing for preventive detention based on reviewable sentencing. A similar Act was passed later in New South Wales that enabled the detention of an offender named Gregory Wayne Kable (Community Protection Act 1994), but this was subsequently struck down by the Australian High Court.

Forensic mental health services

Just as the Australian states have substantially different legislation for MDOs, so too do they have different mental health services. This is in part owing to varied geography and population demographics. The population is largely urban. Anyone outside the urban areas is disadvantaged in relation to all aspects of health care, including mental health services.

Two National Mental Health Plans (Australian Health Ministers 1992; Commonwealth Department of Health and Family Services 1998) and a series of meetings including representatives from all states and territories paved the way for a measure of agreement nationally about mental health service provision. With regard to forensic mental health services, key issues identified included the following: location of secure forensic inpatient facilities away from prisons; the need to shift from an exclusive focus on institutional care to outpatient and community care (including both parallel forensic mental health outpatient services and reform of existing general services to accept more forensic patients); diversion of mentally disordered offenders away from the criminal justice system via court-based mental health liaison and assessment services; and better delivery of multidisciplinary care within prisons, including systematic assessment and screening of prisoners on reception (Mullen 2000).

In contrast to arrangements in many other countries, some states provided most of their mental health beds within prison rather than in secure hospitals outside prison. This could be problematic in relation to confidentiality and the authority to control placement and movement of prisoner-patients. Extensive use of private contractors to provide both prisons and health services to prison may compound these difficulties. In Sydney, 90 of the 120 Long Bay Prison Hospital beds are still designated psychiatric beds, but this arrangement is to end soon. There will be an increased number of medium secure beds available in outside psychiatric hospitals, although the intended location of one new hospital is immediately outside the secure perimeter of the prison.

By contrast, South Australia, Queensland, the Northern Territory and Tasmania provide all secure hospital beds outside their prison systems. Most were designated high secure, but increasingly medium and low secure beds have been included.

Despite the historical emphasis on institution-based services, there is an increasing recognition that community-based forensic services are equally important when the needs of mentally disordered offenders are considered in the round. At the millennium, an Australia-wide survey of community (forensic mental health) services reported them as present in all states and territories except New South Wales, whereas Western Australia's were described as limited (Mullen 2000). As an indication of the pace of development, both New South Wales and Western Australia now have well-developed community-based forensic services (K.P. O'Brien 2007 personal communication).

Serious personality disorder and sex offenders

Historically, persons with a primary diagnosis of personality disorder or substance misuse have not usually fallen within the provisions of relevant mental health legislation, or within the remit of forensic mental health services. Thus, Garry David (supra) was not detainable under Victorian mental health legislation, whereas he could have been detained under the 1983 English Mental Health Act if considered treatable. The emphasis has always been on the treatment of the seriously mentally ill.

Sex offenders have also not been regarded as falling within the remit of mental health services, although, increasingly, forensic mental health services do provide therapy, particularly for paedophiles. As in other parts of the world, treatment programs tend mostly to be provided by psychologists and counsellors employed directly by prisons and community-based correctional services.

Aboriginal and Torres Strait Islanders' mental health

The health of Aboriginal Australians is poor compared to that of non-Aboriginal Australians, and worse than their indigenous counterparts in New Zealand, Canada and the United States (Ring and Firman 1998). Although only 2.4% of the overall population, Aboriginal and Torres Strait Islanders constitute 22% of the national prison population, and 30% of women in full-time custody are indigenous (Corben 2004). Problems including high rates of smoking, alcohol abuse, illicit substance misuse, violence and abuse have been documented repeatedly over many years. In 1991, a Royal Commission into Aboriginal Deaths in Custody made more than 300 recommendations regarding social, health and judicial issues, those concerning mental health being focused mainly on suicide risk following incarceration (Johnston 1991).

There have, however, been few publications on the mental health of Aboriginal people in custody. A recent study was the first to compare in detail the mental health of Aboriginal and non-Aboriginal offenders in Australia. Few differences in the prevalence of mental illness in male prisoners were found, although depression and psychological distress were higher in the non-Aboriginal group. Aboriginal women prisoners were more likely than their non-Aboriginal counterparts to be given diagnoses of psychosis, depression and obsessive compulsive disorder (Butler et al 2007).

Conclusion

The complexity of Australia's system of states and territories raises intriguing questions of equity in both criminal justice and mental health terms. At present, the legislative framework owes something to its colonial ancestor but has developed in significant and diverse ways. At the same time, the number and plight of ethnic minority offenders in Australia resonate with concerns raised in both the United Kingdom and other European countries.

Key points

- Forensic psychiatry has only recently been established in Australia
- There has been rapid growth and development in forensic mental health
- States and territories in Australia have separate systems
- The indigenous population continues to be disadvantaged

References

Australian Health Ministers Conference. 1992 National Mental Health Policy. National Mental Health Strategy, Commonwealth Department of Health, Housing and Community Services. Canberra: Australian Government Publishing Service.

Butler, T., Allnut, S., Kariminia, A. and Cain, D. 2007 Mental Health Status of Aboriginal and Non-Aboriginal Australian Prisoners. Australian and New Zealand Journal of Psychiatry 41: 429–435.

Commonwealth Department of Health and Family Services 1998 Second National Mental Health Plan. National Mental Health Strategy, Commonwealth Department of Health and Family Services. Canberra: Australian Government Publishing Service.

Connelly, C. and Williamson, S. 2000 A Review of the Research Literature on Serious Violent and Sexual Offenders. Scottish Executive Central Research Unit.

Corben, S. 2004. NSW Inmate Census 2003: Summary of Characteristics, Statistical Publications No 25. Sydney: NSW Department of Corrective Services.

Eastman, N.L.G. 1999 Public Health Psychiatry or Crime Prevention. British Medical Journal 318: 549–551.

Fox, R.G. 1999. Competition in Sentencing: The Rehabilitative Model versus the Punitive Model. Psychiatry, Psychology and Law 6: 153–162.

Hansard 1999: Col 601–3, 5 February 1999.

Johnston, E.C. 1991 Royal Commission into Aboriginal Deaths in Custody. National Report. Vol. 1–5. Australian Government Publishing Service.

Mullen, P.E., Briggs, S., Dalton, T., and Burt, M. 2000. Forensic Mental Health Services in Australia. International Journal of Law And Psychiatry 23: 433–452.

Ring, I.T. and Firman, D. 1998. Reducing Indigenous Mortality in Australia: Lessons from Other Countries. Medical Journal of Australia 169: 528–533.

Cases

The Queen v. O'Connor (1980) 146 CLR 64.DPP v. Majewski (1977) AC 443.

Chapter 32

Forensic mental health care in New Zealand

Ceri Evans

Aim

To outline key elements of forensic mental health care in New Zealand.

Learning objectives

- To understand the development of forensic services in the cultural context of New Zealand
- To delineate similarities and differences in mental health legislation in New Zealand and England and Wales

Historical context

New Zealand was relatively late to develop forensic psychiatric services. Prior to 1987, there were no services designated as such; nor was forensic psychiatry even a recognized sub-specialty (Brinded 2000). The main focus for forensic mental health practice before this was a 'maximum security' inpatient unit at Lake Alice Hospital in the North Island. This was commissioned in 1965 and called the 'National Security Unit'. It was originally developed to contain the 54 most violent psychiatric inpatients in New Zealand, but closed in 1999, as policy was redirected in favour of developing regional capabilities.

The impetus for change was caused by the confluence of several adverse clinical events, including an escalating suicide rate in the maximum-security prison at Paremoremo and several homicides by psychiatric patients living in the community. One of these involved the killing of two patients in a community mental health facility by an ex-patient from the National Security Unit with a history of serious violence, who had been refused hospital admission.

These events led the government to establish a Commission of Inquiry and the subsequent report, termed the Mason Report (Mason et al 1988), provided the blueprint for the development of forensic mental health services in New Zealand. The report was pivotal, comparable in influence in the New Zealand context to the impact of the Butler report in the United Kingdom at an earlier stage (Home Office and Department of Health and Social Security 1975). The recommendations of the report focused on establishing mental-health-based facilities to care for mentally disordered offenders and potential offenders, based on six principles:

- Mentally ill offenders had the same right to access mental health services as non-offenders
- Mentally ill offenders were the primary responsibility of the health care system rather than corrections

- A system needed to be developed that could identify mentally ill offenders at any stage of the criminal justice process
- Cultural understanding was seen as clinically essential as well as constitutionally mandated
- There should be a multi-disciplinary approach to patient care
- Security and therapy should be integrated, providing delivery of services close to patients' families where possible but in an accountable manner

This report heralded the building of 5 regional secure units in the main population centres, to serve a national population that passed the 4 million mark during 2004. The secure units act as focal points for forensic psychiatric services, which include secure inpatient beds, outpatient services, court-liaison services and psychiatric clinics within the regional prisons. This set-up is similar in concept and design to those services centred on the regionally distributed medium secure units in the United Kingdom.

If the basic organization and functioning of the New Zealand forensic mental health services is similar to those in Britain, in what ways is it different or progressive? Two main areas mark out the New Zealand version of forensic mental health provision as inherently different from UK practice: (1) the cultural environment and (2) the legislative environment.

Cultural environment

A fundamental aspect of New Zealand society is the nature and importance of cultural issues, not just in terms of the delivery of mental health services but more pervasively in terms of the national psyche. The New Zealand cultural mix is unique: in the 2001 census, approximately 15% of the population identified themselves as Maori and more than 6% identified themselves as Pacific Islanders and 6% as Asian.

The pre-eminent historical reference point for understanding any New Zealand social service, including health care of all kinds, is the Treaty of Waitangi. Signed in 1940, the Treaty formed the basis for the relationship between Maori and Pakeha (New Zealanders of predominantly European ancestry) in New Zealand, in which Maori accepted British sovereignty in exchange for certain guarantees of protection (Orange 1987). The Treaty has significant current implications in terms of concepts such as 'biculturalism' and 'cultural safety' (Durie 1994) and, for example, in the domain of mental health, there is an emphasis on cultural competency.

The requirement for mental health services to address the needs of Maori people, in particular, were met in various ways. Each forensic mental health service employs cultural advisors and workers, some of whom provide input into multidisciplinary team functioning. In most regions, each new inpatient will receive both a clinical and a cultural assessment, which is generally conducted within a framework of four related aspects: Te Taha Tinana (physical well-being and attributes), Te Taha Hinengaro (mental well-being), Te Taha Whanau (family/extended family) and Te Taha Wairua (spiritual well-being). There is an identified need for specific culturally aligned resources to be developed. For example, recently a new prison based at Ngawha in Northland has been built within an area of relatively high Maori population density, which will emphasize the importance of incorporating Maori protocols and procedures into care plans; and at the Mason Clinic Regional Forensic Service in Auckland, a bespoke 12-bed medium secure unit has recently been opened that is available exclusively for those of Maori ethnicity.

Legislation

Although the relevant criminal and mental health legislation covers the areas that any comprehensive forensic mental health system would be expected to address, such as fitness to plead, criminal responsibility and dispositional issues, there are some interesting departures or variations from UK legislation.

First, 'mental disorder', the basis for compulsory detention, as defined within the Mental Health [Compulsory Assessment and Treatment] Act 1992, is based on phenomenology rather than categories of disorder, as given in section 2 of the Act:

Mental disorder in relation to any person, means an abnormal state of mind whether of a continuous or intermittent nature) characterized by delusions, or by disorders of mood or perception or volition or cognition, of such a degree that it

1. Poses a serious risk of danger to the health or safety of that person or of others; or
2. Seriously diminishes the capacity of that person to take care of himself or herself

In contrast to practice in England and Wales:

♦ Patients are detained based on phenomenology, rather than categories of mental disorder. Patients with personality disorder, although generally not intended to be detained under the Act, have been compulsorily detained based on a disorder of volition

♦ The Act allows for compulsory care of mentally ill patients both within inpatient units and also in the community with the use of community treatment orders

♦ There is a requirement within the Act that family and caregivers be consulted unless there is good clinical reason not to do so or it is impractical

♦ Although the threshold for initiation of assessment under the Act may be lower in practice than in England and Wales, there are more frequent procedural checks and assessments, particularly in the early stages of assessment and treatment

Second, significant *recent legislation* has been enacted to modernize the way in which mentally impaired people are dealt with by the justice system and to address a specific gap in terms of a lack of provision for the particular needs of people with an *intellectual disability*. The Criminal Procedures (Mentally Impaired Persons) Act 2003 is designed to work 'in tandem' with the Mental Health [Compulsory Assessment and Treatment] Act 1992, and the new Intellectual Disability (Compulsory Care and Rehabilitation) Act 2003, with the latter two acts providing the detail of the dispositional options that are made available to the Court through the Criminal Procedures (Mentally Impaired Persons) Act 2003 (New Zealand Ministry of Justice 2004).

Third, section 38 of the Criminal Procedures (Mentally Impaired Persons) Act 2003 allows the court to request that a *psychiatric report* be prepared on a person charged or convicted of an offence; this assessment can take place on bail, within prison, or as a psychiatric inpatient. This represents a marked difference in practice between New Zealand and some parts of practice in the United Kingdom: part of the core work of consultant forensic psychiatrists is that they routinely prepare court reports on behalf of the forensic service.

Fourth, although legislation concerning *unfitness to stand trial* is similar conceptually to that in England and Wales, the court-ordered report system means that the issue is addressed more routinely and rigorously than in the United Kingdom. As many findings of legal disability are made in New Zealand per year as there are in the United Kingdom despite the marked difference in populations.

Fifth, the threshold for a finding of *insanity* is conceptually lower in New Zealand than in England and Wales because, as defined within section 23 of the Crimes Act (1961), it requires:

[The individual was] labouring under natural imbecility or disease of the mind to such an extent as to render him incapable (1) Of understanding the nature and quality of the act or omission; or

(2) Of knowing that the act or omission was morally wrong, having regard to the commonly accepted standards of right and wrong.

(s.23 The Crimes Act 1961)

This places emphasis on knowing that the act or omission was 'morally wrong' as opposed to 'legally wrong' (as in the United Kingdom). New Zealand does not have legislation in relation to diminished responsibility (other than for infanticide).

Finally, in terms of pre-sentence reports and dispositional issues, although New Zealand does not have 'dangerous offender' legislation, *preventive detention*, an indeterminate, lifelong sentence, has been available for repeat or severe offenders for many years, and has required obligatory psychiatric or psychological reports since 1993 (A.I.F. Simpson 1998). It is currently defined by sections 87 and 88 of the Sentencing Act 2000. It is intended for use with the highest-risk offenders, whose offences may have been of either a violent or a sexual nature. A prisoner subject to preventive detention may not be released into the community if they are still considered to pose a risk to the community after a minimum non-parole period, and those released may be recalled at any point for the rest of their lives. Therefore, in New Zealand law, forensic psychiatrists and psychologists routinely provide the courts with reports, which are considered by the courts in determining whether individuals will be subject to preventive detention, a situation that may cause some practitioners ethical discomfort.

Adequacy of services

Given the rapid development of community-based mental health services, reviews of forensic services have been conducted by the Ministry of Health to gauge how services had developed since the Mason report (e.g. Ministry of Health 2001). Several areas of concern have been identified, including inadequacy of forensic facilities for women and long-term patients; inappropriate placement in forensic settings of people with intellectual disability; ineffective screening for mental illness in prisons; the lack of step-down or community-based residential facilities for forensic clients and a series of major issues in terms of Maori, including lack of participation, lack of Maori frameworks leading to integration and high proportion of Maori in the forensic population.

The provision of adequate mental health services in New Zealand prisons is a particularly pressing problem. Well-designed epidemiological research has established that, like other Western countries, there is a greater prevalence of psychiatric disorder in New Zealand prisons than in the community (Brinded et al 2001). Currently, these mentally ill prisoners are not being identified effectively, a problem compounded by the rising national prison muster and the high rate of imprisonment in New Zealand (in April 2005, the national muster reached approximately 6,800 inmates, representing a high rate of imprisonment of 155 inmates per 100,000 population for 2003/2004, higher than comparable countries other than the United States (Department of Corrections 2005)). A national mental health screening programme is currently being implemented in an attempt to improve identification of those in need of mental health assessment.

Conclusion

Overall, New Zealand has a small but energetic and responsive forensic mental health community, characterized by the importance of cultural issues, a multi-tiered approach to patient advocacy (Brinded 2000) and an increasingly comprehensive legislative system.

Key points

◆ Forensic mental health services developed in the context of concerns about prison suicides and 'psychiatric homicides' in the community

◆ Cultural awareness is a well-established and integrated element of mental health work in New Zealand

◆ Mental health and criminal legislation in New Zealand has similarities to but also important differences from that of England and Wales, for example, different legal understandings of mental disorder

References

Brinded, P. 2000. Forensic Psychiatry in New Zealand. A Review. International Journal of Law and Psychiatry 23: 453–465.

Brinded, P., Simpson, A., Laidlaw, T., Fairley, N. and Malcolm, F. 2001 Prevalence of Psychiatric Disorders in New Zealand Prisons: A National Study. Australian and New Zealand Journal of Psychiatry 35: 166–173.

Department of Corrections. 2005 Statement of Intent 1 July 2005–30 June 2006. Wellington: Department of Corrections.

Durie, M. 1994 Wairoa: Maori Health Development. Auckland: Oxford University Press.

Home Office and Department of Health and Social Security. 1975 Report of the Committee on Mentally Abnormal Offenders Butler Report Cmnd 6244. London: HMSO.

Mason, K., Bennett, H. and Ryan, E. 1988 Report of the Committee of Inquiry into Procedures Used in Certain Psychiatric Hospitals in Relation to Admission Discharge or Release on Leave of Certain Classes of Patients. The Mason Report. Wellington: Department of Health.

Ministry of Health. 2001 Services for People with Mental Illness in the Justice System. Framework for Forensic Mental Health Services. Wellington: Ministry of Health.

New Zealand Ministry of Justice. 2004 Guide to the Criminal Procedure (Mentally Impaired Persons) Act 2003. Wellington: Ministry of Justice.

Orange, C. 1987 The Treaty of Waitangi. Wellington: Allen and Unwin.

Simpson, A.I.F. 1998 Psychiatrist's Role in Preventive Detention: New Zealand Legislation for Indefinite Detention. Psychiatry, Psychology and Law 5: 87–93.

Chapter 33

Care and treatment of mentally disordered offenders in India

Jaydip Sarkar

Aim

To outline mental health legislation in India and its application to the mentally disordered offender, with particular reference to human rights issues evident in service delivery.

Learning objectives

- Introduction to mental health law in India
- Diversion of Mentally Disordered Offenders (MDOs) from criminal justice system
- Health care delivery to MDOs
- Human rights issues

Introduction

India, the largest democracy in the world and one of the new burgeoning economies, lags behind many of the liberal democratic societies of Europe and North America when it comes to providing safe 'and acceptable services to mentally disordered offenders (MDOs). The following paragraphs will introduce mental health law in India, the diversion of MDOs from the criminal justice system and the nature and extent of health care delivery to this group of individuals.

The status and relevance of forensic psychiatry in any country is largely dependent upon two things: law and ethics. The former establishes the statutes that must be adhered to, whereas the latter involves a discourse of the *shoulds* and *musts* that goes beyond statutory law. Absence of reasonable statutes, lack of their implementation where these do exist and the relative lack of a socio-political environment where the ethical implications of actions (or inaction) can be openly discussed and debated, will militate against an acceptable standard of forensic psychiatry in that country.

Mental health legislation in India

India has a tradition of documented, ancient knowledge of mental disorders within a framework of herbal and traditional medicine. However, law about the care and treatment of those with mental disorders appeared only after the arrival of the British in the eighteenth century. Mental asylums were established, the first of which was in Calcutta (now Kolkata) in 1787. The overriding purpose of such asylums was custody rather than care (Shah 1999). This was aided by a slew of legislation, all of which prioritized custodial care over liberal treatment of the mentally ill in a humane manner. The procedural complexities, in conjunction with legislative uninterest, meant that successive mental health legislation perpetuated the status quo.

The current act, the Indian Mental Health Act 1987 (IMHA 1987), is the first one legislated in free India. Although an improvement on its predecessors, IMHA 1987 remains paternalistic, resting all decision-making powers on the judiciary, even for civil cases, with psychiatrists merely making recommendations to the courts. The act continues to prioritize custody over therapy. There is no provision of independent tribunals, valid consent to treatment and second opinions in the act. This allows little protection of the patients' autonomy and human rights. Furthermore, the act establishes similar legal controls for *both* voluntary and involuntary patients. Thus, if a person wishes to seek admission on a voluntary basis he or she would still have to be 'detained' under the Act. The Act is also thought to be discriminatory towards non-governmental institutions of psychiatric care (Trivedi 2002). Consequently, it is not user-friendly, either to patients and their carers or to mental health professionals. An illustration of apathy towards the act was reflected in its non-implementation in many Indian states six years after it came into pragmatic being in 1993 (NHRC 1999).

The apparent unfairness of the act, coupled with lack of proper implementation, further compounded by poor functioning and accountability of regulatory bodies (the regional mental health authorities), has contributed to a worrying disregard of the law. This has culminated in the widespread practice of admitting and treating patients against their wishes, most often based only on proxy consent provided by carers, friends and relatives. By falling outside the purview of an act that in itself does not provide adequate protection of their human rights, patients remain powerless and open to abuse (Sarkar 2004). Effective management of patients is further compromised both by poorly developed primary care services and communication difficulties among different government agencies as well as between private and government psychiatrists (Das et al 2002).

Mental illness and criminal law

The IMHA 1987 defines a mentally ill person as one who is 'in need of treatment by reason of any mental disorder other than mental retardation'. However, the terms 'lunatic' and 'person of unsound mind', legacies of a bygone era (Indian Lunacy Act 1912), continue to be used within both civil and criminal law in India. The term 'lunatic' was defined as 'an idiot or person of unsound mind' but the terms 'idiot' and 'unsound mind' were left undefined in the said Act. The Indian Penal Code (IPC 1860), however, which forms the legal basis of India's criminal justice system, defines 'unsoundness of mind' as a state of mind in which an accused is 'incapable of knowing the nature of his act' or 'knowing that what he is doing is wrong or contrary to law' (Ratanlal and Dhirajlal 2002). This definition is derived from the M'Naghten Rules. The burden of proving *unsoundness* rests on the accused (Chetia v. State of Assam 1976) and a successful insanity defence can lead to acquittal. However, unless a direct link between mental illness and future risk of serious harm can be demonstrated (Marfatia 1972), an insanity defence is likely to fail. Unlike in the United Kingdom, no other mental state defences such as diminished responsibility, provocation and duress are available in India.

Although a completed act of suicide is not considered a crime, s.309 of IPC makes both attempted suicide and abetment and assistance of suicide punishable. The survivor of an 'unsuccessful' suicide attempt must therefore both be punished *and* treated for his condition. This strange paradox was maintained by India's apex court, the Supreme Court (State of Delhi v. Sanjoy Bhatia 1985), which ruled that a person suffering from *any mental disorder* may be detained in a psychiatric hospital for treatment under the IMHA 1987 but may not escape punishment for attempted suicide!

The mental condition of accused persons is dealt with under Chapter 25 of the Criminal Procedure Act 1973 (Ratanlal and Dhirajlal 1992). It concerns the judiciary in two situations: at the time of commission of offence and at the time of trial. If an accused was a person of unsound mind *at the time of offence*, a finding is recorded accordingly and can lead to acquittal following a successful insanity defence. The patient is, however, detained in a place of 'safe custody', the 'place' being often a prison, sometimes a psychiatric hospital or even 'in charge of relatives' in the community (Kuttapan v. State of Kerala 1986). When no longer thought to pose a risk of injury to self or others, the patient is discharged or handed over to the care of a relative or friend who acts as the guardian (Ratanlal and Dhirajlal 1992). As capital punishment still exists in India, it is not uncommon for a prisoner to make a spurious insanity plea when facing serious charges such as murder or treason (Shah 1999).

If an accused is of unsound mind *at the time of inquiry or trial* (based on psychiatric evidence) and therefore deemed *incapable of making his defence*, a court may release him on the assurance that he will be 'received for care', usually in a hospital. In the absence of such assurance from relevant hospital authorities, or if the accused cannot be bailed, he is detained in 'safe custody'. There is no 'trial of facts' while the accused receives care and treatment in 'safe custody', and the trial resumes only when the accused becomes mentally sound. 'Incapable of making a defence' is synonymous with the concept of *fitness to plead* in the United Kingdom.

Mentally disordered offenders in prisons

Prison code for the mentally ill

Mentally ill prisoners are dealt with under the Prisoners Act 1900 and Chapter 33 of the West Bengal Jail Code 1967. Four categories of prisoners with mental disorders are recognized within prisons: (1) remand prisoners with possible mental disorder, (2) those incapable of making their defence (unfit to plead), (3) those not guilty by reason of insanity and acquitted but detained in 'safe custody', and (4) convicted prisoners who become ill following reception into prison (West Bengal Jail Code 1967). Until recently, a fifth category also existed: the 'non-criminal lunatic' (NCL), described as persons who 'wander at large or are dangerous' (unproven by facts in most cases) by reason of mental illness and require to be taken into custody by the police under powers enshrined in Indian Lunacy Act 1912 and IMHA 1987. For years, NCLs were received and detained in prisons, which acted as places of 'safe custody' (Ramanathan 2003), although by definition they were not MDOs.

Service structure

Prison-based mental health services are usually unheard of in India, although many prisons do provide psychotropic medications to MDOs. They are managed within very basic general health facilities that are staffed by nurses, attendants and medical officers. Some prisons receive the services of visiting psychiatrists as part of pilot projects, but these arrangements are often local and not part of a national or state strategy, and consequently little data regarding psychiatric morbidity are available. The situation is compounded by excessive prison overcrowding. Psychiatric facilities at a premier high-profile prison during a 3-month pilot project consisted of an enclosure of 20 cells which housed 30 to 35 inmates, many of whom were kept locked for long hours in the cells, often without proper observation. A single junior doctor was responsible for their care and management in addition to weekly specialist input from a consultant psychiatrist (Chaddha and Amarjeet 1998). A national survey on the extent and quality of mental health care *in psychiatric hospitals* found that the subhuman living conditions in some of them were a stark violation of human rights of the patients. Regrettably, the commission did not visit psychiatric 'wards' of any prison (National Human Rights Commission 1999), where conditions are far worse.

Prevalence rates

Only two notable studies relating to rates of psychiatric morbidity within prisons have been identified. Chaddha and Amarjeet (1998) assessed the psychiatric morbidity in a large prison in Delhi over a 3-month period. Seventy-six inmates were diagnosed over a 3-month period, which leads to an annual prevalence rate of 3.4%. This is likely to be a gross underrepresentation of the actual morbidity as the sample was effectively self-selected, with referrals being made by non-psychiatrists, such that only the most severe and therefore obvious cases were likely to have been referred. Schizophrenia (26%), unspecified psychotic disorder (19%) and depression (18%) were the three most common diagnoses. Schizophrenia and depression were the two main diagnoses found in patients involved in 'major' crimes that included murder, attempt to murder and terrorist activities. The majority of patients with schizophrenia were implicated in homicide cases. The authors characterized offences like culpable homicide (equivalent to manslaughter in the United Kingdom), sexual offences (rape, sexual assault and paedophilia), and robbery as 'minor offences', and found that the main diagnoses in this group were unspecified psychotic disorder (31%), depression (19%), substance abuse (17%) and schizophrenia (14%). More than 80% of patients were remand prisoners and more than one-third of all patients were suffering from a psychiatric illness before committing the alleged offences. Such findings indicate an urgent need for diversion from prisons into mental health facilities.

The situation of the non-criminal lunatic (NCL) detained in prisons is even more grim. Although not offenders by definition, it is nonetheless relevant to discuss their numbers and predicament as they happen to be detained in prisons and are considered by the larger society as offenders. Their numbers were so many that in one state 98% (1,242 out of 1,267) of mentally ill 'prisoners' in 1982 were non-offenders (Shah 1999). The situation had been expected to alter drastically after the highest court in India made such detentions unlawful (Sheela Barse v. Union of India 1989), but that did not happen. Gross violations of law and the human rights of detainees were evident in a survey of records of 22 penal institutions in one Indian state (West Bengal), which found 815 NCLs, including 239 women, under detention (Dutt A.B. v. State of West Bengal & others , 1989, Unlock the padlock 1993). Sixty-two percent of them had been in detention for 6 months to 12 years and 16% for 13 to 34 years. Nearly two-thirds (60%) of detention orders had been made by unauthorized persons (not magistrates as required by law) (Dutt 1996). All of the detention orders had been made under incorrect sections of the Act. Dutt (Dutt A.B. v. State of West Bengal & others 1989) also found that 10 mentally ill remand prisoners, most of them facing minor charges of theft, breach of trust and trespass and sent to prison between 1956 and 1987, were still languishing there.

Transfer to hospital

A mentally ill prisoner can be detained in a psychiatric hospital under only the aegis of IMHA 1987 (Malik 1974). Section 27 of IMHA 1987 provides for admission, detention and eventual discharge of a *mentally ill prisoner* into and from any psychiatric hospital or psychiatric nursing home under orders of the court. The mental and physical condition of the patient in hospital should be monitored by a range of professionals who report back to the court that made the order. The court requires regular reports by the treating psychiatrist, the Inspector General of Prisons (high-ranking police official), state-appointed visitors, including at least one social worker, and a state-empowered psychiatrist, or medical officer where a psychiatrist is unavailable (The Mental Health Act with State and Central Rules 1990). Although such mechanisms aim to protect the rights of the patient, in reality these regulations are often not implemented. In one high-profile case, a person was found to have spent 14 years in prison after being found incapable of making his defence, and continued to remain there, untried, despite having been declared fit by psychiatrists (Ramanathan 2003). Another man remains on remand 24 years after his arrest, and has for the last 12 years been thought to be suffering from mental illness but has neither been transferred to hospital nor received any treatment in prison (Asian Human Rights Commission 2004).

Mentally disordered offenders in psychiatric hospitals

Available figures suggest that 1.4% (Channabasavanna et al 1981) to 1.7% (Sen Gupta and Chawla 1969) of all patients in psychiatric hospitals in India are criminals. No special arrangements exist for the care of MDOs who are transferred to psychiatric hospitals. They are managed in general wards along with non-offender patients who may therefore be vulnerable to exploitation. There are no systematic procedures for gathering information on risk behaviours, and the assessment and management of risk in hospitals is often limited to merely helping the patient to become free of symptoms of serious mental illnesses. Furthermore, staff receive no special training in terms of relational and procedural security measures, care and responsibility procedures (physical restraint of violent patients) or more psychological and emotional issues such as transference and counter-transference. Physical security for forensic patients is either provided by prison officers (this might include two or more officers escorting the patient at all times inside the wards, raising issues of lack of patient confidentiality, or for patients to be handcuffed to metal beds) or given over to nursing staff who are ill-trained in such procedures. MDOs are returned to prisons once they are asymptomatic to serve out their sentences, and mental health services have no responsibility in managing them in the community.

Conclusion

For those who have been trained in the principles and practice of forensic mental health care in Europe or North America, many of the stark and often frightening realities of such care, and more often the lack of it, in other parts of the world may be an eye opener. In India, forensic mental health care still needs to evolve. For India's democracy to be fruitful, respect for each individual is paramount. If a nation's treatment of its socially and economically disadvantaged groups is a marker of its maturity and humanity, then India has still a long way to go. Currently, India's treatment of its mentally ill is open to the same kinds of political campaigns as have been waged on both the former states of the USSR and on China. It could be argued that international organizations should highlight the gross violation of human rights of India's mentally disordered generally, and her MDOs specifically, and that this might facilitate lasting improvements.

Key points

- Current levels of care of MDO are poor
- India's mental health law, especially related to diversion of MDO, must be updated
- Greater coordination and integration to facilitate seamless care and management across departmental boundaries
- Increased awareness of mental health needs of prisoners by the criminal justice system
- Respect for individual autonomy and human rights

References

Asian Human Rights Commission – Urgent Appeals Program 2004. India: A Detainee Waiting for Trial for 24 Years Develops Mental Illness. Available on 16 June 2004. www.ahrchk.net/ua/mainfile. php/2004/703/

Chaddha, R.K. and Amarjeet 1998 Clinical Profile of Patients Attending a Prison Psychiatric Clinic. Indian Journal of Psychiatry 40: 260–265.

Channabasavanna, S.M., Subrahmanya, B., Gangadhar, John, C.J. and Reddy, V. 1981. Mental Health Delivery System in India – A Brief Report. Indian Journal of Psychiatry 23: 309–312.

Das, M. Gupta, N. and Dutta, K. 2002 Psychiatric Training in India. Psychiatric Bulletin 26: 70–72.

Dutt, A.B. 1996 Protection against Violation of Human Rights of the Mentally Ill Persons: An Experiment with the Magistrates. Abstracts, Regional Conference of Royal College of Psychiatrists, Hyderabad, India.

Malik, P.L. 1974 The Criminal Court Hand Book, Chapter XXV of the Criminal Penal Code. Lucknow (India): Eastern Book Company.

Marfatia, J.C. 1972 State v. Raman Raghav. Bombay High Court Confirmation Case No 20 of 1969 in Psychiatry & Law, Bombay: Popular Prakashan.

The Mental Health Act 1987. Lucknow: Eastern Book Company.

The Mental Health Act 1987 with Central & State Rules 1990. Delhi: Delhi Law House.

National Human Rights Commission (NHRC). 1999 Quality Assurance in Mental Health – A Project of the National Human Rights Commission. New Delhi: National Institute of Mental Health and Neurosciences.

Ramanathan, U. 2003 Human Rights in India: A Mapping. International Environmental Law Research Centre Working Paper No. 2001–3. Retrieved from www.ielrc.org/Content/W01031t__4.html, in December 2004.

Ratanlal, R. and Dhirajlal, K.T. 1992 Code of Criminal Procedure, 14th Edition Ch. XXV: Revised by Hidayatullah M. Nagpur, India: Wadhwa and Company.

Ratanlal, R. and Dhirajlal, K.T. 2002 The Indian Penal Code, 29th Edition. (Chandrachud Y.V. and Manohar, V.R. Editors) Nagpur, India: Wadhwa and Company.

Sarkar, J. 2004. A New Mental Health Act for India: An Ethics Based Approach. Indian Journal of Psychiatry 46: 104–114.

Sen Gupta, S.K. and Chawla, D.R. 1970 Mental Health in India, CBHI Technical Studies, 51. New Delhi, India: Central Bureau of Health Intelligence.

Shah, L.P. 1999 Forensic Psychiatry in India, Current Status and Future Development. Indian Journal of Psychiatry: 43: 179–185.

Trivedi, J.K. 2002 The Mental Health Legislation: An Ongoing Debate. Indian Journal of Psychiatry 44: 95–96.

The West Bengal Jail Code, Home Department, Calcutta 1967.

Unlock the Padlock. 1993. Report of the Supreme Court Commission on Mentally Ill in the Jails of West Bengal, Vol. I.

Law reports

Dutt, A.B. v. State of West Bengal & others, Public Interest Litigation, Calcutta High Court, C.O. No. 5775 (W) of 1989.

Kuttapan v. State of Kerala 1986 Cr LJ 271 (Ker).

Sheela Barse v Union of India, W.P.(Crml) No. 237 of 1989 (1993) 4 Supreme Court Cases 204.

State (Delhi) v. Sanjoy Bhatia1985 Cr LJ 931.

Tabu Chetia v. State of Assam 1976 Cr LJ 1416.

R. K. Ghosh v. Secretary, Indian Psychoanalytical Society, A.I.R. 1963 Cal. 261.

Chapter 34

Reflections on the ethical complexities of medical life in apartheid South Africa

Trudie Rossouw

Aim

To illustrate how oppressive states can generate complex ethical dilemmas for the helping professions.

Learning objectives

- To understand, in outline, recent political and societal changes in South Africa
- To use an understanding of the South African apartheid state to consider the moral and ethical dilemmas than can arise for health professionals from an oppressive political system
- To consider the impact of state oppression on the mental health of a population

Introduction

South Africa is a country of extraordinary natural beauty, but it bears the deep scars of the apartheid system that sanctioned the abuse of human rights, repression, racial segregation, forced physical removal, laws preventing interracial marriages, violence, poverty and malnutrition. Apartheid was also a social–economic system based on the exploitation of Black labour. The small minority of 4 million White people were given rights to own land, vote and have access to good schools and other services, whereas 40 million of the rest of the population were denied most of these rights.

This chapter explores the impact of such a system on the mental health of the society and considers some of the ethical issues that emerged for those in the helping professions.

Historical context

State-sanctioned racial oppression and abuse in South Africa predate the apartheid system and goes as far back as 1913 when the Land Act was introduced, restricting Black people to what was known as 'native reserves'. These 'reserves' occupied 13% of the land in the country and were in remote areas, often drought-stricken and poor. Families resettled in these areas, trying to make humble lives from agriculture. Poverty, drought and the absence of infrastructure made it hard for communities to be self-sufficient. Subsequently, most men in their early adulthood moved to the cities to work in mines. This disrupted and destroyed traditional family life. Children grew up without their fathers, and their fathers often had more than one family, one back home and one in the city.

In 1976, high school children in Soweto held a peaceful demonstration against the forced use of Afrikaans in their schools. Five hundred were shot dead by the police. They were all shot in the back as they were running away. In the years after 1976, the anti-apartheid struggle intensified. Some left the country to enrol in military training, others joined in grass roots, underground, political organisations (Hayes 2000). In response to the uprising of political resistance and the increase in violent attacks against state institutions and symbols, the state itself became increasingly violent and controlling. The army or security forces were frequently sent in to disrupt meetings with teargas or gunfire. Beyond the borders of the country, secret forces of the army were regularly sent in to destroy entire villages in the belief that the village was housing African National Congress (ANC)[1] members, or that it was an ANC training camp.

In 1985, the state declared a 'state of emergency'. The police had the power to arrest and detain people they suspected of political crimes without the need for a trial. They had the right to detain people in two ways. Detainees who were not going to be charged, in other words where there was no evidence that could be brought against them, could be held in detention, without trial and legal representation, for an indefinite period of time. The second group of detainees were those against whom the police brought charges and who were awaiting trial. The police had the right to detain them in solitary confinement for 6 months prior to trial. In solitary confinement, they did not have the right to speak to a solicitor or any relative. Their only human contact was with their interrogating officer, their guard, and when they were ill, a doctor employed by the state.

In the author's experience, when prisoners were ill owing to abuse they sustained in the process of 'interrogation', they saw a doctor only when there was no longer any visible evidence of the abuse. Not only did the police enjoy greater freedoms to arrest and detain, but they also had greater freedom to act in brutal and violent ways. Pumla Gobodo-Madikizela (2003), a professor in clinical psychology in Cape Town, who was also a member of the Truth and Reconciliation Committee (TRC), gave a moving account in her book of what it felt like to be a child during those years. She referred to an example she remembered vividly when she was five years old, standing outside her house looking at grown men running wildly like animals through the street. They were followed by army vehicles and the sound of gunfire. Men were shot in front of her and she described the smell of gunfire and blood and the memory of seeing the street full of blood, lined with dead bodies. When she became a member of the TRC, she had access to the archives that contained a description of the events of that night. She was horrified when she discovered the records referred to the death of only one person. She did not believe the record and inquired from her fellow ANC and PAC colleagues, who confirmed the account recorded in the archives. She said (2003: pp 10):

> I can only suggest that when the safe world of a child is shattered by the violent invasion of police, the intensity of the moment is something that the experience of a five-year-old cannot absorb. She lacks the psychological capacity to contain the brutality before her eyes, and certainly has no language with which to re-present the traumatic events. *Blood*, *bodies*, and *death* are the only meaningful words that can capture the image of what she cannot truly articulate through language.

In a community survey in 1997 (Ensink et al 1997), in one of the townships outside of Cape Town, 60 children were interviewed for evidence of exposure to violence and prevalence of

---

[1] The ANC was a political organization committed to ending the apartheid regime and went on to take over government from the White minority. It remains in power, Thabo Mbeki having succeeded from the first Black president of South Africa, Nelson Mandela, a former prisoner on Robben Island.

post-traumatic stress disorder (PTSD). Ninety-five percent of the children interviewed had witnessed violence, 56% had experienced violence themselves. Forty percent met the criteria for DSM-III-R diagnoses and 21% met the criteria for PTSD. In a similar, nationwide survey of 16- to 64-year-olds, 23% of the population had been exposed to one or more violent events (Hirschowitz and Orkin 1997). The difference between the incidence of exposure to violence in the two studies quoted could be explained by the fact that the latter was a nationwide study and the former was a study conducted in a violent area.

The climate of state-sanctioned abuse and torture, and the disruption of the protective stability of families and communities through the detention of large numbers of people, must have implications for the mental health of a society. A psychoanalytic framework can help. Where the state is not protective but intrusive and coercive, it is easy to see that fear, terror and loss can be regular emotional experiences for many people. In such a troubled society, it is also hard to know exactly how many people were affected in this way. Psychodynamically, these experiences could be organized by the individual, and collectively by the group, into compartments of good and bad, friend or enemy. High levels of suspicion and fear were operating in all communities. This affected both White and Black communities, and both communities adopted primitive defence mechanisms to defend themselves against these anxieties.

The White community showed high levels of denial and claimed not to have been aware of what was happening. Studies have also shown high levels of arrogance, superiority and omnipotence in some White communities (Dommisse 1987). Some of the White communities idealized the police and their brutality. This can be seen as result of their capacity to see themselves as superior and to dehumanize the 'other'. Once a group of people is dehumanized, guilt is redundant. As in Nazi Germany, atrocities can be perpetrated on a group without raising anxiety or alarm (Hoffman 1998: 201–240; Richmond 1995: 449–458). An NGO called Organisation for Appropriate Social Services in South Africa (OASSSA) provided therapeutic services to affected Black communities. They commented on similar levels of denial in the Black communities, especially in activists who came out of detention, who denied any emotional vulnerability or pain. Instead, they became triumphant and aggressive, and rejoined the struggle with greater vigour. Fighting was a favoured coping mechanism, preferable to being overwhelmed with pain and loss. In a society organized around these defensive mechanisms, violence can escalate; the traumatic impact of violence may itself breed more violence.

These issues affect the wider society as a whole but have specific implications for the helping professions operating within the state. Neither the Psychological Association nor the Medical Association spoke up against apartheid. It explains how the health care system in one hospital (White) would have one code of ethics and in another hospital (Black) would operate under a different ethical code. A large percentage of helping professionals fell prey to powerful forces of denial and splitting, allowing and supporting the abusive system to continue.

The following personal testimony is written to illustrate, in the first person, how the ethical tensions experienced by many at this point in South Africa's evolution were played out in the life of one doctor, the author.

The personal account of a police doctor

I was employed by the State as a police doctor (the term for it was district surgeon, although it had nothing to do with surgery) in 1988. My role involved twice-weekly visits to Robben Island and to police cells when prisoners or detainees became ill and needed to see a doctor.

It was particularly the plight of the detainees in solitary confinement that struck me. They were detained in small cells that had three brick walls and one wall made of thick wire mesh fencing. Inside their cell was a small bed, a basin and a toilet. A bright, stark light in the middle of the ceiling burnt day and night. Outside the cell a policeman was on 24-hour guard. The only person detainees had contact with on a daily basis was their interrogating officer.

Detainees were stripped of both privacy and dignity; they had no contact with their attachment figures and the outside world; the boundary between night and day was dissolved. Prisoners were regularly told that their children or parents were detained too, and would die or be tortured if the prisoner did not speak.

I was deeply disturbed when I met the first detainees in solitary confinement shortly after my appointment. I saw young people in despair, no longer filled with terror, they seemed to have succumbed to an utter sense of hopelessness. They were reminiscent of the 'musulmen' described in Nazi concentration camps (Levi 1989). They also saw no help in meeting me, as I too was White and seen as part of the system. Being naïve and new in post, I thought I may be able to make a difference by objecting to the way the prisoners were treated, but my objections fell on deaf ears. I felt I was employed to help and at the same time prevented from doing so.

It took some time before I realized that I was employed to help the police in a perverse manner: namely to maintain the appearance that medical facilities were available to the prisoners as long as that did not interfere in the abusive practices.

Although I knew I could not change the system, ethically and morally I could not sleep knowing about the suffering of the prisoners. Slowly, over time, I became involved in smuggling letters between prisoners and their families, which was the only contact they had with one another. Even though this contact was limited, in many cases it was enough to maintain a sense of reality and hope to protect against deep depression. To do this was to place my own life at risk, but seeing the suffering and succumbing to passivity was to place my psyche at risk. I felt I was left with no choice.

I had letters hidden in any imaginable place in my office, for example, neatly rolled up next to batteries in my examining set. I never knew when I was going to see which prisoner. At least one policeman was always in the consulting room with me and the patient so the only moment when letters could be exchanged, and at times written, was when I examined patients behind a drawn curtain. The tension is hard to describe. I resigned after one year. At the same time as my resignation, I was also informed that I was being watched by the police.

Towards reconciliation

In 1990, Mandela was released, and in 1994, South Africa became a democratic country. The Truth and Reconciliation Commission (TRC) was formed in the aftermath of independence to form a non-judicial forum to assist the transition to a nonracist, democratic society (see also Adshead et al this volume (Chapter 9, pp 113–128)). The aim was to acknowledge the truth in the hope that it would restore the dignity of the victim rather than implement revenge and justice on the perpetrator. The events around the TRC are unique to South Africa, perhaps unprecedented in human history. It was introduced by the government to document human-rights violations under the apartheid regime, to establish the fate of the victims and to restore their human and civil dignity by recommending reparation procedures (Van Zyl 1999).

In the hearings, the perpetrators described abusive acts they had committed. This time, abuse was no longer sanctioned by the state and neither was one group of people dehumanized. This resulted in the perpetrators – although this is not true for all – having to see in the pain of the victims or their families, the horror of what they did. They were confronted with the possibility of feeling guilt. They moved psychically from functioning in what can be called a paranoid–schizoid state of inner organization, to a depressive state (Van Zyl 1999). In the paranoid–schizoid state, the background emotional tone is of fear, terror, hate and violence; a world clearly demarcated by friends and enemies; a world where unpleasant awareness of the other's suffering is denied. In the depressive state, a person is able to see the destruction and pain they have inflicted on someone else and is *unable* to deny the painful awareness of that.

For the victims, however devastatingly painful it was to hear the details of the abuse described, the detail affirmed their reality. Noticing the pain and guilt of the perpetrator helped them to feel that their pain was acknowledged and heard, that they were no longer dehumanized. It reduced the fear and hate of the other, but affirmed their loss, which increased their pain. Some victims, often mothers who lost their sons in the struggle, had endured a double pain; they had the original loss of a child, followed by an intensifying of the struggle in the aftermath of the death, which left no time for their private pain and sense of loss to be acknowledged by their communities. The TRC became the first platform where their pain and loss could be publicly recognized, not only by the perpetrators, but also by their own communities.

In some cases, however, victims and their families made a distinction between national and personal reconciliation (Van Zyl 1999). Although they could see that the TRC brought national reconciliation, owing to their own pain and loss, it did not bring personal reconciliation.

Conclusion

As a member of a society we are like a leaf on the ocean, influenced by the currents beneath; we may be swept along without examining the ethical basis of our decisions. As doctors, or other health professionals, we are required to question the society in which we live and the institutions in which we work.

From a forensic perspective, the literature on conduct disorder and the origins of violence suggest that the formative years of a child are crucial in terms of their adult life. A child growing up in a country torn apart by violence and abuse, with parents imprisoned, abused or participating in violence themselves, is at greater risk than others of developing a range of psychopathology. The TRC tried to bring reconciliation and integration. It hoped to influence the developmental path of the country by altering individual lives in a public way. It intended South Africans to learn from their violent past so that the next generation would benefit from stability and security.

Key points

- State sponsored violence in apartheid South Africa affected both the White and Black populations
- A psychodynamic framework of understanding can be used at the level of the individual and the group to consider responses to violence
- South Africa pioneered a radical approach in the aftermath of apartheid, favouring public acknowledgement and reconciliation rather than legal redress

References

Dommisse, J. 1987 The State of Psychiatry in South Africa Today. Society of Science and Medicine 224: 749 –761.

Ensink, K., Robertson, B.A., Zissis, C. and Leger, P. 1997. Post Traumatic Stress Disorder in Children Exposed to Violence. South African Medical Journal 87: 1526–1530.

Gobodo-Madikizela, P. 2003. A Human Being Died that Night. Cape Town:Davidphillip.

Hayes, G. 2000. The Struggle for Mental Health in South Africa: Psychologists, Apartheid and the Story of Durban OASSSA. Journal of Community and Applied Social Psychology 10: 327–342.

Hirschowitz, R., Orkin, M. 1997. Trauma and Mental Health in South Africa. Social Indicators Research 41: 169–182.

Hoffman, E. 1998 Shtetl: The History of a Small Town and an Extinguished World. London: Secker and Warburg

Levi, P. 1989 The Drowned and the Saved New York: Viking.

Richmond, T. 1995 Konin: A Quest. London: Jonathan Cape.

Van Zyl, S. 1999. An Interview with Gillian Straker on the Truth and Reconciliation Commission in South Africa. Psychoanalytic Dialogues 9: 245–274

Chapter 35

Scottish forensic psychiatry

John Crichton

Aim

To describe the key elements of recent Scottish Mental Health Legislation and the way in which they relate to historical and recent service development for Mentally Disordered Offenders (MDOs).

Learning objectives

- To understand the distinctive legal and service characteristics of Scottish forensic psychiatry
- To understand the development of forensic psychiatry in Scotland

---

Introduction

Specific services for MDOs did not develop in Scotland at the same pace as in England. This was despite the fact that Scottish legislation closely mirrored that of England and Wales until devolution. This chapter outlines the recent impetus for service development and the evolving and increasingly different legislation for this group of offenders. It also touches on the distinctive Scottish approach to public safety.

Service development

Although other parts of the United Kingdom developed specialist institutions for MDOs in the nineteenth century, it was not until after the Second World War that Scottish patients were moved from the Criminal Lunatics Department, a wing of Perth Prison, to the newly built State Hospital at Carstairs railway junction next to an isolated moor, halfway between Edinburgh and Glasgow. The development of medium secure forensic services seen in England following the Butler Report (Home Office 1975) did not occur in Scotland.

Mirroring the Reed Report in England (DH 1994), Scotland launched its own policy document regarding a spectrum of services for mentally disorder offenders in 1999 (Mel (5)99; Scottish Office 1995), which is widely referred to as the 'McReed' Report. Implementation of that policy initiative have been slow with Scotland's first medium secure unit, the Orchard Clinic, opening in 2000 and its second, Rowanbank, in 2007; there remains patchy provision for the range of MDO services elsewhere. In 2003, the Forensic Mental Health Services Managed Care Network (The Network) was formed to advance the MDO policy, and now there is a substantial momentum for development of services, spurred by the implementation of the Mental Health (Care and Treatment) (Scotland) Act 2003.

Legal context

Although Scotland was joined with England under one monarch at the beginning of the seventeenth century, and had an amalgamated parliament from the beginning of the eighteenth century, a separate system of jurisprudence was retained. Although there were broad similarities with the English common law, Scots common law remains distinct. In particular, there continues to be the notion of legal principle that may be contributed to by a range of appropriate legal cases, not simply the most recent judgement of the most senior court. In particular, the common law defence of necessity is poorly developed, with some commentators even querying its existence as part of Scots law (Crichton 2000). District Courts only deal with the most minor criminal offences. In any criminal matter where the accused is suspected to have a mental health problem, the case is transferred to the Sheriff Court. The majority of criminal cases are, in any case, heard in the Sheriff Court, but serious violence, rape and murder are reserved for the High Court. The Court of Criminal Appeal is the final criminal appellant court in Scotland, whereas the House of Lords remains the final civil appellant court.

Following the Scotland Act 1998, which created modern devolution, the European Convention on Human Rights became part of Scottish domestic law. Disputes between the UK Parliament and Scottish Parliament regarding the scope of respective powers may be referred to the judicial committee of the Privy Council for legal ruling.

Criminal responsibility, law and mental health

Like other jurisdictions, Scotland has specific law designed to take into account the impact of mental health problems on responsibility for criminal acts. One export of the Scottish legal system to the world is the partial defence of diminished responsibility (Crichton et al 2004). In Scotland, this was originally used to reduce the seriousness of a range of offences. Now, it is restricted to reducing a charge of murder to one of culpable homicide. This provides the sentencing judge with a range of disposals rather than a statutory life sentence for murder. It was the Scottish Law on diminished responsibility that was exported to the English Homicide Act 1957. Until recently, the scope of defence was narrower than that allowed in England; following the Galbraith case (2001), the defence is open to a broader variety of circumstances. It is no longer simply applicable when the state of mind of an accused is 'bordering on insanity'. The Scottish Law Commission (2004) has recommended that the defence should be broadened to include psychopathic disorder, which currently is a diagnosis of exclusion for the defence, as is voluntary intoxication. Both these warrant comparison with the Australian system (see Ferris, this volume: pp 363–368).

Responses to dangerous offending

Scottish forensic psychiatry has not been influenced by the homicide inquiries in England of the 1990s. They have never been a requirement in Scotland. However, the double homicide committed by two personality-disordered patients who escaped from the State Hospital in 1977 cast a long shadow over the development of services (Darjee and Crichton 2003; Scottish Home and Health Department 1977). Scotland has always had a more sceptical position with regard to personality disorder than England. Although it has always been possible to detain someone with treatment of personality disorder under Scottish legislation, it remained innominate, that is, referred to by a description of behaviour rather than warranting a diagnosis per se.

Despite this philosophical distinction, in 1970, 25% of patients at the State Hospital had a primary diagnosis of personality disorder. This was similar to the proportion of such patients in English special hospitals. Following the escape and double murder in 1977, there was a substantial tightening of security at the State Hospital, together with a change in admission practice. By the early 1990s, only 6% of patients at the State Hospital had a primary personality disorder diagnosis; almost all of these were either very long-term patients or had been initially admitted under a mental illness or learning disability primary diagnosis (Thomson et al 1997).

The political context in which offenders who continue to pose a high risk of dangerous re-offending were considered was therefore very different in England and Scotland. In England, the Dangerous and Severe Personality Disorder (DSPD) category was generated by government on the back of the Michael Stone Case (Prins 2007). In Scotland, the McLean Committee, considering similar issues, recommended the creation of the new legal disposal of an Order of Lifelong Restriction (Darjee and Crichton 2002). This disposal was essentially the rebranding of discretionary life sentences for those found to be at high risk of serious future offending. A court can make such an order only after a period of formalized risk assessment. The Risk Management Authority has been created in Scotland to oversee the development of such services and to approve risk management strategies for individual offenders. It is possible for an MDO to be subject to an order of lifelong restriction if linked with an initial hospital disposal. Such a hybrid hospital order is termed a 'hospital direction'.

The Mental Health Care and Treatment (Scotland) Act 2003 was therefore enacted without controversy. This was very different from the atmosphere in England generated by the proposals both for 'DSPD' service development and a new Mental Health Act. The Mental Health Care and Treatment (Scotland) Act 2003 established a partial capacity test for civil detention. This has also underpinned the management of detained patients with a set of guiding principles. For patients detained civilly in Scotland, there must be significantly impaired decision-making ability because of mental disorder. This partial capacity test is solely for civil detention and is specifically excluded as necessary for courts sentencing MDOs to mental health disposals.

The new legislation did retain an important piece of emergency legislation. This was, in fact, the first legislation passed by the newly constituted parliament: the Mental Health (Public Safety and Appeals) (Scotland) Act 1999 (Crichton et al 2001). Noel Ruddell, a restricted patient, was released having appealed against his detention on the grounds that he was suffering from a personality disorder that was not treatable. He had originally been detained suffering from a psychotic illness but this transpired to be a drug-induced psychosis. At the State Hospital there had been poor development of services for the small number of patients with a primary personality disorder. In a judgement that had repercussions in the English context, the House of Lords ruled that a patient with personality disorder that was not amenable to treatment had to be released (Darjee et al 1999). Emergency legislation was then enacted in Scotland so that a restricted patient with personality disorder could continue to be detained, irrespective of treatability, should they pose a risk of serious harm to the public. Failure to challenge this successfully given its incompatibility with the European Convention on Human Rights has revealed the limits of human rights legislation (Darjee and Crichton 2005).

Future plans for services

Paradoxically, perhaps, the Mental Health (Care and Treatment) (Scotland) Act 2003 also includes a provision that is promoting the development of forensic services; the Act provides for appeals against excess security. A Mental Health Tribunal can rule that a patient is held in excessive security and requires a Health Board to provide care at a lower level of security. If the Health Board does not comply with its statutory duty after two extensions permitted by the tribunal, a summary application can be made to the Court of Session (the senior civil court) with the possibility of fines and criminal sanctions for failure to comply. This can be compared with the situation in England, where many patients languished in unnecessary high secure care, for long periods of time, in the absence of long-term medium secure facilities, and with little practical assistance from the available legislation (Bartlett et al 1996). In response to this new piece of Scottish legislation, the Forensic Network has commissioned a range of expert groups to help further plan forensic services in Scotland. This would define levels of security in the Scottish context. Plans include the development of a spectrum of women's services, learning disability services, adolescent services and new personality disorder services, particularly focusing on interagency working with patients in the community. One of the most exciting proposals is the development of a school of forensic mental health care that would be required to help prepare the projected expansion in workforce.

Forensic psychiatry in Scotland may once have been considered underdeveloped, especially viewed from a southerly direction, but current innovations promise the delivery of a world-class forensic service, and forensic mental health care continues to be a priority for the Scottish government.

Key points

- Medium secure hospital units were developed only recently in Scotland
- Scotland is part of the United Kingdom but has a separate system of jurisprudence
- Recent Scottish legislation has developed very differently from England in key areas, that is, serious offending and where an individual's capacity is in question

References

Bartlett, A.E.A., Cohen, A., Backhouse, A., Highnet, N. and Eastman, N.L.G. 1996 Security Needs of South West Thames Hospital Patients: 1992 and 1993. No Way Out? Journal of Forensic Psychiatry 7: 256–270.

Crichton, J.H.M. 2000 Mental Incapacity and Consent to Treatment: The Scottish Experience. The Journal of Forensic Psychiatry 11: 457–64.

Crichton J.H.M., Darjee R. and Chiswick D. 2004 Diminished Responsibility in Scotland: New Case Law. Journal of Forensic Psychiatry and Psychology 15: 552–65.

Crichton, J.H.M., Darjee R., McCall-Smith A. and Chiswick D. 2001 Mental Health (Public Safety and Appeals) (Scotland) Act 1999: Detention of Untreatable Patients with Psychopathic Disorder. Journal of Forensic Psychiatry 12: 647–661.

Darjee, R. and Crichton, J.H.M. 2002 The MacLean Committee: Scotland's Answer to the 'Dangerous People with Severe Personality Disorder' Proposals? Psychiatric Bulletin 26: 6–8.

Darjee, R. and Crichton, J.H.M. 2003 Personality Disorder and the Law in Scotland: A Historical Perspective. Journal of Forensic Psychiatry and Psychology 14: 394–425.

Darjee, R. and Crichton, J.H.M. 2004 New Mental Health Legislation. British Medical Journal 329: 634–635.

Darjee, R. and Crichton, J.H.M. 2005 Reid v. the United Kingdom: Restricted Patients and the European Convention on Human Rights. The Journal of Forensic Psychiatry & Psychology 16: 508–522.

Darjee, R., McCall-Smith A., Crichton J.H.M. and Chiswick, D. 1999 Detention of Patients with Psychopathic Disorder in Scotland: Canons Park Wrongly Decided? Journal of Forensic Psychiatry 10: 649–658.

Department of Health 1994 Review of Health and Social Services for Mentally Disordered Offenders and Others Requiring Similar Services. (Reed Report). London HMSO.

Galbraith v H.M. Advocate 2001 SCCR 551.

Home Office, Department of Health and Social Security. 1975 Report of the Committee on Mentally Disordered Offenders. Cmnd 6244. London: Butler report.

Prins H. 2007 The Michael Stone Inquiry: A Somewhat Different Homicide Report. Journal of Forensic Psychiatry and Psychology 18: 411–31.

Scottish Law Commission. July 2004 Report on Insanity and Diminished Responsibility, The Stationery Office, Edinburgh.

Thomson, L.D.G., Bogue, J.P., Humphreys, M.S., Owen D.C. and Johnstone, E.C. 1997 The State Hospital Survey: a Description of Psychiatric Patients in Conditions of Special Security in Scotland. Journal of Forensic Psychiatry 8: 263–284.

Chapter 36

Diminished responsibility as a cultural phenomenon

Emma van Hoecke

Aim

To illustrate the relevance of the philosophical underpinnings of law and psychiatry to forensic mental health work in Holland and the UK.

Learning objectives

- To understand the Dutch and English concepts of diminished responsibility
- To understand the Dutch approach to expert evidence in criminal courts

Introduction

Dutch and English cultures are distinguishable by many things, including the philosophical basis of their legal and mental health systems. The concept of diminished responsibility, a legal defence to certain criminal charges, is a useful vehicle to explore this and to delineate the contrasting characteristics of forensic mental health practice in the Netherlands and England and Wales.

Models in legal and mental health work

Eastman (1992), an English lawyer and forensic psychiatrist, remarked that law and psychiatry and psychology used different models of 'man', and that this conceptual clash was apparent in the forensic field, where it had implications for an understanding of legal responsibility for criminal acts. Eastman explored the nature of each model and argued that the degree of disjunction varied. He argued that law should better reflect both psychiatric and psychological realities. He stated that a graded approach to responsibility was favourable to a binary approach, although he did not propose a model for a graded approach in his article. Eastman suggested that one way to avoid the problem of the incongruity of the three models was to withhold the psychiatric evidence until the disposal stage of criminal justice proceedings. However, he also regarded this as an unfair way of proceeding. He argued that expert advice to the courts ought to be reliable and valid. This demanded that it be based either on psychiatric phenomena or on psychometry and not on psycho-understanding informed by psychodynamic theory.[1]

---

[1] In a later paper (Eastman, N. and Campbell, C. 2006), Eastman continued to explore the law's difficulty dealing with external evidence, in this case from neuroscience. He suggested that because mental health experts use their expert knowledge to explain the actions of the criminal individual, in fact, courts are likely to find this more digestible than population- and biology-based science, so-called hard science.

Mooij (2004), a Dutch professor in psychiatric aspects of legal practice, prefers a psycho-understanding (empiristic–hermeneutic) model as the basis for the assessment of offending behaviour. In his opinion, it was crucial to place an action in its context to understand its significance for the individual and to assess his or her intention and capacity for reflection. He felt that one should draw on multiple sources of information to construct the personal significance of an offence. This approach attaches less importance to psychometric predictions of recidivism. Mooij felt that his approach started from a broader perspective, that is, the person's experience of offending behaviour, instead of a reductionistic approach, where classification is king. He urged caution with regard to someone having a wholly determined identity, feeling that it was essential in forensic discourse to distinguish between the person who was an offender in the past or at the time of the offence and the potential he or she has in the present for self-realization. In his opinion, all these dimensions should be reflected in the opinions expressed by expert witnesses advising the courts.

Diminished responsibility in England and Wales

These different approaches were reflected in the different evolutions of the psychiatric defence of diminished responsibility in the two countries. In England and Wales, diminished responsibility can be invoked only in murder cases where the charge can be reduced to manslaughter. Reznek (1997) argued that medical perceptions of mental illness were different from both the legal concept of abnormality of mind (a component of the diminished responsibility defence as defined in statute law) and mental responsibility – the one did not necessarily imply the other. Eastman and Campbell (2006) added that the law has its own purpose and that there is little coherence in its understanding of mental disorder. This occurs because it is using mental health evidence only when *it* has a question to answer, which is itself framed as a legal matter. Reznek (1997) commented that psychiatrists might be best placed to apply medical concepts, but insanity and diminished responsibility were matters for the jury. The adversarial system in English courts can put juries into the unenviable situation of having to choose between differing experts. Mackay (2003) argued that the current diminished responsibility plea should be reformed, abolished or applied to all offences.

Diminished responsibility in the Netherlands

In the Netherlands, the diminished responsibility plea can be applied to any type of offence, and the extent to which responsibility is diminished is assessed on a sliding scale. British law is not so subtle, seeing it as present or absent. The Dutch system was developed in the aftermath of the Second World War. Koenraadt (2004) described how a large number of Dutch lawmakers were incarcerated during the German occupation. Their experiences informed their own prison system, and they suggested that it required considerable modernization with an increase in procedural safety.

Van Mulbregt and Sierink (2004) explained that Dutch law requires the expert witness to prove a relationship between a mental disorder and the charge. In Dutch law, if the offender suffers from mental disorder, it does not prove anything with respect to his or her offending behaviour. It is therefore crucial that a clear distinction be made between the patient, their illness and, thus, that the patient not be reduced to his or her disorder alone. A patient is not determined by his or her illness, but retains a degree of freedom of choice while being ill.

The crucial question for the court is whether the mental disorder has compromised the free will of the offender so that his or her insight and options were limited at the time of the offence. For example, if a patient with schizophrenia shoplifted because he or she was hungry, on one hand his or her motive could be considered as opportunistic, or, on the other hand, as behaviour secondary to their illness because of their inability to claim state benefits during a psychotic breakdown. If the patient shoplifted because he or she thought that a camera, which observed him or her, was hidden in the food he or she stole, there is an immediate link between his or her illness and his or her offending behaviour. In the first case, the patient would be considered responsible for his or her behaviour. In the second case, the patient would be deemed to have been in a state of diminished responsibility for the offence because of a serious impairment and an inability to organise his or her life in a practical sense. In the third scenario, he or she will not be considered responsible for his/her offence.

The same principles are applied to Dutch patients with a personality disorder whereby the limitations of their coping skills are taken into consideration. Van Mulbregt and Sierink (2004) highlighted the case of an offender with an antisocial personality disorder, arguing that the defect in the development of his conscience did not necessarily compromise his free will. Patients with this disorder are considered to have a sense for law and order and to be able to choose to resolve their problems via strategies other than their own opportunistic ones.

Five degrees of responsibility are used in the Netherlands: an offender is held to be fully responsible for his or her offence when there is no diagnosed disorder or no relationship between the disorder and the charges. He or she is considered to be of mildly diminished responsibility only if there is a disorder and the disorder had a minor or no influence on the offending behaviour. If an expert witness considered an offender to have mildly diminished responsibility, he found a link between the offence and the disorder, but the suspect was, according to the expert witness, to a large extent 'free' to act differently. This degree of responsibility is also used when the available information does not permit the establishment of a stronger link between the disorder and the offence.

If the degree of diminished responsibility is used, there is a strong link between the seriousness of the disorder and the offence. This is often used for offenders with a personality disorder, as their limited coping skills seriously reduce their options to resolve the situation that eventually resulted in their offence. But in such cases, there is no distortion of reality and therefore the offender is considered to have been in a state of diminished responsibility in relation to the offence.

To be considered to be in a state of strongly diminished responsibility, the offender often suffers from a combination of disorders, whereby his or her choices to resolve a situation are strongly compromised. This degree of strongly diminished responsibility is also applicable when the behaviour of an offender is seriously limited by a psychosis, but there is no proof that the offender acted only upon the basis of his or her psychotic beliefs.

The fifth degree is similar to the British 'not guilty by reason of insanity'. Offenders are not held responsible for their offence if they suffered from serious distortion of reality and/or their behaviour was completely controlled by their psychosis at the time of the offence.

Expert evidence in the Netherlands

Although the application by expert witnesses of a sliding scale system may be expected to be inconsistent, it has been demonstrated that in general there is a strong consistency in the application of these concepts in the Netherlands. Dutch expert witnesses work only for forensic departments and report exclusively from that position to the courts. Furthermore, Dutch forensic services offer training for expert witnesses. All reports are written in the same national format. In the design of that format, the utmost care was taken to ensure that expert witnesses could not interfere with evidence pertaining to their cases and that they answer a standard set of questions for the court. Each report is supervised by the forensic departments, at least by a peer psychiatrist or a peer psychologist, and a lawyer before they are sent to court. If a recommendation has major implications for the offender, such as a TBS recommendation, a joint report must be written by a psychiatrist and a psychologist before such a recommendation can be made. Their advice is discussed at meetings, where several peer professionals and a lawyer are present. This protocol endeavours to ensure that any differences in opinion among peer professionals are resolved, prior to court submissions, a process that is organized in an inquisitorial, not adversarial manner.

It is important to note that this fundamental difference in principle results in two other major cultural differences between British and Dutch forensic practice. The discourse of risk has a limited place in Dutch forensic reports. Psychologists use risk assessments such as the PCL-R and the HCR-20 only as checklists, because their assessments are designed to stress the individual clinical presentation of an offender, including their psychological problems, ability to learn, support systems and perspective. Van Deutekom and Koenraadt (2004) claimed that scoring is considered to be arbitrary. From a legal point of view, Van Mulbregt and Sierink (2004) argued that a risk assessment score does not answer the relevant questions regarding the cause, its seriousness, the level of danger or the actual responsibility of the offender for his or her behaviour, although recent research might challenge that view (Gray et al 2008).

Another major difference between the two cultures is that of the Dutch concept of ongoing responsibility of the offender both at the time of his or her offence and afterwards. In Great Britain, to protect society the choice was made to take over that responsibility when it was felt that the offender posed a serious threat. For example, the courts can make restriction orders and delegate the responsibility for the treatment of the offender via the Ministry of Justice to forensic psychiatrists, referred to as Responsible Medical Officers (RMOs). This promotes cautious decision-making, whereby safeguarding society takes precedence over the individual rights of the offender. In the Dutch context, it is rarely considered that an offender is not responsible for his or her act and even if this is the case, he or she is still expected to behave responsibly during both punishment and treatment. Offenders also know that they will be held accountable if they re-offend. This creates a context in which mentally ill offenders are held more accountable for their behaviour than their psychiatrists; as a result, the threshold at which they may be sent back into society is lowered.

We are products of our culture, and it is interesting to consider the connections between a culture's favoured artistic styles and other spheres of activity, in this case the very different approaches to decision-making in the forensic field in England and in the Netherlands. Bacon, a very English painter, specializes in publicly exposing the unpleasant depths of the human mind. Humanity is depicted, beautifully, in all its ugliness. Just as the forensic experts are preoccupied with horror and risk, societal fears of further trauma through recidivism are evoked in his work. Piet Mondriaan, a Dutch artist, is a polar opposite. His work is known for its precision in which he uses clear black lines and purity of colour. The forensic analogy being the demarcations used in the definition for a graded concept of responsibility and the clarity in the Dutch style of decision-making which emulates the clarity of Mondriaan's beloved primary colours.

Conclusion

The differences in forensic approaches are not just an academic diversion. They are of considerable practical importance with the regular exchange of foreign nationals between EU and other countries. It is essential that these cultural differences between the Dutch and the British forensic fields be taken into consideration when dealing with this kind of issue. Equally, within forensic policy development, an appropriate understanding of equivalence, for example, of high secure care, can be limited. What is required is a more profound grasp of the styles of forensic case processing that generate detained populations in particular jurisdictions.

Key points

- In Dutch law there is a sliding scale of responsibility for criminal acts
- Diminished responsibility can apply to any offence in the Netherlands, whereas in English law it is restricted to murder
- The Netherlands uses a inquisitorial court system where expert wtnesses will peer review their opinions prior to court proceedings. In contrast, the adversarial system in use in England requires expert evidence to be tested in court

References

Eastman, N. 1992. Psychiatric, Psychological and Legal Models of Man. International Journal of Law and Psychiatry 15: 157–169.

Eastman, N. and Campbell, C. 2006 Neuroscience and Determinants of Criminal Responsibility Nature Reviews Neuroscience 7: 311–318.

Gray, N.S., Taylor, J. and Snowden, R.J. 2008 Predicting Violent Recidivism using the HCR 20 British Journal of Psychiatry 192: 384–387.

Koenraadt, F. 2004. Historische wortels en recente ontwikkelingen 155–177 in De persoon van de verdachte. Deventer: Kluwer.

Mackay, R.D. 2003. Some Thoughts on Reforming the Law of Insanity and Diminished Responsibility in England. The Juridical Review, part 1: 57–80.

Mooij, A. 2004. Toerekeningsvatbaarheid: Over handelingsvrijheid. Amsterdam: Psychiatrie en Filosofie Boom.

Reznek, L. 1997. Evil or Ill? Justifying the Insanity Defence. London: Routledge.

Van Deutekom, C.M. and Koenraadt, F. 2004. Het psychologisch onderzoek. De persoon van de verdachte. Deventer: Kluwer.

Van Mulbregt, J.M.L. and Sierink, H.D. 2004. Conclusie en advies 117–140 In De persoon van de verdachte. Deventer: Kluwer.

Chapter 37

Forensic mental health in Switzerland: philosophy and services

Madleina Manetsch

Aim

To outline the current structure of Swiss forensic services.

Learning objectives

- To understand the development of Swiss forensic services and their relation to the wider political system
- To understand the role of forensic psychiatrists within Switzerland

Introduction

Switzerland sits in the middle of Central Europe. It shares much of its history and culture (four national languages spoken in different regions) with its neighbours Germany, Austria, Italy and France. However, it does not belong to the European Union (EU), but has special agreements (bilateral negotiations) with the EU.

Forensic psychiatry, as elsewhere in Central Europe, is a developing and comparatively young discipline. It faces an ongoing task to define its role; it operates as part of the health system as well as providing experts for the justice system. From an external point of view, clients or patients will have to find an understanding both of their mental health issues and of the political landscape in which they are living. As in other European countries, there is a contemporary debate about appropriate punishment for offenders, reduction of risk and public safety.

This chapter aims to provide an introduction into forensic psychiatry services in Switzerland. Current practice will be contextualized by Switzerland's history, its size and population, its political institutions and criminal law as well as the country's development of psychiatric institutions.

Swiss history and its political systems

Setting a 'date of birth' for Switzerland depends on the interpretation of the term 'Switzerland'. Archaeology shows that Stone Age hunters had been living in the region before the last Ice Age (approximately 350,000 BC). However, Switzerland's official Latin name, 'Confoederatio Helvetica', goes back to a Celtic tribe called the 'Helvetians'. Switzerland's history is very much intertwined with the events in the Holy Roman Empire in Western Europe of about 400 AD. In the first days of August 1291, three cantons signed an Everlasting Alliance to make a stand against the Habsburg Empire, and this signifies the beginning of the 'Old Swiss Confederation'. The three-canton core expanded over the years and, after the Swabian War in 1499, the Swiss

Confederation could establish its independence from the Holy Roman Empire. In 1648, the Peace of Westphalia granted the Swiss official neutrality and recognition of their independence from the Austrian Habsburg Empire. Swiss independence was again challenged by Napoleon. However, after his defeat at Waterloo, the Congress of Vienna (again) officially recognized Swiss neutrality. Besides 1291 and 1648, 1848 is the most important date in the history of the Swiss Confederation, as this was when the modern Federal Constitution (with total revisions in 1874 and 1999) was established.

Switzerland's political system is that of a direct democracy with a seven-seat Federal Council (Bundesrat), a cabinet-like board, which is elected every four years by the Federal Assembly. The Federal Assembly consists of the Council of States (Staenderat) and the National Council (Nationalrat), elected directly and every four years by the Swiss public. The two Councils are on an equal level (Das Schweizer Parlament). In contrast to many Western European parliaments, the Swiss Federal Assembly is not made up of professional parliamentary deputies. The members of both chambers exercise their mandates as an accessory activity. The two chambers of Switzerland's national parliament meet several times annually for parliamentary sessions over several weeks, and between these periods prepare meetings in numerous commissions. There are features of direct democracy that grant an unusually high level of participation to ordinary citizens. There are frequent referenda on new or changed laws and popular initiatives, where ordinary citizens may propose changes to the constitution, if they can find a number of supporters (100,000). It is not the mere existence of direct democratic instruments (federalism is widespread and referenda are not unknown to other democratic systems) but rather the frequent use of them that seems uniquely Swiss. This is encouraged by Switzerland's Constitution and practised with enthusiasm by the citizens. Switzerland comprises 26 cantons, which are member states of the Swiss Confederation. They enjoy a large degree of autonomy. The Country's governments, parliaments and courts all operate on three levels; a federal, cantonal and communal one.

Population and culture

The population of Switzerland is strikingly varied. There are four official national languages (German, French, Italian, Romantsch), 26 cantons (states) and about 7.5 million people live in the country. Twenty percent come from a different cultural background (Bundesamt für Statistik 2006).

The cantons have considerable legal autonomy. There is a national regulatory act of civil and criminal law. However, executive tasks are devolved to each canton. Thus, court rulings, powers of imprisonment and treatment of patients/prisoners are decided locally. Switzerland is a small country (41,284 km²), and it can be easily crossed in a few hours (the journey from North to South in a car and on the motorway takes about four hours). Switzerland's location is right in the middle of Europe, but at the same time it is not part of the European Community, and it is therefore independent of the pan-European agenda.

Facilities, prisons, forensic psychiatric hospitals

The Swiss Federal Statistical Office concluded in October 2007 that there were 115 institutions, which can hold people on remand, incarcerate sentenced prisoners or hold people under a hospital order. In all, there exist 6,654 places. This number represents the overall capacity in the whole of Switzerland. These places are located in seven closed institutions and 22 half-open institutions. For offenders between the ages of 18 and 22, four psychosocial institutions exist. There are five centres for compulsory patient commitment, three institutions for those on hospital orders, and 79 prisons and two police stations for the imprisonment of offenders.

As of September 2005, 53% of 6,111 incarcerated people were serving their sentence and/or detained under a hospital order; 9% were awaiting sentence; 31 percent were on remand; and 6% were awaiting deportation. The remaining 1% consisted of people held back in police stations or section under civil law.

Five percent of this total population of 6,111 individuals were women. Seventy percent of these 6,111 individuals were foreign nationals (Bundesamt für Statistik 2005).

Legal issues, criminal law, sentencing, court orders and court reports

The current criminal law of Switzerland (Schweizerisches Strafgesetzbuch) has been developed from that prepared in 1937 and implemented on 1 January 1943. Before this date, criminal law and its execution were the responsibility of each canton. Although this is no longer the case (Article 123 of the federal constitution appoints the constitution as being responsible for criminal justice), there is still no federal criminal justice code. The jurisdiction and execution of the law continue to fall within the power of each canton (Stratenwerth 1982). The criminal law is constantly changed and amended through referenda and popular initiatives. It consists, essentially, of three so-called 'books'.

The first book outlines general regulations and issues, such as self-defence or negligence and the special procedures for children and adolescents. In the second book, all punishable offences are defined. To make it intelligible, this book is sub-divided into 20 'titles' (e.g. offences against body and life, offences against personal means, bribery etc.). In the third book, issues such as jurisdiction and rules of court procedures are regulated. This legal framework has been subject to a lengthy review. Issues such as a special criminal law for children and adolescents, the specific offences of omission, and more severe sentencing (and long detention) for so-called high-risk offenders have been addressed. From 1 January 2007, the new law for children and adolescents (punishable from the age of 10) has been separated from the general criminal law for adults, and consists now of a book of its own.

Swiss law relies on the principle of proportionality, so that the severity of punishment and restriction of freedom is related to the gravity of the crime; it is commensurate with the need for reprisal and appropriate compensation for the offence (Keller 1998). This leads to individual allocation of blame following conviction. Furthermore, the intention is to reduce the risk of re-offending. This is done as follows: first, through the deterrence of a defined punishment according to the offence written down in the criminal law; second, through the punishment, with its emphasis on resocialization and improvement; third, through security measures for offenders with a high risk of recidivism.

Responsibility for the carrying out of the sentences lies with the various cantons (Bundesamt für Justiz 2007). For practical reasons of scale and cost, the 26 cantons work with three concordats (North-West and Central Switzerland, Eastern Switzerland and Concordat Roman), each of them running institutions with different ethos and security levels (Graf, DGPPN 2005, unpublished). There are two different sentencing options; the first approach is a loss of liberty, sometimes including imprisonment; the second approach is welfare- and treatment-orientated. Imprisonment is imposed for security reasons but includes the idea of rehabilitation. Under this first category are various potential restrictions on an offender's liberty, such as conventional prison, less-secure institutions that allow the offender to continue to work, community rehabilitation orders or electronic monitoring. The second category defines measures, ordered by the judge and mostly supported by a report from an expert (psychiatrist, forensic psychiatrist, forensic psychologist). The measures are defined as treatment of mentally disordered offenders (Article 59 of the criminal law), offenders with a drug or alcohol dependency (Article 60 of the criminal law), socio-educational and therapeutic measures for young offenders (defined as aged between 10 and 22, Articles 12–15 of the (new) child and adolescent criminal law) and finally, custody for repetitive and high-risk offenders (Article 64 of the criminal law).

Forensic psychiatric practice: treatment, changes and developments

Psychiatry is a branch of medicine. It relies on empiricism and is informed by other academic perspectives, notably psychology, philosophy and sociology. It is distinct from the law (Freyberger and Stieglitz 1996).

As a forensic psychiatrist in Switzerland there are two major tasks. The first is to be therapeutic and empathic, the second is to assist the court. The second obliges the expert (forensic psychiatrist) to be objective and instruction-orientated. The main task in writing a (court) report is an analysis of an individual offender and his or her influence on the offence on the basis of the expert's psychiatric knowledge. Most often, the expert in a criminal law case is asked by the court to establish the offenders's ability to control his or her actions, soundness of mind, fitness to plead, possible disposal and prognosis in relation to the risk of further offences (in case of a relapse). In a civil law case, one might be asked to examine a person's ability to conduct business or his/her responsibility in relation to marriage or other family matters.

Forensic psychiatry is mostly practised in university psychiatric hospitals. In Switzerland, however, there exist many cantonal forensic services (in cantons without a university). There are 116 registered forensic psychiatrists in Switzerland (Jahresbericht des Praesidenten, SSFP). This is too small a number for the yearly requests of 3,000 to 5,000 reports in the criminal justice system alone. Prosecution and courts are completely free to choose their experts. However, in general, a court report should only be written by a consultant (forensic) psychiatrist or under their close supervision.

Switzerland's forensic institutions and practice today, as well as the different ways of disposal, have to be seen in conjunction with an event that took place near Zurich in 1993 (Nedopil 2001). Erich Hauert, an inmate at one of the prisons, brutally raped and murdered a young girl while on his weekend leave. At that time, he had already been convicted and sentenced for two prior sexual offences and many other minor offences. A shockwave went through the country, and suddenly the spotlight was on the criminal justice system, scrutinizing sentencing, probation, so-called life imprisonment and the practice of forensic psychiatrists, including risk assessment and recommendations for disposal. With the 'murder on the Zollikerberg' all the weak points of the criminal justice system and related agencies between 1970 and 1990 were revealed. Some rather odd and paradoxical practices had been used over the years. For example, offenders with 'a life sentence' were more or less automatically released after 15 years. This happened without further discussion of risk; even if some sort of therapeutic input had taken place, it was often only sporadically documented. Sentences of 'lifelong detention' were not recommended any more, for fear that the offender would be released early owing to good behaviour without any risk assessment (as happened often before the events in 1993). Instead, the courts tried to get as long a sentence as possible with the thought, in the back of their minds, that the longer the sentence the longer the public would be safe from a dangerous offender. Such cases and their sequelae are not restricted to Switzerland. However, what happened after 1993 is perhaps very typical of Switzerland (Urbaniok 2003). A wide socio-political discussion took place throughout the country. This ended in a public initiative ('Verwahrungsinitiative'). It was decided that Switzerland needed more 'forensic beds', and a cantonal decision was taken to enlarge one of the specified forensic clinics with a high security unit.

Although important, this case was only one of the factors that have led to the increasing professionalization and better coordination of forensic mental health services. One sign of this drive towards a professional, country-wide forensic service can be seen in the foundation of the Swiss Society for Forensic Psychiatry (SSFP) in 2007.

Outlook

Forensic psychiatry in Switzerland is faced with the same advantages and disadvantages as the country itself. The size, the complex and multicultural mix of people, the different official languages and its political system, as well as Switzerland's location, all contribute to the above system.

The advantages include fast and often personal communication (owing to the small number of forensic psychiatrists), little travelling, the ability to remain focused and responsible and a strong sense of compromise. All these provide a high-quality forensic psychiatric service. The same qualities, however, can very quickly change and become obstacles (in that forensic psychiatry becomes isolated, too complex and not able to keep up with the speed of neighbouring countries). As a forensic psychiatrist working in Switzerland, the author is alert to the benefits but also the potential pitfalls of the current system.

Key points

- Swiss citizens are able to participate directly in their democracy through frequent referenda and the devolution of state power to cantons

- Forensic psychiatry, as elsewhere, has duties both to patients and to the legal apparatus of the state

- As elsewhere in Europe, there is evidence that high-profile criminal cases have driven and redirected criminal justice policy and practice

- In the recent foundation of the Swiss Society for Forensic Psychiatry (SSFP), the aim for a further professionalization of forensic psychiatry is apparent

References

Bundesamt für Justiz, Sektion Straf- und Massnahmenvollzug. Oktober 2007 Der Strafvollzug in der Schweiz, Bern.

Bundesamt für Statistik. 2005 Kapitel 1: Bevolkerung. Kapitel 19: Kriminalitat, Strafrecht. www.bfs.admin.ch

Bundesamt für Statistik 2006 Federal Statistical Office, www.bfs.admin.ch "topics> population >Migration and integration> 2006".

Freyberger, H.J. and Stieglitz, R-D. (Hrs.) 1996, 10. Auflage. Kompendium der Psychiatrie und Psychotherapie 446–469. Karger: Basel.

Herausgeber Bundeskanzlei, Schweizerisches Strafgesetzbuch, 2004.

Keller, P. 1998 Betreuung im Schweizer Frauenstrafvollzug, Das Betreuungskonzept der Frauenstrafanstalt Hindelbank. Sociology of Crime and Law Enforcement, Online Publication.

Nedopil, N. 2001. Forensische Psychiatrie, Klinik, Begutachtung und Behandlung zwischen Psychiatrie und Recht, 318. Thieme, Stuttgart.

Stratenwerth, G. 1982 Schweizerisches Strafgesetz, Allgemeiner Teil I: die Straftat 16–22. Bern: Verlag Staempfli & Cie AG.

Swiss Society of Forensic Psychiatry (SSFP). 2007/2008 Jahresbericht des Praesidenten.

Urbaniok, F. 2003, Was sind das für Menschen, was sollen wir tun? 137–139. Bern, Zytglogge Verlag.

Chapter 38

Legal models and treatment approaches for the MDO: United States of America

Sameer P. Sarkar

Aim

To describe legal models and treatment approaches to mentally disordered offenders (MDOs) in the United States.

Learning objectives

- To describe legal approaches to the MDO in the United States and to compare and contrast this jurisdiction with the British system
- To outline the development of forensic services in the United States and their relation to the wider political system

---

Introduction

Much of extant American law has roots in English common law; there is so much similarity in the basic premises of law that the legal system is often described as the Anglo-American legal system. As a true federal state (which is one of the most robust aspects of American identity), the United States has varying jurisdictions, each with its unique jurisprudential flavour. As the laws that deal with mentally disordered offenders (MDOs) operate across at least 51 jurisdictions, attempting to identify them would be like trying to find a needle in a haystack. Apart from the US Constitution, against which the validity of any legislation is judged, there is no universally accepted and adhered-to legal philosophy. Different states have both different mental health laws and different service-provision models. In some states, the mental health law may not even cover MDOs; in these cases, the MDO will be dealt with through the ordinary criminal justice system or appropriate juvenile justice system.

Despite this legal diversity, there are some common themes that emerge, and the procedural aspects of law that provide the safeguards to all also protect the rights of the MDO. This chapter will outline the major areas of commonality among these diverse jurisdictions, as well as highlight their differences from the British system.

The size of the MDO problem: whose baby?

US governmental agency, The Bureau of Justice statistics (Ditton 1999) found that, in mid-1998, there were an estimated 283,800 mentally ill offenders in the nation's prisons and jails, amounting to 16% of the incarcerated population. In addition, a further 16% (over half a million) of the nation's probationers had a mental condition or required hospital admission at some point in their lifetime. Even this self-reported, official estimate indicates that offenders who have a mental disorder constitute a sizeable problem. It is perhaps unfair to suggest reasons as to how this situation developed without having an intimate knowledge of local politics, sensibilities and history, but one obvious hypothesis is that there has been a lack of funding for this essentially public service sector. It is felt by many that legislators often failed to provide adequate funding, support and direction for the community mental health systems that replaced the large mental hospitals that were shut down in the 1960s as part of policy to decrease institutionalization (Izumi et al 1996; Lamb et al 2001; Lamb and Weinberger 2005).

A Presidential Commission on Mental Health (2003) described the US mental health system as being 'in shambles'. The Commission found that people with serious mental illnesses (with or without co-morbid untreated drug or alcohol problems), especially those who were also socially disadvantaged, often failed to obtain the mental health treatment they needed. 'Untreated and unstable', they entered the criminal justice system when they offended, although many of the offences were relatively minor public order or nuisance offences. It is sometimes said, with some irony, that many mentally ill people only get access to mental health treatment by entering the criminal justice system.

Although the United States operates a different social welfare system to Britain there is also a different societal attitude towards offenders. It is a common, and some would say not unreasonable, feeling among the lay populace that criminal offenders, whether mentally disordered or not, should not have claim to a higher level of service than that available to non-offender citizens. Local politicians are acutely aware of the strength of this public feeling (Jenkins 2008), which in turn influences budgeting decisions for mental health services (Cuffel et al 1994). A further fundamental difference from the British position lies in the perception of culpability. In every jurisdiction, a person is assumed to be responsible for his or her actions, regardless of whether he or she is suffering from a mental disorder. As a result of the stringent American approach to due legal process and fairness, the very basis of this assumption is tested at the outset, in the form of a determination of competence to stand trial (CST).

Competence to stand trial

The incompetence doctrine has its origins in seventeenth century English common law. It is based on the premise that a person who is unable to plead cannot put up a defence, and thus it is inherently unfair to put him or her on trial. The modern version of the competency standard was spelt out by the US Supreme Court in Dusky v. United States, and it emphasizes both cognitive and communicative capacity. The standard set, at least for federal cases, in Dusky was, 'Whether the defendant has sufficient present ability to consult with his lawyer with a reasonable degree of rational understanding and whether he has a rational as well as factual understanding of the proceedings against him.'

With minor variations, the Dusky standard is used in most jurisdictions.

Although traditionally raised at arraignment (the formal reading of the charges against the accused), CST can be raised at any stage by any individual involved in the legal proceedings, including the defendant's lawyer, the prosecutor, the arresting officer, family and friends, jail officer or even the presiding judge. An estimated 60,000 criminal defendants a year undergo a CST (Bonnie and Grisso 2000). Once it is decided that an evaluation is necessary, experts, usually forensic psychologists, but also psychiatrists, and in the minority of cases mental health professionals from other disciplines (Warren et al 2006), are appointed by the court to carry out the evaluation, which can take place as an outpatient or as an inpatient. As well as providing an opinion regarding the defendant's CST for defendants who are considered incompetent, the expert must give an opinion regarding the restoration of competence if the person is provided with the appropriate 'restoration services' (Jackson v. Indiana 1972). Although, in theory, lawyers can be present during the evaluation, in practice, this is rarely the case. Case law across all jurisdictions has consistently indicated that such an evaluation does not violate the Fifth Amendment right against self-incrimination.

The determination of trial competence is a legal rather than a clinical decision, and as such is determined by the judge, although some jurisdictions allow jury determination (much like fitness to plead in England and Wales). The burden of proof differs between jurisdictions and is almost equally divided between defence and prosecution. The standard of proof is usually 'preponderance of evidence', which is slightly higher than the civil 'on balance of probability' (roughly about 75% certainty). Although the Court is not bound to follow the expert's recommendation, disagreement is rare (Cruise and Rogers 1998). Over a 10-year period, clinicians found that 19% of defendants evaluated were found to be incompetent to stand trial (IST) and considered 23% of these unlikely to be restored to competence (Warren et al 2006).

If the defendant is deemed competent to stand trial the criminal proceedings are resumed. If the defendant is found incompetent, he or she is remanded for treatment to restore competence. Although, in theory, treatment could be done as an outpatient, it generally involves automatic hospitalization. The mandatory treatment that the court orders to restore the defendant's competency is limited to that purpose only, and is primarily aimed at curing the defendant's mental disorder. These defendants' right to treatment, or indeed right to refuse treatment, is not automatically derived from existing law, and the laws relating to treatment and consent to such treatment differ across jurisdictions. Similarly, the right to be treated in the least-restrictive alternative is also evolving and not yet settled law. How long a defendant should stay in hospital is also not settled, but in the landmark case of Jackson v. Indiana, the Supreme Court said that such defendants must be restored to competency and remitted to trial within a reasonable time, or else be civilly committed or released. The Court also added that the civil commitment standards in such cases must follow the State's ordinary civil commitment procedures. The time spent hospitalized is credited against sentence in most jurisdictions.

Acquittal by reason of insanity

Anglo-American criminal law is based on the premise that an individual who chooses to do an illegal act is morally blameworthy. The severely mentally ill defendant is not so blameworthy because he does not have the free will to form the intent to commit a criminal act. If the defence can show that the defendant was severely mentally ill at the time of the offence then he may be found 'not guilty by reason of insanity' (NGRI). All modern American versions of the insanity test are essentially derived from the nineteenth century English M'Naghten Rules (Rollin 1996) (see Chapter 19). Although in theory the NGRI verdict results in an acquittal, in practice, the acquittees are always sent to psychiatric facilities, often without limit of time, and suffer the dual stigma of being mad and bad.

Although infrequently pleaded, and even less frequently successful, the public perception of acquittal on the grounds of NGRI has never been favourable, leading to attempts, some successful, to abolish this defence or modify it to 'guilty but insane' in some jurisdictions. Whether it is called an acquittal or 'guilty but insane' (or, in some states, guilty but mentally ill or GBMI), the disposition is mandatory indeterminate commitment, which, in part, explains the relative unattractiveness of this defence among defendants. Furthermore, many states have more stringent release criteria for NGRI patients than ordinary civilly committed patients, or view NGRI commitment as a form of preventive detention, focusing solely on dangerousness. Both the sanity and the dangerousness criteria are used in the decision to release, disadvantaging the NGRI defendant. In some jurisdictions, there is the further complication that the release decision has to be made by a criminal judge (as if it were an extension of the original crime). Consequently, the standard of proof used is the criminal standard of 'beyond reasonable doubt' as opposed to the civil 'on balance of probability' or the slightly more onerous quasi-criminal standard 'preponderance of evidence'.

In addition to the problems relating to the ease of commitment (acquittees are automatically committed to psychiatric facilities under civil statute) and the stringent discharge criteria, insanity acquittees have been traditionally housed in maximum security wards or institutions. However, in many jurisdictions, recent case law has altered the emphasis of the verdict away from criminal to civil. Several states now treat the NGRI acquittal as no more than a civil commitment, with all the accompanying procedural safeguards, including rights about conditions of confinement. Although many states have more favourable dispositional alternatives, there still remains a need for an overarching reform of both commitment and release criteria as well as the conditions of confinement.

Special dispositional alternatives for 'abnormal offenders'

The two categories of mental health disposal described are indirect modes of disposal. The first, IST, is invoked before guilt or innocence is considered, and the second, NGRI, assumes lack of criminal responsibility and thus guilt or blameworthiness. A third and more direct route is increasingly being used to divert a group of offenders whose guilt is established by trial, but, instead of standard penal sentencing, they are committed to special mental health programs. Originally devised for the 'defective delinquents' who were thought to be unable to benefit from the rehabilitative potential of indeterminate sentencing, this route was initially unpopular, but it went on to pave the way for the more popular programmes for the sexually dangerous. The first of these 'sexual dangerous statutes' was passed in 1937 in Michigan, and their popularity, at least among the lawmakers, is reflected by the fact that currently at least 15 states have laws governing civil commitment of sexually violent predators (SVP). Some authors (Rogers and Jackson 2005) have classed this group of patients as 'SVP detainees', pointing out that the primary objective seems to be incapacitation rather than treatment. The triggering conditions vary from jurisdiction to jurisdiction but most require there to be a sexual aspect of the conduct. Although claimed to be a form of civil statute (and a form of civil commitment), the statutes are often criticized for having a variety of drawbacks, including the lack of requirement on the state to provide an effective treatment programme (Sarkar 2003). Despite being the focus for protracted litigation with respect to procedural or constitutional matters, these statutes have survived repeated Supreme Court challenges, and look set to proliferate among other jurisdictions.

Treatment options for the mentally disordered offender

In Britain, MDOs are meant to be treated in specialist mental health services or hospitals, outside of the penal system, but in the United States almost every state treats their MDOs in prison or prison hospitals. Separate and sometimes cumbersome laws govern prison-to-hospital transfers and are reserved for serious cases. Prison transfers are viewed as an extra limitation on liberty and are protected by additional procedural safeguards, ranging from a report from a physician or psychologist to a full-blown commitment-style hearing before a quasi-judicial panel.

Most of the treatments for MDOs, once they have been adjudicated to be competent to stand trial and convicted, are delivered in hospital wings within prisons. Such facilities are often run by generic therapists or psychiatrists, and posts are often vacant. The correctional institutions have never been popular places of employment for experienced psychiatrists, and one study (Harry et al 1990) found that less than 10% of the members of the American Academy of Psychiatry and the Law (AAPL), the country's foremost professional body for forensic psychiatrists, provide service to prisons or secure hospitals. Although there is no survey on the working preference of forensic psychiatrists in the United States, experience suggests that often the most experienced psychiatrists limit their involvement to the assessment phase of the criminal process. More recently, services for MDOs are being developed within the generic mental health system in the community (Lamb and Weinberger 2005).

In broad terms, states provide services for those who are found to be either IST or NGRI in psychiatric facilities within the mental health system. For those offenders who become mentally disordered while in prison, treatment is provided in prison psychiatric wings, usually under the management of the Department of Correction. The more seriously ill offenders are usually transferred out of prisons to maximum or even super-maximum secure hospitals, which are again run by the mental health system of the state. Various versions of these arrangements are found across America. However, the growth in prison population has resulted in some states building sophisticated psychiatric hospitals, with varying degrees of security, which, although outside the correctional setting, are still managed by the prison system.

The usual forensic patients (individuals found to be IST and NGRI) are sent to state forensic facilities that utilize a three-tier security classification – maximum, medium and minimum – the level of security usually being determined by the charge. Resource implications, especially in small rural communities, may mean that many of these facilities are centralized and far from a patient's family and social support network. Many states also lack specialized services for women or young offenders.

A prisoner's right to treatment

The right of a prisoner to have treatment was derived from the US Constitution's Eighth Amendment ban on cruel and unusual punishment, the issues of which were embodied in the landmark case of Estelle v. Gamble (1976). Once state deprives a person of liberty, by definition, that person is unable to obtain the basic needs for human survival without help from his or her captors. These needs include medical care without which a person in captivity will suffer needlessly and may even die. The *Estelle* judgement held that a prisoner cannot make a claim for violation of their rights under the Eighth Amendment with respect to alleging acts or omissions sufficiently harmful to evidence deliberate indifference to serious medical needs, and that medical malpractice does not arise to the level of 'cruel and unusual punishment' simply because the victim was a prisoner. Subsequent decisions that have interpreted the Eighth Amendment have further eroded a prisoner's right to mount a claim of violation of this Amendment.

Most prisons have small health or psychiatric wings that can only manage acute psychiatric episodes. Prisoners who have chronic or more severe psychiatric disorders are sent to special forensic facilities or maximum-security prison hospitals. Although there are many local variations, the predominant culture is to offer treatment in small psychiatric units attached to major prisons or prison hospital, thus avoiding the legal minefield of a prison transfer (see above).

The standard of care in these units is comparable, for better or worse, with similar non-prison state psychiatric facilities. Offenders, whether they are within the state hospital system or the prison health system, have similar rights to consent or to refuse treatment, and broadly the same right to treatment. To forcibly medicate someone, the state has to prove that a mental disorder exists and that the treatment is in the patient's best interest. The state does not have an absolute right to impose treatment, and the prisoner does not have an absolute right to resist treatment. Disagreement in this area is resolved by administrative or, in some cases, by judicial hearings. Prisoners also have certain procedural protection to resist a transfer for treatment from a prison to state hospital. In reality, the problem is often not one of the prisoner resisting transfer but of how to access a hospital bed when there is often a severe resource shortage.

Community-based treatment programmes

Causes of criminality in the mentally ill are multiple, and to date there is no gold-standard intervention that prevents recidivism. It is sometimes erroneously thought that providing mental health services to the mentally ill at an individual level will reduce involvement with the criminal justice system (Dvoskin and Steadman 1994; Lamb et al 2001; Mullen et al 2000). Based on this belief, a wide variety of interventions have been designed that target MDOs. Some of these are pre- or post-booking 'jail diversion' programmes that move offenders from a 'criminal justice track' to a 'mental health track'. Mental Health Courts have been operating with variable degrees of success in some parts of America as well as in Britain (Griffin et al 2002; James 1999; Kondo 2003; Lamb et al 2001; Watson et al 2001). In addition, 'in-reach' programmes or specialized case management programmes ease the transition of the prison inmate back into the community treatment system. Although matching people with appropriate services that may have previously been unavailable to them can only be a good thing, one criticism of this approach has been that many of these services are returning offenders to the same system whose previous involvement failed to prevent them entering the criminal justice system.

The case management model

Initially, the case management model was regarded as a generalist service that brokered specialized services on behalf of their clients (Burns et al 2001; Catty et al 2002). It was soon recognized that given the complexity of the patients' needs, more supportive and direct services were required. Although various case management models are operating across America, the assertive community treatment (ACT) approach appears to be the most comprehensive and well-thought-out model. This model aims to transfer all functions from the hospital to the community, using multi-professional teams. As it is an expensive model, it tends to be reserved for the patients with the most complex needs. Experience has shown that patients can transfer from the ACT programme to less-intensive programmes within a reasonable time.

Swartz's study (Swartz et al 2001) suggested that community treatment reduced recidivism. Although this finding was not replicated in a more recent study (Kisely et al 2004), the findings by Swartz and colleagues heralded a golden age for mandated community treatment, but the criticism remains that criminal acts committed by the mentally disordered cannot be equated with criminal acts committed while mentally ill. In their early paper, Dvoskin and Steadman (1994) described how ACT (or intensive case management) helped reduce violent offending. The Mental Illness Offender Treatment and Crime Reduction Act (MIOTCRA 2005) authorized the Justice and Mental Health Collaboration Program. This grant funded programme is designed to increase public safety by both facilitating collaboration across the criminal and juvenile justice systems and mental health treatment and substance abuse services, and by improving access to treatment for people with mental illnesses who are involved with the justice system.

Other factors, such as the development of atypical antipsychotic drugs and compliance with medication regimes, have also made a valuable contribution to how patients are managed in the community. Similarly, mandated outpatient treatments have also had a positive impact on recidivism and readmission rate. Whether the relatively small gains are worth the extra limitations a patient will face, and whether these gains are sustained, only time will tell (Lamb et al 2001).

Conclusion

At a time when American health services are going through wide-ranging transitions in the way they are funded and accounted for (Lamb et al 2001), the service provisions for MDOs cannot be immune to the funding challenges. How much society will spend on services for what some may regard as its least attractive members is a serious question. Although it is easy to criticize one system in preference to other, especially from a distance where the realities may not be easily discernable, the uncomfortable reality may be that both the US and UK systems of treatment for MDOs have a great deal in common. The essential and age-old conflict between welfare and justice would, at first glance, seem to be more acute in the American courts and prison hospitals, but there is no reason to believe that it is uniquely so. As our societal norms and jurisprudence are essentially similar, the tension is as acute here as it is over the Atlantic. Mental health activism and more innovative health care delivery models may make things better in the short term for the mentally disordered offender, but ultimately the citizenry will decide if a major paradigm shift is needed in how we deal with this subgroup of offenders.

References

Bonnie, R. and Grisso, T. 2000 Adjudicative Competence and Youthful Offenders 73–103 in Youth on Trial (Grisso, T. and Schwartz, R. Editors) Chicago IL: University of Chicago Press.

Burns, T., Knapp, M., Catty, J. et al 2001 Home Treatment For Mental Health Problems: A Systematic Review. Health Technology Assessment 5, 15: 1–139.

Catty, J., Burns, T., Knapp, M. et al 2002 Home Treatment for Mental Health Problems: A Systematic Review. Psychological Medicine 32: 383–401.

Cruise, K.R. and Rogers, R. 1998 An Analysis of Competency to Stand Trial: An Integration of Case Law and Clinical Knowledge. Behavioral Sciences & the Law 16: 35–50.

Cuffel, B.J., Wait, D. and Head, T. 1994 Shifting the Responsibility for Payment for State Hospital Services to Community Mental Health Agencies. Hospital Community Psychiatry 45: 460–465.

Ditton, P.M. 1999 Mental Health and Treatment of Inmates and Probationers. BJS Special Report, US Bureau of Justice Statistics. NCJ 174463. Washington, DC: US Bureau of Justice Statistics.

Dvoskin, J.A. and Steadman, H.J. 1994 Using Intensive Case Management to Reduce Violence by Mentally Ill Persons in the Community, Hospital & Community Psychiatry 45: 679–684.

Griffin, P.A., Steadman, H.J. and Petrila, J. 2002 The Use of Criminal Charges and Sanctions in Mental Health Courts Psychiatric Services 53: 1285–1289.

Harry, B., Maier, G.J. and Miller, R.D. 1990 American Forensic Psychiatrists Who Work In State Institutions. Bulletin of American Academy of Psychiatry Law 18: 99–106.

Izumi, L.T., Schiller, M. and Hayward, S. 1996, Corrections, Criminal Justice, and the Mentally Ill: Some Observations about Costs. San Francisco, California: Mental Health Briefing, Pacific Research Institute.

James, D. 1999 Court Diversion at 10 years: Can it Work, Does It Work and Has It a Future? Journal of Forensic Psychiatry 10: 507–524.

Jenkins, C.L. 2008 Va Shortchanged Fairfax. Falls Church Officials Say Share of Mental Health Funding is Questioned. World Psychiatry.

Kisely, S.R., Xiao, J. and Preston, N.J. 2004 Impact of Compulsory Community Treatment on Admission Rates: Survival Analysis Using Linked Mental Health and Offender Databases. British Journal of Psychiatry 184: 432–438.

Kondo, L. 2003 Advocacy of the Establishment of Mental Health Speciality Courts in the Provision of Therapeutic Justice for Mentally Ill Offenders. American Journal of Criminal Law 28: 255–336.

Lamb, H.R. and Weinberger, L.E. 2005 The Shift of Psychiatric Inpatient Care from Hospitals to Jails and Prisons. Journal of the American Academy of Psychiatry and the Law 33: 529–534.

Lamb, H.R., Weinberger, L.E. and Gross, B.H. 2001 Community Treatment of Severely Mentally Ill Offenders under the Jurisdiction of the Criminal Justice System: A Review. New Directions for Mental Health Services 90: 51–65.

MIOTCRA. 2005 The Mental Illness Offender Treatment and Crime Reduction Act of 2004.

Mullen, P.E., Burgess, P., Wallace, C., Palmer, S. and Ruschena, D. 2000 Community Care and Criminal Offending in Schizophrenia, Lancet 355: 614–617.

Rogers, R. and Jackson, R.L. 2005 Sexually Violent Predators: The Risky Enterprise of Risk Assessment. Journal of the American Academy of Psychiatry and the Law 33: 523–528.

Rollin, H. 1996 Forensic Psychiatry in England: A Retrospective in 150 Years of British Psychiatry Vol. 2, The Aftermath (Freeman, H. and Berrios, G.E. Editors) Athlone.

Sarkar, S.P. 2003 From Hendricks to Crane: The Sexually Violent Predator Trilogy and the Inchoate Jurisprudence of the U.S. Supreme Court. Journal of the American Academy of Psychiatry and the Law 31: 242–248.

Swartz, M.S., Swanson, J.W., Hiday, V.A., Wagner, H.R., Burns, B.J. and Borum, R. 2001 A Randomized Controlled Trial of Outpatient Commitment in North Carolina. Psychiatric Services 52: 325–329.

Watson, A., Hanrahan, P., Luchins, D. and Lurigio, A. 2001 Mental health Courts and the Complex Issue of Mentally Ill Offenders. Psychiatric Services 52: 477–481.

Warren, J.I., Murrie, D.C., Stejskal, W. et al 2006 Opinion Formation in Evaluating the Adjudicative Competence and Restorability of Criminal Defendants: A Review of 8,000 Evaluations. Behavioral Sciences & the Law 24: 113–132.

Cases

Dusky v. United States. 1960 362 U.S. 402.

Estelle v. Gamble. 1976 429 U.S. 97.

Jackson v. Indiana. 1972 406 U.S. 715.

Suggested reading

Stone A.A. 1984 Law, Psychiatry, and Morality: Essays and Analysis. Washington, DC: American Psychiatric Publishing.

Appelbaum, P. 1994 Almost a Revolution: Mental Health Law and the Limits of Change. Oxford: Oxford University Press.

Gutheil, T.G. and Appelbaum, P. S. 2000 Clinical Handbook of Psychiatry and the Law 3rd Edition. Baltimore: Lippincott Williams and Wilkins.

Grisso, T. 2004. Double Jeopardy: Adolescent Offenders with Mental Disorders. Chicago: University of Chicago Press.

Website

www.bazelon.org

Index